THE 1982 YEAR BOOKS

The YEAR BOOK series provides in condensed form the essence of the best of the recent international medical literature. The material is selected by distinguished editors who critically review more than 500,000 journal articles each year.

Anesthesia: *Drs. Kirby, Miller, Ostheimer, Saidman, and Stoelting.*

Cancer: *Drs. Clark, Cumley, and Hickey.*

Cardiology: *Drs. Harvey, Kirkendall, Kirklin, Nadas, Resnekov, and Sonnenblick.*

Dentistry: *Drs. Hale, Hazen, Moyers, Redig, Robinson, and Silverman.*

Dermatology: *Drs. Dobson and Thiers.*

Diagnostic Radiology: *Drs. Whitehouse, Adams, Bookstein, Gabrielsen, Holt, Martel, Silver, and Thornbury.*

Drug Therapy: *Drs. Hollister and Lasagna.*

Emergency Medicine: *Dr. Wagner.*

Endocrinology: *Drs. Schwartz and Ryan.*

Family Practice: *Dr. Rakel.*

Medicine: *Drs. Rogers, Des Prez, Cline, Braunwald, Greenberger, Bondy, and Epstein.*

Neurology and Neurosurgery: *Drs. De Jong, Sugar, and Currier.*

Nuclear Medicine: *Drs. Hoffer, Gottschalk, and Zaret.*

Obstetrics and Gynecology: *Drs. Pitkin and Zlatnik.*

Ophthalmology: *Dr. Ernest.*

Orthopedics: *Dr. Coventry.*

Otolaryngology: *Drs. Strong and Paparella.*

Pathology and Clinical Pathology: *Dr. Brinkhous.*

Pediatrics: *Drs. Oski and Stockman.*

Plastic and Reconstructive Surgery: *Drs. McCoy, Brauer, Haynes, Hoehn, Miller, and Whitaker.*

Psychiatry and Applied Mental Health: *Drs. Freedman, Kolb, Lourie, Meltzer, Nemiah, and Romano.*

Sports Medicine: *Drs. Krakauer, Shephard and Torg, Col. Anderson, and Mr. George.*

Surgery: *Drs. Schwartz, Najarian, Peacock, Shires, Silen, and Spencer.*

Urology: *Drs. Gillenwater and Howards.*

1982
YEAR BOOK OF
SURGERY

The YEAR BOOK of

Surgery

1982

Editor

SEYMOUR I. SCHWARTZ, M.D.

Professor of Surgery, University of Rochester School of Medicine and Dentistry

Associate Editors

JOHN S. NAJARIAN, M.D.

Professor and Chairman, Department of Surgery, University of Minnesota Medical School

ERLE E. PEACOCK, Jr., M.D.

Professor of Surgery, Tulane University School of Medicine

TOM SHIRES, M.D.

Professor and Chairman, Department of Surgery, New York Hospital—Cornell Medical Center

WILLIAM SILEN, M.D.

Johnson and Johnson Professor of Surgery, Harvard Medical School; Surgeon-in-Chief, Beth Israel Hospital, Boston

FRANK C. SPENCER, M.D.

George David Stewart Professor of Surgery; Chairman, Department of Surgery, New York University; Director, Department of Surgery, New York University Medical Center and Bellevue Hospital

YEAR BOOK MEDICAL PUBLISHERS, INC.

CHICAGO • LONDON

Printed in U.S.A.

Library of Congress Catalog Card Number: CD38-26

International Standard Book Number: 0-8151-7622-8

Table of Contents

The material covered in this volume represents literature reviewed up to December 1981.

Journals Represented

Acta Chirurgica Scandinavica
Acta Endocrinologica
American Heart Journal
American Journal of Cardiology
American Journal of Clinical Nutrition
American Journal of Diseases of Children
American Journal of Medicine
American Journal of Pathology
American Journal of Physiology
American Journal of Surgery
American Surgeon
Annals of Internal Medicine
Annals of Ophthalmology
Annals of Otology, Rhinology, and Laryngology
Annals of the Royal College of Surgeons of England
Annals of Surgery
Annals of Thoracic Surgery
Archives of Pathology and Laboratory Medicine
Archives of Surgery
British Journal of Plastic Surgery
British Journal of Surgery
British Medical Journal
Burns
Canadian Journal of Surgery
Cancer
Cancer Research
Circulation
Clinical Pharmacology and Therapeutics
Contemporary Surgery
Diabetologia
Digestive Diseases and Sciences
Diseases of the Colon and Rectum
European Surgical Research
Gastroenterology
Gut
International Journal of Cancer
International Surgery
Investigative Radiology
Journal of the American Medical Association
Journal of the American Osteopathic Association
Journal of Bone and Joint Surgery (American Volume)
Journal of Clinical Investigation
Journal of Hand Surgery
Journal of Immunology
Journal of Laboratory and Clinical Medicine
Journal of the National Cancer Institute
Journal of Neurology, Neurosurgery and Psychiatry

Journal of Otolaryngology
Journal of Pediatrics
Journal of Pediatric Surgery
Journal of the Royal College of Surgeons of Edinburgh
Journal of Surgical Research
Journal of Thoracic and Cardiovascular Surgery
Journal of Trauma
Journal of Urology
Kidney International
Lancet
Mayo Clinic Proceedings
Metabolism
New England Journal of Medicine
Plastic and Reconstructive Surgery
Proceedings of the National Academy of Sciences of the United States of America
Radiology
Reviews of Infectious Diseases
Scandinavian Journal of Plastic and Reconstructive Surgery
Science
Southern Medical Journal
Surgery
Surgery, Gynecology and Obstetrics
Thorax
Topics in Emergency Medicine
Transplantation
World Journal of Surgery

Annual Overview

General Considerations—Acute surgical pain in patients with sickle cell anemia is relatively common. An algorithm for differentiating between abdominal pain due to sickle cell crisis and pain associated with surgical illness is presented. Sickle cell anemia necessitates specific considerations concerning anesthetic management.

A large review points out the current state of the art in the management of hemophiliac patients undergoing major surgical procedures. In the face of available replacement therapy, most operations should be uncomplicated. The present cryoprecipitate concentrates are the most effective agents for use in replacement therapy. In the future, the oral administration of factor VIII-loaded liposomes may prove to be useful.

Fluid, Electrolytes, and Nutrition—Newer technology continues to elucidate the role of internal movement of fluids and electrolytes in response to various forms of injury. The time-honored Starling equation and Starling forces are now beginning to be extended significantly. It is clear from an examination of the thermodynamics of the Starling equation that several variables have not been measurable in the past. These include the very important changes in capillary permeability and, consequently, flux rates of both ions and larger molecules. Recent studies have been able to address this problem far more adequately, particularly in relation to pulmonary function by simultaneous studies of flow and composition of lymph. The identification of capillary leak and increase in protein flux is a major advance in the understanding of Starling forces and in the ability to handle the pulmonary response to injury, with its attendant change in fluid and electrolyte distribution.

The internal redistribution of fluid and electrolytes locally in response to injury, the local sequestration or "third-space" phenomenon, is being better understood than in years past. It is quite clear now that replacement of the operatively induced third-space sequestration is essential if the hormonal response to injury is to be modified. There is little doubt that the response of aldosterone and antidiuretic hormone is minimized if the third-space losses are replaced intraoperatively. These losses are being quantitated to a greater degree despite the fact that equilibration of various molecules differs depending on the steady state and length of time these molecules are allowed to equilibrate. One additional major component of this phenomenon has been studied in several articles this year, the presence of cellular injury in response to local wounding. This cellular compartment for translocation of fluid and electrolytes, which previously has been demonstrated by myself and others in hemorrhagic shock, apparently also will occur to a far lesser degree at the site of an injury. Quantitation of these defects is now being accomplished.

There is a continually impressive number of studies investigating the cause of negative nitrogen balance and breakdown of various tissues after serious injury, starvation, or infection. This year, newer techniques of investigation, such as stable isotopes, confirm that the negative nitrogen balance after severe injury is primarily due to an increased breakdown in muscle protein. These studies also confirm that there are significant alterations in muscle synthesis of protein after injury, but that this synthesis lags behind breakdown for several days. The net effect of these late changes in protein synthesis is dependent in large part on the various types of trauma sustained, severity of the injury, nutritional intake during recovery, and the presence or absence of sepsis. In addition, several studies detail again that the composition of the nutritional intake may make some difference, particularly in the more severely injured patient. For example, branched-chain amino acids may be a preferable substrate for the correction of the amino acid losses in some severe posttraumatic catabolic states. Other studies, however, indicate that any form of augmented parenteral or enteric alimentation will supply the nutritional needs for correction of the catabolic rate induced by severe trauma.

Replacement of the small but significant portion of total calories after injury should be in the form of fatty acids. Essential fatty acid deficiency during total parenteral nutrition has been carefully studied now, and the clinical syndrome that results after approximately 2 weeks of total parenteral nutrition without fatty acids is well documented. It appears at present that when 3% of calories given intravenously, or 15% of calories given orally, are administered as fat, essential fatty acid deficiency will be prevented in patients receiving total parenteral nutrition.

Additional and detailed elegant studies are assessing the alterations in metabolism in patients, particularly in relation to the change in catabolic ratios among the burning of protein, carbohydrates, and fat in response to injury. Specific forms of therapy involving amino acids, whether protein in origin or branched chain, fat, and glucose are being further delineated. It would appear that the sequencing of these metabolic needs will depend largely on the severity of injury and the presence or absence of associated infection. Other articles discuss the complications of hyperalimentation and the safeguards to be used. Specific details in measurement of trace elements needed, such as zinc and copper, are now appearing with increasing frequency and better quantitative methods. These contributions to improving the accuracy and adequacy of total parenteral nutrition now far outweigh articles concerning the potential hazards of this form of therapy. Finally, the measurement of delayed cutaneous hypersensitivity has been evaluated by several investigators, using four or five recall antigens. While a rough correlation does exist between the nutritional state of the patient and the ability of the skin to recognize recall antigens, the overlap is such that this gross measure of immunocompetence clearly no longer will be significantly useful clinically. It should be pointed out, however, that this form of immune testing in severely ill or malnourished patients has led to a variety of elegant studies that measure more sophisticated evaluations of immunoresponsiveness, particularly the various components of white blood cell function.

Shock—Virtually all of the work on shock appearing during this past year has been focused at the cellular and subcellular level. In recent years, the quality of research and the degree of technologic innovation have improved remarkably as many additional methods for measurement of cellular and subcellular performance continue to appear. The forms of shock being studied both clinically and experimentally are still primarily those seen most often in patients, that is, hemorrhagic shock and septic shock. Two elegant studies this past year examined the internal redistribution of fluids in animals based on the cellular response to injury, specifically, the transcapillary refill phenomenon initiated by hemorrhage and shock. The work indicates that transcapillary or plasma refilling increases with a level of hemorrhage up to 30%. Refill after hemorrhage of more than 30% of blood volume, the level at which severe shock is produced, is no faster than refill after hemorrhage of 10% of blood volume. These data confirm, lastly, the gradation of body response to shock injury in that cellular membrane injury and reversal of transcapillary refill trends are not seen until severe shock has been achieved. At that point, once cellular injury has occurred, the movement internally of interstitial fluid into cells begins to limit seriously the plasma refilling that occurs in response to lesser degrees of hemorrhage.

Various papers during the past year emphasize the sophistication needed to achieve standardized shock models and to be able to measure internal redistribution of fluids in response to severe shock injury. Several of these papers show the necessity for a variety of steady-state measurements when any shock preparation is studied. These include long equilibration times; markers that are specifically excluded from a compartment even if the compartment, such as the cell water, is altered by the shock state; definition of shock injury to either include or exclude cellular membrane injury; and reinjection of tracers and markers used to measure body fluid volumes if internal redistribution between interstitial and cell compartments is induced by the model studied. Adherence to basic ground rules will clear the way for common denominators in the study of shock models. In many experiments in past years, shock injury was determined by the level of blood pressure achieved. Obviously, this imprecise definition of the shock state is no longer acceptable when work is being done on internal fluid and electrolyte distribution or cellular function.

Because the cell and subcellular components have been shown to be so sensitive to severe shock injury, many papers advocate a variety of substances to prevent or reverse membrane injury. Several studies indicate some benefit in experimental animals from the injection of adenosine triphosphate (ATP) or ATP-$MgCl_2$ in the shock state. Two other elaborate studies appeared during the year indicating that intravenously injected ATP is degraded completely before the time the substance would reach the cell membrane. Other studies, looking at a model of slow changes in cell membrane and energy function in tissues such as skeletal muscle, detailed the fact that the cell membrane injury occurs before ATP levels in the cell membrane decrease. It would appear that improved survival in animals after the injection of ATP probably is due to a pharmacologic effect other than a resupply of energy to a cell with a damaged cell membrane. Improvement in cell function also has been attempted with the use of opiate antagonist drugs, which can be shown to enhance cardiovascular function in hemorrhagic shock. This interesting approach will bear careful study. In addition, there have been several attempts to improve peripheral oxygen transport and utilization after what is physiologically otherwise adequate resuscitation from shock. These efforts to manipulate vascular and interstitial responses also deserve further investigation.

Two excellent studies of the response of patients to volume restoration appeared during the past year, both based on the experimental results described in previous years. The findings indicate that in the resuscitation of patients from hemorrhagic shock the combination of oxygen-carrying substances, such as red blood cells, and the refill of plasma and intersitial volume with an extracellular mimic such as Hartman's solution appears to be optimal. Human serum albumin or colloid added nothing to this regimen. Because these substances are quite expensive and potentially hazardous, most authors writing on this subject believe there is no indication for the addition of extra colloid in the resuscitation of patients with hemorrhagic shock.

One unique bacteriologic clarification that occurred during the past year relates to studies of toxic shock syndrome. Little question now exists that the syndrome is caused by a new varient of *staphylococcus aureus*. Furthermore, it is clear that this variant may develop in any of several sites within the body and produce the identical syndrome. This identification was made possible by careful phage typing with a new combination of phage types capable of producing pyrogenic exotoxin C.

As is true for hemorrhagic shock, cellular and subcellular studies of septic shock have begun to appear that use close mimics of septic shock in patients. These mimics are certainly more fruitful when injection of live whole organisms is used. The instability of commercially produced endotoxin has virtually precluded its use for meaningful animal studies of the septic shock state. Injury to the cell membrane consistently is shown when live whole organisms are injected. Depolarization of the cell membrane often precedes the onset of deep hypotension, indicating that cell injury is a primary cause of the effects, particularly the internal redistribution of fluids, rather than a result of the shock state.

Additional interesting metabolic data have indicated that during bacteremic shock caused by injection of live *Escherichia coli* organisms, the skeletal muscle in animals becomes insulin resistant, a position that previously has been called the "pseudodiabetic state." Remarkable insulin resistance was shown in studies of isolated skeletal muscle. In a similar vein, adipose tissue lipoprotein lipase activity in infected patients who had sustained injury was demonstrated to be much greater than that in infected patients. These studies confirm the unique and severe cellular effect of sepsis on metabolism.

Several other studies of shock report the lack of effect of administration of steroids, even when given in massive doses to young animals and when used as the only adjunctive therapy. This continues to be a highly controversial topic. Even in septic shock, significant effects are being claimed only when steroids, fluids, and antibiotics are used simultaneously. Additional articles have shown, predictably, that when the malnourished state is abolished, resistance to sepsis and septic shock improves. This is now being shown by indicating a response in immunocompetence after repletion in a nutritionally depleted animal. It would appear that the increasing number of studies in this area will continue to elucidate the primary need for enhanced immunocompetence in sepsis and septic shock.

Trauma—Continued progress is being made in all aspects of the care of the severely injured patient. Because injury usually occurs during the productive years of life, the improvements in the rate and quality of survival after severe trauma are extremely gratifying.

Articles on prehospital care continue to appear with increasing frequency, including additional documentation of the advantages of categorization of hospitals for receiving patients with life-threatening injury or illness. Certainly, as a primary guiding principle for prehospital care, the 10% to 15% of patients in the high-risk categories, including those who have sustained trauma and those with heart attacks, spinal cord injury, neonatal distress, burns or cardiac disease, should be taken to the closest and most appropriate facility. It is interesting how the patterns of categorization of hospitals and transportation of patients vary according to the geographic arrangement of population and the included hospitals. It is pointed out again this year that the adequacy of these lifesaving prehospital emergency care systems is dictated almost entirely at the community level. This is one aspect of medical care that must be initiated, organized, funded, and sustained at the local level. Enhancement at the federal level has been meager and now virtually has disappeared. With the increased attention to prehospital care and regional emergency medical services, articles are beginning to appear that allow sophistication of these efforts. One article, for example, deals with methodologic considerations in determining the outcome after prehospital care and transportation. One such approach is a quick and simple single-page precoded abstracting form containing an alphabetical description for each type of trauma within a body region. Using such methods, a computer algorithm was developed to assign injury severity codes and then determine patient outcome in relation to time in transit, initial support and emergency room efforts, and definitive care. Similar studies can do nothing but improve the prehospital and early hospital phases of care of the traumatized patient.

A number of studies this year relate specifically to organ response to severe injury. Some of these are increasing our understanding of gastric response to systemic trauma, particularly in the form of stress ulceration. This complication now is being prevented more often and managed far better due to increased understanding of hydrogen back-diffusion and greater protection of the patient from mucosal ischemia.

Several excellent articles this year continue to examine the pulmonary response to trauma and shock. Studies show that patients who died after severe trauma, excluding head injury, had minimal and reversible pulmonary injury. When significant and protracted pulmonary injury was present in a series of autopsy studies, patients invariably had systemic sepsis. Several authors this year reinforce the idea that the term "shock lung" should be dropped and "septic lung" substituted. Supporting data for this describe the lack of pulmonary response after massive doses of steroids early in the treatment of the seriously injured patient. In fact, some evidence of reduction in pulmonary function was documented. This study complements those in the past 2 years that showed no benefit from the addition of steroids in the resuscitation or early treatment of severely injured patients.

One other study appeared this year to validate several recent papers concerning the selective use of ventilatory therapy in patients with flail chest injury. It is becoming more obvious that even with an anatomical flail chest, "internal stinting" will be needed with mechanical ventilatory assistance only in approximately half the patients. Fully half of the patients presenting with paradoxical movement of a segment of the chest wall can be handled without endotracheal intubation.

One of the primary advances in the management of the trauma patient is the use of the abdominal computed tomography (CT) scan. Several articles detail quite well the indications for the use of the CT scan in the diagnosis of severe abdominal trauma. It appears that the liver, spleen, kidney, and pancreas are all well visualized on emergency CT scans and the degree of injury often can be assessed. At least two categories of patients have been identified: (1) those with significant abdominal injury who are stable, and yet in whom there is suspicion of significant injury, and (2) those who have sustained multiple injury but in whom a clinical sign cannot be demonstrated at present because of central nervous system depression, injury, or similar factors. These two groups appear to be prime candidates for emergency CT scanning.

In the surgical management of one of the more significant and serious injuries, that is, severe injury to the liver, the exact role of local control as opposed to resectional debridement, hepatic resection, and hepatic artery ligation is still evolving. Each form of therapy has its advocates. However, resection for the massively bleeding liver is assuming an increasing role in view of the use of hepatic clamps that immediately control bleeding and permit quick, easy, and relatively bloodless resection after hepatic injury. The percentage of direct control, arterial ligation, and sublobar or lobar resections will almost certainly vary with the type of injuries sustained and the experience of the surgeon concerned. This is a severe injury, and it is not surprising that arguments about the role of the various approaches continue to appear.

One interesting new technique, namely, electromicroprobe analysis, was used to measure cell swelling in vivo after renal ischemia. This study showed that with this new technique there is reversible injury to the cell membrane, with loss of sodium chloride and water inside the cell and movement of potassium and phosphate outside the cell. This is an interesting model because it showed the reversibility of this significant cell membrane defect, which in this instance was produced by direct injury, that is, renal ischemia, rather than by renal ischemia as a part of systemic shock.

Additional attempts are being made at early detection of the compartment pressure syndrome, and articles this year detail the use of a polyethylene split catheter. This looks like a promising early diagnostic technique. Several articles also describe the remarkable advances and advantages in the use of arthroscopic surgery of the knee after injury. Certainly, in time, electrocoagulation and laser through the arthroscope will largely replace open knee surgery. The use of the arthroscope is a striking development in the management of major joint injuries.

Wound Healing—Additional experience with amniotic membrane as a temporary allograft to close large wounds has made it clear that amnion is just as good as skin allografts and better than zoografts. Because amnion has negligible cost, does not require special storage techniques, and is readily available on a daily basis in most hospitals, it seems now to be the temporary cover of choice. For approximately 50 years, an adhesive glycoprotein called "fibronectin" has been identified ubiquitously in healing or regenerating tissue. Recent studies suggest that fibronectin is an important precursor to the fibrous stage of wound healing. The ability to control fibronectin synthesis and deposition could, therefore, be pivotal in the biologic control of surface and deep scarring. Prevention of intestinal adhesions, particularly, may be possible through the manipulation of fibronectin deposition.

Advances in the biologic control of surface scar continued in phase III (human) trials in 1981. Colchicine and lathyrogenic agents such as β-aminopropionitrile and penicillamine were used successfully to limit net collagen synthesis and deposition in patients with large keloids. In phase II experiments (laboratory animals), colchicine also was shown to be an effective inhibitor of myofibroblast function during wound contraction. Studies on the bacteriologic aspects of wound healing showed again how the surface of virtually all permanent suture material provides protection for bacteria. Such studies emphasized the importance of utilizing predictably absorbable sutures when the danger of infection exists. Inferior healing in diabetic patients may be improved by administering vitamin A; data from animal experiments showed significant improvement in the healing of diabetic rats. New studies on gain of tensile strength in an intestinal anastomosis demonstrated the importance of sutures and healing in the submucosal layer. The technique of placing sutures and the type of suture material are not as important as location of sutures in the submucosal plane. Segmental limb blood pressures measured by Doppler ultrasound and digital photoplethysmography were used to predict healing in below-the-knee amputations. Although some useful information can be generated from such studies, hemodynamic indices were shown not to be completely reliable in predicting the outcome of amputation for arterial insufficiency. Multiple sinus tracts in infected perineal skin were shown to be improved most expediently by excision and allowing secondary healing by epithelialization and wound contraction to occur naturally; skin grafting in the perineal area does not seem efficacious in patients with "pus-pot" perineal infections.

Infections—Experience in 1981 evaluating computed tomography (CT) as a diagnostic tool for detecting intra-abdominal collections of pus indicates that ultrasonography and radionuclide scanning are superior techniques for most patients. A possible exception is the upper abdomen where, occasionally, subdiaphragmatic collections of pus are more clearly demonstrated by a CT scan. It appears that, with more experience, computerized axial tomography scanning will be reserved primarily for the head while ultrasonic and nuclide scanning will become the major techniques for detecting lower abdominal pus. Ultrasound diagnosis of amebic liver abscess has become so accurate that if needle aspiration does not confirm the radiologic diagnosis, open operation is indicated. Moreover, continued use of ultrasonography appears to be an ideal method for following the progress of treatment. Serum lactic acid levels were shown to be an accurate adjunctive test (to direct and indirect scanning) in the search for intra-abdominal pus. As might be expected, improved accuracy of radiologic localization of pus in the abdomen has been followed by the demonstration that catheters can be inserted under radiologic control to drain pus out of the abdomen. Most surgeons are not ready yet to recommend that drainage by insertion of catheters under radiologic direction is better than open drainage. Another method reported in 1981 for evaluating treatment of intra-abdominal infection is measurement of chemotaxis, migration, and chemoluminescence of neutrophils. Such tests proved to be early indicators of recurrent or inadequately treated body cavity infections. A 1981 review of agents used to disinfect skin suggested that the agent of choice now is chlorhexidine. Data to support such a conclusion did not appear convincing to reviewers. Similar problems still exist in evaluating topical providone-iodine as a treatment or preventative of wound infection. Enthusiasm remains high; data to support enthusiasm are not convincing. The eternal search for practical immunization of patients against nosocomial infection continued in 1981. Early results of new trials seemed encouraging, but a major breakthrough does not seem to have occurred. Progress was reported in the development of techniques to measure tissue levels of antibiotics. In most patients, these levels are much lower than might have been predicted by serum levels.

Burns—The question of whether intravascular administration of protein is of any measurable value in the treatment of burned patients during the first 24 hours was not answered in 1981. Apparent improvement in patients treated with albumin does not appear to be due necessarily to retention of albumin within the vascular space; adequate controls, such as the effect of H_2-blocking agents, have not been described. Although studies reporting superiority of low volumes of fluid and, in some patients, the use of hypertonic salt solutions suggest improvement in treatment of burn shock, the major cause of death is not shock. Infection and energy depletion are causing most fatalities, and readjusting the volume of water or concentration of salt, or both, simply does not make a significant difference in the death rate of patients with large burns. Similarly, claims that respiratory distress is practically always the result of overhydration or unrecognized sepsis still seem incomplete and oversimplified. Fatal respiratory distress is a complex phenomenon, and the problem of the stiff lung has not been solved by the use of albumin and antibiotics. Studies in 1981 reveal that prolonged anesthesia in small children who are undergoing dressing of burns results in a significant energy loss to replace heat. That loss can be reduced by attention to such details as the duration of anesthesia and dressing techniques. Parenteral alimentation continues to make a major contribution to preservation of immunologic responses and prevention of infection. Assays of biologic reactions such as lymphocyte responsiveness and the presence of serum suppressors were shown to predict accurately the prognosis in patients with major burns. Diagnosis of viral infections can be made in burned children and may contribute to the patient's recovery. When control of bacterial and viral infections has been successful, relatively harmless fungi such as *Candida* can become dangerous pathogens in the burn wound or blood. The mesh graft has proved so useful in treating large burns that it seems to be used indiscriminately, and perhaps unwisely, in small burns. The most important research in wound management produced advances in the development of artificial skin. Cultures of human epithelium and grafting of cultured cells on a collagen substrate were major laboratory advances. Small grafts of cultured epithelium on human wounds showed promise that cultured skin may become a pragmatic answer to the major problem for the burned patient—shortage of skin.

Transplantation and Artificial Organs—During the past year, the major impact on the transplantation scene has been the greater use of either polyspecific or donor-specific pretransplant blood transfusions, along with an increasing use of cyclosporin A as an immunosuppressive agent. Cyclosporin A continues to improve the results in all categories of transplantation—kidney, liver, heart, pancreas, and combined heart-lung grafts.

In the field of tissue typing and tissue matching, there is continued interest in the importance of matching class I and class II antigens and the resultant kidney transplant survival. The role of the class I antigens (HLA A and B) is well accepted and, with increasing use of DR and mixed leukocyte culture reactivity, the added benefit of the class II antigens is becoming more apparent. In addition, immunologic monitoring has made a great step forward, specifically with the use of monoclonal reagents capable of identifying T cell subsets. These reagents will allow for the fine tuning of immunologic monitoring and may provide new insights into immunosuppressive management.

Polyspecific third-party transfusions before transplantation continue to be accepted as beneficial for successful transplantation. The current data illustrate that the more transfusions the better; 10 pretransplant transfusions, however, seem to be adequate. The blood should be given as packed red blood cells, probably not leukocyte poor or frozen, and can be given in small intravenous quantities before transplantation. Corry and Birtch have noted a beneficial effect even with perioperative transfusions; however, these reports have not been confirmed. The use of donor-specific transfusions may represent an important advance in living-related-donor transplantation. The results reported by Salvatierra and others show an improvement of graft survival in those patients who do not become sensitized to donor-specific transfusions and eventually receive that specific donor kidney. The question arises, however, whether the 35% of patients that become sensitized to their donors and eventually must require cadaveric transplantation, coupled with the 15% of patients who reject their transplants, would have results better than those reported for polyspecific transfusions and for immunosuppressive therapy with antilymphocyte globulin (ALG), azathioprine, and prednisone. More work is needed in this field to determine the precise contribution of donor-specific transfusions.

Antilymphocyte globulin continues to be used at many transplant centers. Monoclonal ALG has been made available for both prophylactic trials and treatment of rejection episodes. Cosimi and co-workers have shown that the use of OKT3 monoclonal antibody was effective against acute rejection episodes, as is polyclonal ALG. Unfortunately, many of the patients who have responded to OKT3 monoclonal antibody have shown a subsequent rejection episode. This material creates sensitization and cannot be used a second time. Perhaps if the anti-OKT3 reagent were administered with prednisone, as is the current practice with polyclonal ALG, monoclonal ALG also might be used repeatedly.

In general, thoracic duct drainage has been discontinued as a method of immunosuppression because of its cumbersome technique. In its place has been substituted cyclosporin A, which appears to be an effective immunosuppressive agent, especially when used with small doses of steroids, as described by Starzl and his co-workers. Our own prospective double-blind randomized study at the University of Minnesota includes more than 60 patients treated with cyclosporin A and prednisone, as compared to 60 patients receiving standard therapy with azathioprine, prednisone, and ALG. At present, there have been less rejection episodes with cyclosporin A and fewer kidneys have been lost, although the figures are not statistically different from those of our standard triple therapy. The most striking finding has been the decrease in the number of infections, both viral and bacterial, that are present in the patients receiving cyclosporin A alone. The long-term toxicity of cyclosporin, however, still needs to be tested. The nephrotoxicity seems to be controllable by using alternate-day dosage of cyclosporin; the hepatotoxicity is also equally managable and reversible. The real problem is the development of lymphomas that may be of concern over the long term. We have only seen one such lymphoma in our series. The randomized prospective trial will continue at our institution until the clinical efficacy of cyclosporin has been determined.

Immune monitoring with cyclosporin reveals several interesting facts. The first is that it is important to maintain the presence of cyclosporin in the blood to sustain immunosuppression; when the drug is stopped, rejection seems to follow shortly thereafter. In addition, immunologic monitoring shows no decrease in T cell number but a definite decrease of T cell responsiveness to concanavalin A, phytohemagglutinin, and third-party mixed leukocyte culture. This effect seems to be mediated by the plasma that contains cyclosporin; once the patients' cells are removed from that plasma and placed in normal plasma, the effect is gone.

Segmental pancreas transplants are continuing to be done in increasing numbers. There have been more than 200 pancreas transplants reported to the Pancreas Transplant Registry, directed by Dr. David Sutherland at the University of Minnesota. Our own experience includes more than 47 transplants in 44 patients, and 17 of those transplants are currently functioning. The present operative technique includes either drainage into a Roux-en-Y jejunal segment or blockage of the pancreatic duct with silicone rubber. Both of these techniques appear to be working well and, with the use of cyclosporin and a decreased need for prednisone, the results continue to improve. Islet cell transplantation is done strictly as an autotransplant in patients who require pancreatectomy for chronic pancreatitis. Allotransplantation of islets have been discontinued because of the exquisite sensitivity of islets to rejection.

The results of both liver and heart transplantation have improved since the use of cyclosporin A was begun.

Finally, in the field of artificial organs, an internal pump has been developed by Buchwald and his colleagues at the University of Minnesota. This pump has been used for the continuous infusion of heparin and chemotherapeutic agents during the past 3 to 4 years. Within the past year, this pump also has been used to administer insulin continuously to patients with type II (adult onset) diabetes, with salutary results. It is now being tested on some type I (juvenile onset) diabetics as well. In addition to this internal pump, there are many external pump devices that deliver insulin either intraperitoneally or subcutaneously. In general, these pumps have been helpful in modulating glucose excursions in diabetic patients, particularly those with adult-onset diabetes. Both internal and external pumps, including an implantable artificial heart pump which is being developed by the group in Salt Lake City, are showing promise in preliminary clinical trials.

Oncology and Tumor Immunology—Multimodal cancer treatment with operation, radiation therapy, chemotherapy, hyperthermia, and immunotherapy continues to be explored in both the laboratory and the clinic. Unfortunately, the major breakthroughs that were predicted a decade ago have been infrequent. Gradual progress in multimodal therapy of sarcoma, however, has become apparent recently. Immunotherapy has added much, thus far, and both systemic and local hyperthermia are too new to even conceive of their ultimate role in the treatment of the surgical patient. Nevertheless, certain promising trends are apparent in surgical oncology.

Local hyperthermia using radiofrequency devices appears to be a promising adjunct to chemotherapy in the treatment of certain cancers, especially those metastatic to the liver. Systemic hyperthermia has become increasingly safe; with careful hemodynamic monitoring and rapid fluid replacement, it now carries a very low mortality. On the other hand, cures have not been observed, and this modality must be combined with chemotherapy. The combination of hyperthermia with subsequent local resection, or with radiotherapy for extensive local disease, has not been tried. A mechanism by which tumor cells seem more susceptible to heat is not yet clear. Both vascular events and cell biologic responses are certainly responsible.

Several years ago, Salmon and Hamburger reported that tumors could be cloned in vitro, thereby offering the opportunity to study in vitro sensitivity of the tumor to a variety of chemotherapeutic agents. There is no reason why sensitivity to hyperthermia or radiation therapy also should not be studied in vitro. These techniques initially were used to select agents to which the tumor could be expected to respond. In fact, the negative selection of agents to which the tumor would not be expected to respond appears even more promising. The first studies are emerging in the use of the clonogenic in vitro chemotherapy assay to determine sensitivity of solid tumors commonly seen by surgeons. These results also appear promising. There is a high degree of negative selection and some degree of positive selection. Unfortunately, establishing clonogenic assays is time-consuming and expensive and requires a vast commitment of facilities. Therefore, it may be some time before sensitivity studies of tumors become routine, similar to the studies used by medical microbiologists for determining sensitivity of bacteria to antimicrobial agents.

The role of limited operation with supplemental, but curative, radiation therapy in the treatment of stage I cancers is gaining some ground. The early, admittedly incomplete, results that compare combined local tumor excision plus radiation therapy to radical or modified radical mastectomy demonstrate little difference in the projected outcomes. Despite the enthusiasm for this approach, thereby sparing the patient considerable insult to her self-image, most authorities, including radiotherapists, agree that total mastectomy with axillary node dissection is still the current standard treatment for stage I breast cancer.

The advent of monoclonal antibody technology has been embraced enthusiastically by tumor immunologists and nonimmunologic oncologists alike. Basically, this technique involves fusion of a sensitized antibody-producing cell with a myeloma cell. A single antibody is then produced that is highly specific for a single determinant. The clutter of antibodies in response to polyantigens thus is eliminated. By careful screening of a number of these hybridomas, certain immortal cell populations can be selected that will produce antibodies of a given specificity and a given type. For example, antibodies can be selected (1) that react with some but not with other antigens on the tumor cell surface; (2) that react with antigens on a tumor cell surface that will not react with the native tissue from which the tumor arose; or (3) that react with tumor antigens that can bind complement, therefore exerting a direct destructive effect against the antigenic tissue. Antibodies can be labeled in various ways and used to detect small tumor metastases. Antibodies can be labeled with toxic materials and used to carry these toxins, radioactive or otherwise, directly to the tumor without exerting toxic effects on other tissues. Antibodies can be used to analyze tumor antigens on cell surfaces for the subsequent selection of antigens to make new antibodies. One must remember, however, that polyclonal antibodies may have many more functions than do monoclonal antibodies in clinical medicine. Collection of pure, highly specific, antibodies may, in fact, eliminate certain aspects of the multimodal, i.e., polyspecific antibody mixture, attack on a tumor cell. Nevertheless, monoclonal antibodies allow one to analyze and dissect the immunodiagnostic and immunotherapeutic potential of these new discoveries.

Hand—Enthusiasm for replanting amputated digits continued in 1981. Most experienced surgeons conclude, however, that replantation of a single digit, particularly the index finger, is not advisable in most patients. Arterial shunting as a temporary means of revascularization while bone, tendon, and nerve repairs are performed was recommended to reduce cool ischemia time, although it appears from isolated case reports that cool ischemia time for a distal digit can be as long as several days without producing irreversible changes that make replantation unsuccessful. Function after digital replantation has not been optimal for many patients; it seems that more replantations are done now than will be performed after psychological, social, and economic factors are considered. A technical improvement introduced in 1981 uses a neurovascular bundle transfer from an adjacent uninjured digit to avoid interposition grafts for vessels or nerves in the replanted digit. Veins accompanying digital arteries are not reliable, however; neurovascular transfers probably will be most useful for artery and nerve deficits. Local sympathectomy still is being recommended by some hand surgeons for digital ischemia caused primarily by spasm. The prevailing opinion among most hand surgeons is that proximal sympathectomy of the entire upper extremity is required for severe spastic disorders. A randomized prospective study performed as objectively as possible for subjective factors concluded that there were no measurable advantages to performing fascicular rather than conventional epineural neurorrhaphy on digital nerves. Because there are significant theoretical and practical disadvantages to fascicular repair, this study should result in a return to conventional epineural neurorrhaphy. Previous studies revealing that partial lacerations of flexor tendons probably should not be repaired in most patients were challenged by the report of complications occurring in some patients with unrepaired partial lacerations. Most of the reported complications should have been anticipated, however; the majority of partial lacerations of flexor tendons probably are handled best by not introducing suture material into the tendon. Attenuation of tendon junction scar was shown to be preventable by exacting technique, including adequate debridement of tendon ends, correct placement of sutures, and careful supervision of early motion. Failure of carpal tunnel decompression to relieve signs and symptoms was shown to be the result of inadequate exposure and identification of carpal canal structures. The recurrence rate of 12% after surgical excision of wrist ganglia is a marked improvement over previous studies that revealed a 30% to 40% long-term recurrence. Wide excision of all redundant dense connective tissue around the joint rather than enucleation of a single cystic structure seems to be responsible for improved results.

Breast—Early diagnosis of breast tumors was attempted in 1981 by the use of CT mammography. Although there may be some advantages over other types of mammography for special high-risk patients, the need for infusion of an iodinated contrast medium and the relatively high cost make CT scanning inappropriate now as a general screening tool. Although scintiscanning of the breast with ^{99m}Tc-diethylene triamine penta-acetic acid appears accurate in the early diagnosis of primary breast tumors, lymphoscintigraphy, in general, still is not a reliable method of diagnosing minimally involved axillary lymph nodes. Better epidemiologic surveys than previously available showed in 1981 that there was not a significantly increased risk of breast cancer in women with most types of fibrocystic disease. Although the final answer to the important and still perplexing problem of the relation of fibrocystic disease to breast cancers still is not clear, it seems increasingly certain that previous studies indicating a high incidence of breast cancer associated with benign disease were flawed. Additional evidence was reported in 1981 that microscopic breast cancer is multifocular in many patients. The biologic significance of this type of breast cancer is still not certain; it is too early, therefore, to use such data as a basis for abandoning present studies on conservative management of breast carcinoma. Additional data were accumulated showing that quadrant excision of the breast for small cancers, limited axillary dissection as a sort of staging procedure, and postoperative radiation can produce control rates for at least 7 years that are as good as those after more radical extirpative surgery. More aggressive institution of early shoulder rotation and abduction after axillary dissection was shown to be efficacious without significant risk. Early motion is even more satisfactory when a limited dissection is performed, one in which only the lower level of lymph nodes is removed. An important study by the National Adjuvant Study Group revealed that removal of the lower two levels of axillary lymph nodes provides information just as accurate for subsequent treatment as does removal of all lymph nodes. Such studies argue strongly that regional lymph nodes primarily are indicators of the biologic characteristics of breast carcinoma and are not instigators of distant disease. Data reported in 1981 raise again the question of whether pregnancy affects the prognosis of postmastectomy patients. The most recent study suggests that pregnancy does not present an added risk factor for most patients. Studies on social, psychological, and financial aspects suggest that adjuvant chemotherapy probably is being used a little more often than is desirable for some patients. Reconstruction of the breast after mastectomy continues to improve; a new method featuring transfer of redundant abdominal fat, skin, and muscle to the amputation site, thus eliminating the need for a prosthesis, produced the standard for 1981.

Head and Neck—An article in 1981 raising the question of the need for relatively aggressive versus relatively conservative surgical extirpation of benign parotid tumors seems to have overlooked the concept of simultaneous nerve-tumor dissection without regard for whether the resulting procedure turns out to be aggressive or not so aggressive. The basic principles established over 50 years ago seem to hold despite repeated analysis and redefinition of the problem presented by a potentially dangerous, yet histologic benign, tumor when it is adjacent to an important motor nerve. Ultrasonography and CT scanning may have improved preoperative diagnostic evaluation of the spread of malignant tumors a little, but the data offered in 1981 were not convincing that any major improvement has occurred. Evaluation showed that statistical methods used in predicting microscopic spread in a neck with clinically negative findings also were not impressive when compared to historical and biologic analyses of tumor characteristics. Additional evidence that a bilateral neck dissection can be performed safely in one stage appeared in 1981, but the need to perform a bilateral complete (both internal jugular veins) neck dissection in most patients was not convincing. A superb study, one of the very few and certainly one of the best, if not *the* best, randomized prospective study on the value of preoperative irradiation for head and neck cancers should put to rest the theoretical notion that a combination of surgery and radiation is superior to the best of each performed alone. New advances in palliative care feature primarily significant improvement in the control of pain. Advanced neurosurgical and neurophysiological electric stimulation techniques have achieved significant control of the pain of head and neck cancer. Demineralized bone, similar to the protein substrate developed by Urist over 20 years ago, was shown in 1981 to provide a useful scaffold for osteogenesis in cranial reconstruction. Severe exophthalmos was shown to be correctable to a greater extent than previously possible by the simultaneous decompression of at least three sides of the orbit. Recent techniques in craniofacial reconstruction for congenital anomalies have been used in the most extensive enlargement of the orbital cavity yet attempted.

Thorax—The article by Tepas et al. concerning 74 tracheostomies in infants, 48 of whom were newborns, supports the fact that, properly performed, tracheostomy in a newborn can be virtually free of complications. The report by Boyd and his co-workers on reconstruction of chest wall defects may be quite significant because the increased stability of the chest wall with the use of myocutaneous flaps may make the introduction of foreign material such as Marlex or Lucite unnecessary.

Progress in the treatment of bronchogenic carcinoma remains disappointingly small. Some encouragement has appeared in studies finding that survival is significantly improved in patients with small cell carcinoma treated with the combination of chemotherapy, radiation, and operation.

Finally, the role of radiation in superior sulcus tumors has been resurrected, with the report by Komaki et al. suggesting that radiation is the method of choice. This contrasts sharply with Paulson's carefully reported series spanning a period of years in which preoperative radiation was combined with resection.

Congenital Heart Disease—Only seven abstracts were selected for this chapter, as reports concerning congenital heart disease have been less abundant than in previous years. Sixty-six patients older than age 60 years had an atrial septal defect closed at the Mayo Clinic, with only 4 deaths resulting, all unrelated to pulmonary vascular resistance. Aziz et al. describe the use of two-dimensional echocardiography for evaluating patients after a Mustard operation. This may prove to be a useful noninvasive method for follow-up for late complications, such as obstruction of the superior vena cava or pulmonary veins. Finally, the review from the Mayo Clinic of procedures for the univentricular heart is sobering, indicating that only about 25% of 45 patients had a satisfactory result.

Valvular Heart Disease—Eight articles were selected for review. The series from Detroit of 61 patients who had tricuspid valvulectomy during a period of 10 years is probably the largest in the world. The data indicate that this is the procedure of choice with endocarditis, although the authors' conclusion that long-term absence of the tricuspid valve is satisfactory remains dubious.

The article by Gallo et al., which focuses attention on the technical problem of removal of a large left atrial thrombus, is significant. With proper operative technique, the removal may be quite satisfactory. Otherwise, several disasters can occur, such as operative or postoperative catastrophic embolization.

Debate continues about indications for and durability of the porcine valve. Morrow's group at the National Institutes of Health has changed its policy of routine use of the prosthesis and now limit it to selected patients. The group at Stanford University reports their experiences with over 1,400 patients.

The unusual but grim problem of rupture of the left ventricle after replacement of the mitral valve with a prosthesis is described by Gosalbez et al. Because of the lethal nature of this complication, I have discussed this report in some detail.

Finally, the report by Macmanus and his co-workers on the frequency of thromboembolism after replacement of the mitral valve is quite surprising, because more than 90% of mitral ball-valve prostheses implanted after 1973 remain free of emboli after 5 years, as compared to less than 70% before that time. The reason for the improvement is unknown.

Coronary Artery Disease—The Coronary Artery Surgery Study, described by Kennedy et al., followed the course of 25,000 patients after coronary arteriography and will be a landmark study in determining the natural history of coronary artery disease. Data thus far available indicate the grim prognosis with the combination of triple-vessel disease and significant impairment of ventricular function—a 4-year mortality of nearly 50% with medical therapy.

The rationale for the use of sequential bypass grafts is discussed in the report by O'Neill et al. Use of these grafts is increasing rapidly with the improved techniques of myocardial preservation and the feasibility of complete coronary revascularization. The influence of bypass on longevity, the crucial question with the operation, continues to be discussed. Loop and his co-workers from Cleveland describe 5-year survivals of between 88% and 93% in different groups.

A most significant field of study is the treatment of ventricular arrhythmias, especially in association with left ventricular aneurysms. The group in Philadelphia led by Harken and the group at Duke University led by Coxe have had exciting results with endocardial mapping followed by surgical excision of the trigger zone.

Radionuclide studies have made serial evaluation of left ventricular function after bypass grafting possible and indicate that the abnormalities in left ventricular function may be significantly improved.

The controversial report by Berg et al. of 10 years' experience with emergency operation for acute infarction in 227 patients presents thought-provoking data: an operative mortality of less than 2%, an impressive 1-year survival, and excellent results found on repeat catheterization. The role of emergency operation remains experimental, but may become a significant form of therapy, perhaps in conjunction with infusions of streptokinase.

Finally, Loop et al. describe the results of a second coronary bypass operation, required because of either progressive atherosclerosis or occlusion of the previous grafts. Mortality was only 4%, and significant benefit was achieved in 86% of the patients.

Miscellaneous Cardiac Disease—The papers selected for this chapter cover a wide variety of subjects. These include techniques of preoperative care, operative management, and postoperative care; pacemakers and artificial heart and cardiac transplantation; and diseases of the great vessels.

The article by Culliford et al. on noncardiogenic pulmonary edema is particularly important, defining a syndrome that probably has been described in different forms for years. The exact mechanism is unclear, but almost certainly represents an allergic reaction between a blood product and the pulmonary endothelium. It is almost indistinguishable from left ventricular failure unless left atrial pressure is measured. The difference is crucial, for the disease is quickly lethal without prompt therapy, but with steroids, positive-pressure ventilation, and diuretics, full recovery may occur between 24 and 72 hours.

The role of emergency thoracotomy in the intensive care unit is well described in 64 patients by Fairman and Edmunds; the data show that a prompt, unsterile thoracotomy saves far more lives than delaying operation until the patient can be returned to the operating room.

Separately, the report by Gielchinsky et al. indicates that myocardial edema may be so extensive that closure of the sternum can be lethal. Some patients may be salvaged by leaving the sternum open for 24 to 72 hours, followed by delayed closure.

The article by Culliford and co-workers on the lack of correlation between activated clotting time and plasma heparin focuses attention on the question of the best measurement of effective anticoagulation during bypass. An activated clotting time above 400 seconds seems to be the best measurement at present.

Progress continues in the field of cardiac transplantation, with an article by Gaudiani et al. and one by Watson et al. The 5-year actuarial survival at Stanford University since 1975 has been about 40%.

The report by Glassford et al. on pulmonary embolectomy, an area of little clinical activity at present, raises the serious question of the advisability of routinely performing a pulmonary embolectomy if arteriography demonstrates that more than 50% of the pulmonary arterial tree is obstructed. The safety of pulmonary embolectomy in these circumstances would support its more widespread use.

Two papers describe further experiences with perforation of the pulmonary artery by a Swan-Ganz catheter, discussed in the overview in the 1981 YEAR BOOK. Increasing data support the importance of a precise technique in the use of these catheters.

Progress continues with surgical treatment of dissection of the thoracic aorta, with the remarkable report by Turley et al. of operations in 21 patients in 5 years with only 1 operative death. The article by Crawford and Saleh is especially significant because the mortality usually associated with transverse aortic arch operations is well over 50%. Techniques for periods of circulatory arrest with hypothermia, described in this article, are most encouraging.

Finally, two papers describe experiences with the grim problem of aortic graft-enteric fistulas. Diagnostic studies are accurate in only about 50% of patients and the ultimate survival remains well under 50%.

Arteries—Recently, it has been shown that antithrombin deficiencies may be the cause of otherwise unexplained thrombotic episodes. The presence of antithrombin deficiency has been estimated to be 1 in 2,000. Heparin resistance is common in these patients, but treatment can be effected with fresh-frozen plasma and warfarin. The antiplatelet effects of prostaglandins, which are also vasodilating drugs, have been responsible for effective therapy in patients with distal arterial diseases. A review focuses on mycotic emboli of the peripheral vessels, a lesion that undoubtedly will increase in the future. Aggressive therapy is advised, but the results generally have been poor.

Local antibiotic irrigation has been effective in the management of arterial grafts and infections and has obviated removal of a graft in certain circumstances. There has been an ever-increasing spectrum of disorders for which selective embolization of arteries has proved effective. The primary indication remains acute or recurrent bleeding.

Arterial embolization has been assessed; the most common source is cardiac. Within a range of 8 hours to 7 days, the delay in treatment had a linear relationship to the severity of ischemic changes and deterioration. Anticoagulation reduced the rate of recurrence and the early and late morbidity and mortality. A study has demonstrated the need for close monitoring of objective hemodynamic responses in establishing the proper role of percutaneous transluminal angioplasty for lower extremity ischemia. A study of factors contributing to recurrent lower limb ischemia focuses on the importance of progressive atherosclerotic occlusion involving the inflow and outflow tract. Another series emphasizes the need for an aggressive surgical approach toward popliteal aneurysm. The importance of the morphological structure of the pedal arch and its relationship to the patency of crural vascular reconstruction has been established, as has the role of antiplatelet therapy in patients with gangrene of the toes.

Veins and Lymphatics—In patients without risk factors for bleeding, the intermittent administration of heparin for deep venous thrombosis is considered preferable because of fewer recurrences and little increase in hemorrhagic complications. In patients with a high risk of bleeding, conventional doses of heparin given continuously reduce the rate of hemorrhagic complications, but are associated with more recurrences. A functional assessment of the postthrombotic leg in patients receiving streptokinase demonstrates little improvement after this therapy for deep venous thrombosis. Additional data indicate that the Greenfield vena caval filter represents the preferable device, because it is associated with the highest patency rate. It has been shown that femoral valve reconstruction performed alone for venous stasis is not sufficient, and it must be accompanied by conventional therapy of the distal perforators in the superficial system. Primary lymphedema continues to be managed conservatively in all but a few cases, and it has been shown that further spreading of lymphedema occurs rarely after the first year and is almost unknown after 5 years. Patients without pelvic lymphatic obstruction had good prognoses even if the distal lymphatics were obliterated. Surgical therapy generally is used in those with obstruction of the pelvic lymphatics. Microsurgical techniques have been applied with success to the treatment of lymphedema of the limbs.

Esophagus—The very common problem of gastroesophageal reflux has continued to occupy the attention of investigators during the past year. The important role of the lower esophageal sphincter in preventing reflux has been reaffirmed. It appears now that measurement of lower esophageal sphincter pressure, which for the past few years has taken a backseat to 24-hour esophageal pH determinations, is about to become an acceptable—if not pivotal—test once again if the volume of acid introduced into the stomach that will produce reflux is measured concurrently. In other words, there seems to be a very strong and direct correlation between lower esophageal sphincter pressure and the volume of 0.1 N HCl instilled in the stomach before reflux occurs. In my opinion, the latter test, namely, the introduction of acid into the *stomach,* probably ultimately will replace both the measurement of lower esophageal sphincter pressure and the 24-hour monitoring of esophageal pH.

The controversy as to whether fundal wraps can safely be left within the thorax after Nissen fundoplication continues, not because the antireflux mechanism fails in the chest, but, rather, because the supradiaphragmatic pouch seems to cause some delay in emptying and to become the site of ulceration. My suspicion is that the major value of the Collis gastroplasty will ultimately be to obviate these complications rather than to provide an intra-abdominal esophagus that, for ethereal reasons, provides a better antireflux mechanism.

There is a resurgence of interest in a multidisciplinary approach to the treatment of squamous cell carcinoma of the esophagus, and it appears that combination chemotherapy, radiation, and surgery may indeed improve survival. At the same time, some surgeons such as Akiyama and his collaborators have shown that extensive mediastinal lymph node metastases, far removed from the primary site, are often present in patients with this disease. For this reason, they have advocated and carried out total esophagectomy with radical mediastinal lymph node dissection, and they have achieved remarkably low mortality rates and surprisingly good long-term survival. Whether such can be achieved in a less carefully selected group of patients remains to be seen.

Stomach and Duodenum—The problem of postoperative reflux gastritis remains with us, especially in regard to its diagnosis. Recent studies suggest that perhaps it is intestinal content rather than bile salts or alkaline pH that causes the symptoms. Instillation of the patient's own intestinal juice seems to reproduce symptoms more reliably than bile salts or alkaline pH. To our knowledge, however, no one has developed sufficiently strict diagnostic criteria that are universally acceptable. For this reason, large numbers of Roux-en-Y diversions are being done, many of which may not be warranted. That these diversions are not without problems is evident by the recognition that a surprisingly high percentage of these patients (about one-fourth to one-third) develop delayed gastric emptying after the Roux-en-Y diversion. The mechanism for such delay is not clear.

Even though upper gastrointestinal endoscopy has become almost commonplace, a very fine controlled trial by Peterson and his colleagues has now shown that endoscopy does not alter outcome in any way in the patient who enters the hospital with upper gastrointestinal hemorrhage but who stops bleeding spontaneously and stabilizes. It is interesting that, in this study, urgent operation was carried out with the same frequency in both the endoscopy and the no-endoscopy groups. Whether outcome would have been altered in this study had the knowledge of the importance of the "visible vessel" in the ulcer crater been available to the endoscopists is not apparent, because no mention of this criterion for early operation was made. In another randomized trial, however, the importance of the "visible vessel" as a predictor of an increased chance of rebleeding has been clearly demonstrated. Hopefully, the mortality rate of upper gastrointestinal hemorrhage will be reduced to some extent by this finding, because patients who will require operation can be identified at a very much earlier stage.

The criteria for the diagnosis of gastrinoma are becoming sharper, so that we now have data to show that secretin will not cause the serum gastrin concentration to rise more than 40 pg/ml in vagotomized patients in the absence of gastrinoma. In addition, the use of bombesin may help distinguish between duodenal and pancreatic gastrinomas.

Small Intestine—This has been a year of reassessment for investigations pertaining to the small intestine, rather than a period during which major new breakthroughs have been accomplished. The enthusiasm for use of the Doppler monitor to assess viability of precariously viable intestine has been tempered by an excellent trial that clearly demonstrated the superiority of the use of fluorescein over the Doppler monitor. The entity of intestinal angina remains relatively rare, and it is still unclear as to why angina does not occur in some patients with vascular occlusions of the same magnitude as patients with angina. There is now almost unanimous agreement that compression of the celiac axis does not cause chronic abdominal pain and that operative decompression of the celiac axis is not indicated unless it is part of a larger operation designed to improve overall splanchnic blood flow, although it rarely will be needed even in these circumstances.

Reevaluation of the use of the Baker tube or the Leonard tube to prevent recurrent intestinal obstruction in patients in whom operation has produced extensive and frequent serosal denudations indicates that such stenting is probably of little, if any, value. The incidence of complications may be increased with the use of such intraluminal stents.

Colon and Rectum—The interest in provision of continence to patients who necessarily must undergo panproctocolectomy continues. Since Parks revived the use of ileoanal anastomosis, many different types of pouches have been used proximal to the anal sphincter. The abnormal rectal mucosa is difficult to remove, and the incidence of complications remains fairly high. In addition, diarrhea and nocturnal incontinence are relatively common. Finally, it is likely that the "pouchitis" that has afflicted the Kock continent ileostomy will also involve these pelvic pouches, although reports of such have not appeared as yet. A new entity of colitis in the rectum distal to a colostomy or ileostomy has been described by Glotzer et al. and has been called "diversion colitis." The clinical importance of the recognition of this entity is obvious, as failure to do so has resulted in unnecessarily radical operations because of the false attribution of the inflammation in the rectum to either ulcerative colitis or Crohn's disease.

Carcinoma of the rectum has a high incidence of local recurrence within the pelvis, whether after abdominoperineal resection or low anterior resection, and such recurrences are often the cause for much discomfort as well as death. Administration of postoperative radiation in patients with residual disease at the time of the original resection has recently produced very encouraging results, suggesting that perhaps the use of this adjunct might be extended. For rectum and distal sigmoid severely injured by radiation, Bricker and his associates have developed imaginative new methods of repair using uninjured proximal colon.

Hemorrhoidectomy may become an extinct procedure. Dissatisfaction with the long-term results of this operation, together with the recognition that multiple injections of sclerosing solutions or rubber-band ligations provide excellent results, has contributed to the less frequent use of hemorrhoidectomy.

Liver and Spleen—A change in thinking regarding hepatic trauma has evolved. Intra-abdominal packing for control of exsanguination from hepatic hemorrhage has been shown to be lifesaving. There were no instances of rebleeding after removal of the packing in 9 patients. It has been shown that subcapsular hematoma secondary to trauma can be managed nonoperatively. A large series of patients in whom resection of primary solid hepatic tumors was carried out underscores a mortality of less than 3% in experienced hands, and it justifies aggressive treatment of primary hepatic malignancy. An increasing interest in resection of liver metastases from colorectal cancer is noted. The use of carcinoembryonic antigen and alkaline phosphatase to screen patients has provided a reasonable method of assessing those in whom angiographic evaluation, CT scan, and subsequent exploration are indicated.

A large series of cases is the focus of a report of congenital hepatic fibrosis, an autosomal recessive disease causing portal hypertension and cholangitis. Portal systemic shunts obviate future bleeding and are not associated with encephalopathy in these patients. When portal hypertension is a consequence of extrahepatic portal vein thrombosis, it does not represent a life-threatening problem as far as exsanguination is concerned, but repeated episodes of bleeding are well controlled by decompressive surgery, with minimal mortality and no subsequent encephalopathy. The most readily correctable bleeding associated with portal hypertension relates to that in which the hypertension is limited to the left side, usually as a consequence of pancreatic disease and splenic vein thrombosis. The definitive therapy is splenectomy, but transgastric ligation of a bleeding site may be necessary. In cirrhotic patients with bleeding varices, the medical regimen is based on lavage, Pitressin, balloon tamponade, or a combination of these. Bleeding was controlled in 69% of cases and permitted surgical treatment with an improved Child's score. In a prospective study, the incidence of portal systemic encephalopathy after emergency shunting procedures was 31.5%, with severe encephalopathy in 7% of survivors. In long-term (10 years or more) survivors, encephalopathy was virtually absent. The 1981 literature contains the definitive article concerning the technique of selective transsplenic decompression of varices. There is also a study suggesting that the distal splenorenal shunt, with gastrosplenic mesenteric disconnection, loses its selectivity a few months after surgery, as evidenced by a decrease in portal flow at that time. It is the authors' contention that the distal splenorenal shunt does not appear to differ hemodynamically from side-to-side shunts. The occurrence of hypersplenism in control cirrhotic patients and patients with prophylactic portacaval anastomosis was assessed, and no significant difference in the incidence of hypersplenism was noted. Additional success with portacaval shunts to reduce serum cholesterol levels in patients with heterozygous type II hypercholesterolemia was reported. These patients with portal hypertension who underwent portacaval shunt showed no evidence of postshunt encephalopathy. The mechanism of action of the peritoneovenous shunt used in the management of intractable hepatic ascites remains unclear, but it has been noted that peritoneovenous shunting in selected patients partially reverses the sodium retention. Sodium retention is multifactorial, with both the renin-aldosterone system and possibly portal hypertension playing a role.

Conservative, nonoperative management and preservation of the injured spleen continue to be championed. One of the pitfalls of this approach in reference to blunt trauma is the possibility of missing concomitant serious abdominal injuries. Successful selective management of the injured spleen has been reported, particularly in the pediatric literature. In a series of children with this disorder managed since 1977, splenic salvage was reported in 86%. This technique has also been applied in an adult series. In 33 patients, no subphrenic abscesses developed, and delayed rupture of the spleen could not be established.

Splenectomy continues to provide the best results for patients with immune idiopathic thrombocytopenic purpura. Complete remission occurred in 77% of patients, and 85% benefited from the procedure. A reported series showed a predictive correlation in the response to corticosteroids in these patients.

The uncommon circumstance of thrombosis of the portal vein after splenectomy was reported in 5 of 28 patients undergoing excision of the organ for myeloid metaplasia. This did not correlate with thrombocytosis.

Splenectomy is being performed with increasing frequency for patients with lymphomas and chronic lymphocytic leukemia. It represents a valuable adjunct because patients are palliated in regard to symptoms related to the splenomegaly and hypersplenism. The operation should be considered at the first suggestion of splenic overactivity.

Biliary Tract—Hepatobiliary isotope scanning has represented a significant addition to the diagnostic armamentarium and is particularly applicable to the diagnosis of acute cholecystitis. It is to be emphasized, however, that the scans probably will not replace contrast radiology in the diagnosis of chronic gallbladder disease. The surgical section of the American Academy of Pediatrics surveyed 188 cases of choledochal cysts and emphasized the importance of early surgical attention and an increasing tendency to resect the lesion in order to obviate the development of carcinoma. It has been reported that primary repair of biliary enteric fistula usually can be performed in patients without obstruction. However, when intestinal obstruction results as a consequence of gallstones, that lesion should be treated initially and the fistula should be corrected at a later time. Choledochoscopy has been shown to have a significant impact on the management of choledocholithiasis. Additional stones were noted in 24% of patients in whom initial exploration was negative. Retained biliary stones can be dissolved, and a new agent, Capmul 8210, has a distinct advantage over sodium cholate because it is more powerful and has fewer side effects.

The argument continues as to whether patients with gallstone pancreatitis should have early operative intervention. A recent series indicated that early surgery was as safe as delayed surgery and resulted in savings of both time and money. Chiba needle cholangiography has been applied to the diagnosis of possible acute pancreatitis associated with cholelithiasis; it helps separate patients in whom the elevated amylase level is a consequence of pancreatitis from those in whom the elevation results merely from obstruction of the bile duct. The National Cooperative Gallstone Study has reported the results of chenodeoxycholic acid for dissolution of these stones. Complete dissolution of the stones was confirmed in 13.5% of patients given high-dose therapy. Dissolution was more frequent in women, thin patients, and patients with small or floating gallstones or a serum cholesterol level of 227 mg/dl or above. Sphincteroplasty has proved a satisfactory operation in patients with primary cholangitis; more than 80% were asymptomatic after discharge. It has been shown that choledochoduodenostomy and choledochojejunostomy or sphincteroplasty should not represent competitive operations; when they are used under appropriate circumstances, they provide equivalent results.

Biliary tract surgery in patients with cirrhosis is associated with increased mortality and morbidity. A more conservative approach to elective cholecystectomy in the cirrhotic patient is indicated. If an operation is performed, increased bleeding should be anticipated and extensive intrahepatic dissection avoided, and intraoperative infusion of vasopressin and an antifibrinolytic agent should be considered.

There has been little improvement in the results of surgery for patients with carcinoma of the gallbladder even when radical procedures are carried out. The best prognosis in patients with bile duct carcinoma is associated with lesions of the lower third, and there is general dissatisfaction with aggressive management of lesions of the confluence of the right and left hepatic ducts. Nonoperative measures may be indicated, including percutaneous drainage using a stent to allow the bile to enter the bowel. The role of radiotherapy in the management of this tumor remains to be established. Cholangitis is a frequent presenting symptom in patients with malignant obstruction of biliary outflow. These patients may be palliated by drainage.

Percutaneous transhepatic biliary decompression lowers operative morbidity in patients with obstructive jaundice, particularly if the bilirubin concentration is greater than 6 mg/dl. Long-term percutaneous decompression of the bile duct has proved a satisfactory treatment for poor-risk patients. Internal drainage is to be preferred, but external drainage should be performed for a period of time before conversion to internal drainage. Recent data enforce the statement that biliary tract operations performed in conjunction with other abdominal procedures can be carried out with a relatively low morbidity and mortality rate. It is also reasonable to perform definitive surgery for most gastrointestinal diseases discovered incidental to planned cholecystectomy.

Pancreas—The increasing use of endoscopic retrograde cholangiopancreatography (ERCP) is beginning to give us a better understanding of some of the heretofore so-called idiopathic cases of pancreatitis. For example, isolated distal pancreatic ductal stenoses have been identified preoperatively with greater frequency and have responded well to surgical treatment. Great interest has been generated in instances of pancreas divisum, although whether this congenital anomaly (present in about 10% of all people) in reality predisposes to pancreatitis—as some have suggested—is not clear. The natural history of chronic alcoholic pancreatitis as it affects the ductal system is also being elucidated by ERCP. It has been shown that the ductal changes in alcoholic disease may be progressive even if the intake of alcohol is discontinued, whereas such is not the case in gallstone pancreatitis.

The dismal outlook for patients with adenocarcinoma of the pancreas continues despite heroic attempts to carry out the most radical of procedures, such as resection of the celiac axis and port vein. Studies now also have shown that total pancreatectomy does not increase salvage, so that its only advantage is avoidance of the pancreaticojejunal anastomosis, a gain that is offset by the imposition of diabetes.

Transhepatic superselective catheterization of the venous drainage of the pancreas for measurement of hormone levels continues to occupy the attention of some investigators, who hope to localize pancreatic endocrine tumors, especially insulinomas, more precisely. In my opinion, the results are far from superb, and this procedure will be of great practical value only rarely.

Endocrine Glands—A new disorder called "familial hypocalciuric hypercalcemia" has been identified and must be kept in mind as a disease that easily can masquerade as primary hyperparathyroidism. It could account for some cases of previous misdiagnosis of primary hyperparathyroidism. Ultrasonography has been proposed as a method for preoperative identification of enlarged parathyroid glands. It is attractive because it is noninvasive, but it has limited value in the patient previously operated on, and its ultimate benefit must await further experience. For patients previously operated on or in the case of mediastinal adenomas, CT scanning is probably more useful. Several studies have now confirmed the fact that "double adenomas" do indeed occur in about 3% of patients with primary hyperparathyroidism. For that reason, unilateral cervical exploration probably should never be done, except perhaps in patients previously operated on in whom normal glands clearly have been identified on the contralateral side.

Serum thyroglobulin levels probably will replace repeated radioactive iodine scans in the postoperative evaluation of patients with thyroid cancer. The advantages of avoiding a prolonged period without thyroid replacement are obvious, and the accrued data suggest that the serum thyroglobulin levels while the patient is taking thyroid replacement are at least as accurate as the radioactive iodine scan in identifying patients with persistent or recurrent carcinomas.

The enthusiasm for transcervical thymectomy for myasthenia gravis is waning as the long-term results are becoming available. It seems clear that total thymectomy has a very real advantage in terms of outcome, and it is also evident that such is not so readily achieved by the transcervical operation as the original reports suggested. More radical operations to clear the entire anterior mediastinum of all thymic tissue are becoming increasingly popular.

1. General Considerations

1-1 **Acute Surgical Illness in Patients With Sickle Cell Anemia.** Acute abdominal pain is common in sickle cell crisis, and the clinical picture may simulate acute surgical illness. Kenneth A. Kudsk, Robert F. Tranbaugh, and George F. Sheldon (San Francisco) determined the incidence of acute surgical problems in 81 patients with hemolytic anemia and abdominal pain, seen in 1963–1980. Only 7 patients were operated on during the review period. Six of them had sickle cell anemia, and 1 had sickle hemoglobin C disease. Clinical data are presented in the table. Five patients had had an average of 2½ admissions annually for sickle crisis. Six patients had an admission diagnosis of sickle crisis. Four had biliary tract disease, 1 had an infected intrauterine device, and 1 had appendicitis. In 1 patient admitted with a diagnosis of appendicitis, the laparotomy findings were negative. Three of the patients with biliary disease had colicky, sharp pain rather than the diffuse upper abdominal pain characteristic of sickle crisis. Routine laboratory tests were helpful in distinguishing surgical illness from sickle crisis in these cases. The serum bilirubin level was not helpful except in the context of previous patterns of illness.

The cause of abdominal pain associated with sickling is unknown. The pain may be associated with peritoneal irritation, and can mimic diseases such as appendictis and cholecystitis. Some patients fail to improve with hydration and supportive care. Medical records are critical in differentiating sickle crisis from surgical conditions; deviation from a characteristic pattern should suggest that illness is caused by a problem other than sickle cell crisis. Biliary tract disease has been the most common cause of intra-abdominal infection leading to surgery. All patients with sickle cell anemia who intermittently hemolyze red blood cells should have annual evaluation of the biliary tract by sonography or oral cholecystography. Incidental appendectomy is

DATA ON SEVEN PATIENTS OPERATED ON

Case	Hemoglobin-opathy	Age (yr)	Admissions (n)/Years	Frequency of Crisis	Abdominal Pain	Hemoglobin/ Hematocrit	Disease
1	SS	11	12/6	10–15/yr	Yes	7/25	Acute edematous cholecystitis
2	SS	18	5/3	1–2/yr	At age 7 only	8/22	Acute edematous cholecystitis
3	SC	26	None	2–3/yr*	Yes	11/31	Infected IUD
4	SS	23	7/3	4–6/yr	Yes	7/22	Negative appendix
5	SS	27	None	None	No	7/22	Stone impacted in common bile duct
6	SS	18	20/5	8–10/yr	Yes	9/28	Appendicitis
7	SS	24	21/9	10–15/yr	Yes	7/19	Stone impacted in ampulla with cholecystitis

*None since age 21 years.
Note: IUD indicates intrauterine device; SC, sickle cell/hemoglobin C disease; SS, sickle cell anemia.

(1–1) Am. J. Surg. 142:133–117, July 1981.

rational in patients with sickle cell disease, but prophylactic appendectomy may not be warranted, because the incidence of appendicitis in these patients is low.

▶ [The authors provide an extremely helpful algorithm for differentiating between abdominal pain due to sickle cell crisis and pain associated with surgical illness. Sickle cell anemia necessitates specific anesthetic consideration. Hypoxia is always to be avoided because a crisis can ensue and adequate oxygenation is required during the postoperative period. Wound healing may be affected adversely in patients with SS hemoglobin genotype, by virtue of intravascular thrombosis during sickling crises. In patients with AS hemoglobin genotype, there is no particular problem in wound healing. Sickle cell disease is an important cause of splenic infarct and must be considered in any patient who complains of pain in the left upper area of the abdomen. It is also an etiologic factor in the formation of the rare primary splenic abscess. In several series, thrombosis of the splenic vessels with infarction was a constant factor in the evolution of splenic abscesses (Schwartz et al.: *Tropical Surgery,* McGraw Hill, New York, 1971, p. 355).—S.I.S.] ◀

1-2 **Major Surgery in Hemophilia** is discussed by Witold J. Rudowski (Warsaw, Poland). Surgery in hemophilia always carried a high risk of bleeding and hemorrhagic complications. The development of factor VIII concentrates was a breakthrough in performing major surgery on hemophiliacs. A total of 131 operations were done on 110 patients with hemophilia and other clotting disorders in 1961–1979. Eighty-five patients with hemophilia A underwent 104 operations. A large majority of patients had major abdominal and orthopedic procedures. The mortality was 4.55% (3.8% of procedures). Two patients died after severe hemorrhagic complications. The overall incidence of hemorrhagic complications was 11%. These were less frequent in severe than in mild cases. More than one third of urologic procedures were followed by hemorrhagic complications. The incidence after abdominal surgery was 22% and that after orthopedic surgery, 10.5%.

The plasma factor VIII levels should be elevated to 40%–50% of normal until wound healing is complete. The only effective approach is the administration of antihemophilic globulin preparations. The basic product in replacement therapy for patients with hemophilia A is fresh frozen plasma, but in severe cases, plasma infusions are ineffective. At present, cryoprecipitate concentrates and "Cryodex" (CI fraction) are the most effective agents for use in replacement therapy for patients with hemophilia A. The development of circulating inhibitors of factors VIII and IX is a major problem. Inhibitors tend to develop in patients with severe hemophilia who have received multiple units of factor VIII preparations. Life-threatening bleeding can be controlled with large doses of antihemophilic globulin. Where the inhibitor titer is too high, exchange transfusion, plasmapheresis, or immunosuppressive drugs may be necessary. Recently, patients with circulating inhibitor have been given concentrates of prothrombin complex and the Feiba fraction. Oral administration of factor VIII-loaded liposomes may prove to be useful.

▶ [Rudowski's contributions to the field of surgical hemotology have been significant, and it is appropriate that he present this Moynihan lecture, because Lord Moynihan made major contributions to the field of surgical hematology and hemostasis. This report presents a view of the current state of the art and incorporates a large

---

(1–2) Ann. R. Coll. Surg. Engl. 63:111–117, March 1981.

experience at a single institution. In the modern age of replacement therapy, most operative procedures should be uncomplicated. Therapy is based on the appreciation that approximately half of the posttransfusion activity of factor VIII disappears within 4 hours. After major surgical treatment of a hemophiliac, replacement of factor VIII should be continued for at least 10 days. If sutures remain, transfusion should be reinstituted prior to their removal. As pointed out by Rizza (*Clinics in Hematology,* W. B. Saunders Co., Philadelphia, 1976, pp. 113–133), for any patient undergoing major surgery, the level of factor VIII desired in the blood of the patient immediately after transfusion should be 80% of normal, which necessitates 40 to 50 units per kg body weight as a dosage.—S.I.S.] ◄

2. Fluid, Electrolytes, and Nutrition

2-1 **Protein vs. Electrolytes and All of the Starling Forces.** Richard M. Peters and Alan R. Hargens (Univ. of California, San Diego) point out that hemodilution-induced reductions in intravascular protein concentration in patients and animals with intact capillaries do not lead to pulmonary edema, despite a significant increase in extravascular water in the systemic interstitial space. The protective factors include a fall in the extravascular protein concentration, a rise in interstitial tissue pressure, and an increase in lymph flow. Pulmonary or peripheral edema may occur when the lymphatic pump fails to keep ahead of fluid-filtered high-output failure. If the capillary endothelium is damaged, protein leaks into the extravascular space, and protein infusion has a decreased effect on fluid exchange across the capillaries. Preventing an increase in capillary hydrostatic pressure is the chief means of preventing pulmonary edema, whether the capillaries are intact or injured.

A number of workers have recommended the use of hyperosmolar sodium solutions of 450 and 500 mOsm in order to avoid administering large amounts of electrolyte solutions. Hypertonic fluids may provide a useful means of limiting the total amount of fluid infused and reducing cell swelling following blood loss. Some workers have reported an improved clinical course in burn injury patients when solutions containing up to 240 mEq of sodium with 120 mEq of chloride and 120 mEq of lactate are used. The present authors are completing a study comparing Ringer's lactate and hypertonic sodium lactate solutions for fluid replacement in patients undergoing aortic surgery. Preliminary analysis indicates that only half as much fluid is needed in the group given hypertonic solution. Further studies are needed to determine whether the use of hypertonic fluids with a reduced net gain of fluid in muscles, especially heart muscle, will lower the diffusion path length for blood gases to increase gas exchange and improve cellular function and whether hypertonic mannitol or hypertonic salt solution is preferable.

▶ [This nice review of the Starling forces and their effects on capillary transfer of fluids from the plasma to interstitial fluid is contained in a volume that many of us participated and that was developed as a festschrift to the late and great Dr. Sam Powers, of Albany, New York.

While no new data are presented in this article, it is certainly a thoughtful and well-written review of some of the historical development of the Starling forces as well as current interpretations and extensions of the Starling formula. It also indicates some directions for future research in terms of fluid and electrolyte movements within the body.—T.S.] ◀

(2-1) Arch. Surg. 116:1293–1298, October 1981.

2-2 **Total Body Water in Malnourished Infants After Surgical Treatment.** Children with protein-calorie malnutrition have a large increase in body water content and a reduction in lean tissue mass. S. Tsingoglou, Harriet Phillips, and A. W. Wilkinson thought that similar alterations might occur in surgical patients with postoperative vomiting or diarrhea caused by infection or disaccharide intolerance who cannot be fed adequately by mouth. Total body water was measured in 29 infants with severe complications after surgery for congenital abnormalities of the alimentary tract. Nine had been operated on more than once. All the infants were younger than age 6 months and were severely malnourished. Nineteen had persistent vomiting, 8 had diarrhea, and 5 had evidence of severe systemic infection. Eight infants had been inadequately fed intravenously. Eight patients died, 5 of malnutrition and infection.

Mean total body water content was significantly higher in study patients than in normal infants of the same age and was also higher than in neonates with uncomplicated intestinal obstruction. Total body water decreased as the infants were fed satisfactorily by mouth and gained weight, but it remained high for weight and age. Total body water correlated negatively with body weight. All but 4 infants were below the third percentile for weight at the time of study. Total body water, as percentage of body weight, did not change significantly during administration of amino acid solution and fat emulsion. An increase occurred during administration of glucose and electrolyte solutions.

Infants with prolonged starvation, assessed after surgery and infection, have an increased total body water content despite body fluid losses and apparent clinical dehydration. An infant recovering from severe, prolonged malnutrition requires 150 calories per kg of body weight daily. The use of 10% or 20% solutions of dextrose or fat emulsion is necessary to avoid overloading them with water. Lost sodium must be replaced accurately when large extrarenal losses of body fluids occur, in order to maintain the extracellular fluid volume and an adequate actively circulating volume of blood.

▶ [These data on total body water in infants suffering from severe malnutrition and complications after surgical treatment of congenital abnormalities of the alimentary tract are extremely valuable, as these infants are all younger than age 6 months. As anticipated, the mean total body water content was significantly higher in surgically treated patients with malnutrition than in normal infants of the same age. This increased total body water decreased as the infants were fed satisfactorily by mouth and gained weight. One extremely interesting finding from this patient population would have been the measurement of distribution of this increased total body water among cell water, extracellular water, and intravascular water in plasma. Certainly, there would have been variations if some of these patients were also sodium depleted from frequently associated diarrhea, vomiting, or associated infection. One would guess that the extracellular fluids were high in many instances and yet were functionally distributed in such a way as to be ineffectual. Nevertheless, these are interesting baseline data in human subjects.—T.S.] ◀

2-3 **Influence of High and Low Sodium Intakes on Postoperative Antidiuresis.** S. F. Tindall and R. G. Clark (Northern Genl. Hosp.,

---

(2-2) J. R. Coll. Surg. Edinb. 26:272–277, September 1981.
(2-3) Br. J. Surg. 68:639–644, September 1981.

Sheffield, England) examined the effects of isovolumetric regimens with a high sodium content and with no sodium on the fluid balance and extracellular fluid composition in two groups of 6 men, aged 35–60 years, who underwent vagotomy, alone or with pyloroplasty, or uncomplicated cholecystectomy. No patient was taking medication other than antacids. None had an operative blood loss of more than 200 ml. The groups received identical volumes of intravenous fluids as either 450 mmoles of NaCl daily in 0.9% saline solution or 5% dextrose solution containing no sodium. Neither group received potassium supplements.

The saline group gained weight, while the dextrose group maintained weight initially and then lost it. Urine volume increased more rapidly in the dextrose-treated patients. Saline-treated patients showed a strongly positive water balance during the 4-day study period, in contrast to the dextrose-treated patients. The saline-treated patients had a strongly positive sodium balance, while the dextrose-treated patients were in negative balance. Potassium losses tended to be greater in the saline group. Negative free water clearance was observed in the saline group and positive clearance in the dextrose group. The plasma sodium level fell to 131.8 mmoles/L in the dextrose group, and plasma osmolality also decreased. The fall in plasma potassium was similar in the two groups. Plasma water content rose significantly in the saline group and moderately in the dextrose group. The estimated extracellular fluid volume rose substantially more in the saline-treated patients.

These findings confirm the importance of the sodium content of intravenous fluids in both the early development of hyponatremia and the water and salt balance in the later postoperative period. As recovery progresses, the "third space" contracts and an "autoinfusion" occurs, which may have to be taken into account if third-space losses were initially thought to have been large.

▶ [This interesting article shows how balance studies and body weight will simply not determine the internal redistribution of fluid and electrolytes in response to injury. While saline-treated groups show a positive water balance during and after the operative procedure, obviously this was not related to third-space sequestration, nor was the third-space measurement performed in these patients. As shown previously, the development of hyponatremia after administration of sodium-free solutions during an operatively incurred third-space sequestation was as predicted. Certainly, the use of water without salt in this situation will result in hyponatremia and may not correct the third-space sequestration enough to prevent the elevations of aldosterone and antidiuretic hormone, as has been shown previously by other investigators. Previous results are clear, and the historical development of fluid and electrolyte therapy, as reviewed by many authors, reveals that the volumes that are necessary to replace third-space intraoperative sequestrations can now be quantitated rather accurately.—T.S.] ◀

2–4 **Influence of Injury and Nutrition on Muscle Water and Electrolytes: Effect of Elective Operation.** Water and sodium are retained in the post-traumatic state, masking the loss of body tissue, but the effects of surgical injury on the tissue composition of various organs have not been thoroughly studied. Jonas Bergström, Peter Fürst, Bo Holmström, Erik Vinnars, Jeffrey Askanasi, David H. Elwyn,

(2–4) Ann. Surg. 193:810–816, June 1981.

Christopher B. Michelsen, and John M. Kinney performed percutaneous biopsies to analyze changes in muscle composition and the effects of nutritional intake in 28 patients undergoing colectomy and 22 having total hip replacement surgery. The colectomy patients received total parenteral nutrition with varying nitrogen intakes. Those having hip replacement received 5% dextrose, 3.5% amino acid solutions, or both. Muscles remote from the area of surgical injury underwent biopsy before and 3 or 4 days after operation. Eight healthy subjects kept at strict bed rest for 4 days, 4 of whom received 5% dextrose solutions, also were evaluated.

The healthy subjects showed small reductions in muscle potassium and intracellular water content, but there were no significant changes in levels of intracellular potassium, total water, or muscle sodium or chloride. Preoperative nutrition with Vivonex for 4 days (energy, 120 kjoule/kg, and nitrogen, 100 mg/kg daily) led to significant reductions in total, extracellular, and intracellular water and in total sodium and chloride levels in the patients with colonic carcinoma. Muscle glycogen content increased markedly. Potassium values did not change when related to glycogen- and fat-free solids. Patients given only glucose and fat showed no significant change in muscle water or electrolyte values postoperatively, but those given amino acids as well showed increases in extracellular water, sodium, and chloride and a slight reduction in muscle potassium related to fat-free solids. Muscle glycogen content was at baseline 3 days after colon resection. A slight loss of muscle potassium as related to glycogen- and fat-free solids was noted postoperatively. Magnesium values did not change significantly. Hypocaloric infusions in hip replacement patients had no significant effects.

These changes in muscle water and electrolytes appear to be related to the severity of trauma. Major changes in intracellular electrolyte values were not observed.

▶ [This study really is related more to the influence of nutrition on injury in muscle than to fluid and electrolyte movements. No measurements were made on acute cellular injury, and, consequently, a significant change would not be expected in the distribution of sodium, chloride, potassium, or energy-rich compounds under these circumstances. As pointed out by the authors, the calculation of distribution of water and electrolytes between the extracellular and intracellular fluid in muscle tissue is based on the old chloride method, assuming the transmembrane potential to be normal. As is again indicated by the authors, it is known that sick patients with metastatic carcinoma, uremia, acute injury such as severe shock or sepsis, and other debilitating conditions have a decrease in muscle cell membrane potential that makes the assumption invalid. If any changes in muscle membrane potential could have been demonstrated in the current study, these would have to have been shown in areas of direct injury such as in the site of injury or under a surgical retractor. Because these measurements were not performed in these patients, no assumptions were made by the authors, nor should any be inferred, concerning the distribution of fluid and electrolytes between the cells and extracellular fluid under these highly specialized circumstances.

All of this notwithstanding, the data on nutritional intake are extremely interesting. There was no effect of varying levels of nitrogen intake in patients undergoing standardized injury such as colectomy or total hip replacement. Consequently, with the level of injuries studied, the effects of varying the nitrogen intake were relatively minor.—T.S.] ◀

2-5 **Whole Body Protein Metabolism due to Trauma in Man as Estimated by L-(^{15}N)-Alanine.** The direction of changes in whole body protein synthesis and breakdown rates due to stress appears to depend on the severity of the stress. Ronald H. Birkhahn, Calvin L. Long, David Fitkin, Malayappa Jeevanandam, and William S. Blakemore (Med. College of Ohio, Toledo) evaluated the whole body protein turnover of 4 patients given a hypocaloric, protein-free diet after accidental trauma and of 5 control subjects given the same nutritional regimen. Protein turnover was estimated using a single pulse of L-(^{15}N)-alanine, followed by computer modeling. Isotopic decay data were computer curve-fitted to obtain the best estimates for 8 parameters of a 4-pool model; ^{13}C-urea also was administered.

The trauma patients excreted nearly 5 times as much urinary nitrogen as control subjects (Fig 2–1) and utilized one third more energy. Trauma expanded the "active metabolic nitrogen" pool and the transfer rates of nitrogen into and out of a "slow turnover protein" pool. Whole body protein synthesis of the trauma patients was 37% above normal, and protein breakdown was 79% above normal. The findings were in accord with those obtained using a ^{14}C-leucine continuous infusion technique.

It appears that trauma accelerates nitrogen flow, protein synthesis, and protein breakdown. The mechanism for negative nitrogen balance is consistent with that found for other severe stresses but differs from that associated with milder stresses such as elective surgery. In the group of trauma patients, the metabolic pool was expanded, the urea pool tended to be expanded, and both protein synthesis and pro-

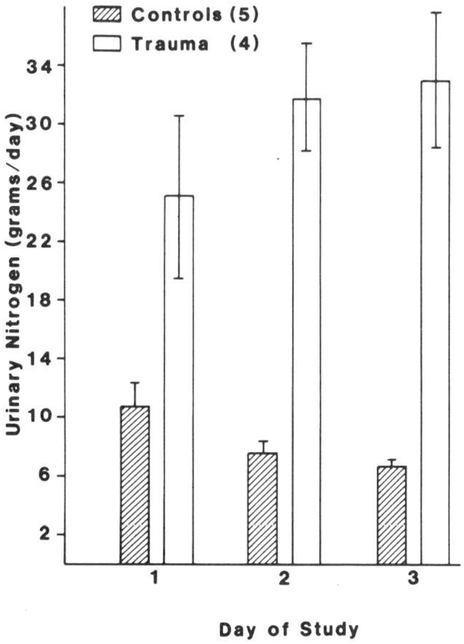

Fig 2–1.—Daily urinary nitrogen excretion for healthy control subjects and for trauma patients during 3-day course of protein-free, hypocaloric diet. (Courtesy of Birkhahn, R. H., et al.: Am. J. Physiol. 241:E64–E71, July 1981.)

(2–5) Am. J. Physiol. 241:E64–E71, July 1981.

tein breakdown were increased. The validity of the findings was supported by independent measurements.

▶ [The details of whole body protein metabolism due to trauma in man was examined in this study by utilizing stable isotopes, namely, ^{15}N-labeled L-alanine. While body protein turnover in severely injured patients and 5 control subjects given a hypocaloric protein-free diet was measured after a single pulse of ^{15}N-labeled L-alanine, followed by computer modeling. It is extremely interesting that trauma patients excreted nearly 5 times as much urinary nitrogen as control subjects and utilized one third more energy. It appears from these studies that trauma accelerates nitrogen flow, that is, both protein synthesis and protein breakdown. The mechanism for negative nitrogen balance in this study is consistent with that found for other severe stresses, but is far greater than that associated with mild stress such as elective surgery. The metabolic pool in the present group of injured patients was expanded, as was the urea pool, and both protein synthesis and protein breakdown were increased significantly. These values were further validated by using a continuous infusion method of ^{14}C-tagged lucine.—T.S.] ◀

2-6 **A Comparison of the Effects of Skeletal Trauma and Surgery on the Ketosis of Starvation in Man.** The relationship between ketosis and protein metabolism in healthy subjects is poorly understood, and it is an unknown factor in sepsis and trauma. In a previous study of skeletal trauma patients, it was found that hyperketonemic subjects had smaller nitrogen losses and a better clinical course than normoketonemic subjects. Ronald H. Birkhahn, Calvin L. Long, David L. Fitkin, Antonio C. Busnardo, John W. Geiger, and William S. Blakemore (Med. College of Ohio, Toledo) examined the response to total fasting of 20 patients with skeletal or soft tissue trauma who received a carbohydrate-free diet for 3 days and then a diet including carbohydrate for 3 days. The patients appeared to have been in good nutritional condition prior to trauma and did not have diabetes or sepsis. The control subjects were 10 postoperative patients and 2 healthy subjects who received a similar diet.

The resting metabolic expenditure was 21% greater for tested trauma patients than for tested control subjects. The surgical patients averaged 7% higher than predicted by the Harris-Benedict equation, while the trauma patients averaged 15% higher than predicted. Trauma patients generally lost twice as much nitrogen as control subjects. Both groups showed a fall in plasma glucose and insulin levels during the fasting period, but the initial glucose level was much higher for trauma patients. Serum levels of free fatty acids were lower in the trauma group. Fasting control subjects had rapidly increasing ketonemia, in contrast to the sluggish increase in ketones of fasting trauma patients (Fig 2–2). The low nonprotein respiratory quotient of trauma patients suggested that fat contributed about 61% of body energy expenditures on the third day of fasting, compared to 83% for control subjects.

These findings indicate that fat is utilized by trauma patients, but their fat metabolism is abnormal compared to that seen in starvation of mildly stressed patients or healthy subjects. Further studies of ketosis and its interaction with protein metabolism are needed, especially with reference to protein-wasting conditions.

(2–6) J. Trauma 21:513–519, July 1981.

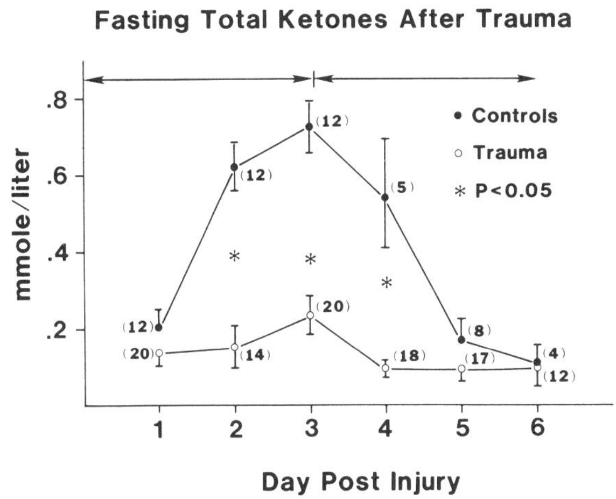

Fig 2–2.—Comparison of total plasma ketone body (sum of acetoacetate and 3-hydroxybutyrate) concentrations for trauma patients and control subjects during 3-day fast and subsequent 3-day carbohydrate intake. Each point is mean of number of subjects listed; bar = SEM; asterisk = significant ($P \leq .05$) difference. (Courtesy of Birkhahn, R. H., et al.: J. Trauma 21:513–519, July 1981.)

▶ [This carefully done metabolic study examined the response to total fasting of 20 patients with skeletal or soft tissue trauma who received a carbohydrate-free diet for 3 days, followed by a diet including carbohydrates. Controlled studies also were done in patients sustaining mild trauma and healthy subjects on similar diets. The resting metabolic expenditure was 20% greater for the trauma patients tested than for the control subjects. Trauma patients generally lost twice as much nitrogen as control subjects. Both groups showed a fall in plasma glucose from insulin during the fasting period. The levels of free fatty acids were lower in the trauma group than in the fasting control subjects. Ketonemia increased much more rapidly in the fasting control subjects, as compared with the slowly increasing ketone level seen in the fasting traumatized patient. The low nonprotein respiratory quotient of trauma patients suggested that fat contributed about 60% of body energy expenditures, whereas 83% was contributed by fat in the control subject. These findings indicate that fat is utilized by trauma patients, but their fat metabolism is abnormal compared to that seen in starvation of mildly stressed or healthy persons.

This is an interesting study of the difference in the way patients sustaining severe stress and trauma respond in terms of metabolic needs to the increased demand for energy after injury.—T.S.] ◀

2–7 **Contribution of Skeletal Muscle Protein in Elevated Rates of Whole Body Protein Catabolism in Trauma Patients.** Increased protein catabolism and metabolic energy expenditures are observed in seriously ill and injured patients, but the contribution of muscle protein to whole body protein breakdown following skeletal injury in the adult is unknown. Calvin L. Long, Ronald H. Birkhahn, John W. Geiger, and William S. Blakemore (Med. College of Ohio, Toledo) evaluated muscle protein breakdown rates, using the excretion of 3-methylhistidine (3-MEH), and whole-body protein synthesis and breakdown rates, using L-^{15}N-alanine, of 7 patients with multiple fractures and 8 control subjects, all of whom received a hypocaloric, protein-free diet of intravenous 5% glucose solution.

(2–7) Am. J. Clin. Nutr. 34:1087–1093, June 1981.

Blood urea nitrogen levels were significantly elevated in the trauma patients. The resting metabolic expenditure was significantly increased in the trauma group (28.7 vs 21.9 kcal/kg/day). Urinary excretion of 3-MEH was increased following trauma, to about the same extent as net protein breakdown as measured by urinary nitrogen excretion. The estimated contribution of myofibrillar muscle protein in the whole body catabolic rate was 15.9% for male and 14.1% for female control subjects. Male and female trauma patients had values of 26.3% and 21.1%, respectively. Assuming that the catabolic rates of myofibrillar and sarcoplasmic muscle proteins are the same, the contribution was 40.4% for male and 33% for female trauma patients.

The disproportionate increase in muscle protein breakdown observed in this study of patients with skeletal injury is consistent with muscle protein metabolism being most seriously affected by severe injury. Final validation of the contribution of myofibrillar muscle protein to whole body protein breakdown in normal and diseased states requires comparison of whole body turnover rates with measured catabolic rates of myofibrillar muscle protein in animal studies.

▶ [This is another of the elegant studies by this group to examine the source of the increase in energy requirements demonstrated in the severely injured patient. In this particular investigation, the contribution of skeletal muscle protein in response to injury was assessed. As expected, the resting metabolic expenditure was greatly increased in the trauma group. On detailed measurement of the protein contribution to this energy expenditure, a disproportionate increase in muscle protein breakdown was observed. It would appear from this study that protein metabolism is most severely affected by severe injury, with muscle protein breakdown being quite remarkable. It certainly appears from this study that this disproportionate increase in muscle protein breakdown is probably the most seriously affected pathway after a severe injury.—T.S.] ◀

2–8 **Reliability of Skin Testing as a Measure of Nutritional State.** A relation between immune competence and nutritional status has long been suspected, but malnutrition has not been proved to be related causally to impaired immunocompetence. R. Armour Forse, Nick Christou, Jonathan L. Meakins, Lloyd D. MacLean, and Harry M. Shizgal (Montreal) correlated responses to skin testing with nutritional status, as determined by measurements of body composition, in 257 patients given total parenteral nutrition (TPN). A total of 459 studies were performed at 2-week intervals in 141 men and 116 women. Most patients received solutions containing crystalline L-amino acids and 25% dextrose. Some received a significant portion of nonprotein calories in the form of 10% Intralipid. Delayed cutaneous hypersensitivity was evaluated by tests with five recall antigens.

Patients with normal skin test responses had a mean body composition only slightly different from normal but anergic patients had findings consistent with severe malnutrition, including a reduced body cell mass and an expanded extracellular mass. There was, however, considerable overlap in body composition between the normal, reactive, and anergic patients, and 43% of normally reacting patients were malnourished. Body composition deteriorated in patients who became anergic after TPN and improved in others who converted from the

(2–8) Arch. Surg. 116:1284–1288, October 1981.

anergic to the reactive state during TPN. Patients who remained anergic showed insignificant improvement in body composition after TPN. Infections occurred in anergic patients, even those who became reactive during TPN. Neoplastic disease was more common in anergic patients who failed to convert.

Skin testing with recall antigens is an excellent means of identifying patients with increased mortality and complications. Malnutrition is an important factor in development of the anergic state. Since many other factors are involved, however, skin testing with recall antigens cannot be used to assess a patient's nutritional state accurately.

▶ [The reliability of skin testing to five recall antigens as a measure of the nutritional state was determined in 257 patients receiving total parenteral nutrition; the patients were simultaneously and repeatedly evaluated by skin testing with the five recall antigens at 2-week intervals. There was clearly a response to parenteral nutrition in the reactivities to skin testing. However, the overlap between the reactive and nonreactive patients were so great that the presence or even the persistence of the anergic state is not an accurate assessment of a person's nutritional status.

This study confirms many previous criticisms of the skin testing recall antigen technique for measuring immunocompetence. It is very clear that there are a host of factors, including nutrition and immunocompetence, as well as other variables, that influence the anergic state of skin reactivity. While this test was developed as a measurement of immunocompetence and has pointed the road toward more intensive study of specific immune responses, it is clear that this is a very nonspecific test and probably will not prove useful clinically in the long run.—T.S.] ◀

2–9 **Effect of Nutritional Support on Immune Competency in Patients Suffering From Trauma, Sepsis, or Malignant Disease.** Nutritional support has been recommended by some as a means of improving host defenses in surgical patients. Timothy J. Mullin and John R. Kirkpatrick (Detroit) studied the effects of nutritional support on immune functions in 39 consecutive patients requiring such support. Fourteen were moderately malnourished and immunologically competent, whereas 25 had trauma, sepsis, or malignancy as well as varying degrees of malnutrition. Seven of the latter patients were immunologically competent, 6 were competent except for anergy, and 12 had immunologic incompetence in association with severe malnutrition. Protein-calorie support was nearly identical in the various groups; 41.6 calories/kg and 1.28 gm of protein/kg were provided daily. The mean length of treatment was 15 days.

The 14 control patients were in significant negative nitrogen balance initially, but all achieved positive balance during treatment and had satisfactory weight gain. The same was true of the immunologically competent study patients. Significant changes in T and B cells were noted in individual cases. The anergic patients responded similarly to nutritional support. Only 2 patients converted from negative to positive skin tests. The severely malnourished, immunologically incompetent patients achieved positive nitrogen balance by the time nutritional support was well under way. Lymphocyte counts responded to treatment, but no significant T or B cell changes were observed. Four patients converted from negative to positive skin tests. Anergy was initially present in 72% of this group.

(2–9) Surgery 90:610–615, October 1981.

The clinical course was similar in the three management groups. All patients survived. No biochemical differences were observed except in urea, which was significantly higher in the amino acid-treated patients. Nitrogen balance was less markedly negative in this group. On day 8, these patients had lost an average of 45 gm of nitrogen more than supplied, compared to a net loss of 84 gm in the glucose-treated group and 95 gm in the glucose-fat-treated group. No significant group differences in serum osmolality were observed. There were no significant differences in total protein or albumin levels during the study.

Improvement in nitrogen balance was associated with administration of amino acids to multiply injured patients in this study. The improvement was probably chiefly due to an increase in protein synthesis. Measurements of serum enzymes, especially alanine aminotransferase, offer a means of estimating the degree of tissue damage in and the general state of severely injured patients.

▶ [This is a comparison of the effect of three different isocaloric parenteral nutritional regimes on recovery in 19 patients with severe multiple injury as measured by their clinical course, biochemical analyses, and nitrogen balance. The three groups received either glucose and insulin, fat and glucose or fat, glucose and an amino acid nitrogen. All patients survived, and the clinical course was similar. However, recovery in nitrogen balance was more rapid in the group given amino acids, glucose, and fat compared to the other two groups, probably mainly due to an increase in protein synthesis. These authors concluded that, at least in the type of patient studied, the specific composition of the isocaloric parenteral nutrition regimens made little difference in terms of the measurable parameters, and primarily in clinical recovery from multiple trauma. This is an interesting study with obviously interesting clinical implications. However, this kind of investigation will not reveal insights into the changing energy requirements supplied from protein, carbohydrate, and fat in response to the stress of severe trauma, as previously reported in this YEAR BOOK.—T.S.] ◀

2–12 **Total Parenteral Nutrition in the Cancer Patient** is discussed by Murray F. Brennan (Natl. Cancer Inst., Bethesda, Md.). Total parenteral nutrition (TPN) is a lifesaving method of nutritional support for patients who are unable to ingest, digest, or absorb sufficient nutrients. While TPN has proved useful in the treatment of cancer patients, it is not yet clear whether it can reverse the nutritional and metabolic defects accompanying malnutrition nor has it been established whether TPN affects tolerance to treatment. Some cancer patients can achieve a positive nitrogen balance and weight gain with TPN. Suppression of gluconeogenesis from alanine is accompanied by an increased rate of glucose recycling. Data on possible effects of TPN on tumor growth in human beings are lacking. Most patients are adequately managed with a subclavian venous catheter. A caloric source and an amino acid source are necessary, as well as essential electrolytes and vitamins. Small amounts of iron are also recommended.

Nutritional indices, function, and well-being have been restored by TPN before, during, and after treatment of cachectic cancer patients. Improved serum albumin levels and decreased postoperative weight loss have been reported. Patients with esophageal and gastric cancer who were given TPN had fewer surgical complications. No change in

(2–12) N. Engl. J. Med. 305:375–382, Aug 13, 1981.

tolerance of radiotherapy has been observed in cases of advanced neoplastic disease. Many studies have failed to show improvement in response to treatment. Routine nutritional support does not appear warranted for patients undergoing aggressive treatment, but TPN can be recommended for nutritional support until the patient recovers from the side effects of antineoplastic therapy when response rates and nutritional morbidity are high. The theoretical advantages of utilizing the obligate glucose need and high glycolytic activity of tumors while providing host tissues with alternative substrates, such as ketones or glycerol, are being assessed in animal studies.

▶ [This interesting assessment of the use of total parenteral nutrition in the cancer patient is timely. Certainly, there is evidence that nutritional indices, function, and well-being have been restored by total parenteral nutrition in cachectic cancer patients before, during, and after treatment. Improvement can be seen in the serum albumin level, and decreased postoperative weight loss has been reported. Surgical complications have been reduced in patients with upper gastrointestinal cancer given total parenteral nutrition. However, no change in tolerance to radiotherapy has been observed in patients with advanced neoplastic disease. Most studies have failed to show improvement in response to treatment after total parenteral nutrition. Consequently, the fair judgment following such data is that routine nutritional support does not appear warranted in patients undergoing aggressive treatment, but can be recommended until patients recover from the side effects of the antineoplastic therapy, when response rates and nutritional morbidity themselves are high. This article seems to be a sensible state-of-the-art review regarding the effect of total parenteral nutrition in patients with serious tumors. Other interesting questions are raised by the author, such as the effect of total parenteral nutrition on tumor growth itself. Data on this problem in human beings, as the author points out, are lacking, but this does not appear to be a serious problem at present. Consequently, this study seems to be a current statement of the art.—T.S.] ◀

-13 **Zinc and Copper Replacement During Total Parenteral Nutrition.** Prospective studies have shown progressive reductions in blood zinc and copper levels during total parenteral nutrition (TPN), but little is known of proper replacement levels of these trace elements for intravenously fed patients. Stephen F. Lowry, J. Cecil Smith, Jr., and Murray F. Brennan undertook a prospective study of zinc and copper replacement in 29 courses of TPN in 20 tumor-bearing patients. Urinary excretion of zinc and copper was also studied prospectively in 8 of these patients. Four patients given no supplementation of trace metals during TPN served as a control group. Seven study patients had had surgery within 2 weeks of the start of TPN. Parenteral nutrition was continued for at least 2 weeks. A solution of Freamine II in 20%–25% dextrose was used, as well as 10% Intralipid. Study patients received zinc, about 4 mg/day, and 2.8 mg of copper, as well as MnS_{O4} and NaI in the TPN solution.

Both zinc and copper levels declined progressively over 4 weeks in control patients, but in patients given supplementation the levels remained within normal ranges. Patients with initially lower zinc levels had greater increases during supplementation; these patients also had lower urinary zinc excretion levels than the others. Serum copper levels increased most markedly in initially depleted patients, and a trend toward lower urinary losses of copper was noted in this group.

(2–13) Am. J. Clin. Nutr. 34:1853–1860, September 1981.

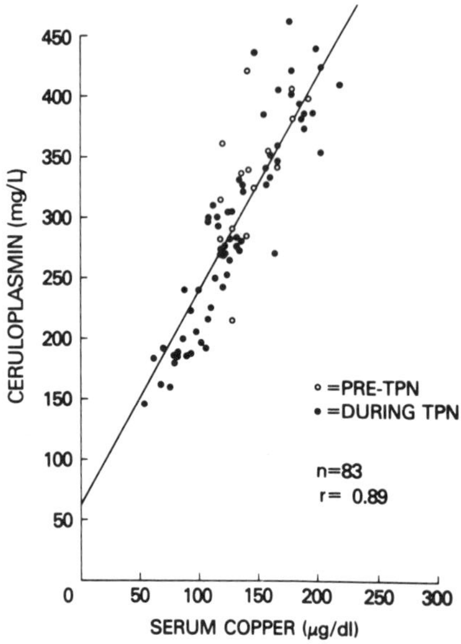

Fig 2–4.—Relationship of plasma ceruloplasmin level to serum copper concentration before and during TPN in patients who underwent intravenous copper supplementation. (Courtesy of Lowry, S. F., et al.: Am. J. Clin. Nutr. 34:1853–1860, September 1981.)

The serum copper and ceruloplasmin levels correlated significantly before and during copper supplementation (Fig 2–4).

The parenteral zinc supplementation rate suggested by these findings is in accord with observations in patients on TPN with extensive gastrointestinal losses. Recent recommendations for stable adult patients on TPN include 2.5–4 mg of zinc, 0.5–1.5 mg of copper, 10–15 μg of chromium, and 0.15–0.8 mg of manganese daily. Adjustments for fecal and fistulous losses are necessary. It seems likely that other TPN-related deficiencies of trace elements will ultimately be recognized.

▶ [The time course of reduction of zinc and copper levels during total parenteral nutrition (TPN) has been carefully assessed in this study. Furthermore, the study has quantitated the levels of zinc and copper supplementation necessary in stable adult patients receiving TPN. They include 2½ to 4 mg of zinc, 0.5 and 1.5 mg of copper and 10 to 15 μg of chromium as well as 0.15 to 0.8 mg of manganese daily. It seems that these TPN-related deficiencies in trace elements are now very well quantitated and should be used clinically.—T.S.] ◀

2–14 **A Prospective Study of Infant Zinc Nutrition During Intensive Care.** Recommendations have been made for zinc supplementation in parenteral nutrition solutions for infants, but the adequacy of suggested levels has not been proved. James W. Thorp, R. L. Boeckx, Sandra Robbins, Sherill Horn, and Anne B. Fletcher evaluated the zinc nutritional status of 55 infants during intensive care in order to determine effective means of monitoring zinc status and to assess the effects of zinc supplementation for deficiency. Most infants received a modified cow's milk formula containing 6.6 mg of zinc per 100 kcal.

Initial plasma zinc values were significantly higher for infants whose gestational age was less than 28 weeks (mean, 134 μg/dl) than for

(2–14) Am. J. Clin. Nutr. 34:1056–1060, June 1981.

those of greater gestational age. Serum albumin levels were relatively constant, whereas serum alkaline phosphatase levels were quite variable. Zinc levels fell more rapidly in the more premature infants. Zinc levels of 45 μg/dl or below occurred at about age 6 weeks in 14 of 39 premature infants. Two premature infants had true zinc deficiency, with increased gastric residuals, poor sucking, and decreased growth, but neither infant had cutaneous or gastrointestinal features of zinc deficiency. One of the infants had received 7 days of parenteral nutrition and 39 days of enteral nutrition before symptoms occurred; the other had received parenteral nutrition for 53 days and enteral nutrition for 21 days. Symptoms resolved within 4 days of the start of oral zinc acetate administration in a dosage of 2 mg/kg of body weight daily.

Zinc status should be monitored for 6–8 months for all premature infants, and supplementation should be given when indicated. Zinc deficiency should be considered if signs of poor growth or poor appetite are noted, even for infants given enteral nutrition soon after birth. Parenteral nutrition should be routinely supplemented with zinc; currently recommended amounts may be inadequate. The amount of zinc in currently available formulas also may be inadequate, but further work is needed to determine the amount that is necessary.

▶ [This is a study very similar to one reported previously, but in this instance the investigation was confined to the need for zinc trace element supplementation in parenteral nutrition in infants. The authors apparently have adequately documented the zinc deficiency in the newborn, particularly in the premature infant undergoing intensive care and parenteral nutrition. Consequently, it appears that additional zinc trace element will have to be added to parenteral nutrition in infants.—T.S.] ◀

2–15 **Effect of Various Nutritional Formulations on Candidiasis in a Hyperalimented Rat.** *Candida* is a major cause of catheter-associated infections in patients receiving total parenteral nutrition (TPN), but the precise mechanisms involved are unclear. Maarten F. von Meyenfeldt, H. Stephen Bjornson, Bengt W. Jeppsson, Robert Rolfes, and Josef E. Fischer (Univ. of Cincinnati) examined the role of various standard parenteral alimentation formulations in augmenting disseminated candidiasis in a hyperalimented rat model. A strain of *C. albicans* obtained from the blood of a patient with fatal disseminated candidiasis was utilized. Inocula were delivered into the internal jugular vein of male Sprague-Dawley rats, and the kidneys were removed after 1 week.

In surviving catheterized rats, positive kidney, blood, and urinary bladder cultures were more frequent than in noncatheterized control animals. Kidney cultures were positive after 1 week in 35 of 50 rats infused with standard TPN solutions and in 5 of 15 control rats. The mean change in body weight correlated significantly with the percentage of positive kidney cultures in the rats given TPN solutions (Fig 2–5). Infusion of lipid or solutions containing a high glucose concentration significantly augmented proliferation of *Candida* in the kidneys.

This animal model simulates disseminated candidiasis in human

(2–15) J. Surg. Res. 30:287–292, March 1981.

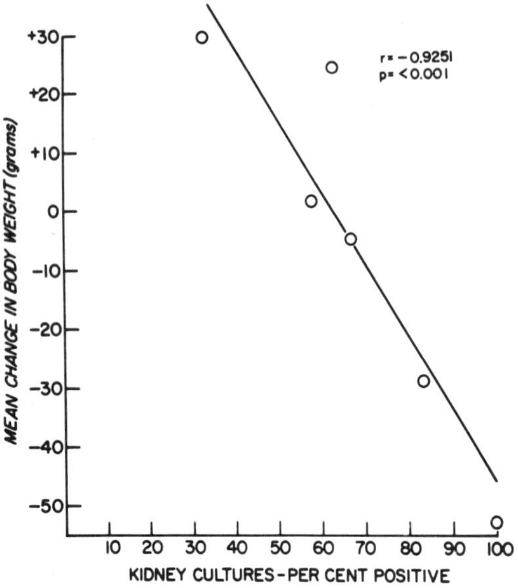

Fig 2–5.—Correlation between the mean change in body weight and the percentage of positive kidney cultures for the catheterized and noncatheterized rats. (Courtesy of von Meyenfeldt, M. F., et al.: J. Surg. Res. 30:287–292, March 1981.)

beings with central catheters in place. The nutritional status of the catheterized animal appeared to be a determining factor in the development of disseminated candidiasis after the intravenous injection of *C. albicans*. Changes in host defenses may have contributed to an increased incidence of disseminated disease in rats given inadequate nutritional support. Once *Candida* has colonized the kidneys, proliferation may be facilitated by a high dextrose level or Intralipid.

▶ [This is an investigation of the role of various standard parenteral alimentation formulas in augmenting disseminated candidiasis in an animal model. Interestingly, the study showed that an infusion of lipids or solutions containing high-glucose concentration appeared to augment significant proliferation of *Candida* in the kidneys of these animals after an intravenous injection of *C. albicans*. Obviously, this could have clinical implications if similar findings can be shown in patients with candidiasis during total parenteral nutrition.—T.S.] ◀

2–16 **Essential Fatty Acid Deficiency During Total Parenteral Nutrition.** Clinically significant essential fatty acid (EFA) deficiency has become a problem with the increasing use of fat-free total parenteral nutrition (TPN). Louis H. Barr, G. Dewey Dunn, and Murray F. Brennan attempted to determine the minimal fat requirements for patients given continuous TPN. A prospective study was made of 77 patients given 97 courses of TPN lasting 2 weeks or longer. The age range was 8–68 years. All patients but 8 had malignant disease. Nine patients with malignancy who were not receiving TPN also were evaluated. No patient was EFA-deficient prior to the start of TPN. The TPN solution consisted of 20% dextrose and 4.25% Freamine II

(2–16) Ann. Surg. 193:304–311, March 1981.

with supplemental electrolytes, trace metals, and vitamins and was given through a superior vena caval catheter. Patients received no fat supplementation, a 10% soybean oil emulsion intravenously, fat from an oral diet, or both intravenous and oral fat. The soybean oil emulsion contained 54% linoleic acid. The oral diet was assumed to contain about 7.5% of fat calories as linoleic acid.

More than two thirds of the 19 patients given no fat during TPN developed biochemical EFA deficiency within 2 weeks, as reflected by an abnormal triene-tetraene ratio; 18 were EFA deficient within 3 weeks. Up to 3% of nonprotein calories as intravenous fat delayed the onset of EFA deficiency for up to 6 weeks, and more than 3% prevented EFA deficiency in all instances but 1. The log of the final triene-tetraene ratio correlated closely with the daily percentage of nonprotein calories given as intravenous fat (Fig 2–6). No abnormal values occurred when intravenous fat constituted at least 3.2% of total calories. No deficiency occurred in patients given more than 15% of calories as fat by mouth, and the log triene-tetraene ratio also correlated with the percentage of calories given as oral fat.

At least 15% of calories given orally or 3.2% given intravenously as fat prevents EFA deficiency in patients receiving TPN. The 7.7 gm

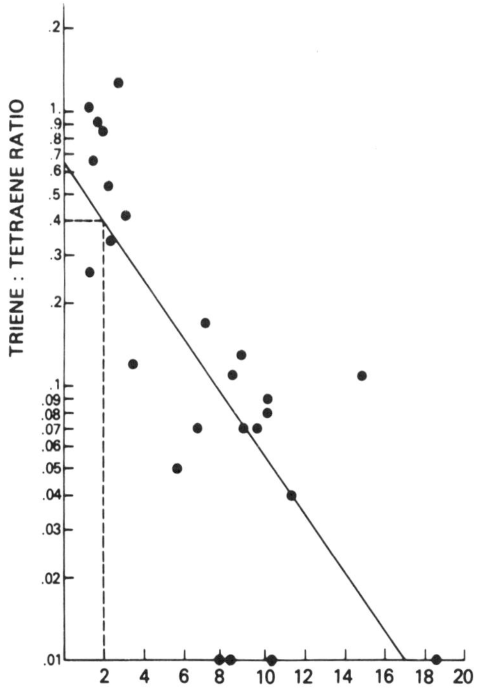

Fig 2–6.—Correlation of percent of total nonprotein calories given as intravenous fat with the triene-tetraene ratio at the end of each TNP course. A ratio of ≥0.4 defines biochemical EFA deficiency. No abnormal ratios are noted when at least 3.2% of calories is given as intravenous fat. N = 25, r = .7514, P <.001. (Courtesy of Barr, L., H., et al.: Ann. Surg. 193:304–311, March 1981.)

of linoleic acid per day provided in 1 L of 10% soybean oil emulsion per week provides enough fat to prevent EFA deficiency.

▶ [This interesting study in a large patient series was designed to establish the minimal fat requirements for patients given continuous total parenteral nutrition (TPN). The study also examined the need for fat calories to maintain stability when all sources of calories were given orally. The quantitative conclusions were that at least 15% of calories given orally or 3.2% of calories given intravenously as fat totally prevented essential fatty acid deficiency in patients receiving TPN. This is an interesting baseline figure and was largely supported by these studies in that more than two thirds of 19 patients given no fat during TPN developed biochemical essential fatty acid deficiency within 2 weeks. Consequently, it appears this baseline minimal fat caloric requirement should be adhered to in patients receiving TPN.—T.S.] ◀

2–17 **Nitrogen-Sparing Mechanisms of Singly Administered Branched-Chain Amino Acids in the Injured Rat.** Recent in vitro studies suggest a regulatory role for branched-chain amino acids (BCAA) in muscle protein metabolism. Herbert R. Freund, J. Howard James, and Josef E. Fischer (Univ. of Cincinnati) attempted to determine what properties ascribed to BCAA are responsible for the improved nitrogen conservation observed postoperatively. Rats undergoing laparotomy and jugular vein cannulation received infusions of 1.5% solutions of valine, isoleucine, leucine, and valine in 5% aqueous dextrose in a mean daily dose of 0.85 gm of amino acid. Tyrosine labeled with ^{14}C was added for the last 24 hours of infusion.

All groups of rats were in negative nitrogen balance, but animals given amino acids were in less negative balance than control animals given 6.5% dextrose in water. There were no significant differences among the amino acid-treated groups. All animals lost weight during the study. The fractional synthesis rate of mixed liver protein was increased significantly in all BCAA-treated groups. Only valine infusion significantly increased muscle protein synthesis. Total body protein breakdown rates were similarly reduced in all amino acid-treated groups and correlated with nitrogen balance.

It is concluded that the protein-sparing properties of the BCAA in the posttraumatic period are mediated through a reduction in whole body protein breakdown and by increased protein synthesis in both liver and muscle protein. The findings appear to be specific for BCAA, since isonitrogenous amounts of alanine did not have the same effect. The increase in fractional synthetic rate of muscle protein and decrease in total body protein degradation seen with BCAA infusion are important in view of the muscle protein catabolism caused by injury. The increase in fractional synthetic rate of liver proteins may be equally important for survival after injury.

▶ [The conclusion from this examination of the nitrogen-sparing mechanism of singly administered branched-chain amino acids in injured rats, that the protein-sparing properties of branched-chain amino acids in the posttraumatic period are mediated through a reduction in whole body protein breakdown and by increased protein synthesis in liver and protein, is obviously of potential clinical significance. The findings appear to be specific for branched-chain amino acids, because isonitrogenous amounts of alanine did not have the same effect. These data are extremely interesting clinically as providing a source for repletion of the increased protein breakdown occurring after a severe injury.—T.S.] ◀

(2–17) Surgery 90:237–243, August 1981.

3. Shock

3-1 **Colloid or Crystalloid in Resuscitation of Hemorrhagic Shock: A Controlled Clinical Trial.** Gerald S. Moss, Robert J. Lowe, Jane Jilek, and Harry D. Levine (Chicago) compared the results of fluid resuscitation with human serum albumin (HSA) and Ringer's lactate (RL) in patients with a systolic arterial pressure of 80 mm Hg or less at admission or before operation or who required 5 or more units of washed red blood cells (RBCs) before surgery. Ringer's lactate, alone or with 50 gm of 25% HSA solution, was administered until the systolic pressure was above 80 mm Hg, the pulse was under 100 beats per minute, and the urine output exceeded 30 ml/hour. Red blood cells were given to maintain the hematocrit reading at 30%.

Twenty of the 36 study patients received RL alone, and 16 received HSA. The groups were clinically comparable; most patients in both groups had penetrating injuries. The median resuscitation volume was 8 L for both groups, and the amounts of RBCs transfused were similar. One patient in the RL group died of sepsis 3 days postoperatively. Two patients in each group required mechanical ventilation for longer than 24 hours. No patient had overt pulmonary edema. Serial pulmonary function tests showed no important differences between the groups. The total protein level was significantly reduced in the RL group on the first day. No group differences in base deficit were noted.

The circulating blood volume of severely injured patients can be restored, without incurring pulmonary dysfunction, by means of an inexpensive colloid-free regimen of RL and RBC concentrates. Serum albumin is not necessary for the safe and effective resuscitation of hypotensive trauma patients. Considerable savings can be effected by not using albumin in this setting.

▶ [This clinical study confirms the opinion of most American investigators examining the need for extra colloid in the initial resuscitation of patients with hemorrhagic shock. It shows that using washed red blood cells with an extracellular mimic in the form of Ringer's lactate solution was as good as the same volume of washed red blood cells with Ringer's lactate and 4% human serum albumin added to the solution. In this series, the restoration of the circulating blood volume and the subsequent recovery of patients without significant complications revealed no important differences between the two treatment groups. Pulmonary dysfunction did not occur with any more frequency in patients in the group that received Ringer's lactate and red blood cells without albumin. The authors conclude that serum albumin is not necessary for safe and effective resuscitation of hypotensive trauma patients; in addition, significant economies can be achieved by not administering albumin in this setting. It is most interesting that detailed monitoring was not used, and, in fact, the usual clinical parameters of return of blood pressure, urinary output, and pulse rate were the end points of successful resuscitation. This study lends credence to the developing concept that detailed Swann-Ganz monitoring in the usual patient with hemorrhagic shock, in whom resuscitation is possible and the cause of the shock correctable, is simply not necessary.—T.S.] ◀

(3–1) Surgery 89:434–438, April 1981.

3-2 **Impaired Restitution of Blood Volume After Large Hemorrhage.** Complete restitution of blood volume in the later posthemorrhagic phase is necessary for cardiovascular stabilization. Donald S. Gann, Drew E. Carlson, Gerard J. Byrnes, J. Carl Pirkle, Jr., and Catherine F. Allen-Rowlands (Providence, R.I.) examined the changes in blood volume, protein levels, and osmolality accompanying hemorrhages of 10%–40% of initial blood volume in 42 adult conditioned mongrel dogs. Both anesthetized and awake animals were subjected to hemorrhage of 7.5, 15, or 22.5 ml/kg, 3 weeks or longer after splenectomy.

Restitution of blood volume at 12 and 24 hours was significantly greater for hemorrhages of 15 ml/kg than for hemorrhages of 7.5 ml/kg. Restitution after hemorrhages of 22.5 ml/kg did not differ from that in either of the other groups. Similar findings were obtained for restitution of plasma protein levels, except that restitution was less after bleeding of 22.5 ml/kg than after bleeding of 15 ml/kg. The findings are illustrated in Figures 3–1 and 3–2. The increase in plasma

Fig 3–1 (top).—Blood volume restitution at 24 hours plotted against total hemorrhage for individual dogs. *X,* anesthetized; *solid circle,* awake.

Fig 3–2 (bottom).—Plasma protein restitution at 24 hours plotted against total loss of plasma protein for individual dogs. *X,* anesthetized; *solid circle,* awake.

(Courtesy of Gann, D. S., et al.: J. Trauma 21:598–603, August 1981.)

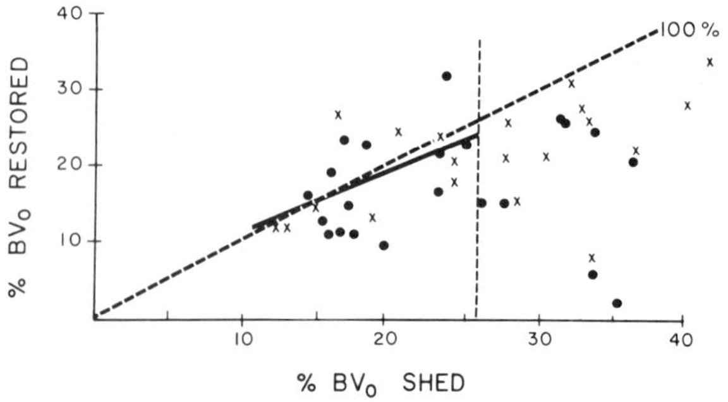

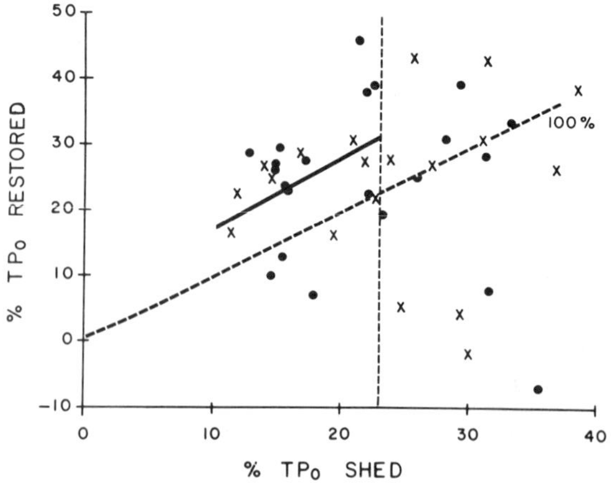

(3–2) J. Trauma 21:598–603, August 1981.

osmolality after hemorrhage was larger for larger bleeds. The change in osmolality correlated positively with the restitution of plasma protein and with the restitution of blood volume for hemorrhages less than 26% of initial volume, but correlated negatively after greater hemorrhages.

It seems likely that a fluid shift out of cells in response to increased osmolality after hemorrhage is offset by shifts into cells as the magnitude of hemorrhage increases. This failure of homeostatic restoration of blood volume, with resultant failure of cardiovascular stabilization, may be an early event in the development of hemorrhagic shock.

▶ [This experimental study describes the restitution of blood volume after significant and increasing degrees of hemorrhage. Serum osmolality increased with larger hemorrhages, providing an increasing driving force for restoration of plasma volume. The breakpoint in this cycle occurred after 30% hemorrhage, which is interesting in that restitution of blood volume was no greater after 30% hemorrhage than after 10%. This confirms previous reports of fluid shifts into damaged cells after a greater than 30% hemorrhage associated with decreased membrane potential, indicating cellular injury. As these authors point out, it appears likely that a fluid shift out of body cells occurs in response to moderate blood loss and increased osmolality, but this is offset by fluid shifts into cells as the magnitude of the hemorrhage becomes significant, producing shock and cellular injury.—T.S.] ◀

3–3 **Transcapillary Refill in Hemorrhage and Shock** is discussed by William R. Drucker (Univ. of Rochester), Christopher D. J. Chadwick (Univ. of Ottawa), and Donald S. Gann (Brown Univ.). The relationship between circulatory function and body fluid volumes is a far more important feedback regulatory system for defense of the circulation than the combined effects of autonomic reflexes, hormonal systems, and most other accessory regulatory factors. Transcapillary exchange of fluid between the plasma and interstitium is a major determinant. In the absence of trauma, hypovolemia alone can lead to hemoconcentration after initial compensatory hemodilution if the hypovolemia is profound or persistent. The direction of fluid movement between the plasma and interstitium is determined by hydrostatic pressures on each side of the capillary membrane, the protein osmotic pressures of plasma and tissue fluids, and the physical properties of the capillary membranes in their role as a mechanical filter.

Plasma oncotic pressure is a direct function of the protein concentration. Lymph flow is an essential means of preventing accumulation of protein in the tissue spaces, with resulting edema. In addition to the central factors controlling capillary hydrostatic pressure, most vascular beds have an intrinsic capacity to compensate for moderate changes in perfusion pressure by alterations in vascular resistance, so that blood flow remains relatively constant. Interstitial volume is the result of fluid movements into and out of the interstitium. Restriction of renal salt and water excretion does not have a major role in blood volume restitution after hemorrhage. Early reflex vasoconstriction and hormonal adjustments are followed by the restitution of albumin with fluid from the interstitium. Hyperosmolality may contribute to the mobilization of cellular fluid for restoring interstitial volume. The mechanism by which glucose may aid the restitution of

(3–3) Arch. Surg. 116:1344–1353, October 1981.

plasma volume remains controversial. In the reversal of capillary fluid exchange after prolonged shock, it is possible that mechanisms leading to hyperosmolality may act on cells to reduce the effectiveness of the sodium pump, permitting the movement of fluid into the cells and offsetting the normally homeostatic effect of extracellular hyperosmolality.

▶ [This is an elegant review of current and previous thinking on circulatory function and body fluid volumes in response to hemorrhage and shock. The authors discuss in great detail the reasons for the increased transcapillary exchange, or movement of fluid from cells to interstitial fluid to plasma, in response to moderate degrees of blood loss. All the Starling forces are reviewed and appear to be operative in this setting. However, the authors' studies also show that at increasing degrees of hemorrhage and severity of shock, the normal operating forces tend to be overcome by the cessation of transcapillary refilling. This correlates precisely with the degree of shock previously shown to be necessary to produce a cellular injury. As pointed out in this article, the initial transcapillary refill forces are aided greatly by hyperosmolality. However, as the severity of shock increases, this phenomenon is overcome by the need for cellular uptake of fluid and electrolytes from the interstitial fluid.—T.S.] ◀

3–4 **Posthemorrhagic Changes in Plasma Water and Extracellular Fluid Volumes in the Rat.** Some workers have found a reduction in extracellular fluid volume after hemorrhagic hypotension, while others have not. M. Larsson, G. Nylander, and U. Öhman (Stockholm) used ^{125}I-labeled human albumin and ^{51}Cr-labeled EDTA to investigate changes in plasma water and extracellular fluid volume in rats subjected to a standardized hemorrhage. Animals were bled to an arterial pressure of 40 mm Hg and were allowed to recover without retransfusion of shed blood for 10 or 90 minutes. Blood pressure rose exponentially to a mean of 77 mm Hg after 20 minutes and to 88 mm Hg after 90 minutes. Urine production was negligible in all studies.

Posthemorrhagic hematocrit readings and plasma water volume were reduced in both groups of animals, but extracellular fluid volume was not decreased significantly. The biologic half-life of EDTA in the recovery phase was 58 minutes, compared with 41 minutes in control studies. In the 10-minute recovery group, tissue plasma water volume was reduced in the spleen, large bowel, and subcutaneous fat. Extracellular fluid volume was decreased in the liver, spleen, and subcutaneous fat. In the 90-minute recovery group, plasma water volume was reduced only in the liver, and this organ also had a reduced extracellular fluid volume.

A standardized hemorrhage to an arterial pressure of 40 mm Hg in the rat, involving withdrawal of 35%–40% of the total blood volume, is followed by a phase of rapid spontaneous restitution of the plasma water volume, half of the loss being restored within 10 minutes. The extracellular fluid volume of the whole animal was unchanged after bleeding. Of the 11 tissues examined, only the liver, spleen, and subcutaneous fat showed a reduction in extracellular fluid volume 10 minutes after bleeding, and at 90 minutes this effect persisted only in the liver.

▶ [This article points out some of the problems in the study of shock that are due largely to methodological differences. The major methodological difference in this model is that sustained shock, with its attendant cellular injury, was not produced.

(3–4) J. Trauma 21:870–877, October 1981.

The shock preparation in which a given blood pressure is attained by hemorrhage and animals are allowed to recover does not produce a sustained shock model that allows for equilibration of substances across the capillary membrane, much less for the termination of the ability or lack of ability of substances to penetrate into the cell mass. Consequently, attempts to measure changes in plasma water and extracellular fluid volume cannot be assessed because there was no steady state, and the level of shock needed to induce cell injury was neither documented nor, apparently, attempted. To this end, it is apparent that equilibration occurred in many instances at 10 minutes; evidence of cellular injury was not measured. Also, the lack of reinjection technique after equilibration, assuming that cellular injury may have occurred, invalidates the measurements with regard to distribution of extracellular fluid inside or outside cells. In addition, the measurements of regional distribution must be challenged because analysis of the distribution of plasma water to various organs requires tagging of red blood cells in those organs to determine how much of the plasma water loss was, in fact, due to blood lost locally from the tissues.

Although the data obtained are undoubtedly reproducible, this model of shock, which is extremely variable and induces in effect, minimal shock injury, makes this study one of measuring volume changes in response to hemorrhage. This is in contrast to the more significant challenge of a model of shock sustaining cellular injury, which is associated with entirely different mechanisms of refill, as outlined in the two preceding articles.—T.S.] ◀

3–5 **Alterations in Cell Function With Ischemia and Shock and Their Correction** are discussed by Irshad H. Chaudry, Mark G. Clemens, and Arthur E. Baue (Yale Univ.). Decreased blood flow due to shock or ischemia results in reduced oxygenation and impaired removal of waste products. Activation of the neuroendocrine system leads to fluid shifts and extracellular fluid and intercellular matrix changes. Cell transport processes are altered, and the transmembrane potential difference eventually declines, leading to increased lactate and hydrogen ion production within cells and a decrease in pyridine nucleotides. With the entry of Na^+ into cells and the egress of K^+, the Na-K-ATPase system is activated, mitochondria produce more energy, and cyclic adenosine monophosphate levels and activity are reduced. Altered responsiveness of the adenyl cyclase system may modify the effects of various hormones, especially insulin and glucagon. Cell swelling occurs as volume regulation of the cell is impaired, accompanied by mitochondrial swelling. Regulation of calcium ion is compromised, and phospholipase may be activated with resultant effects on the altered membranes. All these changes lead to a decreased metabolic capability and may contribute to a cycle of enzyme release and toxic effects on cells.

Cold chemical cardioplegia has been a major advance in myocardial preservation. Measures to prevent cell swelling and maintain cell energy levels and membrane integrity have prolonged the time that kidneys can be preserved before transplantation. A major problem in sepsis and multiple organ failure is metabolic failure of the liver, skeletal muscle, and perhaps the entire energy apparatus of the individual. Support with nutrients, substrates, and cellular energetic activities appears to be of critical importance in mobilizing host resistance to infection and providing for metabolic activities and survival. The use of substrates, polarizing solutions, hyperosmotic solutions, and energy sources such as adenosine triphosphate with $MgCl_2$ may

(3–5) Arch. Surg. 116:1309–1317, October 1981.

well have clinical applicability during and after low-flow states and ischemia. Hypertonic mannitol infusion has led to increased oxygen delivery in patients with the acute respiratory distress syndrome. This and the increased blood flow and decreased resistance observed suggest an increase in oxygen diffusion capacity in peripheral tissues, perhaps related to decreased tissue swelling.

▶ [This is basically a review of the pathophysiology of cellular and subcellular function in response to shock. As these authors point out, the underlying mechanisms shown by several investigators now reveal common denominators of cellular injuries, failure of the membrane to function adequately with movement of fluid and sodium inside the cells and loss of potassium. A logical argument is made for the use of ATP-magnesium chloride as an attempt to supply energy to a cellular membrane that has been injured by the shock state. However, as indicated by the authors, several recent studies, including those of Schloerb and this editor, have shown that this particular approach does not seem to affect cellular function in response to shock.

The authors correctly point out that many successful attempts at arresting cell metabolism during low-flow states have been developed. One of those, of course, is cold chemical cardioplegia, using potassium to stop the heart and provide myocardial preservation while the coronary circulation is occluded for valve replacement and coronary artery bypass grafting. There is no question that cold cardioplegia does decrease cellular metabolism and preserve membrane function during cessation of the heartbeat. Similarly, the prevention of cell swelling and the maintenance of cell energy levels and membrane capability have prolonged the time that kidneys can be preserved for transplantation.

The authors rightly conclude that an appropriate way for decreasing or reversing cellular injury in vivo in response to the injury of hemorrhagic shock must be developed.—T.S.] ◀

3–6 **Red Blood Cell Sodium, Potassium, and ATP Levels During Hemorrhagic Shock.** It has been suggested that a generalized defect in active transport of Na^+ across cell membranes occurs in hemorrhagic shock. If the red blood cell membrane also is altered, this would be a valuable model in which to study the cellular lesions of shock. David J. Kreis, Jr., Irshad H. Chaudry, Sarah Schleck, and Arthur E. Baue (Yale Univ.) examined the effects of mild and severe hemorrhagic shock and blood transfusion on red blood cell Na^+, K^+, and adenosine triphosphate (ATP) levels in the rat. Either the blood pressure was reduced to 40 mm Hg and allowed to rise to about 70 mm Hg within 30 minutes or a pressure of 40 mm Hg was maintained for 2 hours. Some animals in the latter group received whole blood that had been stored in ACD buffer at 4 C for 6 days.

No changes in red blood cell Na^+ or K^+ were found in the animals whose blood pressure rose to 70 mm Hg, but the others showed significant, though small, reciprocal changes in red blood cell Na^+ and K^+ levels. Red cell ATP levels decreased from 1.51 to 1.27 mmoles/L of red blood cells during shock in this group. Transfusion of stored blood led to a rise in red blood cell Na^+ from 3.5 to 8.4 mmoles/L and a reduction in K^+ from 100.3 to 85.0 mmoles/L. A 62% increase in red blood cell Na^+ occurred when blood stored for 3 days was infused. The red blood cell Na^+ level of stored blood itself increased over time, and a significant decrease in red blood cell K^+ was observed with cold storage of blood.

Severe hemorrhagic shock produces small changes in red blood cell

(3–6) J. Surg. Res. 31:225–231, September 1981.

Na^+ and K^+ levels. Large changes in cation levels are observed when stored blood is transfused to animals in hemorrhagic shock. The reciprocal cation changes associated with severe hemorrhagic shock are in accord with the possibility of red blood cell Na^+ pump inhibition during shock. The changes probably are not related to a decrease in ATP levels. The large changes in red cell cation content reported in patients in shock appear to be due to the transfusion of stored blood rather than to shock itself.

▶ [An attempt is made in this study to detail further the previously shown effects of hemorrhagic shock on red blood cell transport of sodium and potassium. There is no question that some changes in response to shock were shown in the red blood cells of the experimental animals used and that the infusion of transfused blood aggravated the measurement of the existing cellular defect. However, as others have shown previously and as was mentioned in the 1981 YEAR BOOK, such a cellular defect in anesthetized animals has been extremely difficult to measure. Similarly, it recently has been shown that a significant defect in red blood cell sodium-potassium exchange is also difficult to show in man, unless the shock has been severe and sustained for more than 2 hours. However, it is clear from this study and the others mentioned that severe hemorrhagic shock does produce changes in red blood cell sodium and potassium levels if the shock state is significant, severe, and prolonged. The differences in the significance and degree of these changes probably are related to the species of animal studied and the presence and absence of anesthesia. It would seem that added proof of the defect is provided by the demonstration once again that the effect of transfusion of stored blood is certainly significant, as compared to the transfusion of stored blood in the nonshock state.—T.S.] ◀

3–7 **Intravenous Adenosine Triphosphate (ATP) in Hemorrhagic Shock in Rats.** Energy is accepted as a limiting factor in survival from hemorrhagic shock, and levels of ATP and other high-energy metabolites have been found to be reduced in the tissues of animals in severe hemorrhagic shock. Some reports have suggested improved survival with parenteral ATP administration. Paul R. Schloerb, Lynette Sieracki, A. James Botwin, John M. Winblad, and M. Helen Maguire examined the utility of intravenous ATP in elevating lowered tissue ATP levels in shocked rats. The distribution of radioactiv-

TISSUE ATP LEVELS IN HEMORRHAGIC SHOCK RATS WITH AND WITHOUT INTRAVENOUS ATP-$MgCl_2$ TREATMENT AND IN SHAM-OPERATED RATS*

	n	iv Infusion	ATP Levels, μmol/g: Blood*	Pect major	Kidney	Liver	Heart
Hemorrhagic shock	7	6.25 μmol ATP-$MgCl_2$	0.7 ±0.1	5.6 ±0.1	1.5† ±0.1	2.9 ±0.2	3.5 ±0.2
Hemorrhagic shock	7	0.85% NaCl	0.6 ±0.1	5.8 ±0.2	1.5† ±0.2	2.8 ±0.3	3.7 ±0.2
Sham-operated	7	None	0.6 ±0.02	6.2 ±0.2	2.0 ±0.2	3.0 ±0.2	3.7 ±0.1

*Values are means ± SE. Hemorrhagic shock and sham-operated rats were prepared and maintained in the awake state for 2.5 hours. Shock rats received 0.25 ml of infusion solution followed by return of any remaining shed blood; 5 minutes after infusion, rats were stunned and their tissues were sampled for ATP measurements. Tissues of sham-operated controls were obtained similarly. Blood levels are in μmoles of ATP per milliliter of blood.

†$P < .05$ vs. sham-operated.

(3–7) Am. J. Physiol. 240:R52–R60, January 1981.

ity was determined in components of the adenine nucleotide pools of tissue in animals given 8-^{14}C-ATP-$MgCl_2$ intravenously. Study animals were initially bled to a mean arterial pressure of 40–50 mm Hg by removing 25% of the blood volume; a total of 40% was removed within 35 minutes. A dose of 0.25 ml of 25mM ATP-$MgCl_2$ was administered.

Mortality was 50% in shocked rats treated with ATP-$MgCl_2$ and 53% in saline-treated control rats. Tissue ATP levels in treated animals did not differ from those in saline-treated shocked rats or control animals that had sham operation (table). The tissue distribution of activity was similar in shocked, sham-operated, and nephrectomized rats. Activity in the heart, lungs, kidneys, and liver of shocked and sham-operated rats was present almost entirely as nonphosphorylated 8-^{14}C-ATP catabolites.

Administration of ATP-$MgCl_2$ did not improve survival or enhance tissue ATP levels in rats in rats subjected to hemorrhagic shock. The administered ATP was rapidly and extensively degraded. Extensive degradation of intravenously administered ATP accounts for the lack of benefit from this treatment in animals in hemorrhagic shock.

▶ [This article examines the hypothesis that reversal of the cellular membrane defect produced by hemorrhagic shock might be produced by supplying exogenous ATP, particularly when it is complexed with $MgCl_2$. In this study, significant and sustained shock was produced and half of the animals were treated with ATP-$MgCl_2$ and the other half with saline. Tissue ATP levels in animals treated with ATP-$MgCl_2$ did not differ from those in the saline-treated shocked rats or the control animals with sham operations. The tissue distribution of activity was similar in the two groups, and the activity in the heart, lungs, kidneys, and liver of the shocked and sham-operated rats was present almost entirely as nonphosphorylated ATP catabolites. The conclusion is that the administered ATP was rapidly and extensively degraded. Consequently, the ATP administered simply did not have any effect at the cellular level insofar as its ability to supply energy is concerned.

It would appear from these studies, and others published even more recently, that the exogenous administration of ATP-$MgCl_2$ in its present form does not have a significant energy-supplying effect on the cellular injury of hemorrhagic shock.—T.S.] ◀

3–8 **Defects in Peripheral Oxygen Utilization Following Trauma and Shock.** Analysis of a large series of injured patients showed an unexpected correlation between whole body oxygen consumption and oxygen delivery, suggesting that tissue hypoxia continues despite successful resuscitation. The patients also exhibited lactic acidemia and decreased reactive hyperemia in the peripheral circulation. Dhiraj M. Shah, Jonathan C. Newell, and Thomas M. Saba (Albany Med. College) hypothesized that injured patients have an impaired oxygen diffusion capacity between the capillaries and mitochondria due to an increased distance for diffusion. Microcirculatory disturbances during initial tissue ischemia may persist after resuscitation. They may be due to increased tissue edema, microembolus-induced closure of capillaries, or a reperfusion syndrome in which tissue edema and/or endothelial cell swelling block the capillaries.

Studies were done on an isolated canine hind limb as a model of the peripheral circulation. Interstitial edema was induced by infusion of buffered saline infusion. Hypoperfusion and reperfusion were car-

(3–8) Arch. Surg. 116:1277–1281, October 1981.

ried out, and microembolization was produced by injecting polystyrene microspheres. Interstitial edema alone did not reproduce the defect in peripheral oxygen utilization, but both reperfusion and microembolization reproduced the response. Hypertonic mannitol and imidazole reversed the defect after either reperfusion syndrome and microembolization, respectively. The restoration of oxygen utilization to normal by imidazole after microembolization suggested that microembolization not only plugs capillaries, but also leads to the release of vasoconstrictor agents that accentuate ischemia in the vicinity of the emboli.

Defective oxygen utilization in patients who have incurred major trauma may be responsible for deterioration in organ function after successful resuscitation. Defects in peripheral oxygen utilization related to microembolization, reperfusion, and tissue edema may be treated by specific means.

▶ [The hypothesis examined by these authors is that, for some reason, patients with hemorrhagic shock have an impaired oxygen diffusion capacity between the capillaries and the mitochondria; however, no definitive recommendation for control is delivered. This hypothesis was developed because of continued tissue hypoxia despite successful resuscitation in animals and patients after significant trauma and shock. The unanticipated correlation between whole body oxygen consumption and oxygen delivery suggested continued tissue hypoxia despite successful resuscitation as evidenced by high cardiac output and high mixed venous Po_2. This is an interesting explanation of a diffusion defect for oxygen caused by the initial injury. The authors' conclusion that the defect is related to the effects of reperfusion, edema, and microembolization on the peripheral vascular bed is certainly to be considered speculative at present. Reversal of some of these phenomena by the use of drugs is terribly nonspecific and may well be associated with other, more fundamental, physiologic changes than demonstrated in this study.—T.S.] ◀

3–9 **Opiate Receptors and Endorphins in the Pathophysiology of Hemorrhagic Shock.** Endorphins or opiate receptors may be involved in the pathophysiology of hemorrhagic shock. Naloxone has improved cardiovascular performance and survival in a canine model of hemorrhagic shock. Nelson J. Gurll, Thomas Vargish, David G. Reynolds, and Robert B. Lechner (Univ. of Iowa) examined the role of this system in cardiovascular function in anesthetized adult dogs bled to a mean arterial pressure of 45 mm Hg for 1 hour and then given either 0.9% saline or naloxone. Naloxone was given in an initial bolus of 0.5, 1, or 2 mg/kg, followed by an infusion of 0.5, 1, or 2 mg/kg/hour for 3 hours.

About 70% of the estimated blood volume was removed. Cardiac output, stroke volume, and pulmonary artery pressures declined in the first hour of hypovolemic shock. The heart rate rose, and the left ventricular contractility (LV dp/dt max) decreased at first and then gradually increased. Steady cardiovascular deterioration occurred in saline-treated animals, which died within 45 minutes. The mean arterial pressure, cardiac output, stroke volume, and LV dp/dt max all increased slightly with the lowest dose of naloxone, but deteriorated after 90 minutes. With the intermediate dose, cardiovascular improvement persisted in the second hour of shock, and with the highest dose even better results were obtained. Survival at 72 hours was re-

(3–9) Surgery 89:364–369, March 1981.

lated to the dose of naloxone administered. All 5 animals given the highest dose survived to 72 hours, and they probably would have lived longer if permitted to do so.

Naloxone therapy improved cardiovascular function and survival in dogs subjected to hemorrhagic shock in this study. Fluid therapy should not be withheld from patients in shock, but naloxone may be an important temporizing measure or a useful adjunct to fluid resuscitation. The findings implicate opiate receptors and possibly endorphins in the pathophysiology of hemorrhagic shock.

▶ [This is one of the first of only a few published articles indicating some benefit from the use of opiate receptor blockade with naloxone. In these studies of significant hemorrhagic shock in dogs, the cardiovascular response to replacement of volume with saline was greatly enhanced by the use of the specific opiate receptor antagonist naloxone. Because naloxone has minimal effect on cardiovascular function in dogs without shock, these results do implicate opiate receptors, perhaps endorphins, in the cardiovascular pathophysiology of hemorrhagic shock. These studies are in concert with my previous studies indicating that there may well be a central nervous system-mediated hormone that significantly influences sodium and potassium cellular transport in response to hemorrhagic shock. As stated by the authors, these results suggest that opiate receptors, possibly endorphins, may be intimately involved in the pathophysiology of shock.—T.S.] ◀

3–10 **Studies of the Staphylococcal Causation of Toxic Shock Syndrome.** Over 1,100 cases of toxic shock syndrome have been reported in the United States and Canada. *Staphylococcus aureus* has been recognized as the likeliest etiologic agent. W. A. Altemeier, Sue Lewis, P. M. Schlievert, and H. S. Bjornson carried out a blinded study of 159 *S. aureus* isolates obtained from patients with toxic shock syndrome and 86 isolates from other clinical sources, such as infected wounds, normal vaginal tracts, and nasal cultures. Isolates were obtained from patients at various institutions.

The group 1 phage type 29 was the dominant strain of *S. aureus* in toxic shock syndrome. It was present, often in association with type 52, in 59.1% of cases. Type 52 accounted for another 5% of cases. This complex was present in only 10.5% of control cultures. About one fourth of toxic shock syndrome isolates were untypable, as were 35% of control isolates. Nearly all toxic shock syndrome isolates of phage type 29 gave a positive C toxin test. The results of antibiotic resistance studies are given in the table.

Group 1 phage type 29 was the dominant strain of *S. aureus* associated with toxic shock syndrome in this study. It was found alone or in frequent combination with type 52. The finding that most of these strains were capable of producing pyrogenic exotoxin C supports their etiologic importance in toxic shock syndrome. The high rate of nontypable isolates suggests that another important phage type may be present. The findings emphasize the versatility of *S. aureus* and its ability to produce different pathogenic strains capable of causing different or new clinical infections.

▶ [As pointed out by the authors, in over 1,000 cases of toxic shock syndrome reported in the United States and Canada, *S. aureus* has been recognized as the most likely etiologic agent. These authors investigated the characterization of *S. aureus* isolates obtained from patients with toxic shock syndrome as well as isolates from

(3–10) Surg. Gynecol. Obstet. 153:481–485, October 1981.

ANTIBIOTIC RESISTANCE STUDIES OF 159 TOXIC SHOCK SYNDROME *Staphylococcus aureus* ISOLATES COMPARED WITH 86 CONTROLS*

	Pencillin				*Ampicillin*				*Tetracycline*				*Erythromycin*				
	R		*I*		*R*		*I*		*R*		*I*		*R*		*I*		
Phage type	*No.*	*Per cent*	*No.*	*Per cent*	*No.*	*Per cent*	*No.*	*Per cent*	*No.*	*Per cent*	*No.*	*Per cent*	*No.*	*Per cent*	*No.*	*Per cent*	*Total tested*
29+, inc. 52 . . .	84	89.4	6	6.4	82	87.2	8	8.5	3	3.2	0		6	6.4	0		94
52+, not inc. 29 .	5	62.5			4	50.0	1	12.5									8
Other group 1 . .																	1
Total group 1 . .	89	86.4	6	5.8	82	79.6	9	8.7	3	2.9			6	5.8			103
Group 2																	0
Group 3	7	100.0			7	100.0			1	14.2			1	14.2			7
Miscellaneous . .	8	100.0			8	100.0			1	12.5							8
Nontypable	26	63.4	5	12.1	24	58.5	7	17.0	1	2.4					1	2.4	41
																	159
NONTOXIC SHOCK SYNDROME ISOLATES—CONTROLS—86 STRAINS																	
29+, inc. 52 . . .	5	55.6	2	22.2	5	55.6	2	22.2	2	22.2							9
52+, not inc. 29 .			1	100.0			1	100.0									1
Total group 1 . .	5	50.0	3	30.0	5	50.0	3	30.0	2	20.0							10
Group 2	4	100.0			4	100.0											4
Group 3	9	64.3	2	14.3	8	57.1	3	21.4	2	14.3			1	7.1			14
Miscellaneous . .	26	92.9	1	3.6	25	81.3	2	7.1	3	10.7			1	3.6			28
Nontypable	20	66.7	4	13.3	18	60.0	6	20.0	3	10.0			2	6.7			30
																	86

*R, resistant; I, intermediate.

other clinical sources, including infected wounds, vaginal tracts, and nasal passages. The group 1 phage type 29 was the dominant strain of *S. aureus* in toxic shock syndrome. The complexes isolated were present in only 10% of the control cultures and about 60% of the toxic shock syndrome cases. Nearly all toxic shock syndrome isolates of phage type 29 gave a positive C toxin test result. This finding, that most of these strains were capable of producing pyrogenic exotoxin C, supports their etiologic importance in toxic shock syndrome. These findings emphasize the versatility of the *S. aureus* organism, which has been around for many many years, and its ability to vary its type and produce different pathologic and pathogenic strains capable of causing different or new clinical infections.—T.S.] ◀

3–11 **Membrane Defect and Energy Status of Rabbit Skeletal Muscle Cells in Sepsis and Septic Shock.** Cell membrane depolarization in hemorrhagic shock has been attributed to failure of an active, energy-dependent Na-K pump, the activity of which is directly dependent on the adenosine triphosphate (ATP) concentration. The cellular defect in skeletal muscle in septic shock is similar to that observed in hemorrhagic shock. Hana P. Illner and G. Tom Shires (New York Hosp.-Cornell Med. Center) investigated the causes of this defect in an animal model of septic shock caused by live *Escherichia coli.* Levels of ATP and creatine phosphate (CP) in rabbit skeletal muscle were correlated with changes in cellular function as indicated by alterations in measured transmembrane potential difference (PD). A suspension of live *E. coli* was injected intra-arterially to induce deep septic shock associated with metabolic acidosis.

The skeletal muscle PD was reduced 10–15 mV from baseline at the start of shock. All animals had a PD below 75 mV 2 hours before death, and reductions to 60–65 mV occurred in the last hour. Muscle biopsy specimens obtained when the mean systolic blood pressure was 55.5 mm Hg and the mean PD was 61.1 mV showed a small, insignificant increase in ATP and a decrease in CP.

Depolarization of the cell membrane, indicating cell swelling, preceded the onset of deep hypotension in this model. The findings suggest that cell injury is a primary cause rather than a result of shock. The lack of significant abnormality in levels of high-energy phosphates in skeletal muscle in the terminal stages of shock reduces the possibility of an energy deficit as a factor in cell membrane malfunction in septic shock. The possibility of an endotoxin effect on cell membrane permeability to Na^+, resulting in a reduction in measured PD, could not be evaluated in this study.

▶ [This study utilized live whole organism infusion of *E. coli* to produce a septic shock model in animals. The septic shock preparation resulted in significant cellular injury, measurable by transmembrane potential difference, similar to the cellular injury observed in skeletal muscle in hemorrhagic shock. In this septic shock model, depolarization of the cell membrane preceded the onset of deep hypotension, suggesting that cell injury is a primary cause rather than a result of the consequences seen in shock due to sepsis. The lack of a significant abnormality in high-energy phosphate in skeletal muscle cells in the terminal stages of septic shock reduced the possibility of primary energy deficit as the major factor in cell membrane malfunction. Whether this might, in fact, be due to a specific effect of the endotoxin produced by the live whole organism as opposed to the shock state could not be resolved in the present study.—T.S.] ◀

(3–11) Arch. Surg. 116:1302–1305, October 1981.

3–12 **Skeletal Muscle Insulin Resistance During *Escherichia coli* Bacteremic Shock in the Dog.** Changes in carbohydrate metabolism are known to occur in sepsis and circulatory shock. Insulin resistance has been described in association with disordered regulation of the plasma glucose level. Richard M. Raymond, James M. Harkema, and Thomas E. Emerson, Jr. (Michigan State Univ.) attempted to determine whether insulin resistance in the dog develops in skeletal muscle during bacteremic shock induced by live *E. coli.* The isolated in situ gracilis muscle preparation was used. Insulin was infused into the muscle intra-arterially before and after the induction of shock by a 30-minute intravenous infusion of live *E. coli.* Control animals received physiologic saline over 30 minutes.

Before shock, the glucose uptake by gracilis muscle increased by 395% during insulin challenge. Glucose uptake did not change significantly during insulin challenge at 1, 2, and 3 hours of shock, and there were no significant changes in muscle lactate production or muscle oxygen uptake. Lactate production increased significantly during shock. Arterial pressure declined during shock, but muscle blood flow and muscle venous Po_2 did not change significantly. The arterial glucose level increased initially but then fell to about 45 mg/dl.

These findings support the hypothesis that insulin resistance develops in skeletal muscle during gram-negative bacteremic shock in the dog. Transition from the high-cardiac output, hypermetabolic state of sepsis to the low-cardiac output, hypometabolic state of septic shock may be the result of multiple organ failure due to excessive visceral and skeletal muscle "wasting," which could be a consequence of insulin resistance. Loss of skeletal muscle sensitivity to insulin does not prevent hypoglycemia.

▶ [This interesting study examines the oft-quoted insulin resistance that is supposed to develop in peripheral muscle in response to septic shock. These authors used the technique of insulin infusion to measure muscle glucose uptake before and during shock in an in vitro constant-flow profused muscle preparation. The study confirms the loss of responsiveness to insulin with no change in muscle oxygen uptake, muscle venous Po_2, or muscle blood flow. It is nicely demonstrated that insulin resistance in skeletal muscle developed early during the course of bacteremic shock and that this, in itself, did not necessarily even prevent hypoglycemia. This confirms the previously demonstrated clinical syndrome of so-called pseudodiabetic state in response to sepsis.—T.S.] ◀

3–13 **Lipoprotein Lipase Activity in Surgical Patients: Influence of Trauma and Infection.** The hydrolytic activity of lipoprotein lipase (LPL) is the major means by which circulating triglycerides are cleared from the blood. Arnold P. Robin, Jeffrey Askanazi, M. R. C. Greenwood, Yvon A. Carpentier, Frank E. Gump, and John M. Kinney studied the effects of acute injury and infection on LPL activity in skeletal muscle and adipose tissue. Biopsy specimens were obtained from 17 injured and 11 infected surgical patients and from 11 normal subjects. The patients were evaluated 3–7 days following trauma or surgery after having received only 5% dextrose. Six of the normal subjects were maintained on intravenously administered glucose, 500 kcal daily for 4 days.

(3–12) Surgery 90:853–859, November 1981.
(3–13) Ibid., pp. 401–408, August 1981.

Semistarvation produced a marked fall in adipose tissue LPL activity and a significant decrease in plasma insulin in normal subjects. Adipose tissue weight per unit of protein content decreased, indicating a reduction in adipocyte size. Lipolytic activity in skeletal muscle was unchanged. Trauma patients had skeletal muscle LPL activities similar to those of normal postabsorptive subjects, but their adipose tissue LPL activities were higher than in diet-matched control subjects. Plasma insulin and glucose levels were increased in this group. Infection was associated with adipose tissue LPL activities lower than in uninfected trauma patients. Triglyceride levels were higher than in the other trauma patients or normal postabsorptive subjects. Adipose tissue LPL activity was not related to in vivo lipid-clearing capacity, even after correcting for whole body adiposity.

Increased adipose tissue LPL activity and plasma insulin levels are observed in trauma patients, and low LPL activity is seen in infected patients. Insulin appears to have a major role in the regulation of adipose tissue LPL activity. The hormonal regulation of muscle LPL activity is less well understood.

▶ [These authors compared lipoprotein lipase activity in biopsy specimens from patients who had sustained trauma or infection with that in specimens from normal subjects. The study showed increased adipose tissue lipolytic lipase activity and plasma insulin level in traumatized patients, in contrast to low lipoprotein lipase activity in infected patients. Triglyceride levels were higher in the septic patients than in the other trauma patients or normal postabsorptive subjects. Insulin appears to have a major role in regulation of adipose tissue lipoprotein lipase activity; this interesting measurement needs to be pursued to determine the hormonal or other possible regulation of muscle lipoprotein lipase.—T.S.] ◀

3–14 **Corticosteroid Therapy in Hemorrhagic and Septic Shock in Puppies.** The efficacy of steroid therapy in shock remains unclear, although the rationale for such treatment is sound. Robert H. Connors, Arnold G. Coran, John R. Wessley, Robert A. Drongowski, and William H. Weintraub (Mott Children's Hosp., Ann Arbor, Mich.) attempted to isolate the effects of steroid therapy in hemorrhagic and septic shock in puppy models of *Escherichia coli* shock and hemorrhagic shock. Steroid therapy consisted of the intravenous administration of methylprednisolone sodium succinate, 30 mg/kg.

Shock was delayed in animals pretreated with steroid before *E. coli* administration, but no reversal of the gradual fall in cardiac output was noted, and the same was true of blood pressure. No significant metabolic differences were observed in the steroid-treated and control animals during *E. coli* shock. In hemorrhagic shock, no significant hemodynamic differences were found between the steroid-treated and control groups. Lactate elevations and changes in glucose and lipid levels were unaffected by steroid administration. As in *E. coli* shock, no significant trends in blood gas values were observed.

Steroid treatment failed to produce beneficial effects in these puppy models of hemorrhagic and septic shock. It is possible that the shock was so severe that no single agent could reverse it. Recent studies have suggested that steroids must be used in conjunction with fluid

---

(3–14) J. Pediatric. Surg. 15:790–796, December 1980.

resuscitation and antibiotic therapy in order to obtain a positive response.

▶ [This study attempts to isolate the effects of steroid therapy in hemorrhagic and septic shock in puppies by using an *E. coli* shock model as well as a hemorrhagic shock model. In order to isolate the effects of steroid treatment, no volume or antibiotic therapy was given. In this strict model, metabolic and cardiovascular parameters and survival did not differ between steroid-treated and control animals. Similarly, metabolic measurements, including lactate elevations and changes in glucose and lipid levels, were unaffected by the steroid administration.

It is interesting, as the authors point out, that steroid treatment, when put to an isolated, severe test such as was done in these experiments, produced no beneficial effects in either hemorrhagic or septic shock models in young animals. The significant benefits being reported with a combination of fluid resuscitation, antibiotics, and steroids are being studied by these authors because the isolated effects of each alone are far less impressive.—T.S.] ◀

3–15 **Corticosteroids Block Binding of Chemotactic Peptide to Its Receptor on Granulocytes and Cause Disaggregation of Granulocyte Aggregates In Vitro.** Steroids blunt the responses of polymorphonuclear leukocytes to activated complement components and inhibit granulocyte aggregation. They have been reported to alter surface receptors in immune adherence assays, and altered receptor function has been proposed as a mechanism of high-dose steroid effects on granulocyte responses to complement components. Keith M. Skubitz, Philip R. Craddock, Dale E. Hammerschmidt, and J. Thomas August examined this hypothesis by using the synthetic chemotaxin *N*-formyl-methionine-leucine-phenylalanine (FMLP) as a probe to study the effect of steroids on granulocyte receptor function. Many of the effects of activated complement are mimicked by FMLP, and FMLP-induced granulocyte aggregation is inhibited by the same concentrations of steroids that inhibit C5a-induced aggregation.

With the use of methylprednisolone, hydrocortisone, and dexamethasone, dose-dependent inhibition of FMLP binding to its specific receptor on granulocyte surfaces was observed; the corticosteroid concentrations paralleled the plasma levels achieved with an intravenous bolus of 30 mg of drug per kg of body weight. Methylprednisolone was the most potent, and dexamethasone the least. Receptor numbers were unchanged, but a decrease in the association rate constant for the FMLP-receptor interaction was observed, leading to decreased receptor-ligand affinity. Dissociation kinetics were unchanged by steroid exposure in cold-chase studies. Aggregated granulocytes disaggregated on exposure to steroids, and the same order of potency was observed.

Steroids can displace FMLP from granulocyte surfaces by slowing association while dissociation proceeds. If the same is true for physiologic stimuli, such kinetic changes may be important in the clinical effects of very high-dose steroids, such as those administered to patients in shock. Changes in receptors on other cells for other mediators may also contribute to the efficacy of steroid therapy in various syndromes. The mechanism by which steroids alter the receptor-ligand interaction remains unclear.

(3–15) J. Clin. Invest. 68:13–20, July 1981.

3-16 **Effect of Enteral and Parenteral Feeding in Malnourished Rats With *Escherichia coli*-Hemoglobin Adjuvant Peritonitis.** Some of the gastrointestinal tract defects associated with protein-calorie malnutrition (PCM) persist after intravenous feeding, and increased susceptibility to infection often is associated with PCM. Kenneth A. Kudsk, Gary Carpenter, Scott Petersen, and George F. Sheldon evaluated the role of the route of nutritional support in the maintenance of host defenses in rats fed a 2% agar protein-depletion diet for 2 weeks, followed by total parenteral nutrition solution parenterally or enterally in comparable amounts. An *E. coli*-hemoglobin mixture was injected intraperitoneally after a 24-hour prechallenge fast.

Equal nitrogen balance occurred in the orally and intravenously fed animals, but intravenously fed rats gained significantly more weight. Rats fed a regular diet gained more weight than the orally repleted animals, as shown in Figure 3–3. Intravenously fed animals had lower total body water volumes than the orally repleted animals, and their greater weight gain probably was due to fat deposition. Survival following injection of the *E. coli*-hemoglobin mixture to induce peritonitis was unrelated to the type of oral nutrition provided, whether TPN solution or rat chow. Rats fed intravenously had a significantly greater mortality 24 hours after injection than the orally fed groups. The differences were not significant at 48 hours, but the orally fed animals appeared to recover more rapidly from peritonitis than the intravenously refed survivors.

The resistance to peritonitis of malnourished rats repleted with TPN solution is improved by oral feeding. Whether intravenous feeding impairs the response to peritonitis or fails to reconstitute a PCM-induced immune defect is unclear. The findings suggest, however, that the gut may have a previously undefined role in host defenses.

▶ [This isolated animal study attempts to evaluate the effect of parenteral as opposed to enteral nutrition with the same substance on the ability of animals to respond to septic peritonitis. It is interesting that rats fed intravenously had significantly greater mortality 24 hours after injection of the *E. coli*-hemoglobin adjuvant used to produce peritonitis than did rats fed orally. The orally fed animals also recovered

Fig 3–3.—Weight change per day was significantly greater in rats fed intravenously or with a regular diet than in rats given enteral nutrition. (Courtesy of Kudsk, K. A., et al.: J. Surg. Res. 31:105–110, August 1981.)

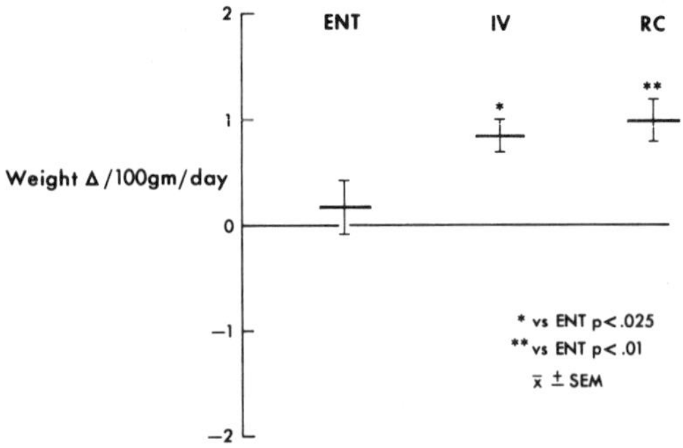

(3–16) J. Surg. Res. 31:105–110, August 1981.

more rapidly from peritonitis than the intravenously fed survivors. Consequently, it appears that the resistance to peritonitis of malnourished rats repleted with TPN solution is improved by oral feeding. If this is borne out, it would indicate that passage of food material through the bowel may have a previously undefined role in enhancing host defenses to infection.—T.S.] ◀

4. Trauma

4-1 **Commitment to Trauma in a Low-Population-Density Area.** Kirk M. Gilmore, Terry P. Clemmer, and James F. Orme, Jr. (Univ. of Utah) conducted a retrospective and prospective study of 202 patients with blunt trauma. The patients were aged 11–92 years and were admitted consecutively in a 14-month period to intensive care units from a low-population-density area in the Intermountain West. Both the Injury Severity Score (ISS) and Glasgow Coma Score (GCS) were used. Patients were managed by an experienced trauma team using a formal resuscitation protocol. Instant communication among the trauma surgeon, emergency department, and field personnel was available, and communications between rural hospitals and transport systems are integrated by the center. A transport team and a special shock and trauma unit are available. An outreach program was conducted to improve the ability of rural hospitals, paramedics, and emergency medical technicians to cope with injured patients.

About two thirds of injuries were caused by motor vehicle accidents. The overall mortality was 14.8%, and 12.9% of patients had persistent morbidity. The mean ISS was 39 for nonsurvivors, 36 for patients with persistent morbidity, and 23 for successfully rehabilitated patients. In the 119 patients with head injuries, the mean GCS was 7 for nonsurvivors, 10 for patients with persistent morbidity, and 12 for rehabilitated patients. The mean hospital stay for survivors who were rehabilitated was about 15 days. Patients with multiple trauma who initially were cared for elsewhere and survived the first 6 hours had an ultimate survival similar to that of patients initially resuscitated at the trauma center.

Regionalization of trauma care is generally advisable, particularly if the volume of cases is low. Community commitment to trauma care is necessary if an impact is to be made. State emergency medical services agencies and trauma centers have a responsibility to educate paramedics, emergency medical technicians, and physicians in rapidly evaluating the risk of vital organ involvement and initiating appropriate resuscitative measures before transporting patients to the closest trauma center capable of dealing with their injuries.

▶ [This interesting epidemiologic report shows the type of community commitment and initiative required to implement regionalized care to improve the management of the traumatized patient. Certainly, patient outcome, in terms of both morbidity and mortality, and the efficacy of a committed system are well documented in this report.—T.S.] ◀

4-2 **Methodologic Considerations in the Use of the Abbreviated Injury Scale in Trauma Epidemiology.** The importance of trauma

(4–1) J. Trauma 21:883–888, October 1981.
(4–2) Ibid., 627–631, August 1981.

severity indices in injury control and outcome evaluation is now acknowledged, but little stringent, systematic testing of these indices has been carried out. J. I. Barancik and B. F. Chatterjee (Case Western Reserve Univ.), in the course of an incidence study of external cause-specific trauma, used the Abbreviated Injury Scale (AIS) and the Injury Severity Score (ISS) to assess the severity of anatomical injuries. Medical records specialists trained in AIS procedures observed notable variations in interpretation of scaling procedures in the AIS dictionary, and this then was replaced by a new single-page (SP) precoded abstracting form containing alphabetical descriptors for each trauma type within a body region. A computer algorithm was developed to assign AIS severity codes, which are not mentioned on the form. Instead, a three-digit identifier was assigned to each descriptor.

Accuracy and precision were markedly improved by eliminating the need to make severity scoring decisions during the AIS coding process. A total of 150 cases were selected serially from emergency department records and were coded twice by 3 medical records professionals. More body regions had AIS-coded injuries with the SP method than with the dictionary-manual (DM) method in cases with more widely dispersed, possibly more complicated, codable injuries. Coding by the DM method took about 28% longer than coding by the SP method.

The SP approach is more productive than the older DM method, and the potential for coder bias is reduced. The need to make severity coding decisions in hospitals is virtually eliminated. More information is provided than with the DM method, because the recorded codes uniquely identify specific anatomical injuries. This can be very important for subsequent analyses. A number of the problems associated with use of the AIS are methodologic in origin, and greater emphasis is needed on the relevance of methodology to conceptual issues in trauma epidemiology.

▶ [This paper is representative of several attempting to improve the study of effects of the prehospital as well as the inhospital care of the severely injured patient. This particular investigation evaluated a shortened and simplified format, a single-page precoded abstracting form to regularize cases insofar as the severity score for injury is concerned. Further development of this type of data is needed to standardize reporting concerning mortality and morbidity among various multiply-injured patients.—T.S.] ◀

4–3 **Evaluation of a Rapid Immunoturbidimetric Assay for Opsonic Fibronectin in Surgical and Trauma Patients.** Plasma opsonic fibronectin, or $_{\alpha 2}$-SB glycoprotein, is a determinant of reticuloendothelial system phagocytic function. The liver slice bioassay for circulating opsonic fibronectin is technically difficult and has limited sensitivity, and electroimmunoassay is a time-consuming procedure. Thomas M. Saba, Winfried H. Albert, Frank A. Blumenstock, George Evanega, Fritz Staehler, and Eshin Cho evaluated the rapid, sensitive kinetic immunoturbidimetric assay for serum opsonic fibronectin, based on measurement of an antigen-antibody reaction. Both this assay and the electroimmunoassay were used to analyze samples ob-

(4–3) J. Lab. Clin. Med. 98:482–491, October 1981.

tained from 14 adult surgical and trauma patients before and after cryoprecipitate infusion. Immunoelectrophoresis was used to verify the monospecificity of the antifibronectin provided in the assay kit.

The immunoturbidimetric assay can be done within 10 minutes, compared to the 24–48 hours needed for the quantitative electroimmunoassay. Only 5 μL of serum or plasma is needed. Samples are prepared from plasma anticoagulated with EDTA and supplemented with aprotinin to inhibit proteolysis. The monospecificity of the commercial antihuman fibronectin was confirmed by immunoelectrophoresis. Ouchterlony double diffusion showed the commercial and laboratory antibodies to be identical. Results obtained by the automated immunoturbidimetric assay and the electroimmunoassay correlated positively. Periods of opsonic fibronectin deficiency and periods of elevation after cryoprecipitate infusion were readily quantified by both methods.

The kinetic immunoturbidimetric assay for opsonic fibronectin is a rapid, highly specific, very sensitive, quantitative method. It also is economical. The assay may have value in patients given replacement therapy and as an indicator of reticuloendothelial system function in septic injured patients.

▶ [This is a report on the general assessment of patients who have sustained trauma and their immunologic ability to respond to such injury after therapy. The new assay for opsonic fibronectin is a more rapid, specific, sensitive quantitative method. Preliminary reports indicate that opsonic fibronectin is at least a parallel indicator of the ability of the reticuloepithelial system to function in septic or injured patients.—T.S.] ◀

4–4 **Stress Ulceration: The Clinical Problem** is reviewed by Charles E. Lucas (Wayne State Univ., Detroit). In 1933, Cushing noted a relationship between stress ulceration and brain tumors. A correlation between serious injury and stress bleeding has been documented more recently. Multiple factors apparently operate in the development of stress bleeding in seriously injured patients, including the presence and severity of hypovolemic shock, the number and site of injuries, associated organ failure, and postoperative complications, particularly sepsis and pneumonitis. Organ failure or sepsis precipitates the progression of erosions in the fundic mucosa. Resolution of sepsis is associated with healing of the mucosal erosions. Abnormal blood coagulation often develops in cases of shock and severe sepsis. Steroid therapy may be a causative agent in stress bleeding.

Effective nasogastric decompression is important in the assessment and management of patients susceptible to stress ulceration. A properly positioned, functioning nasogastric tube reduces active bleeding and helps prevent rebleeding, apparently through both the removal of hydrochloric acid and a reduction in the mucosal surface area. Premature removal of a nasogastric tube has commonly been observed in cases of severe stress bleeding. Intraoperative diagnostic endoscopy permits confirmation of stress ulceration as the source of bleeding, allowing appropriate surgery to be performed. This approach eliminates the need to perform intraoperative gastrotomy, with its attendant problems. Increased mortality is associated with both operative

---

(4–4) World J. Surg. 5:139–151, March 1981.

and nonoperative therapy for established stress bleeding, especially for elderly patients. As knowledge of gastric mucosal metabolism increases, pharmacologic treatments aimed at altering gastric mucosal blood flow and oxygen dynamics can be developed. Better means of preventing and treating sepsis in high-risk patients also are needed.

▶ [This paper is a good summary of the clinical and pathophysiologic status of stress ulceration after multiple injuries. Principles of clinical management, which are often neglected, are again reemphasized, including the use of the nasogastric tube and the use of intraperative endoscopy for diagnosis.—T.S.] ◀

4–5 **Disability After Severe Head Injury: Observations on the Use of the Glasgow Outcome Scale.** B. Jennett, J. Snoek, M. R. Bond, and N. Brooks (Glasgow) analyzed the nature of the neurologic and mental impairments resulting from severe head injury in 150 conscious adult survivors of injury who were recalled at least 1 year later (range, 1–14 years). Mean follow-up was 5.2 years. The mean age at evaluation was 28 years. An acute intracranial hematoma had been evacuated in about half the cases. The distribution of outcome categories at 6 months was similar to that in a series of over 1,000 severely head-injured patients from 3 countries, accumulated prospectively in Glasgow in a 10-year period.

Two observers agreed on the outcome in over 95% of cases evaluated at 6 and 12 months in terms of vegetative state, severe or moderate disability, or good recovery. Ten percent of patients who were severely or moderately disabled 6 months after injury were in the next better category by 12 months. One quarter of survivors had no neurophysical disability. Sequelae were more frequent in patients who had had an intracranial hematoma evacuated in the acute stage. None of 9 patients with a severe cognitive deficit made a good recovery, while none of 45 with good cognitive recovery had severe disability at follow-up. Similar results were obtained for personality change. Some deficit was present in all but 3% of patients. Two thirds had personality change, which in nearly 30% of cases was the only deficit. Over 60% of patients with no or only a mild physical deficit had marked personality change, and the same was true for patients with no or a minimal cognitive deficit. Most patients with marked cognitive or physical deficits also had definite deficits in the other areas. Mental handicap was considered more significant than physical sequelae in contributing to overall disability in more than half the cases, while physical impairment was more significant in fewer than 30% of cases. Patients who emerged from posttraumatic amnesia within 4 weeks were nearly certain to become independent but could be moderately disabled.

The Glasgow Outcome Scale permits a reliable assessment of overall social outcome in most cases of head injury. Relatives or close friends should be interviewed to verify the effect of injury on the patient's life-style. In the present study, mental handicap contributed more significantly than neurologic deficit to overall social disability.

▶ [This article is a critical follow-up and evaluation of the use of the Glasgow Outcome Scale for patients who have sustained severe head injury. This scale has con-

(4–5) J. Neurol. Neurosurg. Psychiatry 44:285–293, April 1981.

tinued to grow in popularity, and its statistical validity is fairly well documented in this article, in which mean follow-up of the patients was 5.2 years. The categories outlined in the Glasgow Outcome Scale are now becoming standardized and they seem to serve a very useful prognostic function for eventual outcome after a given level of head injury.—T.S.] ◀

4-6 **The Lung After Trauma and Shock: Fine Structure of the Alveolar-Capillary Barrier in 23 Autopsies.** Postmortem ultrastructural studies have suggested that adult respiratory distress syndrome (ARDS) results from nonspecific injury to the pulmonary endothelium. G. G. Pietra, J. R. Rüttner, W. Wüst, and W. Glinz examined the ultrastructure of the alveolar septa in the lungs of 23 victims of severe trauma and shock who died within 4 weeks after admission. Ten patients died within a week after injury. Their median age was 44 years. All had sustained multiple fractures, and 5 were in shock at admission. The median survival was 2 days. Thirteen patients with a median age of 32 years lived for a median of 10½ days after injury, and for at least 1 week. These patients had less severe injuries than the first group, but most experienced septicemia or pneumonia and severe arterial hypoxemia that were consistent with ARDS.

The most consistent findings in patients who died soon after injury were interstitial edema and fat emboli. Alveolar edema was observed in 6 of 10 cases. Half of the patients had interstitial and alveolar hemorrhages. Fat emboli were less frequently seen in the patients who died later after injury, but more severe interstitial and alveolar edema was observed in this group. Endothelial injury occasionally was seen in the form of cytoplasmic swelling, cell membrane discontinuity, or cytoplasmic osmiophilia. Hyperplasia of type II pneumocytes was focally present in 6 cases and was extensive in 2 others, in whom it was associated with organization of hyaline membrane and widespread interstitial and alveolar duct fibrosis.

Patients incurring severe injuries and shock are particularly susceptible to fatal infections. The present findings do not support the view that shock, tissue trauma, and resuscitative measures lead to anatomical endothelial damage and permeability edema. The lung lesions observed in trauma victims who die in the immediate postinjury period appear to be self-limited and potentially reversible. Lesions attributed to "shock lung" probably are typical of severe sepsis, not shock per se.

▶ [This is a different approach to the assessment of posttraumatic pulmonary insufficiency. This particular group studied the records of patients who died after severe injury. The most consistent findings in those who died soon after injury were interstitial edema and microemboli. Endothelial injury was occasionally seen with cell membrane discontinuity. The conclusions of the study are extremely interesting in that patients with severe injuries and shock were shown to be particularly susceptible to fatal infections. The view that shock, tissue trauma, or resuscitative measures lead to anatomical endothelial damage and permeability edema was not supported in this study. On the contrary, the view that many, including the editor, have expressed, is sustained: The lung lesions observed in patients who died immediately after injury appear to be self-limited and potentially reversible. The lesions that previously have been attributed to this so-called shock lung were typical of severe sepsis rather than shock. The term for the postinjury pulmonary insufficiency, therefore, is more liable to be correct if "septic lung" rather than "shock lung" is used.—T.S.] ◀

(4–6) J. Trauma 21:454–462, June 1981.

4–7 **Pulmonary Response of Massive Steroids in Seriously Injured Patients.** Many of the physiologic alterations implicated in the development of pulmonary edema in injured hypovolemic patients are thought to be modified or circumvented by early massive steroid administration. Charles E. Lucas and Anna M. Ledgerwood (Wayne State Univ., Detroit) examined the pulmonary effects of massive steroid supplementation in 114 severely injured patients in hypovolemic shock who survived operation and were in stable condition postoperatively. By random selection, 54 patients received 1 gm of methylprednisolone in the operating room, followed by 15 mg/kg/day for 3 days. All patients were resuscitated with balanced salt solution supplemented by fresh frozen plasma. The patients received an average of 13 transfusions, 760 ml of plasma, and 11.7 liters of crystalloid solution.

A significant rise in central venous pressure was noted in steroid-treated patients (Table 1). A rise in pulmonary wedge pressure also occurred. A change in plasma or blood volume was not responsible. The steroid-treated and control patients received similar levels of inspired oxygen at the time of initial postoperative evaluation, but arterial oxygen tension was significantly higher in the control group (Table 2). Physiologic shunting in the lungs was less marked in the control patients. Patients given steroid supplementation required ventilatory support for an average of 5.1 days, compared with 3.0 days for control patients. Seven steroid-supplemented and 2 control patients died. Neither of these differences was significant.

Massive steroid supplementation did not prevent or ameliorate pulmonary failure after hypovolemic shock in this study. In contrast, steroids may aggravate pulmonary failure after shock. Relative impairment in oxygenation was associated with prolonged ventilatory support for steroid-treated patients. Withholding steroids from patients with postinjury or postshock respiratory failure may be beneficial and will be cost-effective. Further studies are needed on the relation between pulmonary function and other organ function after massive steroid therapy in the severely injured patient.

▶ [This was a prospective study of the response of seriously injured patients to massive doses of steroids and included over 100 patients who were in hypovolemic shock and survived surgery. The only difference in resuscitation in the two patient groups,

TABLE 1.—EFFECT OF STEROIDS ON CENTRAL VOLUME DYNAMICS

Mean ± SE	Steroid-treated Patients	Nonsteroid-treated Patients	p Value
Study CVP (cm H_2O)	10.1 ± 1.2	7.4 ± 0.7	<0.05
Study plasma volume (ml)	3,340 ± 207	3,348 ± 139	<0.5
Study blood volume (ml)	4,691 ± 170	4,787 ± 194	<0.5
Theoretical normal blood volume (ml)	5,100 ± 138	5,072 ± 107	<0.5

(4–7) Ann. Surg. 194:256–261, September 1981.

TABLE 2.—EFFECT OF STEROIDS ON PULMONARY FUNCTION

Mean ± SE	Steroid-treated Patients	Nonsteroid-treated Patients	p Value
Physiologic shunting in the lungs (%)	25 ± 3	22 ± 1	<0.10
Study Po_2 (torr)	95 ± 6	112 ± 6	<0.05
Study Fio_2 (%)	36.6 ± 3	37.6 ± 2	<0.5
Study Fio_2/Po_2	0.45 ± 0.05	0.37 ± 0.02	<0.05
Number of days on ventilator (days)	5.1 ± 2	3.0 ± 0.6	<0.10

as both had received a balanced salt solution and whole blood, was the use of 1 gm of methylprednisolone in the operating room followed by 15 mg/kg for 3 days. Interestingly, this massive steroid supplementation did not prevent or ameliorate any evidence of pulmonary failure after hypervolemic shock and multiple injury. In contrast, it was felt that in many instances the steroids aggravated pulmonary failure after shock. The time required for ventilatory support was nearly doubled in the patients who received steroids. These authors conclude that withholding steroids from patients with respiratory failure after injury and shock may actually be beneficial. This is a well-controlled clinical study that tends to contradict some of the in vitro investigations indicating possible benefits for steroids on a theoretical basis in a multiple-injury patient.—T.S.] ◀

4–8 **Selective Use of Ventilator Therapy in Flail Chest Injury.** Mortality from flail chest injuries continues to be 20% to 50%. Steven R. Shackford, Richard W. Virgilio, and Richard M. Peters (Univ. of California, San Diego) utilized mechanical ventilation in a limited manner in the prospective management of 36 patients seen in 1975–1979 with a diagnosis of flail chest, based on the presence of paradoxical movement in a segment of the chest wall. Thirteen patients with clinical respiratory distress or an intrapulmonary shunt of 25% or more (group 1) were supported with continuous positive airway pressure (CPAP), alone or combined with intermittent mandatory ventilation (IMV). Seven patients (group 2) required temporary respiratory support for associated injury but had no evidence of pulmonary dysfunction. Sixteen patients (group 3) had no indications for respiratory support.

The three groups were similar in the degree of insult to the thoracic cage present. Nineteen patients had x-ray evidence of pulmonary contusion within 24 hours of admission. Group 1 patients received ventilatory support for an average of 10½ days. Forty complications occurred in 11 of these 13 patients. Pneumonia occurred in 9 group 1 patients, and 3 patients had barotrauma. Two group 1 patients (15%) died of progressive pulmonary failure complicated by sepsis and myocardial infarction. The average ventilation time in group 2 was under 1 day. Three patients had complications, but none died. One group 3 patient required respiratory support. Four group 1 patients and 2 in group 3 had airway complications.

The respiratory distress and hypoxemia seen with flail chest pri-

(4–8) J. Thorac. Cardiovasc. Surg. 81:194–201, February 1981.

marily result from a pulmonary parenchymal insult caused by pulmonary contusion, rather than paradoxic motion of the chest wall. Patients with respiratory distress and hypoxemia are managed by CPAP, with or without IMV. A more conservative approach is possible if respiratory distress is absent and the arterial P_{O_2} is above 65 torr. Chest physiotherapy and postural drainage are coordinated with periods of maximum pain relief. Patients should not be moved from intensive care until their pain is well controlled, coughing is effective, and the tidal volume is adequate.

▶ [This interesting investigation confirms increasing reports in recent years that the ventilator therapy necessary in patients with flail chest injury is almost always related to the concomitant pulmonary parenchymal insult caused by pulmonary contusion rather than the paradoxical motion of the chest wall. Even with the mechanical flail chest, if respiratory distress is absent and arterial P_{O_2} is greater than 65 torr, chest physiotherapy, postural drainage, and periods of maximum pain relief suffice to maintain pulmonary function. It would appear from this and other reports that at least 50% of patients with flail chest can be managed quite adequately with more conservative therapy than the use of an endotracheal tube and ventilatory support under the so-called internal stability that has been advocated for most flail chest injuries. Endotracheal tube ventilatory support generally will be required only in those patients who have sustained significant parenchymal lung damage.—T.S.] ◀

4–9 **Emergency Abdominal Wall Reconstruction With Polypropylene Mesh: Short-term Benefits Versus Long-term Complications.** Primary closure of abdominal wall defects under tension promotes wound ischemia and predisposes to dehiscence and evisceration. Complex reconstructive methods may involve a risk of invasive infection, and delayed skin grafting over exposed bowel carries a high risk of early enteric fistula formation. C. Randle Voyles, J. David Richardson, Kirby I. Bland, Gordon R. Tobin, Lewis M. Flint, and Hiram C. Polk, Jr. (Univ. of Louisville) reviewed experience with polypropylene mesh (PPM), used to replace the abdominal wall in 31 patients in 1976–1980. Twenty-five patients had necrotizing fascial infections, often with severe intra-abdominal infection. Three had shotgun wounds with extensive abdominal wall loss, and 3 had massive bowel distention that prevented closure. The 23 men and 8 women had a mean age of 42 years. Prosthetic mesh was used most often at reoperation. A single layer of PPM was secured subfascially with polypropylene sutures.

Mesh was placed in a heavily contaminated field in 29 cases. Seven patients died, 6 of uncontrolled infection. In none of the survivors did the mesh appear to promote local infection, and no patient had evisceration. Reoperation was not necessary for fasciitis alone. No early enteric fistulas developed. Two of 6 patients had wound hernias after removal of the mesh and direct closure of the fascia. Split-thickness grafting over the mesh failed in all 9 patients in whom it was tried. Full-thickness skin coverage over the mesh now is used where the PPM is necessary for sustained abdominal wall continuity. Full-thickness flaps may be mobilized to cover granulating mesh. One patient having split-thickness grafting died after experiencing an intestinal fistula that required reoperation.

(4–9) Ann. Surg. 194:219–223, August 1981.

Polypropylene mesh has exhibited significant early advantages in providing abdominal wall integrity, even in the presence of severe infection, but long-term problems have been frequent. If the mesh cannot be totally removed, myocutaneous flap surgery should be strongly considered after the primary condition has resolved.

▶ [In the past 2 years, several articles have appeared concerning acute replacement of the abdominal wall with polypropylene mesh, generally for acute avulsion of the abdominal wall from injury or for extensive abdominal wall infection. This study, like the others, indicates good immediate closure of the abdomen by the acute insertion of polypropylene mesh in extensive defects. Some other articles have reported success with split-thickness skin grafting over the polypropylene mesh after its impregnation with granulation tissue. The current experience, however, indicates a much higher degree of success if myocutaneous flaps are used to cover the granulating polypropylene mesh.

These wounds are very difficult to manage. In some instances, packing has been used with the development of granulation tissue over the exposed bowel, followed by some form of skin coverage. It would appear at present that the predominant form of management in this situation is related to initial insertion of polypropylene mesh.—T.S.] ◀

4–10 **Abdominal Trauma: The Role and Impact of Computed Tomography** are reviewed by Michael P. Federle (Univ. of California, San Francisco). Accidents are the fourth most common cause of death in the United States, and abdominal injuries account for much of the morbidity and mortality. It often is difficult to determine accurately the site and extent of suspected abdominal injuries. Computed tomography (CT) has been performed in patients with a history of abdominal trauma and relatively stable vital signs for whom admission is warranted and in patients with evidence of generalized or abdominal trauma in whom the physical abdominal examination is considered unreliable. Patients with probable indications for surgery also are studied. All patients receive intravenous contrast unless there is a clear history of severe allergy; noncontrast scans are not necessary. Patients also receive 1% aqueous contrast material orally or by nasogastric tube. Only combative adults and young children are sedated.

Computed tomography is a very accurate and simple means of diagnosing subcapsular hematomas of the spleen. It also can clarify the diagnosis of splenic lacerations. The study depicts the entire extent of subcapsular hepatic hematomas, is useful in evaluating patients with hepatic lacerations, and can detect injuries to biliary structures. Computed tomography occasionally may show evidence of duodenal laceration. It is an accurate means of detecting a wide variety of pancreatic lesions due to trauma and now routinely is done whenever pancreatic trauma is suspected.

Urography may fail to show the extent of renal injury accurately in up to a third of cases. Computed tomography, however, can assess a wide variety of renal and perirenal injuries very accurately. It has been used primarily to evaluate patients suspected of having major renal injuries on urographic and clinical grounds. It is done in a clinically unstable patient or if the urogram suggests major injury. The

---

(4–10) Invest. Radiol. 16:260–268, July–Aug. 1981.

study permits more confident nonoperative management of patients with renal trauma and may result in a shorter hospital stay for observation. It also is a convenient means of assessing the results of conservative management. In surgical cases, CT may help predict the need for complete nephrectomy or the appropriateness of more limited repair.

▶ [This is but one of a series of articles advocating the use of computed abdominal tomography in the stable patient with abdominal trauma. The present series shows accurate diagnostic correlation with injuries of the spleen, including subcapsular hematoma, hepatic lacerations, duodenal laceration, and a wide variety of pancreatic injuries. The authors also reported a high degree of success with renal injuries, particularly in the approximately one third that fail to show up on intravenous urography. The two important groups of patients studied in this series are those with a history of abdominal trauma and relatively stable vital signs and those with abdominal trauma in whom the physical examination is felt to be unreliable. Unless the need for surgery was urgent, such patients were studied by computed tomographic scanning. This is proving to be an increasingly useful technique when there is proper patient selection and immediate availability of qualified staff to perform the computed tomography. —T.S.] ◀

4–11 **Computed Tomography in the Evaluation of Blunt Abdominal Trauma: Review of Three Cases.** Computed tomography (CT) may simplify the radiologic evaluation of patients with blunt abdominal trauma. Morten G. Stiris, Johan G. Johansen, and Jan Due (Univ. Hosp., Tromsø, Norway) used CT to evaluate 3 patients with blunt abdominal trauma. In the first patient the CT findings of subcapsular hepatic bleeding were confirmed at exploration. A postoperative scan showed a cystic lesion that also was verified operatively. The second patient exhibited multiple areas of low splenic attenuation and signs of intraperitoneal leakage, and surgery confirmed splenic laceration with hematoma formation. The third patient was not explored, but CT showed a crescent-shaped area of low attenuation on the renal surface after contrast injection, consistent with subcapsular bleeding. The patient did well on conservative management but did not return for follow-up.

Computed tomography can be useful in evaluating patients with possible injury to the liver or spleen or in the retroperitoneal region. The study is noninvasive but not organ specific. It played the major role in evaluation and follow-up of the present patients with blunt abdominal trauma. Both accurate anatomical data and information on dynamic function can be obtained by CT. The study may suggest an immediate surgical or a conservative approach in selected cases.

▶ [Once again in this article, the value of computed tomography in diagnosing injuries to the liver, spleen, and kidney is shown. While pancreatic scanning was not included in this series of cases, it obviously has been a part of major series that were larger than this one.—T.S.] ◀

4–12 **Hepatic Resection: The Logical Approach to Surgical Management of Major Trauma to the Liver.** At present, there is a dangerous trend to not perform resection in emergency cases of liver trauma, but, rather, to use inferior methods of controlling bleeding. Hemorrhage continues to be the chief cause of death in this setting.

(4–11) Acta Chir. Scand. 146:367–370, 1980.
(4–12) Am. J. Surg. 142:580–583, November 1981.

M. Balasegaram and Suresh K. Joishy (Kuala Lumpur, Malayasia) reviewed data on 379 patients treated for liver injury since 1961. Immediate laparotomy for diagnosis is necessary in some instances. Extensive wounds with bleeding and devitalized liver tissue require resection. Subcapsular hematomas with intralobar rupture caused by blunt injury also are resected, as are high-velocity missile wound tracts. Stab wounds may be managed without resection unless extensive internal damage is present. All patients are given broad-spectrum antibiotics intravenously after operation.

Extensive lacerations, tears, and subcapsular hematomas with intralobar rupture of the liver were common in the 206 patients with blunt trauma, and required major resections. Most resections were right-sided and involved hemiresection or extended hemiresection. All but 6 of these 51 patients survived. Twenty-six of 81 patients with high-velocity missile injuries underwent resection, and only 3 died. Seven of 31 patients with stab wounds causing extensive internal shatter injuries of the liver underwent resection, and all survived.

Nonresectional procedures should never replace resection where indicated in patients with liver injuries. The low mortality from major hepatic resections probably is the result of more rapid resection and the achievement of hemostasis by clamping techniques. Resection is a logical first line of treatment for major hepatic trauma. In cases of hepatic venous injury, it is best to gain direct access to the veins after extending the abdominal incision to the chest.

▶ [This article is written by individuals with a remarkable amount of experience in liver resection for various causes, due in part to the geographic location of the surgeons and patients. The authors not only have extensive experience, but also a remarkably high degree of success in managing hepatic injuries. Certainly, the rebuttal by this group to a previous article by Walt (*Am. J. Surg.* 135:12–18, 1978) is well documented. Their technique of liver resection using a modification of the clamps devised both in Japan and in Taiwan deserves some real respect. It should be added that American surgeons are also converting more and more to the use of a hepatic clamping device that will control the massively bleeding liver. With this, one certainly will see more resections performed with lower mortality, as the current experience is revealing. The final resting place of resection as a major aid in the management of hepatic trauma is probably yet to be determined. The authors refer to articles relegating management by hepatic resection to the 2% level, which is perhaps too low, and certainly the level of 30% of all liver injury is too high. Nevertheless, this is an interesting rebuttal from authors with extensive experience with hepatic resection.—T.S.] ◀

4–13 **The Fate of Unruptured Intrahepatic Hematomas.** Liver injury is the second most common form of blunt abdominal trauma and continues to carry high morbidity and mortality. Most injuries are associated with rupture of the liver and intraperitoneal bleeding, but a small number of patients have liver injury from within with an intact capsule and no free intraperitoneal bleeding. The natural course of the intrahepatic hematoma is unclear. W. Peter Geis, Karl A. Schulz, Joseph L. Giacchino, and Robert J. Freeark (Loyola Univ., Maywood, Ill.) reviewed 4 years' experience with intrahepatic hematoma. Of 283 patients with severe blunt torso trauma, 65 had serious hepatic injury, and 16 of these had intrahepatic hematomas. The 9 female and

(4–13) Surgery 90:689–697, October 1981.

7 male patients had an average age of 40 years. All injuries were caused by a direct blow. Many patients had local evidence of injury to surrounding structures.

Two patients had hemoperitoneum. Four required surgery for late complications of the intrahepatic hematoma. All had a presumptive diagnosis of hepatic abscess with sepsis, confirmed at operation. More than half of the patients with intrahepatic hematoma had no abdominal tenderness until 12 hours or longer after injury. In all, 6 patients were operated on for the hematoma. Three patients had an expanding hematoma resulting in life-threatening bleeding. Complications were more frequent in patients with large hematomas more than one-third the size of the right lobe of the liver. Three patients were receiving anticoagulant therapy at the time of injury. Trauma was mild in all of these cases. One of these patients had had an intrahepatic hematoma 6 years before, with a recurrence in the same location.

Liver-spleen scanning is indicated in patients with blunt torso trauma. An intrahepatic hematoma should be managed nonoperatively at first for at least 28 days. Intrahepatic hematoma associated with anticoagulation is highly lethal and must be managed aggressively. Urgent surgery is indicated in patients with progressive abnormalities such as sepsis, peritoneal involvement, blood loss, or expansion of an intrahepatic hematoma.

▶ [This paper is an attempt to justify the inhospital observation of most intrahepatic hematomas after severe blunt abdominal trauma. Of the patients observed for up to 1 month in the hospital, delayed operative intervention was indicated for hepatic abscess with sepsis in 4 patients and expanding hematoma in 2 others. The conclusion that patients admitted with blunt trauma who are stable should undergo some form of liver and spleen scanning examinations cannot be argued. However, the 1-month observation period for nonoperative management can be questioned in view of the extremely high instance of subsequent bleeding or life-threatening complications. One point to be made from this group of patients was that the combination of anticoagulation and intrahepatic hematoma is highly lethal. It would seem that this article does not, in fact, resolve the dilemma of the stable patient with a large intrahepatic hematoma.—T.S.] ◀

4–14 **Computed Tomographic Evaluation of Blunt Renal Injuries.** Computed tomography (CT) has been shown to be of diagnostic value in a wide variety of renal lesions. Carl M. Sandler and Barry D. Toombs (Univ. of Texas, Houston) reviewed experience with CT in 10 patients suspected of having blunt renal injuries. Only 1 had an isolated renal injury. In 5 cases, the urogram had shown an abnormality. Four patients had CT within 24 hours of admission. All patients were examined after the injection of Renografin-60. Scans were obtained at 1-cm intervals throughout the length of the kidneys.

A renal injury was diagnosed by CT in 9 patients. In 1 case, CT showed that the urographic abnormalities were caused by atrophic pyelonephritis. Intrarenal hematomas were shown by CT in 4 cases, 3 of which had extension to the renal capsule or beyond. The hematomas appeared as rounded areas of decreased attenuation with poorly marginated borders. Subcapsular or perirenal hematomas, or both, were present in 2 other patients, and 2 patients had a renal laceration. Two had segmental occlusion of polar arterial branches, with

(4–14) Radiology 141:461–466, November 1981.

sharply demarcated zones of infarction on CT examination. The CT findings were confirmed angiographically in both of these cases. All patients were managed nonoperatively. Seven patients had normal renal function at follow-up. One patient who ordinarily would have been operated on was not because of concomitant chest injuries, and a nonfunctioning kidney was found at follow-up. The 2 patients with traumatic segmental arterial occlusion had permanent cortical scarring in the areas of infarction.

Computed tomography is more specific than more conventional noninvasive studies in showing the nature of blunt renal injuries. Occasionally, an injury is shown only by CT. However, CT should not replace urography or angiography in evaluating suspected renal trauma. It is most useful in defining the specific nature of a urographic abnormality, avoiding the need for angiography in otherwise stable patients or those in whom there is a discrepancy between the clinical and conventional radiographic findings.

▶ [This is another in the series of papers advocating the use of CT for evaluation of blunt abdominal trauma—in this case, renal injuries. The renal injury was diagnosed by CT scan in 9 of the 10 patients in this study, despite the fact that 5 patients had shown no abnormality on the intravenous pyelogram. Certainly, these authors are making the same conclusions as the authors of the preceding article, which is that CT scanning is proving increasingly useful in the diagnosis of significant abdominal injury.—T.S.] ◀

4–15 **Intracellular Electrolyte Composition Following Renal Ischemia.** A marked reduction in renal blood flow, as occurs in circulatory shock or before transplant surgery, is a frequent cause of acute renal failure. Experimentally, temporary interruption of blood flow to the kidney by renal artery occlusion is followed by a persistent impairment in renal function with deficient fluid reabsorption and limited concentrating-diluting ability, as well as decreased inulin clearance. June Mason, Franz Beck, Adolf Dörge, Roger Rick, and Klaus Thurau (Univ. of Munich) used electron microprobe analysis to examine the effects of ischemia on intracellular electrolyte composition in the outer rat renal cortex and the effects of restoring blood flow to the kidney. Renal ischemia was induced by occluding the renal artery with a weak-sprung clip; the kidney was maintained in either air or nitrogen. Ischemia lasted for 20, 60, or 90 minutes, and reperfusion lasted for 2, 20, or 60 minutes or 18 hours.

When the exposed kidney was maintained in air during ischemia, the composition of the surface cells differed little from the control state, and electrolyte disturbance was confined to the deeper-lying cells. In nitrogen, all of the cells exhibited uniform changes in electrolyte composition. Sodium and chloride levels increased in proximal tubular cells after 20 minutes of ischemia in nitrogen, and potassium and phosphate levels decreased, as did the dry weight. In the distal tubular cells, 1 hour of ischemia in nitrogen led to a rise in sodium and chloride levels and a fall in potassium and phosphate levels. On reperfusion, the electrolyte disturbances were rapidly reversed in all cells, virtually completely within 1 hour. Disturbances returned in some proximal tubular cells by 18 hours of reperfusion.

(4–15) Kidney Int. 20:61–70, July 1981.

Disordered sodium and potassium values in ischemic renal cells primarily are caused by inhibition of the sodium-potassium pump, while the changes in chloride, phosphate, and dry weight content result mainly from an influx of extracellular fluid. The disorder is fully reversible within an hour of reintroducing blood flow, but the recovery is short-lived. The deeper-lying nephrons may be chiefly responsible for the functional defects observed after renal ischemia.

▶ [An extremely difficult but highly quantitative technique, electron microprobe analysis, was used by these authors to examine the effects of ischemia on intracellular electrolyte composition in animals. The authors showed reversible changes in the cell membrane in response to ischemia; the changes included the movement of sodium and chloride in water into cells and the exclusion of potassium and phosphate by the injured cells. On reperfusion, the electrolyte disturbances were rapidly reversed. The authors concluded that the inhibition of the sodium-potassium pump induced by ischemia resulted in an influx of extracellular fluid into the cell. This new and unique method of analysis therefore provides an interesting confirmation of cellular injury in response to low flow.—T.S.] ◀

4–16 **Compartmental Pressure Measurements: Experimental Investigation Using the Slit Catheter.** Failure to diagnose and appropriately treat an acute compartment syndrome usually results in a contracted, useless extremity. Irreversible damage may be present by the time there are conclusive clinical signs of a compartment syndrome, and measurements of compartment pressure can be very helpful. Cecil H. Rorabeck, G. S. P. Castle, R. Hardie, and J. Logan (Univ. of Western Ontario, London) describe a new system of measuring compartment pressures utilizing a slit catheter and a pressure monitoring system. The device consists of a 20-cm length of polyethylene tubing with 5 symmetrical slits in the end, extending 3 mm along the length of the tubing. The accuracy of this technique was compared with that of a wick catheter and that of the needle manometer technique in dogs.

Studies were done on the anterolateral compartment of the canine leg as saline was infused to raise the pressure, by increments of 10 mm Hg, to 100 mm Hg. The various methods were compared at a constant compartment pressure of 35 mm Hg. The wick and slit catheters achieved about the same level of accuracy over the range of pressures used, with standard deviations of less than 2 mm Hg for each method. The needle technique was the least accurate, with standard deviations of ±5 mm Hg. The needle method gave falsely high readings at pressures below 50 mm Hg and falsely low readings at higher pressures. The slit catheter was the most accurate of the methods when a continuous pressure of 35 mm Hg was maintained for 24 hours; the standard deviations were less than ±2 mm Hg. The slit catheter did not lose accuracy over time, as did the wick catheter method. A significant scatter of values with large standard deviations was observed with the needle technique.

The slit catheter is at least as accurate as the wick catheter and is more accurate than the needle manometer method in measuring compartment pressures. It appears to be the best of the methods tested for continuous pressure monitoring.

(4–16) J. Trauma 21:446–449, June 1981.

▶ [Acute compartment syndrome after ischemia and trauma is a very severe complication that often results in a contracted, useless extremity. The authors conclude, by using a new system of measuring compartment pressures with a slit catheter and a pressure monitoring system, that compartment compression syndrome can be diagnosed early and definitive therapy applied when it is still effective. The technique used was found to be far superior to that of a wick catheter or a needle manometer. This new technique is simple and may well prove extremely useful clinically in the evaluation of a possible compartment compression syndrome, particularly in an anterior compartment of the leg. If so, definitive surgical procedures can be done early, with resultant removal of the pressure in the anterior compartment.—T.S.] ◀

4–17 **Arthroscopic Surgery of the Knee: History and State of the Art** are reviewed by Conrad T. Fraider (Philadelphia). Arthroscopy has become an integral part of the orthopedic management of knee disorders. Arthroscopic surgery permits more rapid rehabilitation, especially of athletes, than conventional arthrotomy. Most procedures can be done on an outpatient basis. Multiple small incisions are cosmetically preferable to a disfiguring scar. The complication rate is very low. A secondary arthroscopy or other procedure can be done with low morbidity. Arthroscopic surgery presently is in its infancy. The use of laser technology in this setting is not far off. The knee is merely the first of the joints amenable to arthroscopic surgery.

Loose bodies in the knee joint can be removed arthroscopically by either a single- or double-puncture technique. An irrigation technique is most applicable to the removal of cartilaginous loose bodies, particularly those lying in the joint line. A medial synovial plica and medial intra-articular bands and adhesions can be managed arthroscopically. In cases of osteochondritis dissecans, drilling and pin insertion can be performed arthroscopically. Intra-articular shaving under arthroscopic control has given good early results in cases of chondromalacia patellae. Lateral retinacular release can be performed arthroscopically in cases of lateral tracking syndrome. Meniscoresis has been done in patients with parameniscal tears. Meniscectomy or partial meniscectomy probably is the greatest breakthrough in arthroscopic surgery. The overall results have been more than satisfactory, and complications generally have been minimal. Synovectomy has been performed by the Japanese using a modified electric resectoscope.

▶ [This is a review article of the current state and importance of arthroscopic surgery of the knee. As these authors point out, arthroscopic surgery, although it is still in its infancy, is certainly a promising technique. Most of the procedures that previously were carried out through formal arthrotomy of the knee can now be done through the arthroscope. These include irrigation for removal of loose bodies as well as management of intra-articular bands and adhesions. In some instances, drilling and pin insertion can be performed arthroscopically. Meniscectomy or partial meniscectomy is probably the greatest breakthrough in arthroscopic surgery. The overall results have been quite good and complications have been minimal. The use of electric resectoscopes through these arthroscopes, as well as lasar technology, would lead one to believe that this technique will be expanded and improved in the future.—T.S.] ◀

(4–17) JAOA 80:817–822, August 1981.

5. Wound Healing

5-1 **Wound Healing Using Amniotic Membranes.** R. N. Matthews, J. P. Bennett, and W. Page Faulk (Queen Victoria Hosp., Sussex, England) present a case report illustrating the angioneogenic effects of amniotic membrane when applied to wounds.

Woman, 68, with hypertension and cerebral atherosclerosis, sustained severe burns to the head when she fainted and lay unconscious in front of a fire for 2 hours. The burn involved the full thickness of the scalp and partial to full-thickness destruction of the cranium over a wide area. Because of the age and frailty of the patient, surgery was restricted to the drilling of bur holes through the outer table to allow granulation tissue to proliferate over the bare bone surface. Three years later, sequestration of the outer table and a full-thickness portion of the cranium over the vertex was complete. The sequestra were removed and split-skin grafts applied to the exposed granulation tissue and dura mater. Despite repeated grafting over the next 3 years, some areas remained unhealed due to the poor quality of the granulation tissue and the patient rubbing the freshly grafted areas.

A single application of tissue culture-maintained amniotic membrane to the raw areas for 5 days produced a marked clinical and histopathologic vascular response in the granulation tissue and stimulated healing by marginal epithelialization. Split-skin grafts were applied to the remaining raw areas and a protective plaster helmet was fitted. The patient dislodged this device on the second day, upsetting the take of the graft, but one application of stored skin provided complete skin cover.

The pliability of amnion allows it to conform closely to irregular surfaces, and this may be important in its greater effect in reducing wound infection when compared with homografts and xenografts. It has been suggested that amniotic fluid has broad-spectrum antibiotic activity and that extraembryonic fetal tissues contain glycoproteins that block the rejection reaction. These factors, together with its angioneogenic properties, may contribute to the observed vascular response in tissue to which amnion is applied. Amnion, a possibly ideal biologic dressing, deserves further study and use.

► [Amnion is a superb biologic dressing. It is functionally equivalent to allogenic skin and much easier to obtain. Remember, however, the shiny side goes out! In my judgment, surgeons should stop using pigskin as a temporary cover. Expense, storage, and crossing major histocompatibility lines are not necessary when amnion serves equally well for wound closure.—E.E.P.] ◄

5-2 **Control of Wound Healing and Scar Formation in Surgical Patients** is discussed by Erle E. Peacock, Jr. (Tulane Univ.) At present, it generally is necessary for the surgeon to excise offending scar tissue, restore the wound to a prehealing state, and manipulate new scar formation. Present biologic and pharmacologic techniques are only adjuvents to surgery, useful in preventing scar formation during the

(5-1) Br. J. Plast. Surg. 34:76-78, January 1981.
(5-2) Arch. Surg. 116:1325-1329, October 1981.

healing process. Surgical methods have been designed primarily to alter the direction of scar tissue to release tension from muscular pull or joint motion. Scar tissue can be reduced, especially in patients with large keloids, by addition of free skin grafts to release tension. Agents available for controlling scar tissue formation in humans include colchicine, penicillamine, and β-aminopropionitrile (BAPN). All these agents appear to be safe in recommended dosages.

Anticollagen drugs may be most useful in treatment of acute alkali burns of the esophagus. Prevention of recurrent urethral strictures with lathyrogenic agents after dilation or urethrotomy has been less impressive. Scar tissue surrounding the gliding surfaces of repaired or injured tendons can be made lathyritic by administration of BAPN or penicillamine. Control of scar tissue in solid organs, such as the liver, lungs or kidneys, may also be possible with a combination of agents. Control of secondary remodeling of fibrous adhesions to produce tendinous bands causing intestinal obstruction awaits development of a safe and controlled antifibrin or fibrinolytic agent for use in the peritoneal cavity.

The author has obtained good results in 15 patients with keloids or hypertrophic scars by treatment with BAPN or other agents. Some patients, however, developed a moderate hypertrophic scar after several years. No typical keloid has recurred.

▶ [The often repeated Paré statement, "I dressed the wound; God healed it," will not be true forever. The quality and quantity of scar tissue in a surgical incision can be controlled and will become a useful adjunct to surgical therapy.—E.E.P.] ◀

5–3 **Impaired Wound Healing in Streptozotocin Diabetes: Prevention by Supplemental Vitamin A.** Wound healing often is slow in diabetics, and it is complicated by infection more often than in nondiabetics. Goodson and Hunt showed improvement in wound healing in streptozotocin-induced diabetic rats with insulin treatment. Trauma reduces wound healing in rats, and feeding of vitamin A largely prevents the effect. Eli Seifter, Giuseppe Rettura, Jacques Padawer, Frank Stratford, Demetrios Kambosos, and Stanley M. Levenson (Albert Einstein College of Medicine, New York) thought that if impaired wound healing in streptozotocin-diabetic rats is caused by an impaired inflammatory reaction, feeding of supplemental vitamin A should prevent this. Rats were fed a chow containing twice the recommended amount of vitamin A and received streptozotocin, 60 mg/kg. Some animals then received vitamin A, 150,000 units/kg. All animals had 7-cm skin incisions made and polyvinyl alcohol sponge implanted subcutaneously.

Poor wound healing was observed in streptozotocin-diabetic rats, as reflected by the breaking strength of skin incisions and the hydroxyproline content of sponge reparative tissue. Supplemental vitamin A did not influence hyperglycemia or glycosuria, but was associated with increased breaking strength of the incisions in diabetic animals, and with increased sponge hydroxyproline. Similar results were obtained when wounding and the start of supplemental vitamin A were delayed until 28 days after streptozotocin administration. Vitamin A

(5–3) Ann. Surg. 194:42–50, July 1981.

did not influence the decrease in cross-linking of reparative collagen induced by streptozotocin, but the peripheral lymphocytopenia, adrenal hypertrophy, and thymic involution responded to supplemental vitamin A treatment.

Vitamin A supplementation corrects impaired wound healing in streptozotocin-diabetic rats without affecting the disordered carbohydrate metabolism. The effect is attributed to a speeding up of the initial inflammatory events in wound healing. Supplemental vitamin A therapy may prove useful in preventing wound infection and prompting wound healing in surgical diabetic patients, and in surgical tumor patients who are receiving streptozotocin.

▶ [Impaired wound healing, a clinical problem in some diabetic patients, affects injuries of deep organs such as the stomach and duodenum, as well as surface wounds. The effect of vitamin A should be tested in human beings now that controlled experimental data suggest it may be beneficial in rats. Excessive administration of vitamin A should be avoided, but doses in the range used in this study are not toxic and should be used when wound healing problems are anticipated.—E.E.P.] ◀

5–4 **Use of Colchicine to Inhibit Wound Contraction.** Contraction of open skin wounds probably is caused by the myofibroblasts. Ehrlich et al. reported that topical application of colchicine and vinblastine inhibited wound contraction in vivo, and suggested that this might be a result of disruption of microtubules. Ross Rudolph, Irwin Hurn, and Marilyn Woodward (Univ. of California, San Diego) examined the effects of colchicine on wound contraction in rat and rabbit models, using both wound area measurements and electron microscopy. Full-thickness skin wounds were excised in both models. Colchicine was administered systemically using an implanted minipump, orally, and topically. Plastic sheeting was used to prevent drug dispersion into the dressing.

Topical colchicine inhibited contraction to varying degrees in the rat. Vinblastine but not colchicine was effective in the rabbit (Fig 5–1). Systemic colchicine administration did not significantly alter wound

Fig 5–1.—Effect on wound contraction in rabbits of colchicine, 1×10^{-4} M (0.04 mg) per day, and vinblastine, 5×10^{-5} M (0.45 mg) per day. Colchicine did not inhibit wound contraction, but vinblastine did (both with wound infection). Saline solution was used in the control group. (Courtesy of Rudolph, R., et al.: Am. J. Surg. 141:712–717, June 1981.)

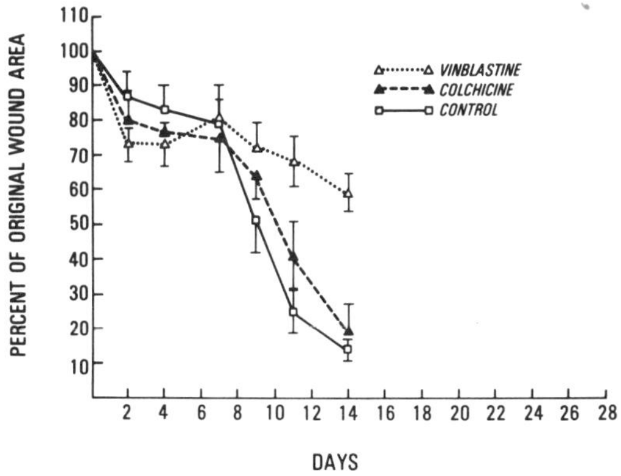

(5–4) Am. J. Surg. 141:712–717, June 1981.

contraction in the rat, and oral colchicine therapy was ineffective in the rabbit. Considerable tissue necrosis was associated with topical colchicine application. Microtubules appeared to be shorter in treated than in control wounds, but this could not be quantitated. Myofibroblasts with microtubules were evident in both control and treated wounds in rats and rabbits.

Topical colchicine application was associated with inhibition of wound contraction in rats and rabbits in this study with full-thickness skin excisions, but at the expense of local toxicity. Systemic colchicine administration had no effect on wound contraction. Colchicine probably inhibits wound contraction through a local toxic effect rather than by specifically inhibiting myofibroblast structures. Colchicine is unlikely to be useful for inhibiting wound contraction clinically, but other agents such as smooth muscle inhibitors may prove to be effective.

▶ [Clinicians now have two agents that will inhibit wound contraction. Topical smooth muscle antagonists and colchicine can reduce or prevent wound contraction without causing undesirable side effects. Patients in whom grafting cannot be performed, for some reason, before wound contracture develops may be candidates for pharmacologic control of the contraction process.—E.E.P.] ◀

5–5 **Influence of Relaxing Incision on Suture Tension in Bassini's and McVay's Repairs.** Raymond C. Read and P. C. McLeod, Jr. (Little Rock, Ark.) measured tension levels at the suture line during inguinal herniorrhaphy and estimated the benefits of a relaxing incision in 135 men having 151 inguinal herniorrhaphies in 1977 to 1979. Patients with recurrent hernia and patients having previous lower abdominal surgery were excluded from study. Studies were performed only on those patients in whom a relaxing incision was to be performed, thus skewing the patient population to the 60% or 70% with larger, especially direct, defects. The larger defects and most direct defects were repaired with the Cooper's ligament (McVay) approach. Measurements were made with a suture tension probe after sutures had been placed from the transverse layer into either Poupart's or Cooper's ligaments.

Overall, tensions were higher both initially and after relaxation when McVay's repair was used, compared with Bassini's repair (Fig 5–2). Similar reductions in tension were noted after the relaxing incision in both repairs, but initial tension was higher with McVay repairs. Maximal tension was not at the lateral end of the Cooper's ligament sutures close to the femoral vein, but, rather, tension was greater medially. In cases of indirect hernia, the relaxing incision was less effective in reducing tension with McVay repair. In cases of direct hernia, a nearly equal amount of relaxation was noted in both groups. In cases of moderate direct hernia, more relaxation was apparent with McVay repairs. Patients who subsequently developed recurrent direct herniation had higher than average tensions before and after relaxation along the suture line.

Suture line tension is greater when inguinal herniation is repaired using Cooper's ligament rather than Poupart's ligament sutures, presumably because of the greater stretch required to reach the former

---

(5–5) Arch. Surg. 116:440–454, April 1981.

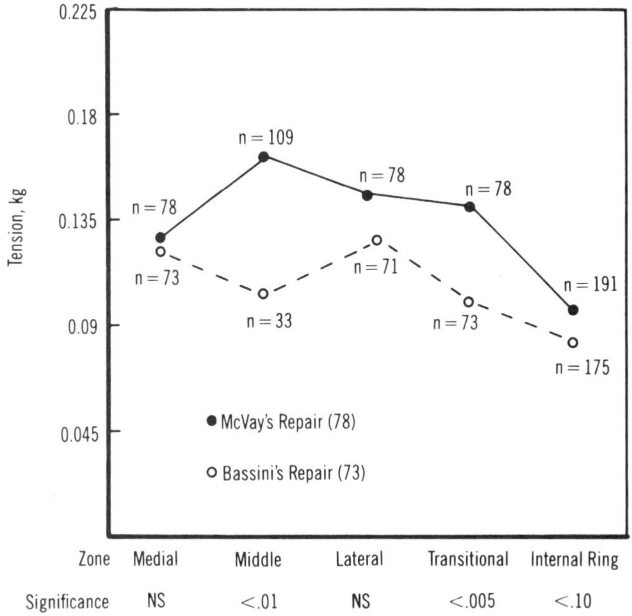

Fig 5–2.—Overall suture tensions measured in 135 patients with 151 unilateral or bilateral hernias. Five suture zones are distinguished medially to laterally along the repair; n indicates number of measurements. (Courtesy of Read, R. C., and McLeon, P. C., Jr.: Arch. Surg. 116:440–454, April 1981; copyright 1981, American Medical Association.)

and because the inguinal ligament is more pliable. The use of artificial mesh may prove to be of value where elevated suture tension is present. Further follow-up is needed to determine whether suture tension at the time of surgery correlates with the risk of recurrence.

▶ [This study is welcomed because it applies quantitative measurements to a very common surgical procedure that has long been in need of serious scientific assessment. To those who have done both types of repairs considered in this paper, it is no surprise that the tensions in the Cooper's ligament repairs are significantly greater than those that use the inguinal ligament. The findings would have been more significant had the authors carried out a randomized study, and this is really the major flaw of this paper. Even though the investigators have made attempts to show that bias was excluded, so long as the operating surgeon has the option to choose one or the other type of repair, bias can never truly be eliminated. I would be very anxious to see long-term studies of patients undergoing hernioplasty in which tensions were consistently measured at operation. Perhaps measurement of tension will become a standard procedure if we are able to identify levels of tension that are sufficiently great to predict a high incidence of recurrence. Under circumstances in which tensions were excessive, the procedure could then be modified at the time of operation.

This is a truly fine contribution. One of the unmeasured variables that is of great importance is the type of anesthetic used for the operative procedure. Differences in amounts of relaxant given during use of general anesthesia could account for very real and significant differences in the tensions generated at the suture line. In addition, spinal anesthetics will clearly produce greater relaxation than general or local anesthesia. It would be important for the authors to exclude these variables.—W.S.] ◀

5–6 **Importance of Apposition of Submucosal Intestinal Layers for Primary Wound Healing of Intestinal Anastomosis.** Anastomotic

(5–6) Surg. Gynecol. Obstet. 152:51–58, January 1981.

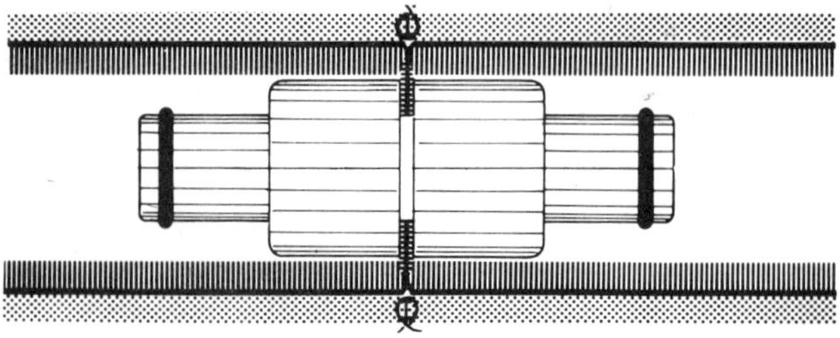

Fig 5–3.—The submucosal and mucosal layers are compressed between the magnetic rings, which results in ideal apposition of the submucosal layer. The seromuscular layers are approximated with 4 to 8 sutures. (Courtesy of Jansen, A., et al.: Surg. Gynecol. Obstet. 152:51–58, January 1981.)

dehiscence and stricture formation often complicate gastrointestinal surgical procedures. A. Jansen, A. E. Becker, W. H. Brummelkamp, J. N. Keeman, and P. J. Klopper (Univ. of Amsterdam) studied the role of the submucosal layers in intestinal healing.

Four anastomoses were performed in the small intestine of each of 18 adult dogs. Two anastomoses were done with a conventional double-layered inverting suture. The other two were performed with an anastomotic apparatus consisting of two rings of polyester-polyethyleneterephtalate containing small Ticonal magnets. This is unlike other mechanical techniques in that only the mucosal and submucosal layers are clasped in the magnets (Fig 5–3). The force between the magnets varied from 0 to 3 newton at distances of, respectively, 15 mm and 0 mm between the rings. After 3–4 days, the rings cut through and disappeared from the anastomosis. The dogs were killed 4 or 10 days postoperatively. The anastomoses were studied morphologically and microangiographically.

In instances of good submucosal apposition, direct bridging of the defect in the submucosal layer was seen with rapid restoration of the villous epithelium and an undisturbed vascular pattern in the anastomotic area (primary intestinal healing). In cases of bad submucosal apposition, indirect bridging of the submucosal layer defect by smaller and longer strands of newly synthesized collagen tissue was seen in the outer intestinal layers, with a collateral circulation from the submucosal plexus to the arterial plexuses in these layers (secondary intestinal healing). In all instances, an epithelial defect still persisted at 10 days.

The magnetic rings produced better circular apposition of the intestinal layers than did conventional techniques.

▶ [The strength of an intestinal anastomosis, regardless of which technique or technical adjuvant is used, lies in the strength of the submucosal layer. For some time, I have been using an end-to-end mucosal approximation to reduce the size of the internal web, and a submucosal suture to provide tensile strength for the anastomosis.—E.E.P.] ◀

5–7 **Bacterial Adherence to Surgical Sutures: A Possible Factor in Suture Induced Infection.** The presence of suture material in a surgical wound has an adverse effect on local tissue conditions and increases the risk of infection. The kind of suture material used is a

(5–7) Ann. Surg. 194:35–41, July 1981.

factor. Shmuel Katz, Mordechai Izhar, and David Mirelman attempted to determine whether differences in bacterial adherence to various sutures could influence tissue susceptibility to infection. Adherence was assessed quantitatively using radiolabeled bacteria including *Staphylococcus aureus, Escherichia coli, Bacteroides fragilis, Serratia marcescens,* and *Shigella dysenteriae.* Both an in vitro assay and an animal model of wound infection in mice were used. In the latter, sutures were implanted into subcutaneous pockets with or without pyogenic staphylococci present. Chromic, Dexon, Ethilon, silk, and Ti-cron sutures were investigated.

The in vitro studies showed that Ethilon bound the least bacteria, and Plain and Dexon bound the most. Even at high concentrations, only 0.5%–4% of bacteria adhered to the incubated sutures. Different types of organisms adhered similarly to the various suture materials. Adherence was markedly enhanced by preincubating sutures with serum or plasma before exposure to radiolabeled bacteria. The suture materials potentiated bacterial growth and caused infection in the mouse model. The degree of inflammation induced correlated well with the in vitro findings. Scanning electron micrographs demonstrated bacterial adherence to various suture materials (Figs 5–4 and 5–5). The ability of bacteria to adhere to sites between the interlacing filaments of braided sutures appeared to increase their adherence to such sutures. Penetration of bacteria to the interstices of a multifilament suture may prevent contact with tissue phagocytic factors.

Fig 5–4.—Composite scanning electron micrograms showing the gross appearance of four surgical sutures: **A,** monofilament nylon; **B,** chromic catgut; **C,** silk; **D,** Dexon; original magnification ×100. (Courtesy of Katz, S., et al.: Ann. Surg. 194:35–41, July 1981.)

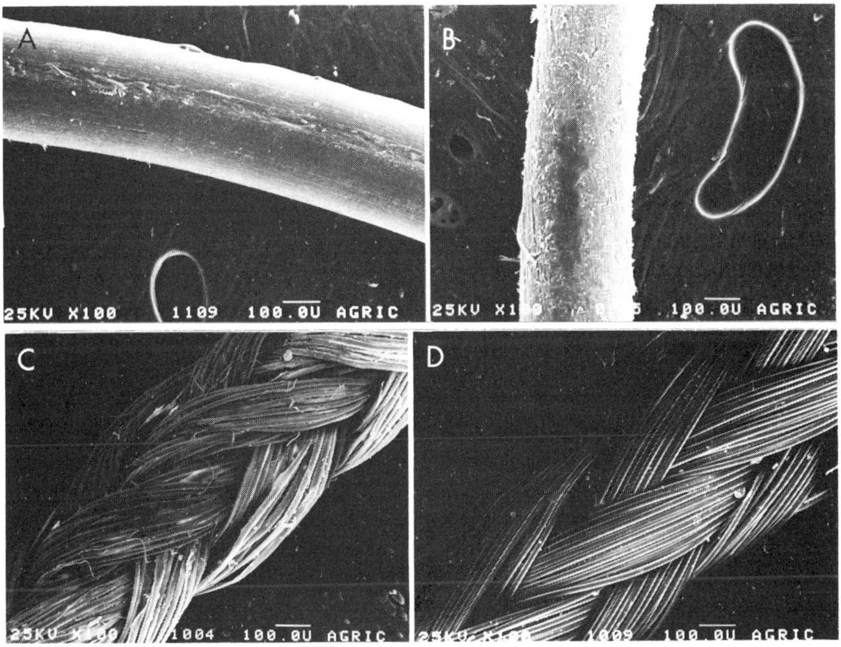

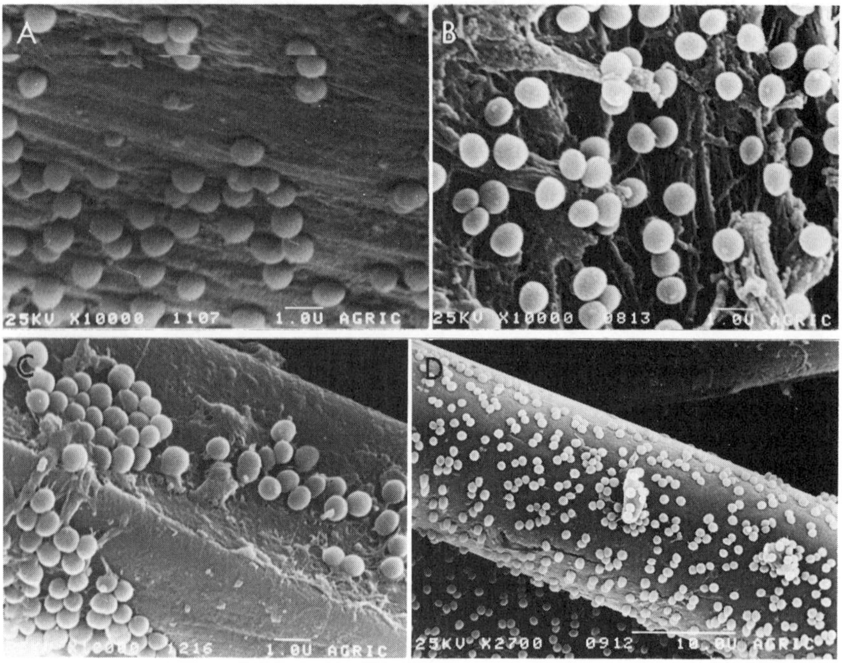

Fig 5–5.—Composite scanning electron micrograms showing staphylococci adhered to surgical sutures: **A,** monofilament nylon (×10,000); **B,** chromic catgut (×10,000); **C,** silk (×10,000); **D,** Dexon (×2,700). (Courtesy of Katz, S., et al.: Ann. Surg. 194:35–41, July 1981.)

Careful suture selection is necessary when wound infection is anticipated. The assay for bacterial adherence to sutures may aid the development of better-designed sutures and minimize their role in the induction of surgical wound infection. The present studies deal only with early postoperative infection; the effect of degradation products of absorbable sutures was not considered.

▶ [It should be remembered that even metal sutures, from a bacteria's eye view, provide a haven of rest in their surface irregularities. Absorbable sutures are always safest if wound infection is a significant danger.—E.E.P.] ◀

5–8 **Fibronectin: A Molecular Glue** is discussed by Jan McDonagh (Univ. of North Carolina). Fibronectin is a group of large, complex, polymorphic proteins having collagen-binding activity. It is distributed widely in tissues and body fluids. It codistributes with collagen in basement membranes and connective tissue. Many cells secrete fibronectin in culture, which then forms a fibrillar, extracellular matrix. Fibronectin is a dimeric protein with a molecular weight of about 440,000. It consists of two subunits held together by one or two disulfide bonds near the carboxy-terminal ends of the chains. The dimeric form of fibronectin is very sensitive to many proteolytic enzymes. The molecule appears to be arranged in several ordered domains connected by extended, flexible, polypeptide regions.

Intracellular fibronectin appears to help maintain normal cellular

(5–8) Arch. Pathol. Lab. Med. 105:393–396, August 1981.

morphologic features. It is related closely to actin in intracellular microfilaments. Fibronectin also is a principal component of the extracellular matrix, and it has a high affinity for collagen. Through its cell-binding property, fibronectin mediates cell-to-substratum binding and cell-to-cell interactions. Cells in culture require fibronectin to bind to collagen. There may be an inverse relation between the expression of extracellular fibronectin and cell transformation. Fibronectin is a plasma protein and has a regulatory role in the blood coagulation process. Fibronectin is a major opsonic protein in plasma. It also has a role in wound healing. Fibronectin is necessary for fibroblasts to interact with fibrin.

A number of diverse functions have been described for both the plasma and cellular forms of fibronectin. Adhesiveness is the general feature uniting these functions, and fibronectin can be described as one of the principal components of the molecular glue. Fibronectin appears to be involved in essentially all physiologic and pathologic processes that require a high degree of adhesiveness.

▶ [Recent studies by Viljanto et al. have shown that fibronectin, an adhesive glycoprotein, is an important factor in the healing of human wounds. The fibrin phase of wound healing has appeared important in the development of intra-abdominal adhesions, as well as in surface wound healing. Measurement of fibronectin and control of fibronectin in the healing wound may be of clinical importance in the years ahead.—E.E.P.] ◀

5–9 **Prediction of Amputation Wound Healing: Roles of Doppler Ultrasound and Digit Photoplethysmography.** Objective measures for selecting the most appropriate distal level of amputation compatible with wound healing are needed. Robert W. Barnes, Brenda Thornhill, Lee Nix, Stanley E. Rittgers, and Glenn Turley (Richmond, Va.) studied the role of Doppler ultrasound and digit photoplethysmography in predicting wound healing in 113 patients, aged 46–88 years (mean, 65 years), undergoing amputation for ischemia of the lower extremity or foot between 1977 and 1979. Forty (35%) patients had diabetes mellitus.

There were 122 primary amputations initially performed, 52 (43%) at the level of the foot, 44 (36%) below the knee, and 26 (21%) above the knee. Segmental limb systolic blood pressures were measured at the proximal thigh, above-knee, below-knee, and ankle levels using pneumatic cuffs and a Doppler velocity detector. Digit pulses were obtained with a photoplethysmograph. The level of amputation was selected by traditional clinical criteria, attempting to preserve maximal limb length to enhance rehabilitation potential.

Of the 122 amputations, 98 (80%) healed primarily or by secondary intention at the original level. The rates of healing were 67%, 84%, and 100% for foot (toe or transmetatarsal), below-knee, and above-knee amputations, respectively. Measurement of sequential limb blood pressures by Doppler ultrasound was a fallible guide to wound healing at either the foot or below-knee level. Although healing failure of a digit or transmetatarsal amputation was more likely if the ankle pressure was below 60 mm Hg, the fact that some foot amputations

(5–9) Arch. Surg. 116:80–83, January 1981.

healed at pressures much lower than this precludes use of such data to dictate the level of amputation. More predictive information was obtained with photoplethysmography, which allowed assessment of digit pulsation and pressure near the proposed foot amputation. Diabetes increased the risk of wound failure at the foot level. Whereas absence of digit pulsatile circulation was compatible with foot amputation healing in nondiabetics, this sign was associated with wound failure in limbs of diabetics. Likewise, the lower limit of digit pressure associated with uniform wound healing was 10 mm Hg in nondiabetics and 25 mm Hg in diabetics. There was no association between segmental limb pressures and the rate of healing of below-knee amputations.

Measurement of limb and digit hemodynamics, while correlating at times with wound healing potential, remains an adjunctive and imprecise index of the outcome of amputation for arterial insufficiency.

▶ [One thing that has been learned through years of trying to predict the success of wound healing in an amputation stump is that a biologic test is still the only sure way. Previously it was thought that below-the-knee amputations would never heal in diabetic or severe arteriolosclerotic patients; we know now that this is not true. Previously it was thought that patients with an absent popliteal pulse would not heal a below-the-knee amputation; we also know that this is not true. Doppler monitoring, ultrasound, and digit plethysmography may make wound healing predictions a little more accurate but, in the final analysis, the only sure test is the actual clinical experiment.—E.E.P.] ◀

6. Infections

6–1 **Agents and Techniques for Disinfection of Skin.** Alan F. Kaul and John Figgis Jewett (Boston) reviewed the literature of the past 75 years relative to preoperative preparation of the hands of the surgeon and skin of the patient. From the wide variety of agents and techniques scrutinized, four major contenders emerge for preferred use.

Hexachlorophene is found in significant levels in the blood of frequent users. Vacuolar encephalopathy has been noted in postmortem studies of premature infants bathed with this agent. It is also suspected of teratogenicity. Hence, hexachlorophene should be removed from general use within hospitals and restricted to use only for specific indications.

Iodophors fail to maintain adequate residual activity and frequently cause skin reactions; also, the rate of release and stability of the complexed iodine vary with time. Thus, iodophors should be replaced whenever agents without these drawbacks are approved and available. However, they might continue to be used for procedures requiring application to large areas of mucous membrane. Lavage of serous cavities with iodophors should be absolutely proscribed.

Benzalkonium should be used, in strict accordance with the Desautels procedure, in preference to all other agents for preparation of the meatus and periurethral area for catheterization and continued care of indwelling catheters. Because of its frequent contamination and misuse with cotton fiber, benzalkonium is not recommended for other surfaces.

A 4% solution of chlorhexidine gluconate in isopropanol is recommended as a standard preoperative scrub and handwash for 5 minutes. Preoperatively, the operative site should be prepared with 0.5% chlorhexidine in 70% isopropanol. Chlorhexidine preparations should not be heat sterilized or diluted because the potential for breakdown to parachloraniline is unpredictable.

▶ [This most recent review suggests that chlorhexidine is superior to other topical agents available for disinfecting the skin. In all previous studies, nothing has been proved to be more satisfactory than alcohol. In my judgment, this review includes no data that contradict the previous conclusion.—E.E.P.] ◀

6–2 **Effect of Topical Povidone-Iodine on Incidence of Infection in Surgical Wounds.** J. A. Walsh, J. Mck. Watts, P. J. McDonald, and J. J. Finlay-Jones (Flinders Hosp., Bedford Park, Australia) conducted a randomized stratified clinical trial of topical povidone-iodine in 314 male and 313 female patients, aged 6–92 years (mean, 43 years), undergoing abdominal surgery (usually appendectomy or biliary tract procedures). Wounds were stratified on the basis of expected bacterial

---

(6–1) Surg. Gynecol. Obstet. 152:677–685, May 1981.
(6–2) Br. J. Surg. 68:185–189, March 1981.

contamination and patient obesity. Within each group, after closure of the peritoneum, patients were randomly allocated to wound spraying with povidone-iodine solution (5% Betadine aerosol spray with 0.5% available iodine) or no treatment. No patient was sensitive to povidone-iodine.

Wounds became infected in 68 patients (11%), including 28 (9%) of 308 in the povidone-iodine group and 40 (12%) of 319 controls. Povidone-iodine reduced the rate of postoperative wound sepsis in female patients, in those receiving subcutaneous low-dose heparin, and during the first quarter of the trial when the infection rate in controls was high. Overall, there was no significant reduction in incidence of wound sepsis after administration of povidone-iodine due mainly to a high infection rate in povidone-iodine-treated male appendectomy patients; in this group, by chance, there was an increased incidence of contamination by *Bacteroides fragilis*. If, for this reason, all male appendectomy patients were excluded from analysis, the overall infection rate became 7% in the povidone-iodine group and 14% in controls ($P < .025$). Povidone-iodine did not influence infection rate within any of the three wound cleanliness categories (clean, potentially infected, dirty).

Use of topical povidone-iodine in addition to appropriate parenteral antibiotics did not increase the protection against infection over that afforded by antibiotics alone. In patients with a wound infection, there was an average decrease in postoperative stay of 5.3 days in those receiving povidone-iodine compared with controls. This significant decrease is indirect evidence that povidone-iodine decreased the severity of wound infection.

Recent evidence indicates that systemic administration of short courses of antibiotics fully effective against aerobic and anaerobic bacteria is the preferred method of prophylaxis of wound sepsis. However, topical povidone-iodine is inexpensive, nontoxic, and free of the problems of induced bacterial resistance. Hence, it offers an additional measure for reducing bacteria in surgical wounds.

▶ [Although the authors present data in support of the use of povidone-iodine in the prevention and treatment of infection in some surgical wounds, I do not agree with their conclusions. The concept that a topical agent such as povidone-iodine could make a significant difference in prevention or treatment of wound infection remains suspect. Data in this paper, in my judgment, support the antithesis more strongly than the thesis.—E.E.P.] ◀

6–3 **Importance of Lactic Acid Levels in Body Fluids in the Detection of Bacterial Infections** is discussed by Itzhak Brook (Naval Med. Res. Inst., Bethesda, Md.). Elevated levels of lactic acid have been described in association with bacterial infections in the cerebrospinal fluid (CSF) and in the synovial, peritoneal, and pleural fluids. Increased levels of lactic acid in the CSF in the wake of a cellular response to bacteria may be a sensitive means of detecting bacterial meningitis. Although the source of lactic acid in the CSF remains unclear, anaerobic glycolysis and tissue anoxia have been implicated. Elevated lactic acid levels in synovial fluid have been associated with

(6–3) Rev. Infect. Dis. 3:470–478, May–June 1981.

septic arthritis, and measurement of lactic acid in ascitic fluid may be useful in diagnosing peritonitis and distinguishing it from other conditions. Elevated levels of lactic acid have been demonstrated in pleural effusion in patients with malignancy and infections of the pleural cavity.

The presence of bacterial infection in a closed body cavity leads to elevated levels of lactic acid, as have been observed in bacterial and fungal infections of the meninges, joints, peritoneum, and pleura. Lactate measurement may be a valuable tool in the early recognition of bacterial infections at these sites and can help distinguish between infectious and noninfectious conditions. False positive results may be obtained in the presence of severe anoxia of the CNS or with peritoneal or pleural irritation by metastases. False negative results can be obtained in gonococcal arthritis. Further work is needed to elucidate the mechanisms that cause changes in lactic acid concentrations at various sites of infection.

▶ [Despite tremendous advances in radionuclide and direct and indirect scanning, detection of bacterial infections in deep body cavities still can produce a diagnostic dilemma. Serum lactic acid levels can provide a useful test in some patients.—E.E.P.] ◀

6–4 **Neutrophils Dysfunction During the Course of Intra-abdominal Infection.** Intraperitoneal infection remains a major cause of death in general surgical patients, often despite apparently adequate drainage and appropriate antibiotic therapy. Depressed delayed cutaneous hypersensitivity reactions have been observed in these patients. Joseph S. Solomkin, Mary P. Bauman, Robert D. Nelson, and Richard L. Simmons (Univ. of Minnesota) examined polymorphonuclear leukocyte (PMN) function in 24 surgical patients recovering from an episode of intra-abdominal infection. The spontaneous and chemotactic movements of the cells were examined, and PMN chemiluminescence was measured. Phagocytic activity was assessed using *Staphylococcus aureus* 502A.

Control subjects having hysterectomy or donor nephrectomy showed transient depression in PMN functions, lasting less than a day. Patients with intra-abdominal infection showed significantly reduced functions before drainage. Antibiotic therapy alone was associated with slight improvement in PMN function in the 4 patients studied. Drainage was followed by markedly depressed function and slow recovery of PMN functions. Recurrent infections were associated with a fall in PMN function before infection was clinically evident. Phagocytosis was adequate in the study patients. Chemotaxis, spontaneous migration, and chemiluminescence could not be correlated with the number of PMNs or the percentage of band forms.

The in vitro oxidative metabolic and migratory responses of PMNs from surgical patients with intra-abdominal infection are grossly compromised, and they are further compromised by operative drainage. Cellular functions are again depressed when infection recurs, and this may precede the clinical diagnosis of infection by several days. A causal relationship has not been proved, but the prolonged period of

---

(6–4) Ann. Surg. 194:9–17, July 1981.

PMN dysfunction may explain, at least partly, the frequent recurrent infections in these patients. Monitoring of PMN functions may aid the early diagnosis of recurrent infection. The restoration or augmentation of various components of the host defense system may be appropriate.

▶ [The idea that monitoring neutrophil function in patients after drainage of an intra-abdominal infection could provide evidence of inadequate drainage or recurrent infection is intriguing. It should be remembered, however, that neutrophil function occasionally is affected by bizarre reactions to antibiotics, particularly topical antibiotics such as Silvadene.—E.E.P.] ◀

6–5 **Immunization Against Nosocomial Infection.** Overwhelming infection with gram-negative bacteremia has become the most serious nosocomial infection in compromised patients. Gram-negative bacteria share a common core lipopolysaccharide, suggesting that a single vaccine or antiserum might control these infections regardless of species. Abraham I. Braude, Elizabeth J. Ziegler, J. Allen McCutchan, and Herndon Douglas (Univ. of California, San Diego) review their work in developing such a vaccine.

A mutant of *Escherichia coli* 0111 (J5) was used that was deficient in uridine diphosphate-galactose epimerase and thus unable to attach "0" side chains, so that core lipopolysaccharide was exposed. A vaccine composed of this mutant produced antibody that gave broad protection against lethal infections by different gram-negative bacteria in immunosuppressed animals. The J5 vaccine protected against 98% lethal doses of *Pseudomonas aeruginosa,* and J5 antiserum improved survival tenfold in animals dying of *E. coli, Klebsiella,* or *Pseudomonas* bacteremia. The protection with vaccine or prophylactic antiserum was undiminished in animals challenged 6 weeks after immunization.

After these encouraging results, a double-blind trial was conducted in 136 patients with gram-negative bacteremia. In those given J5 antiserum, mortality was cut in half and survival from deep shock increased from less than 30% to over 80%. Because of these preliminary results, the study now has been extended to 300 patients with gram-negative bacteremia.

The ability of J5 antiserum to prevent bacteremia in patients predisposed to infection was studied. In this prophylactic trial, neutropenic patients with leukemia and lymphoma were assigned at random to receive either J5 antiserum or preimmune control serum. Each patient received 3 ml of serum per kg intravenously every 21 days while neutropenic. The incidence of febile days was 44% in controls and 18% in patients given antiserum ($P < .005$), suggesting that prophylactic J5 antiserum reduces fever, morbidity, and bacteremia in neutropenic patients with gram-negative infections.

For control of gram-negative bacteremia in hospitalized patients, emphasis should be shifted from administration of antimicrobial drugs to use of immunologic methods.

▶ [For many years, immunologic control of gram-negative infections has been attractive to the surgeon and the physician caring for burned patients. It is important to

(6–5) Am. J. Med. 70:463–466, February 1981.

recognize the difference between a gram-negative bacteremia that causes death and a gram-negative bacteremia that occurs while a patient is dying of burn shock or some other condition. Failure to appreciate this subtle difference has been responsible for previous claims that it was possible to vaccinate patients against gram-negative organisms.—E.E.P.] ◀

6–6 **Pharmacokinetics of Tissue Penetration of Antibiotics** are reviewed by Tom Bergan (Univ. of Oslo). The best models for use in investigating the ability of antibiotics to penetrate into extravascular foci are those measuring lymph and suction-induced fluid in skin blisters. Studies often have lasted only 3 to 4 hours, however, and data on individual animals have not been assessed separately. The extent of penetration of antibiotics into tissue fluid is related to the amount not bound to protein. Protein binding is especially inhibitory to penetration when it exceeds 80%. Penetration ability is best assessed by using the ratio of the area under the concentration curve (AUC) for antibiotic in the peripheral locus to the AUC for serum. Data from each individual are preferable to data derived from curves using mean values. First-order, one-compartment, open models are applicable to the characterization of extravascular concentrations of antibiotics.

The AUC for antibiotic in serum during a given time interval is the factor that determines the amount passing into an extravascular focus. Drug concentrations in tissue are lower than those in serum. Peak concentrations occur simultaneously with the maximal serum levels or shortly afterward. For most antibiotics, elimination from extravascular sites is slower than from the serum; this is especially true of agents with a serum half-life less than 4 to 5 hours. Drug concentrations in extravascular sites can be higher than serum levels toward the end of the dosage interval. Protein at an extravascular site can enhance the local concentration of antibiotic. Multiple doses result in higher extravascular drug levels, even with substances having a low elimination half-life. This tendency is most marked for antimicrobials with high protein binding. The greater penetration of antibiotic given as a bolus is a result of the higher AUC in serum per unit time.

▶ [Progress and treatment of infections has been measured by accurate recognition of the infecting organisms, determination of their sensitivity to antibiotics, and measurement of blood levels of antibiotics. These methods still will not insure successful antibiotic treatment until there is some way to assess the concentration of antibiotics in tissue where the actual battle is being fought. Now, the possibility exists that tissue levels of antibiotics also can be evaluated.—E.E.P.] ◀

6–7 **Computed Tomography in Diagnosis and Localization of Intra-abdominal Abscesses.** Jacob G. Robison and Thomas W. Pollock retrospectively analyzed the outcome in 50 consecutive patients who underwent computed tomography (CT) examination for suspected intra-abdominal abscess in an attempt to assess the accuracy and predictive value of CT in this clinical setting. Transverse scans were generally performed at 1-cm intervals. Contrast medium was often used to facilitate identification of intra-abdominal structures. A scan was considered positive if it demonstrated a localized extra-anatomi-

(6–6) Rev. Infect. Dis. 3:45–66, Jan.–Feb. 1981.
(6–7) Am. J. Surg. 140:783–786, December 1980.

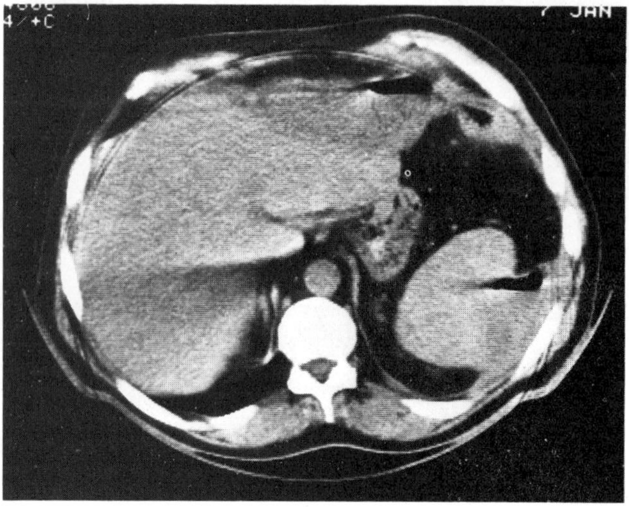

Fig 6–1.—Computed tomographic scan in patient in whom left subphrenic abscess was suspected because of an elevated white blood cell count and low-grade fever after small bowel resection. Large fluid collection is seen anterior to spleen, displacing stomach bubble anteriorly. Posterior to spleen is collection of fluid, which could have been missed at time of exploration. (Courtesy of Robison, J. G., and Pollock, T. W.: Am. J. Surg. 140:783–786, December 1980.)

cal, intra-abdominal fluid collection with a CT number of 0–15 Hounsfield units (Fig 6–1) or showed the presence of extraluminal gas. The presence of an abscess was confirmed in all patients by exploration and drainage, except in 1 patient in whom it was confirmed at autopsy.

The scan results were interpreted as positive in 21 of the 50 patients and negative in 29. Of the 34 patients who had recent abdominal surgery, 17 had negative and 17 had positive findings on scanning. The findings proved to be false positive in 2 of the 21 patients with positive scans, and false negative in 2 of the 29 with negative scans. The overall diagnostic accuracy was 92%. Both the false positive and false negative rates were 4%. The 21 patients who had confirmed clinical abscess and were examined by CT all underwent surgical drainage; none died.

The sensitivity of CT in the diagnosis of intra-abdominal abscess was 0.90 (19 of 21); specificity was 0.93 (27 of 29), prevalence was 0.42 (21 of 50), and predictive value was 90%. The predictive value of 90% encourages confidence in the accuracy of both positive and negative findings in this clinical setting. Computed tomography is a more accurate predictor of the presence of intra-abdominal abscess than gallium scanning, ultrasonography, or other radiologic examinations. It is useful not only in predicting the presence or absence of an intra-abdominal focus, but also in the localization and planning of appropriate surgical drainage.

▶ [Although computed tomography has been of great help in diagnosing intra-abdominal abscess, ultrasonography may be just as effective and is considerably less expensive. There is little question that computed tomography is the most effective diagnostic tool for the head, but its overuse in abdominal diagnosis can be alleviated by the use of nuclear scanning and ultrasonography.—E.E.P.] ◀

6–8 **Diagnosis of Postoperative Intra-abdominal Abscess.** Elizabeth Sonnenwirth-Ozar and Erich W. Pollak (Univ. of Missouri, Kansas City) reviewed the clinical, laboratory, radiologic, and radionuclide findings in 40 patients with surgically proved intra-abdominal abscesses seen in 1976–1980. Seven patients had 2 or more abscesses. Persistent fever of unknown origin and persistent ileus suggested abscess in all cases. In 5 cases, a mass was palpated. Paracentesis was diagnostic in 2 of 3 patients. All patients but 1 had a serially increasing white blood cell count with a left shift. Chest x-ray films were positive in all 14 patients with subphrenic abscess. Fourteen of 33 patients had positive findings on abdominal x-ray films.

Liver-spleen scans showed abnormal findings in 2 of 6 cases. Ultrasound scans detected intra-abdominal abscesses in 9 of 16 patients. Abscesses appeared as sonolucent masses with thick, irregular margins, as acoustic shadowing only, or as densely echogenic masses with acoustic shadowing. Gallium scans gave positive results in 6 of 9 cases. Computed tomography (CT) was positive in 6 of 8 patients. The first and second imaging procedures gave concordant results in 8 of 12 patients, and the results were accurate in 5 cases.

The use of newer radiologic, radionuclide, and ultrasonic methods have been helpful in diagnosing postoperative intra-abdominal abscess, but their usefulness is limited. Sixty percent of the present patients either could not have or did not require such procedures. The tests had a diagnostic sensitivity of 75% or less, and no improvement was obtained by using two consecutive imaging techniques rather than one. Negative findings did not preclude the need for diagnostic celiotomy in patients with highly suggestive clinical findings. The results of CT were better than those obtained with other imaging procedures in this series of cases.

▶ [Increasing enthusiasm over the use of computed tomography for abdominal diagnosis often does not take into consideration that ultrasonic scan, although sometimes more difficult to interpret, is a better diagnostic tool for many abdominal conditions. An exception, of course, is the subdiaphragmatic area. Computerized axial tomographic (CAT) scanning is used most effectively in viewing the head; ultrasonic scanning and radionuclide imaging can be more accurate in certain areas of the abdomen where CAT scanning has produced false negative, as well as false positive, results.—E.E.P.] ◀

6–9 **Treatment of Abdominal Abscesses: Comparative Evaluation of Operative Drainage Versus Percutaneous Catheter Drainage Guided by Computed Tomography or Ultrasound.** Willard C. Johnson, Stephen G. Gerzof, Alan H. Robbins, and Donald C. Nabseth (Boston) have used percutaneous drainage routinely to treat abdominal abscesses since 1976. Percutaneous drainage was performed in patients with a well-established unilocular fluid collection when a safe access route was present and immediate operative backup was available. Both angiocatheter and trocar catheter techniques have been used. Both catheters were sutured in place and managed like surgi-

(6–8) South. Med. J. 74:927–930, August 1981.
(6–9) Ann. Surg. 194:510–520, October 1981.

cally placed drains. Irrigation with saline solution or antibiotics was discouraged.

Twenty-seven patients had percutaneous drainage and 43 had operative drainage, generally by a direct approach. Treatment was successful in 89% of percutaneous cases and 70% of operative cases. Three patients were considered to have inadequate drainage by the percutaneous technique. Nine patients operated on had inadequate drainage, including 4 of 14 patients with postoperative subphrenic abscesses. Five patients in the percutaneous group had enteric communication to their abscesses. One patient had empyema after percutaneous drainage of a left subphrenic abscess. The rate of complications in the surgical group was 16%. The rate of sepsis-related death was 11% in the percutaneous group and 21% in the surgical group. The average period of percutaneous drainage was 17 days, and that of operative drainage was 29 days.

A large majority of intra-abdominal abscesses are amenable to percutaneous drainage. When an abscess is identified and safe access is available, percutaneous catheter drainage under computed tomography or ultrasound guidance is suggested as initial treatment. A concurrent enteric communication to the abscess may be a special indication for percutaneous drainage. Percutaneous drainage avoids intra-abdominal spillage and surgery, and drainage is less prolonged than with operative methods. Inadequate drainage is less frequent with the percutaneous approach.

▶ [These authors, who are real pioneers in this field, have made an extremely important contribution to surgical therapy. This report suffers because the trial was not prospective, randomized, or controlled, and the comparison of the results of percutaneous drainage to operative drainage was done retrospectively for different time periods. It is very unlikely that a proper trial can be carried out now, because it is doubtful that anyone would be willing to do such a study.

I have had a reasonable experience with this method, and I believe that it is an extremely important addition to our armamentarium. It is by no means perfect, as there are complications such as empyema, perforation of loops of intestine, or recurrence of abscesses. However, it would appear from retrospective analysis that the incidence of these complications after percutaneous drainage is slightly lower than after operative treatment. Because we have seen definite recurrences of abscess when the catheter is removed too soon, we inject radiopaque dye into the tract at some reasonable time after percutaneous drainage to assess the extent of shrinkage of the abscess cavity, and we do not remove the percutaneous catheters until the cavity has shrunk to a small tract surrounding the small catheter. Also, we have found that thick material does not drain very well through these small catheters and have, therefore, instituted the practice of irrigating the catheters gently with a small amount of saline solution. We feel that the addition of these two practices will be helpful. In some instances, it is necessary to use not only ultrasonographic localization but also computerized tomography if any question arises as to the location of the cavity to be drained.—W.S.] ◀

6–10 **Percutaneous Catheter Drainage of Abdominal Abscesses: A Five-Year Experience.** Management of intra-abdominal sepsis remains difficult despite the availability of new and effective antibiotics. Stephen G. Gerzof, Alan H. Robbins, Willard C. Johnson, Desmond H. Birkett, and Donald C. Nabseth (Boston) used percutaneous drainage to treat 71 abscesses in 59 male and 8 female patients, aged

(6–10) N. Engl. J. Med. 305:653–657, Sept. 17, 1981.

16 to 77 years, in 1976 to 1981. All the intra-abdominal and retroperitoneal abscesses so treated would otherwise have required surgery. Forty-seven abscesses represented postoperative complications. Most patients had a well-defined unilocular abscess cavity, and a safe drainage route was available. Two patients were poor operative risks. Drainage technique involved use of a pigtail angiocatheter or a trocar catheter. All patients received intravenous antibiotic therapy. Irrigation was used infrequently.

Fifty-eight of 71 abscesses (82%) were managed successfully by percutaneous drainage without operation. The method failed in the 2 poor operative risks with inadequately drained, loculated intraperitoneal abscesses. Three other patients had pancreatic abscesses requiring operative debridement. Forty of the 47 postoperative abscesses (85%) were treated successfully by percutaneous drainage, as were 18 of 24 spontaneous abscesses. Patients tolerated the procedure well with local anesthesia; many were ambulatory within hours of drainage. Six abscesses with enteric communication responded to percutaneous drainage and did not require an additional operation. Mean duration of treatment for all abscesses was 20 days. Four catheter-related complications occurred. Three deaths were considered to be due to inadequate drainage.

Percutaneous aspiration and drainage of abdominal abscesses is at least as effective as surgery, and in many respects is better. Morbidity and mortality are lower than with surgery, and nursing care is easier. The percutaneous approach should be the preferred treatment of intra-abdominal abscesses. Surgery should be reserved for abscesses that are loculated or lack a safe drainage route or for cases where attempted percutaneous drainage has failed.

▶ [Percutaneous aspiration and drainage undoubtedly can accomplish, in some patients, everything that open surgical drainage can accomplish. It is extremely important, however, not to substitute percutaneous catheter drainage for open surgical drainage in all patients at this time. Diagnosis must be precise and patients must be followed with caution to ensure that undiagnosed multiloculated cavities have not been missed. In most institutions, open drainage of a cavity that contains pus is still the safest therapeutic procedure.—E.E.P.] ◀

6–11 **Abdominal Sepsis Managed by Leaving Abdomen Open.** Various methods of drainage may be inadequate if abdominal infection is diffuse and both the wound and peritoneal cavity are involved. John H. Duff and John Moffat (Univ. of Western Ontario) attempted to achieve better drainage by leaving the abdominal incision completely open in 18 seriously ill patients with abdominal sepsis. Diffuse sepsis was present in all except 2 patients, who had necrotizing wound infections. Eight patients had wound infection as well as intra-abdominal sepsis. An upper abdominal incision was left open in 12 cases and a lower abdominal incision, in 6 cases. The wounds were dressed as often as necessary with petrolatum dressings and antibiotics, and adhesions were broken down daily with the examining finger. No retention sutures were used. The wounds were left open until infection was eradicated, and most wounds then were left to heal by secondary

(6–11) Surgery 90:774–778, October 1981.

intention or covered by split-thickness skin. All patients received total parenteral nutrition.

Gram-negative aerobes were isolated most often. Twelve patients had positive blood cultures. Intestinal fistulas were the chief factors contributing to abdominal sepsis in these cases. Mechanical ventilation for an average of 44 days was required in 16 patients. Spontaneous fistulas developed in exposed bowels in 5 patients; the fistulas did not appear to increase the severity of sepsis. Seven patients died, 6 of sepsis and 1 of hemorrhage. Bowel evisceration was a contributing factor to death in 3 instances. Five surviving patients had the wounds skin grafted. Survivors had an average hospital stay of 130 days.

Continuous open drainage of the infected abdomen provides wider and more complete drainage than other methods, and reexploration is not necessary. Evisceration may be difficult to prevent, however, and a giant incisional hernia is unavoidable. In addition, significant fluid and protein losses occur, and there is a risk of spontaneous fistula formation in exposed bowel loops. This radical technique is compatible with excellent recovery if adequate supportive care is available. It is preferable to closing an abdominal wall of questionable viability in the face of severe peritoneal sepsis.

▶ [This article will stimulate much discussion and thought. My fear is that the procedure advocated by these authors will be applied more extensively than it should be. Unfortunately, the series of cases reported by these authors is a mixed bag. Some of the patients had diffuse peritonitis and others had extensive and severe infections of the abdominal wall that required that the abdomen be left open. It is vital that the distinction be made between these two categories, as the outcome probably will differ significantly. Such important distinctions are not clearly evident in this paper. Whereas Duff and Moffat left the abdominal cavity open from the beginning, other authors, such as Maetani and Tobe (*Surgery* 90:804, 1981), have simply opened the abdomen in gradual stages between the second and ninth postoperative days. In neither of these series is it sufficiently clear as to the specific indications for these techniques, and very exceptional circumstances should be present before the procedure becomes commonplace. Unfortunately, many new techniques are swept into practice before full characterization of the indications for them.

From a theoretical standpoint, one can formulate some deficiencies of these methods. First, with the patient lying supine, posterior portions of the abdominal cavity and certainly the pelvis cannot be drained adequately. Testimony to that is the fact that these authors and Maetani and Tobe have indeed found additional abscesses in the peritoneal cavity at autopsy in patients who have died after this treatment. Second, it must be kept in mind that contamination with other organisms from the outside inevitably will occur. Simply opening an abdominal wound, or indeed the peritoneal cavity, does not guarantee freedom from infection. In fact, it exposes the wound to infection by organisms that are already not present and that can produce invasive infection. Third, the nursing and medical management of these patients require big league backup with adequate respiratory therapy, and this technique probably should not be undertaken unless very real tertiary facilities are available. We will be very anxious to see further developments in this interesting method.—W.S.] ◀

6–12 **Surgical Management of "Pus-Pot" Perineum.** "Pus-pot" perineum is a devastating state of chronic draining fistulas, sinuses, abscesses, induration, and scar formation, seen with such conditions as hidradenitis suppurativa, urethral stricture disease, anoperineal fistula, and condyloma acuminatum. Gary L. Berger, Mutaz B. Habal,

---

(6–12) J. Urol. 126:193–196, August 1981.

Ronald W. Sadlowski, Roy P. Finney, and John R. Sharpe (Univ. of South Florida, Tampa) used radical excision and resurfacing with split-thickness skin grafting to treat 10 patients having pus-pot perineum. Seven had biopsy-proved hidradenitis suppurativa; 1 had extensive condyloma acuminatum; 1 had an anoperineal fistula that had been operated on several times; and 1 had long-standing postgonococcal urethral stricture disease. Conservative treatment had given only temporary improvement at best.

All involved tissue in the 10 patients was excised widely, and the defect immediately was resurfaced with split-thickness skin from the thighs. All 7 men required complete excision of the scrotum; the testes were placed in subcutaneous thigh pockets. In 3 cases the penile shaft skin was removed and the penis was resurfaced with skin grafts. In all 3 women the labia majora was excised completely. Four patients received a diverting colostomy. Vascular take of the skin grafts ranged from 30% to 90%. Perineal healing was facilitated by rapid wound contracture in each case. All patients were cured completely. Nine patients have had follow-up for a year or longer, and 1 has had follow-up for 6 months. All 10 have been able to return to their previous work. Carcinoma was found perianally in a patient with rectal adenocarcinoma. The tumor probably was incidental; tumor implants may have seeded in the area of chronic scarring.

Advanced hidradenitis suppurativa of the perineum is believed to be best managed by wide excision with split-thickness skin grafting. This approach also can be useful in patients with pus-pot perineum of other etiologies. A temporary diverting colostomy should be considered if fecal contamination might jeopardize the skin graft.

► [It is not necessary to perform extensive skin grafting procedures in the perineal area. Wound healing by contraction and epithelialization often produces as good a result as grafting, and with considerably less expenditure of time and money. It is also interesting that multiple sinus, chronic skin infections of the buttocks complicating hidradenitis suppurativa can be treated by turning back a thin flap of epidermis and partial thickness of dermis and removing the deep dermis, fat, and skin appendages. The flap then can be reapplied where it usually is revascularized as a free graft. This technique is only suitable for the buttocks; perineal wounds that follow the extensive debridement of infected skin usually are best managed by allowing the wounds to heal secondarily, without using skin grafts.—E.E.P.] ◄

7. Burns

7–1 **Burn Shock** is discussed by Carl Jelenko III (Wright State Univ., Dayton, Ohio). Organ hypoperfusion in shock can result from too little fluid, dilatation of the vascular bed, pump failure, or any combination of these factors. Shock after thermal injury is chiefly due to transudation and sequestration of vascular fluid into the tissues in the region of injury and, in more severe cases, in remote tissues as well. Resuscitation is based on replacement of fluid volume and sodium and must be guided by regular monitoring of hemodynamic function. It is necessary to correct the underlying cause of shock. Resuscitation should be prompt and intensive, but further systemic derangements must be avoided. The author bases resuscitation on the currently available functional vascular space, which depends on both the intravascular volume and the capacity of the vascular bed. The capacity of the vascular bed is under central control by the baroreceptor neuroendocrine mechanism, which is maximally active at a mean arterial pressure of about 60 torr.

When patients with burns of 21%–95% of the body surface were resuscitated with Ringer's lactate solution, colloid-free hypertonic solution, or hypertonic albuminated fluid demand (HALFD) solution to a mean arterial pressure of 60–70 torr, those given HALFD solution required less fluid per unit time and were resuscitated more rapidly than those in the other groups. Patients given HALFD solution also required less total fluid in the first 22 hours after burn and were able to maintain their needs by mouth more rapidly. None required escharotomy to relieve pressure from swelling. Both plasma disappearance from the vascular space and the concentration of serum lactic acid became normal more rapidly in the HALFD group.

The author believes that HALFD solution is optimal for resuscitating burn injury patients and that fluid therapy should be given only in the amounts needed to maintain perfusion of vital organs. Mean arterial pressure should be kept at 60–70 torr.

▶ [The concept that edema in burned patients can be controlled by intravenous administration of protein has never been proved to my satisfaction. Water and salt remain the major components of successful resuscitation after burn injury. Administration of albumin can still be studied, provided patients are not denied adequate salt and water while studies are being performed. Evidence that administration of albumin makes any significant difference during the treatment of a burned patient is still tenuous, in my judgment.—E.E.P.] ◀

7–2 **Low-Volume Burn Resuscitation Regimen: Assessment of Performance by Probit Analysis.** There is agreement that the hypovolemia that often follows burn wounds should be promptly cor-

---

(7–1) Top. Emergency Med. 3:69–73, October 1981.
(7–2) Br. J. Surg. 68:225–228, April 1981.

rected, but there is no consensus on the most appropriate volumes or types of fluid to be used. R. W. Griffiths, N. L. Cross, and J. E. Laing (Wiltshire, England) retrospectively reviewed the results in 1,728 patients admitted between 1969 and 1978 to a burn center. A low-volume colloid resuscitation regimen was used because of concern for the problems of fluid overload. This regimen differs significantly from those used at other major centers where larger volumes of colloid or crystalloid solutions are used.

Blood volume was calculated as 7.5% of admission body weight of the patient. One third of this volume was allocated to the first 8 hours after burn injury and represented the upper limit of colloid infusion considered necessary for this early period. However, the amount of colloid actually infused was judged on the clinical response of the patient rather than on arbitrary parameters. One third of the volume was allocated to the period 8–20 hours after burn injury and the final third to the period 20–36 hours after the burn. This infusion schedule was administered to adults with burns covering more than 20% of the body surface area and to children with burns greater than 10%.

Of the 1,728 patients, 119 died. Most deaths occurred in patients aged 50 years and over, with burns affecting less than 50% body surface area. An investigation of mortality probability was conducted using probit analysis, and the areas of burn injury associated with a 50% mortality probability (LA_{50}) were determined for four age groups. The LA_{50} values were 59% body surface area burn for patients aged 0–14 years, 70% burn for those aged 15–44 years, 38% burn for those aged 45–64 years, and 17% burn for those aged 65 years and older. These figures closely parallel those reported from another large burn center in which a widely different fluid regimen is used.

These results suggest that wide variations in fluid resuscitation regimens, particularly with regard to volume, do little to affect the mortality associated with burn injury as assessed by probit analysis. However, the probit method cannot be used to assess morbidity.

▶ [It does not seem to me that a major frontier now in the treatment of burned patients is adjustment of fluid volume and concentrations. Potentially salvageable patients with major burns usually die from infection, exhaustion, or a combination of the two. Treatment of initial burn shock, including fluid and electrolyte loss, seems to be adequate for most patients now. Data analyzed in this article support such a point of view.—E.E.P.] ◀

7-3 **Fatal Respiratory Distress in Burned Patients.** Lindsay C. Getzen and Erich W. Pollak examined the occurrence of fatal respiratory distress syndrome after massive body burns in a series of 167 major burn cases from Vietnam. All of the injuries occurred in open spaces and were caused by flame-throwing weapons, bombs, or gasoline-related explosions. All patients had second-degree injuries of 30% or more of the body surface. Third-degree injury covered 30%–50% of the body surface in 48 cases and more than half of the body surface in 18 cases. Patients were resuscitated from shock, and burns were managed by the open method. Cardiotonics and steroids were used as indicated. Antibiotics were given only when specifically indicated.

(7–3) Surg. Gynecol. Obstet. 152:741–744, June 1981.

Ten patients died after severe respiratory distress developed, 5 of them within 48 hours of admission. Overhydration had occurred in the latter patients in the presence of severe acute renal failure. One other patient died of overhydration. In the 4 other patients who died 4–12 days after admission, death was due to *Pseudomonas* sepsis and aspiration pneumonia. Mortality from *Pseudomonas* pneumonia was increased significantly in patients having tracheostomy. Eighteen of 24 patients with third-degree burns of more than 50% of the body surface survived. The nonsurvivors had had severe, progressive respiratory failure despite oxygen therapy and mechanical ventilation with positive end-expiratory pressure. Histologic studies at autopsy showed microembolism, intravascular fibrin deposits, and platelet aggregates, as well as interstitial edema and giant macrophage cell infiltration. Areas of congestive atelectasis and hemorrhage alternated with areas of hyaline membrane formation and pneumonitis. Intra-alveolar edema and coagulum formation also were observed.

Preventable causes of fatal respiratory distress were present in all 10 patients in this series. Colloid infusions should be used for burn shock resuscitation, and serial monitoring of pulmonary extravascular water should be carried out. Avoidance of early tracheostomy may help prevent pulmonary sepsis. The concept of idiopathic burn lung syndrome should be replaced by a vigorous search for correctable causes of respiratory failure.

▶ [I do not agree that most patients with respiratory distress syndrome have either been overhydrated or are septic. The idea that respiratory distress syndrome after severe thermal trauma can be controlled in most patients by the use of albumin, aseptic technique, and topical antibiotics is not justified. The problem is still a complex one, and it represents a definable frontier in burn therapy. The problem of the stiff lung must be solved if we are to take advantage of recent advances in general metabolism and wound care; antibiotics and albumin have not solved the problem completely.—E.E.P.] ◀

7-4 **Energy Metabolism in Anesthetized Children With Burns.** Studies of the pathogenesis of hypermetabolism after thermal trauma have given variable results. John H. Crabtree, Bonny H. Bowser, James W. Campbell, Walter S. Guinee, and Fred T. Caldwell (Univ. of Arkansas) evaluated cause and effect relationships between rates of heat production, heat loss, and plasma catecholamine levels when thermoregulatory responses were depressed by methoxyflurane in 10 children, aged 5–12 years (mean, 7 years); all required anesthesia for grafting burn wounds that covered from 1% to 43% (mean, 20%) of the body surface area. The studies were made on postburn day 20–90 (mean, day 40).

Rapid cooling of the burned children was not due to a decreased rate of heat production. Rather, it was due to increased heat loss during the period of anesthesia. Heat production increased significantly, but not enough to counterbalance the increased heat loss, reflecting a block in central thermoregulation by general anesthesia. Mean plasma catecholamine concentrations decreased during general anesthesia (Fig 7–1). Heat production attempted to track heat loss during a period in which plasma catecholamine levels declined.

(7–4) Am. J. Surg. 140:832–835, December 1980.

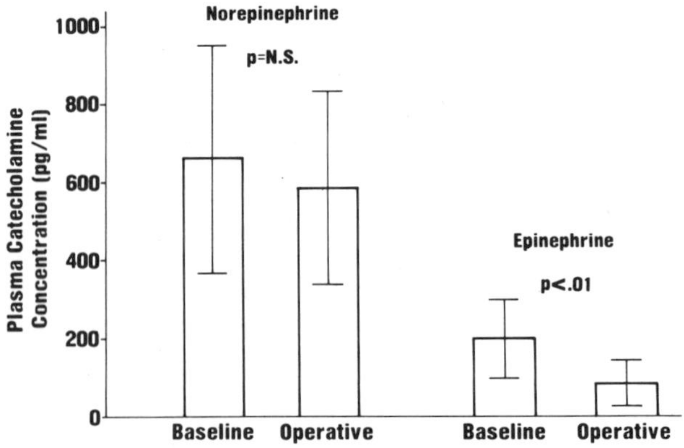

Fig 7–1.—Plasma catecholamine concentrations at baseline and during operative study periods. N.S. = not significant. (Courtesy of Crabtree, J. H., et al.: Am. J. Surg. 140:832–835, December 1980.)

An increased rate of heat loss is apparently the primary stimulus for increased metabolic activity after burn injury.

▶ [Perhaps the most significant clinical reflection to be derived from this article is the importance of using proper dressing and dressing techniques to conserve energy. Although few clinicians would intentionally treat burned children by the exposure method, they may not realize that prolonged anesthesia constitutes a period of exposure with important consequences, such as the one reported in this study.—E.E.P.] ◀

7–5 **Effects of Nutrition on Length of Stay and Survival for Burned Patients.** Hal G. Bingham, Jeffrey P. Krischer, Jonathan J. Shuster, and Irma A. Engelmann (Gainesville, Fla.) analyzed a series of 49 consecutive adults admitted to a burn care center in 1975–1977 to predict the length of hospital stay and survival on the basis of the extent of injury, dietary intake, and age. Thermal injury imposes severe metabolic demands, and adequate nutritional support may enhance wound healing and protect against infection. It has been recommended that burn patients receive 25 kcal/kg plus 40 kcal/% of the body surface burned to minimize weight loss in the acute postburn period.

Thirty-nine of the 49 patients survived. The mean hospital stay was 29 days. Protein intake was negatively correlated with the extent of full-thickness injury and the risk of death, but the average daily caloric and protein intake was related only weakly to patient outcomes. Both caloric and protein intakes correlated negatively with death but positively with the length of stay. Models predicting length of stay for survivors explained 70% of the variation in observed stay, but predictability for all patients was much less. A logit model developed for survival analysis correctly predicted 94% of patient outcomes. An analysis of recommended ideal caloric intake, based on total burn size and patient weight, was not significantly related to patient outcomes.

The relationship between outcome and diet might be strengthened

(7–5) Burns 7:252–257, March 1981.

if the degree of third-degree burn injury was included in calculations of ideal caloric intake. The findings do accord with suggestions of a beneficial association of protein and calorie intake with survival and length of stay in burn injury cases. The risk of death and the expected hospital stay can be predicted quite accurately.

▶ [In my opinion, parenteral alimentation (with or without growth hormone) has made the greatest contribution to the care of burns since the development of topical antibiotics. In addition to wound healing and general metabolism, nothing appears to be more effective in the prevention of infection than the preservation of normal immunologic responses through adequate caloric intake.—E.E.P.] ◀

7–6 **Opsonic Glycoprotein (Plasma Fibronectin) Levels After Burn Injury: Relationship to Extent of Burn and Development of Sepsis.** Deficiency of opsonic α_2-surface binding glycoprotein (plasma fibronectin) occurs after clinical and experimental trauma, especially in association with sepsis. Administration of cryoprecipitate rich in opsonic protein to septic trauma patients reverses opsonic fibronectin deficiency and improves the clinical state with respect to sepsis and cardiopulmonary function. To learn whether the opsonic deficiency in sepsis precedes or follows the septic state, Marc E. Lanser, Thomas M. Saba, and William A. Scovill (Union Univ., Albany, N.Y.) studied the temporal response of plasma opsonic fibronectin, as measured by immunoassay and bioassay, following burn injury in 15 patients. The patients, aged 18–86 years (average, 41 years), sustained second- and third-degree burns of 20% to 90% of the body surface area (average, 40%). The relationship of opsonic fibronectin to both extent of injury and postburn sepsis also was studied.

Immunoreactive opsonic fibronectin was depleted acutely within hours following the burn; maximal depletion occurred at 12 hours. The magnitude of depletion was correlated with body surface area burned. Normal levels were restored at 24 hours after injury. There was a tendency toward rebound hyperopsonemia at 2 weeks, with a slow return to normal over the ensuing weeks. Bioassayable opsonic protein levels generally paralleled those of immunoreactive protein. After restoration of opsonic protein levels, a secondary phase of opsonic fibronectin deficiency developed in those burn patients who became septic. This opsonic fibronectin deficiency actually became apparent prior to the onset of clinical sepsis, although it was maximal during sepsis. Resolution of the septic episode was associated with a return of plasma opsonic fibronectin levels to normal.

Secondary deficiency of immunoreactive opsonic fibronectin may indicate impending sepsis after burn wounds.

▶ [Similar studies have revealed that an assay of lymphocyte responsiveness, and measurement of serum and other suppressors can be used to predict the likelihood of death from major burns. The immunologic response undoubtedly is a complex phenomenon and a critical one in the prevention of death after massive thermal injury.—E.E.P.] ◀

7–7 **Viral Infections in Pediatric Burn Patients.** Bacterial and fungal infections are frequent complications of burn injuries, but the frequency of viral infections is unknown. Calvin C. Linnemann, Jr., and

(7–6) Ann. Surg. 192:776–782, December 1980.
(7–7) Am. J. Dis. Child. 135:750–753, August 1981.

Bruce G. MacMillan carried out a restrospective study of viral antibodies in the serums of 40 pediatric patients admitted to the Cincinnati Shriners Burns Institute. A prospective study then was performed to investigate serum antibodies and viral excretion in 24 children. All subjects in both studies were followed up for at least 2 months.

The 40 children in the retrospective study had an average age of 8 years and an average third-degree burn of 38% of the body surface. Nine of the group (22%) had fourfold increases in cytomegalovirus (CMV) antibodies at an average of 13 weeks. Eight of these patients had prolonged unexplained fevers, 7 had lymphocytosis, and 2 had hepatitis. More extensive burns were present in patients with CMV infection, and more transfusions had been given. Three children had fourfold increases in antibodies to Epstein-Barr virus, 2 in association with fever and lymphocytosis. Three other children had increases in antibody to herpes simplex virus (HSV) without clinical disease. Two children had increases in levels of varicella-zoster virus antibodies. Fifteen children in all had significant increases in viral antibody titers.

The 24 children in the prospective study had an average age of 9.2 years and an average third-degree burn of 28%. Eight of the group (33%) developed CMV infection. Six of the 24 had HSV infection. Four of the group had more than one viral infection during the study. Two of them were the most severely burned children.

Herpesvirus infections, including CMV and HSV, are common in pediatric burn patients. The chief host defense against herpesvirus infection is cell mediated, and cell-mediated immunity is impaired in the postburn period. Cytomegalovirus infection in this setting may represent either primary infection or reactivation of latent infection. Herpes simplex virus infections in burn patients have been reported to cause disseminated disease, burn wound infection, tracheobronchitis, and bronchopneumonia.

▶ [Tertiary medical care at the close of this century will require greater emphasis on detection, classification, and, ultimately, treatment of viral diseases. An electron microscope will be a necessity in the modern hospital laboratory. More accurate and earlier diagnosis of viral infections may make a difference in the treatment of burned patients.—E.E.P.] ◀

7–8 **Candidiasis in Burned Patient.** Topical and intravenous antibiotics used to treat or suppress bacterial infection in burned patients allow emergence of resistant microbes such as fungi, particularly *Candida* species. Michael J. Spebar and Basil A. Pruitt, Jr. examined the spectrum of disease caused by this organism in 1,513 burned patients seen from 1973 to 1978.

Fungi were cultured from 521 (34.4%) of the 1,513 patients; *Candida* species accounted for 452 (86.7%) of these infections. Of the 172 patients with colonization of the eschar by *Candida,* 36 (20.7%) subsequently had invasive candidal sepsis. The wounds in 11% of all burn patients became colonized by *Candida* species; however, only 3.4% of the patients had septicemia and only 2.4% had candidal burn wound invasion. The mortality of *Candida* burn wound infection was 100%

(7–8) J. Trauma 21:237–239, March 1981.

when untreated and 91.6% when treated with aggressive medical-surgical therapy. Of 52 patients with candidemia, 77% died.

Patients with *Candida* burn wound infection were older and more extensively injured than the general burned patient or those with candidemia alone. *Candida* invasion may be a result rather than a cause of a generalized collapse of host defense and homeostatic mechanisms. Control of this lethal complication rests with preventive measures, including aggressive surgical management, expeditious closure of the burn wound before onset of invasive sepsis, and restriction of the use of broad-spectrum antibiotics to the treatment of verified bacterial infection.

▶ [In my opinion, expeditious closure of the burn wound is still the most critical factor in preventing rare and unusual infections. No matter how good the antibiotic therapy and how carefully done the surgeon's dressing technique, sooner or later an open wound will become infected. Candidiasis ultimately will appear, if everything else is controlled.—E.E.P.] ◀

7–9 **Challenge to Resurface Major Burns.** In patients with major burns, resurfacing the wound as early as possible to promote survival is the primary aim, with cosmetic appearance secondary. Ramesh K. Srivastava, Bruce G. MacMillan, and James B. Kahl (Shriners Burn Inst., Cincinnati) resurfaced major burn wounds with large expansion autografts in 10 children aged 1½–13 years (mean, 5 years), with burns covering 70–95% (mean, 77%) of the total body surface (60–90% [mean, 72%] third-degree burns).

After initial resuscitation, the burn wounds were excised by carbon dioxide laser (7 patients) or knife (3). Split-thickness skin grafts of 0.009- to 0.012-in. thickness were obtained with a dermatome, placed on a Dermacarrier, and passed between the rollers of a Meshgraft II Dermatome. For protection of the graft, it was lifted onto a polyethylene sheet and transferred to the burn wound. The meshed grafts were expanded on the wound with saline solution and fixed to peripheral, healthy tissue, if any, by Steri-Strips or suturing with 5-0 Vicryl. Grafts were covered by a layer of coarse-mesh gauze, then by fine-mesh gauze impregnated with a topical antibacterial agent chosen on the basis of the sensitivity pattern of organisms in the burn wounds, then by an occlusive dressing. The dressing was usually changed after 48 hours. Thereafter, the wound usually was dressed with xenografts every day. Epithelialization was completed 10–15 days after grafting, at which time hydrotherapy was started. All patients received pressure dressings and physiotherapy to prevent hypertrophic scar formation and contractures.

Of the 10 patients, 3 died of pulmonary complications in the 4th week after injury, before their burn wounds could be closed. Of the 7 survivors, 2 received 3:1 expansion autografts, 3 received 3:1 and 6:1 expansion grafts, and 2 were resurfaced mainly by 6:1 expansion grafts but with some areas also covered by 9:1 expansion grafts (Fig 7–2). The graft take in all cases was excellent. The 67% survival in the 6 patients with 70% or greater third-degree burns compares with 6% survival of such patients in other hospitals. Factors responsible for

(7–9) J. Trauma 21:307–312, April 1981.

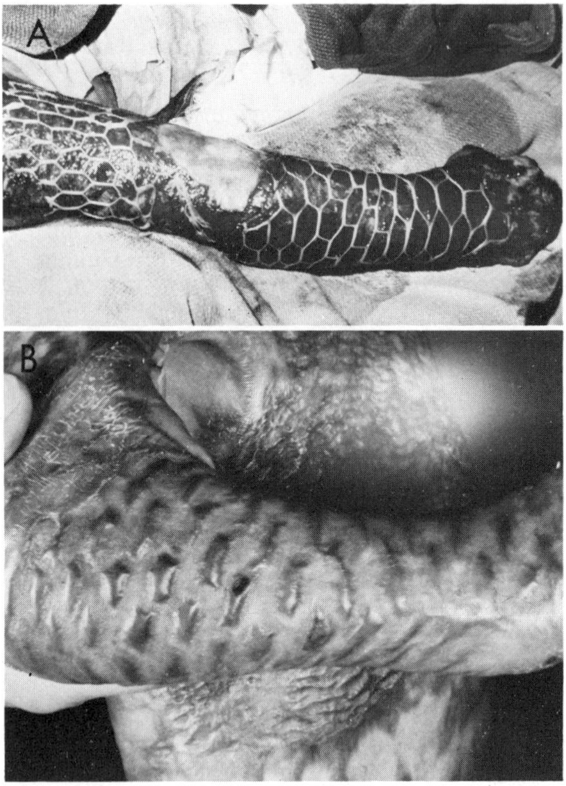

Fig 7–2.—Use of large expansion autografts in boy, aged 2, with 75% total body surface burns, 72% third degree. **A,** upper extremity grafted with 9:1 expansion split-thickness autografts. **B,** grafts 10 weeks old, maturing. (Courtesy of Srivastava, R. K., et al.: J. Trauma 21:307–312, April 1981.)

these good results include early excision, reduction of bacterial colonization from the wounds by topical antimicrobial therapy, aggressive nutritional support, and prompt closure of the burn wound by the expansion autografting technique. Compared with patients treated with 3:1 expansion grafts, those receiving 6:1 and 9:1 grafts needed fewer operative procedures and were covered, on the average, in a shorter period of time. In larger expansion autografts, the epithelium, which grows from the edges and covers the interstices between the ribbons of skin, is thin and requires protection for 3–4 weeks. Later it tolerates the pressure of Ace wraps well, which combats the growth of collagen fibers responsible for hypertrophic burn scars. Results in the 2 patients resurfaced by 6:1 and 9:1 expansion autografts were functionally satisfactory.

▶ [Patients treated in this series demonstrate a valid use for the mesh graft. Although a mesh graft does not cover more burn wound surface than a solid graft, the use of a mesh graft divides the wound into a number of small wounds that can heal by epithelialization and wound contraction more satisfactorily than does a simple large wound. Such a healing process can make a decisive difference in patients who are so critically burned that coverage by other techniques is impossible. The data, however, do not justify the use of mesh grafts in less seriously burned patients, in whom adequate skin is available to resurface the burn wound with unbroken skin.—E.E.P.] ◀

7–10 **Development and Use of a Living Skin Equivalent.** Eugene Bell, H. Paul Ehrlich, Stephanie Sher, Charlotte Merrill, Robert Sarber, Barbara Hull, Takako Nakatsuji, Diane Church, and David J. Buttle fabricated a living skin equivalent consisting of a dermal and an epidermal component, each made with cells taken from a potential graft recipient. It has been used as a wound covering that is accepted, blocks wound contraction, and persists.

A dermal equivalent is prepared first. A small biopsy from the organism that will receive the graft is cut into fragments and cultured. The cells are later removed from their substrate, suspended, and combined with a collagen solution. The collagen comes out of solution in the form of fibrils, forming a gel or lattice through which cells are relatively uniformly distributed. By active compaction of collagen fi-

Fig 7–3.—Epidermal cells on a skin equivalent graft after grafting: **A,** at 9 weeks, ×112; **C,** at 7 weeks, ×56. Normal host epidermis is shown in **B,** ×112. *E,* epidermis; *D,* dermis. (Courtesy of Bell, E., et al.: Plast. Reconstr. Surg. 67:386–392, March 1981.)

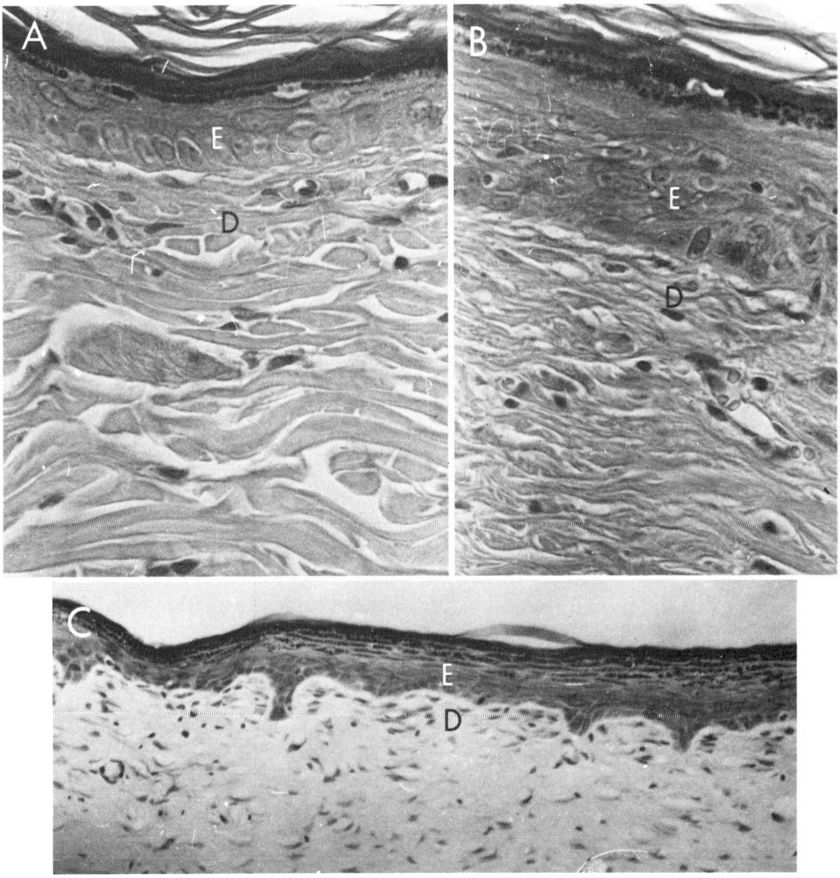

(7–10) Plast. Reconstr. Surg. 67:386–392, March 1981.

brils by the cells, the lattice is transformed into a tissue of firm consistency.

This dermal equivalent provides a substrate for epidermal cells taken from a second biopsy. Epidermal cells dissociated from biopsy fragments are distributed as a suspension on the dermal equivalent. In 2–4 days the epidermal cells form a confluent sheet of cells that covers the dermal substratum and begins to differentiate. As soon as the epidermal cells form a confluent sheet, the living, two-layered tissue is ready for grafting. There is no theoretical limit to the size of graft that can be made.

Skin equivalents have been grafted to many rats. Within 3–5 days, vascularization of the graft begins and continues rapidly with no necrosis or ischemia occurring. The graft almost always inhibits wound contraction. Although some grafts showed a decrease in size with time, most were stabilized by 60 days and none was rejected. Grafts have persisted for up to 10 months. They undergo histologic remodeling with time and in some respects begin to resemble normal skin. The epidermis hypertrophies and, even 10 weeks after grafting, is considerably thicker than adjacent normal tissue; tongues or pegs of epidermis penetrate the dermal equivalent (Fig 7–3). While the grafts acquire a vascular bed equal to that of normal tissue, hair follicles, sebaceous glands, and pigment cells are conspicuously absent.

The key problem in the application of skin equivalent grafts to human beings involves the speed with which they can be fabricated from a biopsy. About 20–26 days are needed to convert 1 sq cm of biopsy tissue to a piece of skin equivalent measuring 100 sq cm. The collagen used to make dermal equivalents has come from rats, and there is evidence that human beings will not reject nonhuman collagens if they are highly purified, but this matter needs further testing.

▶ [This is an obvious next step after the growing of epithelial cells in tissue culture. The frontier for many years has been making cultured epithelial cells attach to a collagen substrate. This problem seems to have been solved, and now the final step is producing artificial skin in sufficient quantities to treat the burned patient.—E.E.P.] ◀

7–11 **Successful Use of a Physiologically Acceptable Artificial Skin in Treatment of Extensive Burn Injury.** Need for a satisfactory, permanent physiologic skin substitute has long been recognized. John F. Burke, Ioannis V. Yannas, William C. Quinby, Jr., Conrado C. Bondoc, and Walter K. Jung (Boston) have evaluated a bilayer artificial skin composed of a temporary Silastic epidermis and a porous collagen-chondroitin 6-sulfate fibrillar dermis, which is not removed. The latter portion is made from bovine hide collagen and chondroitin 6-sulfate from shark cartilage. The artificial skin is stored either as a freeze-dried bilayer membrane or in 70% isopropyl alcohol. The grafting method is essentially the same as that used to autograft an excised burn wound (Fig 7–4). The Silastic epidermis is replaced by autoepidermis when clinically convenient (Figs 7–5 and 7–6).

Ten patients aged 3–60 years with 50% to 90% third-degree burn injuries had an extensive part of their total body surface closed with

---

(7–11) Ann. Surg. 194:413–428, October 1981.

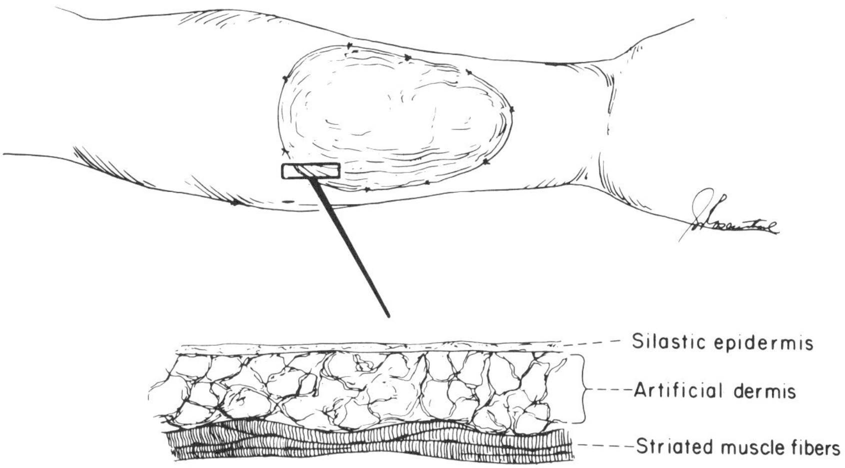

Fig 7–4.—The artificial skin is grafted by conventional techniques and sutured to achieve primary closure. The insert shows that the artificial dermis adheres to the excised bed, whether dermal remnants, subcutaneous tissue, fascia, or muscle, without dead space or fluid collection. (Courtesy of Burke, J. F., et al.: Ann. Surg. 194:413–428, October 1981.)

artificial skin. All had at least 15% of their excised wounds closed with artificial skin; the average area treated in this way was 27.5% of the body surface. The average time of closure with artificial skin was 26 days. Complications included shallow wrinkling of the artificial skin, loosening of the epidermal edge, and, in 1 case, loss of artificial skin over about 3% of the body surface area from hematoma. The overall take of artificial skin approached 100%, and the take of autoepidermis on artificial dermis after removal of the Silastic was 85% to 95%. The healing of meshed autoepidermal sheets proceeded

Fig 7–5.—At time of election, when donor sites are ready for reharvesting, the Silastic epidermis is easily stripped from the artificial dermis with forceps. Insert shows that the artificial dermis is invaded by host cells and vessels and that it is partially replaced by a newly synthesized "neodermis." (Courtesy of Burke, J. F., et al.: Ann. Surg. 194:413–428, October 1981.)

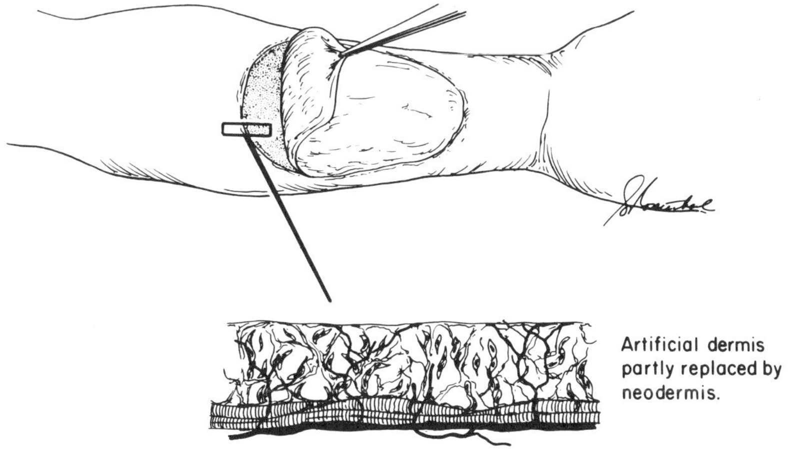

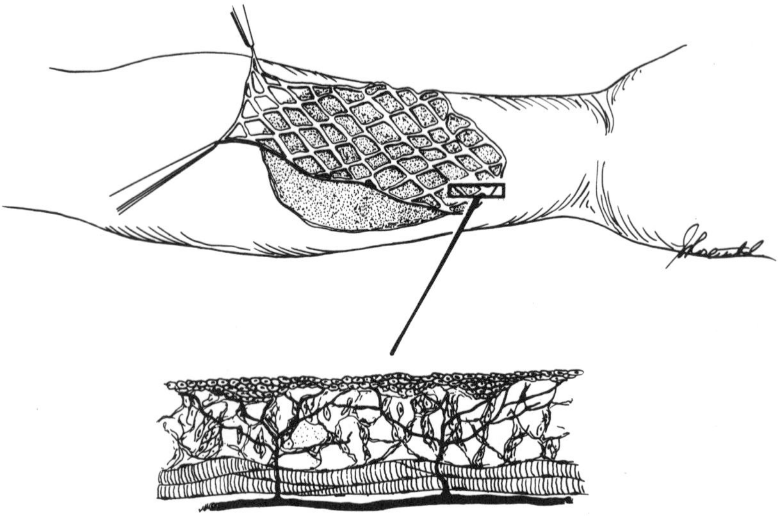

Fig 7–6.—Photomicograph demonstrates grafting of the "neodermis" with a thin epidermal graft directly onto the dermal bed provided by the artificial dermal template. (Courtesy of Burke, J. F., et al.: Ann. Surg. 194:413–428, October 1981.)

normally. Biopsy specimens showed well-healed skin with no remnants of the bovine collagen lattice. The wounds matured rapidly and the final appearances resembled normal skin. No contracture or hypertrophic scar formation has occurred on follow-up for as long as 16 months.

This artificial skin can be produced on a large scale and is immediately available for grafting. Its use promises improved functional and cosmetic results in patients with extensive burn injuries. It may prove feasible to implant epidermal cells in the bilayer material at the time of or close to initial grafting.

▶ [The authors have taken a significant step in the development of biologically useful artificial skin. The theoretical basis of their experiments is brilliant. Practically, however, they have not yet overcome the problems of availability and long-term function of normal dermis and epidermis as a composite tissue organ. The potential is there, but the ability to apply a biologically sound principle to treatment of a large burn is still elusive.—E.E.P.] ◀

7–12 **Grafting of Burns With Cultured Epithelium Prepared From Autologous Epidermal Cells.** Specimens of epidermis as small as 1 sq cm can be disaggregated enzymatically and then cultured. Single cells grow into colonies that then fuse to make a confluent epithelium. Such cultured epithelium, grafted to athymic mice, generated an epidermis that remained of good histologic quality for up to 3 months. Nicholas E. O'Connor, John B. Mulliken, Susan Banks-Schlegel, Olaniyi Kehinde, and Howard Green used cultured epidermal autografts in 2 burned patients: a man, aged 38, with burns of 80% of the body surface area and a man, aged 61, with burns of 40% of the body surface area.

(7–12) Lancet 1:75–78, Jan. 10, 1981.

Within 2 weeks of admission, each patient had two skin samples of 2 sq cm taken for graft preparation. When ready about 5 weeks later, the epithelial grafts with a Vaseline gauze covering were placed on prepared sites with the basal cell layer directed against the recipient bed. The grafts were held in place by a single layer of nonimpregnated fine-mesh gauze and overlaid with a lose layer of coarse-mesh gauze that was changed daily. The fine-mesh gauze and Vaseline gauze usually were removed after 6–10 days and the area redressed with a layer of Vaseline gauze and a loose layer of coarse gauze. These dressings were changed daily for 3–4 weeks. Thereafter, the grafts were left exposed but treated with lanolin ointment daily. The grafts were placed on three different types of recipient bed: early granulation tissue (less than 7 days old), chronic granulation tissue, and areas recently excised down to fascia. Each patient had cultured grafts placed on various burn sites. Each patient was also extensively grafted with conventional meshed autografts.

In the first patient, 3 grafts (primary and secondary cultures) placed on a granulating escharotomy site showed good take by the tenth day and continued to thicken and expand for 3–4 weeks until they became confluent with the surrounding epidermis. Of 8 secondary and tertiary cultures placed on an area of chronic granulation tissue 80 days after the burn, at least 3 took. After 3–4 weeks the epidermis generated from them became confluent with the surrounding meshed split-thickness grafts, and at 6 months the grafts could not be distinguished from surrounding epidermis.

On freshly excised beds, over half of the grafts showed initial take. When they failed to take, or took only temporarily, infection was the most common cause. Thus, for optimal take, beds should be freshly excised and completely covered with grafts. Although takes were obtained from primary, secondary, and tertiary cultures, it is not known whether, over the long term, grafts prepared from later subcultures will perform as well as those of early cultures. Because epidermis taken for cultivation from patients with severe septicemia had very low colony-forming efficiency, skin samples should be taken and cultures started shortly after admission.

▶ [This idea has been tried many times over a long period. The authors may have achieved some success in the laboratory, but growing epithelium alone will not be helpful clinically until cells can be attached to a collagen substrate to produce a more stable surface than epithelium alone. If the techniques reported in this article can be made generally available and will produce grafts large enough to treat major burn wounds, a milestone in burn therapy will have been achieved.—E.E.P.] ◀

7–13 **Treatment of Severe Burns With Widely Meshed Skin Autograft and Meshed Skin Allograft Overlay.** The use of expanded mesh autografts, described in 1964 by Tanner et al., has greatly increased the yield from available donor sites, but a meshed graft with an expansion size of 6:1 or greater often fails to take or is lost through local infection, J. Wesley Alexander, Bruce G. MacMillan, Edward Law, and Dilip S. Kittur (Shriners Burns Inst., Cincinnati) evaluated a method in which a widely meshed autograft is covered by a less

---

(7–13) J. Trauma 21:433–438, June 1981.

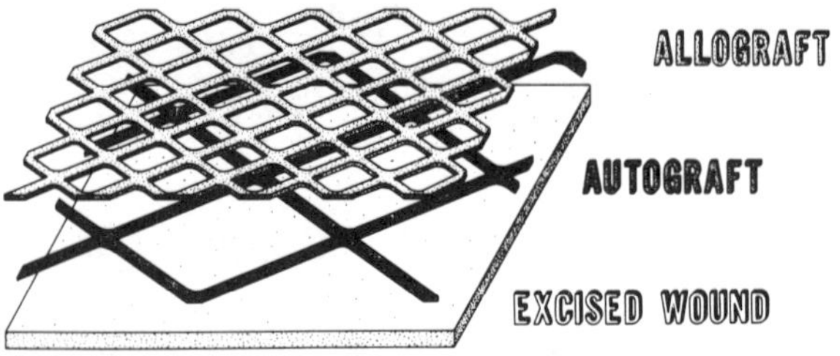

Fig 7–7.—Diagram of a 9:1 expanded mesh autograft with a 3:1 expanded mesh allograft. This was used on the lower leg of a patient at the time of operation B. (Courtesy of Alexander, J. W., et al.: J. Trauma 21:433–438, June 1981.)

widely meshed allograft to enhance take of the autograft. Twenty-two major graft procedures were done in 14 children with burn injuries of 25%–98% of the body surface. The technique is illustrated in Figure 7–7. In 1 instance, the allograft overlay was used to cover postage-stamp grafts. The average size of the grafted region was 6.7% of the total body surface. Eleven operations were done just after excision to fascia, 4 after tangential excision of the wound, and 7 on granulating wounds after debridement. Grafts were expanded to 6:1 to 9:1. Most were held in place with staples and covered with fine-mesh gauze containing a topical antimicrobial agent.

Complete take of the autograft occurred in 19 of 22 procedures, with an average take of 98.9%. Three patients had initial good take but subsequent loss from generalized burn wound sepsis and septicemia. The final cosmetic outcome was acceptable in all cases. Follow-up for up to a year has indicated continued stability of the grafted areas. Hypertrophic scar formation was no greater than is seen with the use of 3:1 meshed autografts. The average time to separation of half of the allografts was 2 weeks. Limited experience with 1.5:1 expansion of allografts suggests superior results because of earlier closure of open spaces by epithelium.

The use of widely meshed skin autograft covered by a less widely meshed allograft provides immediate, complete, and continuous coverage, without a need to regraft the areas when the allografts are rejected. The procedure is done easily and rapidly. Topical antimicrobial agents may be used concurrently. Stable coverage is obtained using a minimum of autogenous donor tissue. The functional and cosmetic results have been satisfactory.

▶ [I have included this article because it presents a new idea, which originated with careful investigators at a superb institution. The concept, however, that interposing allografts and isografts can produce a better take of isografts than conventional techniques, is difficult to follow. One cannot help but wonder if there are not factors other than the use of allografts that have caused the authors to conclude that there are significant advantages to interspersing allografts and isografts.—E.E.P.] ◀

8. Transplantation and Artificial Organs

8–1 **Brain Death Laws and Patterns of Consent to Remove Organs for Transplantation From Cadavers in the United States and 28 Other Countries.** An estimated 20,000 or more Americans die each year under circumstances that could permit the removal of viable organs for transplantation. Frank P. Stuart, Frank J. Veith, and Ronald E. Cranford have analyzed patterns of practice with respect to consent to remove cadaveric organs for transplantation and the legal status of brain death as a basis for declaring death in the United States and 28 other countries.

The Uniform Anatomical Gift Act, adopted throughout the United States, permits either the donor or the family to consent to the removal of cadaveric organs. In no state is consent presumed. The legal status of brain death as a basis for declaring death is established by statute in 25 states (table) and by court decision in 7 others. The model brain death law proposed by the American Medical Association recognizes the equivalence of brain death and death of a person without prescribing the medical criteria or tests used to establish brain death.

Seventeen of the 28 other countries surveyed provide for donor cards similar to those used in the United States. In 15 countries, consent must be obtained from the donor or a family member, and in 6 others the family is notified before proceeding with organ salvage. Brain death is recognized by statute or administrative law in 13 of the 28 countries surveyed. In several countries, medical details and procedures for diagnosing brain death are incorporated into the laws and regulations.

In no country does the number of cadaver organs salvaged meet the needs of potential recipients, and these needs will increase as the clinical outcome of organ transplantation continues to improve. Attempts to introduce presumed consent in any English-speaking country would probably meet much resistance. A consensus is evolving in the United States and elsewhere that brain death can be diagnosed with reasonable certainty and should be recognized by law as a basis for declaring death. Elimination of this uncertainty should increase the salvage of cadaver organs and reduce the ischemic injury incurred before their removal.

▶ [This and the following article highlight the continuing problem of acquisition of organs from cadaver donors. One segment of the transplant community led by the three authors of this article have been working to legalize brain death in order to facilitate organ donation. This article details their progress in having a uniform anatomical gift act adopted throughout the United States. In a similar manner, a President's commission on the problems associated with the definition of death and organ

(8–1) Transplantation 31:238–244, April 1981.

MODELS ADOPTED BY 25 STATES FOR STATUTORY DEFINITION OF DEATH

Kansas model: alternative means for determining death[a]	Capron-Kass model: death is pronounced while heart and lung functions are artificially maintained	American Bar Association model: irreversible cessation of total brain functions equals death	Uniform Brain Death model: Similar to American Bar Association model but emphasizes irreversible cessation of brain stem function
Kansas 1970	Alaska 1974	California[b, c] 1974	Nevada 1979
Maryland 1972	Michigan 1975	Georgia[b] 1975	Wyoming[d] 1979
New Mexico 1973	West Virginia[e] 1975	Oklahoma 1975	
Virginia[b, f] 1973	Louisiana[c] 1976	Illinois[e] 1975	
Oregon 1975	Iowa[b] 1976	Tennessee 1976	
North Carolina[g] 1977	Hawaii[b, c] 1978	Idaho[b] 1977	
	Texas 1979	Montana 1977	
	Alabama[c] 1979	Arkansas[f] 1979	
		Connecticut[b, c, e] 1979	

[a]Specifically allows death declaration on basis of cardiorespiratory failure or brain death.
[b]Use of brain-related criteria to pronounce death requires opinion of two physicians. In Virginia and Hawaii, one of these must be a specialist in neurology or neurosurgery.
[c]Physician who makes determination of death may not participate in removal or transplantation of organs from deceased.
[d]Total brain function is defined as purposeful activities of the brain as distinguished from random activity.
[e]Use of brain-related criteria only to be used for purposes of Anatomical Gift Act, i.e., for purposes of organ donation.
[f]Also requires absence of spontaneous breathing.
[g]As amended in 1979; Capron-Kass-like in some regards.

donation has also issued a report. We continue to maintain our position despite the "right to live" movement and various media presentations that tend to exaggerate the minor differences of opinion in the definition of brain death that exist among neurologists and neurosurgeons. Nevertheless, there is a large consensus, and this continues to be an important problem.

The following article points out the severe difficulties the medical community has in mobilizing its forces to harvest available transplant kidneys. These problems are not easily separable. The major barriers to obtaining cadaver organs are the lethargy and disinterest of the general medical community. Its reluctance to encourage donation is, in part, the result of the failure to define death in such a way that physicians can feel safe from litigation.—J.S.N.] ◀

8–2 **Cadaveric Kidneys for Transplantation: A Paradox of Shortage in the Face of Plenty.** Kenneth J. Bart, Edwin J. Macon, Frederick C. Whittier, Robert J. Baldwin, and Joseph H. Blount undertook a review of in-hospital deaths to determine the potential supply of cadaver kidneys and to define characteristics of potential donors in a prospective effort to improve retrieval of these organs. Medical records of 10,420 of 24,164 patients dying in 67 acute-care hospitals in Georgia, Kansas, and Missouri were retrieved. By center-specific criteria there were 1.7 potential donors per 100 in-hospital deaths, which could make available 109 kidneys per million population. By broad intercenter criteria there were 3.5 potential donors per 100 deaths, which could provide 232 kidneys per million population. By center-specific criteria kidneys from 19.3% of suitable potential donors were retrieved in 1975. The small number of transplantable cadaveric kidneys retrieved was not attributable to a lack of suitable organs, but rather to the failure to identify suitable donors, obtain consent, and retrieve the kidneys.

The typical potential donor by center-specific criteria was a white male, aged 5–55 years, who died in a critical-care unit within 3 days of admission to an acute-care hospital having 350 or more deaths per year and whose death was due to central nervous system trauma, hemorrhage, or tumor. The failure to obtain adequate numbers of transplantable cadaver kidneys represents a failure to make potential donors actual donors. The situation is a paradoxical one of shortage in the face of plenty.

8–3 **Specificities of Antibodies Eluted From Human Cadaveric Renal Allografts: Multiple Mechanisms of Renal Allograft Injury.** Antibodies participate in the destruction of initial renal allografts in some experimental models, but their importance in human renal allograft rejection remains unclear. John J. McPhaul, Jr., Peter Stastny (Dallas) and Richard B. Freemen (Rochester, N.Y.) investigated eluates from 17 surgical biopsies of cadaver grafts exhibiting serious deterioration of function and from 25 nephrectomy specimens obtained after irreversible graft rejection. All patients were on standard immunosuppression at the time of biopsy or nephrectomy. None had received antilymphocyte globulin. No cases of "hyperacute" rejection were included in the study.

Twenty-three of 35 eluates contained immunoglobulin that bound

(8–2) Transplantation 31:379–382, May 1981.
(8–3) J. Clin. Invest. 67:1405–1414, May 1981.

to normal renal tissue. In most instances, smooth muscle, alone or with other structures such as tubular basement membranes and proximal cells, was stained. All 16 eluates tested contained antibodies cytotoxic for cells from normal subjects; 6 were cytotoxic to T cells and 10, to B cell and monocyte-enriched preparations. Antibodies reactive with tubular basement membrane and tubular cells were not removed by absorption of eluates with pooled buffy coat cells, platelet concentrates, and packed, cultured B cells. Two of 5 eluates containing antikidney antibodies bound to rat kidneys in vivo.

These findings suggest that circulating antibodies participate in cadaver kidney graft destruction. Antibodies cytotoxic to mononuclear cells as well as antibodies specific for structural kidney antigens have been identified. Cytotoxic antibodies may be the more important expression of graft-directed humoral immunity. Further studies are needed to characterize the antigens involved and to determine the pathogenic significance of antibodies that can be eluted from allografts undergoing rejection.

▶ [This article takes a traditional immunopathologic approach to the analysis of human renal allograft rejection. Various antibodies are eluted from the renal tissue and used for fluorescent staining against kidney tissue in vivo. Alternatively, various tissues are used for absorption of the antibodies to determine the target of each. The problem with this kind of study is that advanced organ rejection can result during the development of immunity to structural and chemical elements of the grafted organ. These elements have *no* part in the initial rejection reaction, but are simply formed as rejection against alloantigens leads to exposure of other antigenic specificities. These elements may be important to the ultimate destruction of the graft, but they play no initiating role. This intellectual dilemma seems not to be resolved easily. —J.S.N.] ◀

8–4 **Use of Monoclonal Antibodies to T Cell Subsets for Immunologic Monitoring and Treatment in Recipients of Renal Allografts.** Although patient survival has improved in renal allograft recipients, allograft survival has not changed appreciably in the past decade. One problem is the lack of a means of assessing the ongoing effects of immunosuppression other than by the ultimate clinical outcome. A. Benedict Cosimi, Robert B. Colvin, Robert C. Burton, Robert H. Rubin, Gideon Goldstein, Patrick C. Kung, W. Peter Hansen, Francis L. Delmonico, and Paul S. Russell used flow cytometry and monoclonal antibodies to T cell subsets to monitor the peripheral blood lymphocytes serially for at least 2 months in 29 renal allograft recipients. Besides azathioprine and prednisone, 15 cadaver kidney recipients were given antithymocyte globulin (ATG). Two patients who rejected cadaver grafts received OKT3, a monoclonal antibody reactive with virtually all peripheral blood T cells. A dose of 1–2 mg daily was given intravenously for 10 days.

Highly significant correlations were found between changes in T cell subsets and rejection during conventional immunosuppressive therapy. Normal or elevated ratios of OKT4 (helper-inducer) to OKT8 (suppressor-cytotoxic) cells were associated with rejection (Fig 8–1), unless the donor was HLA identical or the total number of T cells was extremely low. Rejection was infrequent in patients with low ra-

(8–4) N. Engl. J. Med. 305:308–314, Aug. 6, 1981.

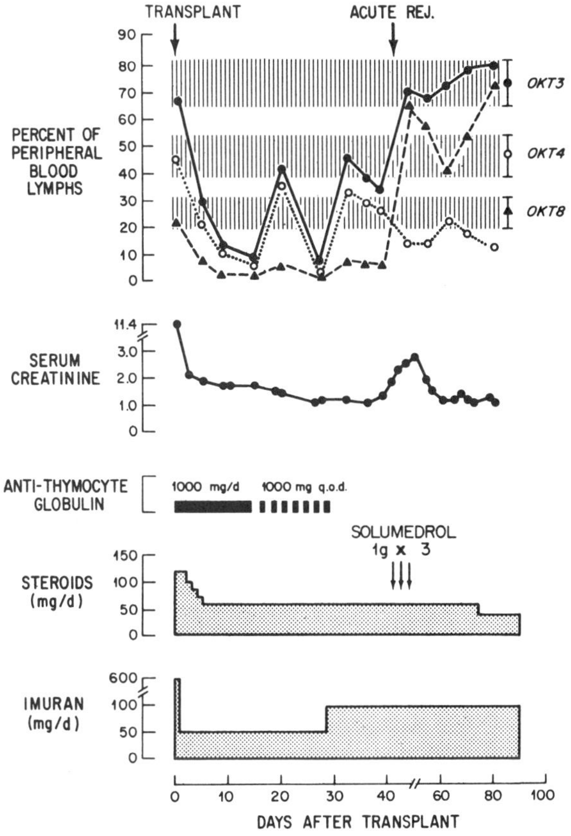

Fig 8–1.—Alterations in T cell subsets in a representative renal allograft patient. Vertical hatchings represent the normal range (mean ± SD) in each lymphocyte population. Note the high proportion of OKT4-reactive to OKT8-reactive cells first appearing when the frequency of ATG administration was reduced to every other day and persisting before the episode of rejection. After successful treatment of rejection, a dramatic inversion of the normal OKT4/OKT8 ratio developed. Treatments included methylprednisolone sodium succinate (Solu-Medrol) and azathioprine (Imuran). Serum creatinine level is measured as mg/dl. (Courtesy of Cosimi, A. B., et al.: N. Engl. J. Med. 305:308–314, Aug. 6, 1981.)

tios. The 2 ATG-treated patients who had rejection may have received an inadequate dose. The patients treated with OKT3 monoclonal antibody for acute rejection showed a rapid disappearance of OKT3-reactive cells from the peripheral blood and prompt reversal of rejection (Fig 8–2).

Monoclonal antibodies may be used in renal transplant recipients to demonstrate changes in T cell subsets that are associated with graft rejection. Monoclonal antibody has immunosuppressive potency in patients with acute rejection of cadaver kidney grafts. The findings show the possibility of specifically manipulating selected T cell subsets in accord with monitoring data.

▶ [The newest technology of monoclonal antibody production and analysis have been used to analyze circulating T cell subsets in many laboratories. Some laboratories have found that rejection can be predicted in increased ratios of OKT4 (helper/indu-

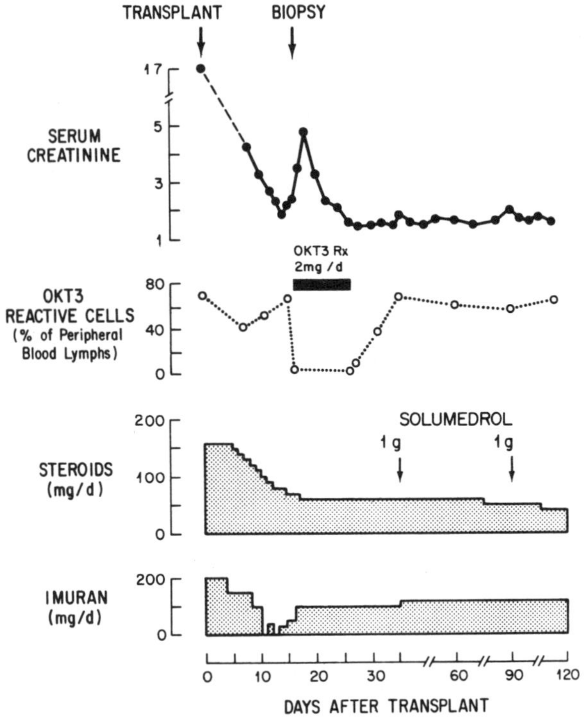

Fig 8–2.—Clinical course in a renal allograft recipient treated with OKT3 monoclonal antibody for acute rejection. Sustained depletion of T cells and return of renal function to normal occurred without the need for increased steroids. In the later period after transplantation, two modest elevations in serum creatinine level were treated with methylprednisolone sodium succinate (Solu-Medrol). Serum creatinine level is measured as mg/dl. (Courtesy of Cosimi, A. B., et al.: N. Engl. J. Med. 305:308–314, Aug. 6, 1981.)

cer) to OKT8 (suppressor/cytotoxic) cells. Other laboratories have shown that reversal of the normal OKT4/OKT8 ratio is associated with graft acceptance. Such studies may be ultimately useful or interesting in determining what degree of adaptation between host and graft has taken place, whether rejection can be expected, and whether immunosuppression is too vigorous or insufficient.

The innovative aspect of this paper is the use of OKT3 monoclonal antibody for the treatment of acute rejection. Antibodies directed against all T cells can be given in small quantities directly into the vein without major toxic effects. The material is, therefore, essentially anti-T lymphocyte globulin that is directed against T cell specificities rather than against many specificities on the lymphocyte that are recognized by the heterologous species in whom the antilymphocyte globulin is made. This work, therefore, finds its place in the mainstream of ALG research. Both the Upjohn preparation currently licensed for use in human beings and the investigational serum made at the University of Minnesota have been shown, in appropriate double-blind randomized studies, to reverse rejection. This study by Cosimi et al. suggests that monoclonal anti-OKT3 antibody is similarly useful. One disadvantage of the anti-OKT3 reagent appears to be the high degree of immunity which the patient develops to the heterologous monoclonal antibody so that second courses of the anti-OKT3 reagent cannot be used. This may be the result of the method of administration and the failure to increase prednisone doses along with the administration of the anti-OKT3 reagent. University of Minnesota immunoglobulin has been repeatedly useful in the vast majority of patients, without development of skin sensitivity, detectable antibodies, or evidence of immune elimination of the antilymphocyte globulin. Whether this useful response is the result of having a polyclonal (rather than a monoclonal) antilymphocyte antibody or whether it is the result of the concurrent increase in prednisone levels or mode of administration is unclear. This practical matter needs to be clarified before the monoclonal reagent is seized upon as a panacea when, in fact, the polyclonal reagent may be the better drug.

Despite years of controversy on the clinical use of antilymphocyte globulins, the recent licensing of at least one product by the Food and Drug Administration for use in the prevention and treatment of renal allograft rejection gives strong support to its ultimate value in conjunction with azathioprine and prednisone. Whether antilymphocyte globulin will be equally useful in combination with cyclosporin or whether such new agents will replace it remains to be established.—J.S.N.] ◀

8–5 **Kidney Transplantation by Use of Splenectomy and Transfusions, Cadaver Haplotype Matching, Suppressor Cell Assays, and T Cell Monitoring.** Walter Severyn, George Kyriakides, Laphalle Fuller, Violet Esquenazi, Cathy Flaa, Les Olson, Carl Goldsmith, and Joshua Miller (Miami, Fla.) used several methods of modulating host immunologic status in an attempt to improve the survival of kidney transplants in 48 consecutive procedures done in 1979–1980. The patients, aged 3–58 years, were followed up for 6–24 months postoperatively. There were 37 transplants from living related donors and 11 from cadaver donors. All patients received at least 2 units of blood preoperatively or perioperatively, and 38 underwent splenectomy. Cadaver donors and recipients were genotyped for 1 HLA A and HLA B locus haplotype. Immunosuppression was adjusted to the preoperative ability to generate mixed leukocyte culture (MLC)-derived suppressor cells versus living-related-donor lymphocyte-defined antigens in both high- and low-MLC-reactive donor-recipient pairs. Therapy also was adjusted to changes in T cell counts and T cell subsets.

Patient and graft survival are shown in Figure 8–3. There were no graft losses from rejection, and the 4 deaths appeared unrelated to rejection or immunosuppressive therapy. Seven of the 8 proved rejec-

Fig 8–3.—Patient and graft survival of 48 cadaver donor and living-related-donor kidney transplant recipients followed up for 6 to 24 months postoperatively. Note that in this series, no graft losses occurred other than in those recipients who died. The numbers at each point indicate the number of patients in the series who have reached that postoperative interval. (Courtesy of Severyn, W., et al.: Surgery 90:364–375, August 1981.)

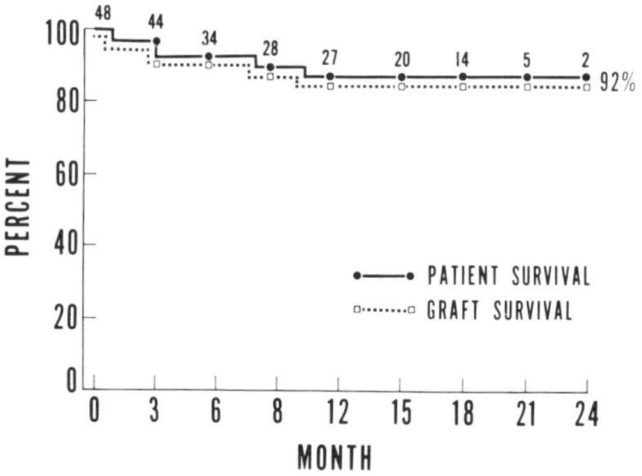

(8–5) Surgery 90:364–375, August 1981.

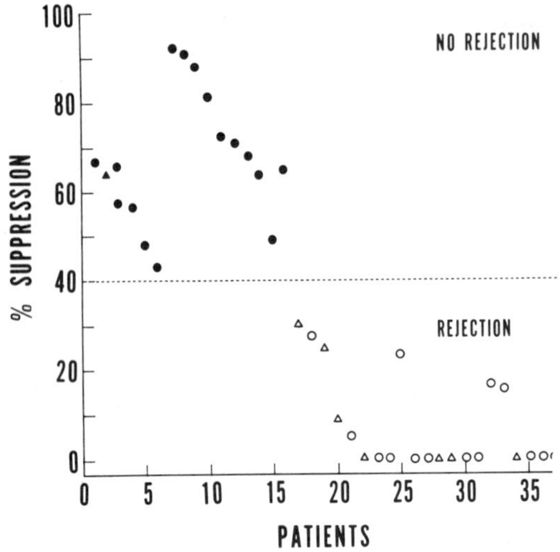

Fig 8–4.—Percentage of suppression of each living-related-donor kidney recipient plotted independently of HLA SD antigen or MLC reactivity. With one exception, indicated by solid triangle (nonsplenectomized patient), in which less than one-third the usual dose of Imuran could be given during the first 3 months postoperatively because of persistent leukopenia, rejection episodes occurred only in patients with less than 30% MLC suppression. Triangles indicate patients who experienced rejection episodes; circles indicate those who did not. (Courtesy of Severyn, W., et al.: Surgery 90:364–375, August 1981.)

tion episodes occurred in living-related-donor graft recipients. Thirteen patients had 22 episodes of infection requiring hospitalization, 9 caused by cytomegalovirus. An inverse correlation was noted between percentage MLC suppression and rejection (Fig 8–4). All cadaver-kidney recipients have normally functioning grafts except 1 who died after revision of a stenotic renal artery. Comparable results were not obtained at other centers using donor kidneys from the same organ retrieval program.

Various immunoregulatory manipulations have improved the results of renal transplantation, but global perturbations of the immune system remain necessary. New immunosuppressive agents such as cyclosporin A appear to hold promise.

▶ [This paper demonstrates that the careful selection and balancing of many immunosuppressive agents can result in exemplary clinical results after transplantation. Each of the modalities utilized, splenectomy, tissue typing, immunologic monitoring, antilymphocyte globulin, and transfusions, appears to offer an additional increment in the spectrum of clinical effectiveness. Herein lies the reason for the growing success of renal transplantation—not in the development of magic bullets designed to solve all the problems of transplantation at once, but in the gradual adoption and manipulation of the entire armamentarium by experienced physicians and surgeons.—J.S.N.] ◀

8–6 **Induction of High Kidney Graft Survival Rate by Multiple Transfusion.** A beneficial effect of pretransplantation blood transfusion on the outcome of renal grafting has been confirmed in many studies, but it is not clear whether transfusion acts by inducing a

(8–6) Lancet 1:1223–1225, June 6, 1981.

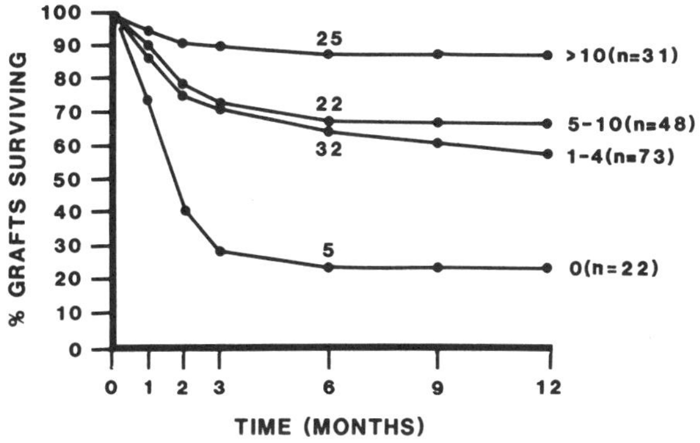

Fig 8–5.—Actuarial kidney graft survival rates according to number of transfusions received before transplantation. Numbers of transfusions are indicated at end of each curve, and numbers of patients are given in parentheses. Numbers of graft survivals for each group at 6 months are as indicated. Number of patients at risk at 6 months is indicated. By weighted regression analysis, $P<.0001$ at 3, 6, and 12 months, indicating that improvement in graft outcome depended on increased number of pretransplantation transfusions. (Courtesy of Opelz, G., et al.: Lancet 1:1223–1225, June 6, 1981.)

state of immune unresponsiveness or by selecting out highly immune-responsive patients. Gerhard Opelz, Beverly Graver, and Paul I. Terasaki (Univ. of California, Los Angeles) obtained evidence that transfusion induced unresponsiveness in patients. A total of 174 patients given cadaver donor kidneys at centers adopting a policy of liberal preoperative blood transfusion were followed. Twenty-two patients received transplants before receiving transfusion. Only packed cells were used in 133 cases.

A striking dose-related increase in graft survival was observed at 1 year, from 23% in nontransfusion patients to 87% in patients given over 10 transfusions (Fig 8–5). An even more marked effect was observed when only patients given nonfrozen blood were considered. Among the 140 patients with no serum cytotoxic antibody reactivity before transplantation, graft survival correlated strongly with number of transfusions given (table). The number of transfusions given during operation did not correlate significantly with graft survival. Sex, age, original disease, duration of pretransplant dialysis, and HLA match were comparable among patients in the various transfusion

Transfusion Effect in Patients Without Cytotoxic Antibodies*

No. of transfusions	No. of patients	Graft survival at 1 year (%±SE)
0	18	28±11
1–4	64	57±8
5–10	38	71±8
>10	20	90±7
Total	140	62±5

*P (regression) <.0001.

categories. None of these findings influenced the results significantly.

This study confirms that preoperative blood transfusions improve the survival of cadaver kidney transplants. Transfusion appears to act not by selection, but by induction of unresponsiveness. Transfusions do not alter the immune response to infectious agents. They are inexpensive and readily available. A policy of transfusion only at the time of transplantation appears to be unwarranted. Further studies are needed to determine whether fresh blood is better than banked blood, what the optimal volume is, and which blood component is the best inducer of unresponsiveness.

▶ [Opelz's original article demonstrating the beneficial effect of multiple transfusions on renal allograft survival is truly the major transplantation discovery of the past few years—rivaling the clinical trials with cyclosporin A. Arguments concerning timing and specificity of the transfusion will continue, but this article once more demonstrates that the more transfusions one receives prior to transplantation, the better. The mechanisms are still unknown, but probably relate to the induction of sensitization against potential donor antigens to which the recipient is likely to become highly immunized, plus the suppression against certain allospecificities to which the recipient can be desensitized.—J.S.N.] ◀

8–7 **Transfusion and Renal Allograft Survival: Beneficial Effect of Transfusions Given on Day of Transplantation.** Transfusions given to patients with renal failure during pretransplantation waiting periods are associated with improved survival of cadaveric renal allografts, but they also cause an increased frequency of histocompatibility antigen presensitization and may delay transplantation or make it impossible for some patients. The problem of presensitization could be avoided if blood given at the time of transplantation were also shown to be associated with improved graft survival.

Lawrence G. Hunsicker, Liem S. Oei, Richard M. Freeman, John S. Thompson, and Robert J. Corry (Univ. of Iowa) reviewed the records of all 180 patients receiving primary cadaveric renal allografts during 1973–78. Of these, 48 received no transfusions, 45 received transfusions on the day of transplantation only, 41 received transfusions only prior to transplantation, and 46 received transfusions both before and on the day of transplantation. Transfusions given at the time of surgery were either of frozen blood deglycerolized by centrifugal washing or of leukocyte-poor washed packed erythrocytes; those given prior to surgery also included unwashed packed erythrocytes and, occasionally, whole blood. There was no set transfusion policy during the study period.

Three-month graft survival in patients transfused only on the day of transplant (73%) was significantly better than that in patients never transfused (54%) and was not significantly different from that in patients transfused during the dialysis waiting period (78%). Graft survival for all 3 groups of transfused patients was significantly better than for patients never transfused up to 4 years after transplantation. The favorable association between transfusion and 3-month graft survival remained significant after stratifying for variables such as patient age, sex, time on a dialysis regimen, frequency of bilateral nephrectomy, pretransplant hematocrit value, original cause of renal fail-

(8–7) Arch. Surg. 115:737–741, June 1980.

ure, year in which the transplant was performed, and presence of cytotoxic antibodies. A single transfusion on the day of transplantation increased 3-month graft survival from 54% to 68%. Maximal beneficial effect was achieved by administration of as few as 2–3 units of blood. The efficacy of frozen or leukocyte-poor blood was at least equal to that of routinely packed erythrocytes or whole blood.

The benefits of transfusion can be obtained while minimizing the risks of presensitization if patients are transfused in the dialysis waiting period only for clear indications; if frozen blood, which is less sensitizing, is used whenever possible; and if patients receive 2–3 units of blood electively at the time of transplantation.

▶ [This study, showing that transfusion can be delayed until the time of transplantation, does not coincide with the reports of others that transfusions are best given prior to transplantation and in larger quantities. If true, delaying transfusion until the day of transplantation would have several advantages, the greatest of which is to avoid sensitization against potential donors. Nevertheless that may be the reason why multiple transfusions are most useful, in that you sensitize patients against allospecificities to which they are likely to respond with vigor and thereby select a donor population to which there is less of a response.—J.S.N.] ◀

8–8 **Technique of Prolonged Thoracic Duct Drainage in Transplantation.** Thoracic duct drainage is useful for immunosuppression in transplantation patients. Maximal benefit requires prolonged lymphocyte depletion rather than temporary diversion. Lawrence J. Koep, Richard Weil III, and Thomas E. Starzl (Univ. of Colorado) describe a method by which thoracic duct drainage for up to 4 months was established in 96% of the patients in whom it was attempted.

TECHNIQUE.—A transverse left supraclavicular incision is made. The clavicular head of the sternocleidomastoid muscle is divided. The internal jugular vein is dissected for at least 2 cm to its junction with the subclavian vein. Small branches of the internal jugular vein are divided and ligated to permit later retraction on the internal jugular. The omohyoid fascia is opened. Dissection is begun along the anterior surface of the subclavian vein and proceeds posteriorly along its superior surface near the angulus venosus until the thoracic duct is identified. The duct is ligated and divided at its venous junction, after which it dilates, facilitating circumferential dissection. Lymphatic tributaries from the left arm and upper part of the neck are ligated and divided from the main trunk, but branches going toward the thorax are preserved. The thoracic duct is dissected for several centimeters until it begins its descent into the superior mediastinum. The descending portion of the main thoracic duct is opened, probed with lacrimal duct probes, and calibrated to accommodate comfortably the largest possible catheter (Fig 8–6). Repeated passage of probes of graded size can rupture obstructing valve leaflets and dilate stricture-like narrowings, two or three of which usually are encountered before the thoracic duct reaches the superior mediastinum. After the probing and dilating maneuvers, the tip of a double-lumen catheter is tunneled into the wound and advanced 3–10 cm down the duct. The mobilized duct is cinched around the catheter with a silk ligature. A large central venous catheter is inserted into a branch of the external or internal jugular vein for lymph return. If the cervical thoracic duct cannot be located or has been used before, a right thoracic approach may be indicated for thoracic duct cannulation (Fig 8–7).

(8–8) Surg. Gynecol. Obstet. 151:61–64, July 1980.

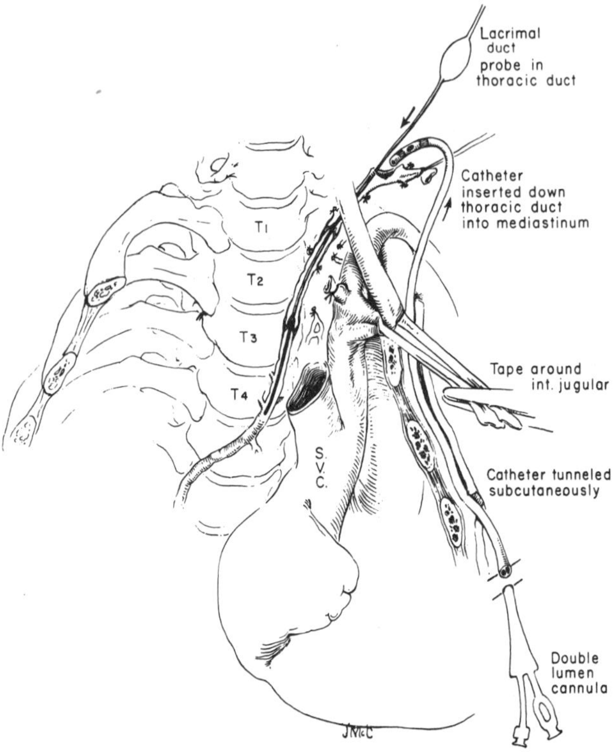

Fig 8–6.—Left cervical approach to the thoracic duct. Division of the duct near its terminus at the angulus venosus permits dissection and probing before insertion of the catheter. (Courtesy of Koep, L. J., et al.: Surg. Gynecol. Obstet. 15:61–64, July 1980.)

The thoracic duct cannula requires prompt and continuous care, beginning before wound closure. Normal saline containing heparin (2 units/ml) is infused at 20 ml/hour to prevent clotting in the catheter. The small side lumen is used for infusion of heparinized saline, while lymph is collected at the larger distal lumen. The wound and catheter exit sites are maintained according to a parenteral hyperalimentation catheter protocol of daily dressings and local antibiotic ointment. Systemic antibiotic prophylaxis for staphylococci is also provided. Lymph is collected in a closed system using blood collection bags prepared without any anticoagulant additives. The lymph bags are centrifuged and the cell-free supernatant is pressed into the appendage bag, refrigerated, and reinfused by the central venous catheter the following day. Most patients on normal diets do not require replacement of the volume disparity between collected and returned lymph. To terminate thoracic duct drainage, heparin irrigation is stopped and the collection bag elevated by daily increments until there has been no flow for a day, after which the catheter is removed.

Thoracic duct drainage was successful for 21–119 days in 86 of 90 patients in whom it was attempted (61 kidney recipients, 26 liver recipients, and 3 heart or pancreas recipients). Average daily lymph output was nearly 5 L in patients with renal disease and even more

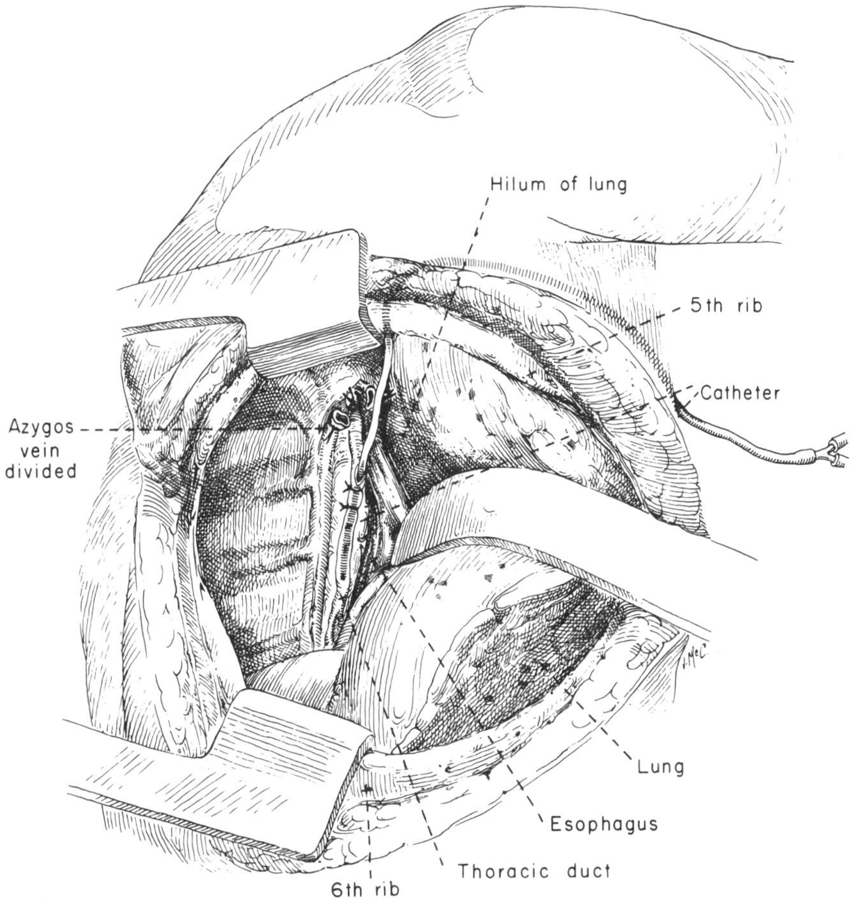

Fig 8–7.—Right transthoracic approach to the thoracic duct. Anterior reflection of the esophagus permits cannulation of the thoracic duct just inferior to the azygos vein. (Courtesy of Koep, L. J., et al.: Surg. Gynecol. Obstet. 151:61–64, July 1980.)

in those with liver disease. About 2 billion lymphocytes were removed daily. Reoperation and revision of the thoracic duct fistula were necessary in 15 of the 86 patients. There was no mortality directly attributable to thoracic duct drainage. Bacterial growth in the collected lymph was documented in 25% of the patients, but septicemia was unusual. Minor complications included local accumulation of lymph in the neck, transient edema of the face or left arm, and temporary Horner's syndrome.

▶ [This and the following two articles may ultimately prove to be of historical interest only. The University of Colorado group instituted a vigorous study to retest the possible role of thoracic duct drainage in clinical transplantation and found it useful, as had the Galveston, Texas, group for many years. Unfortunately, the technique is still cumbersome and, with the licensing of antilymphocyte globulin, the appearance of cyclosporin A, and pretransplant transfusion on the field, the likelihood that thoracic duct drainage will be of widespread use becomes less and less likely. Nevertheless, ancillary benefits may be achieved by such techniques.—J.S.N.] ◀

8–9 **Late Follow-up After Thoracic Duct Drainage in Cadaveric Renal Transplantation.** Thomas E. Starzl, Goran B. G. Klintmalm, Shunzaburo Iwatsuki, Gerhard Schroter, and Richard Weil III (Denver) report the results of cadaver kidney transplantation in 83 patients undergoing prolonged thoracic duct drainage as part of immunosuppressive management. In only 2 instances were there fewer than two mismatches at the A and B loci, and there were no four-antigen matches. Age range was 11–60 years. Azathioprine and prednisone were used for immunosuppression, and 35 patients also received short courses of antithymocyte globulin. Slightly less than half the patients underwent splenectomy. In later cases thoracic duct drainage was performed for periods of 17–58 days before transplantation. Drainage usually was continued for 3 or 4 weeks after transplantation.

Early rejection was not markedly altered by starting thoracic duct drainage at the time of transplantation. With pretreatment for 4 weeks or longer, rejection occurred within the first 3 months in only 4.5% of cases. The relation of graft survival to thoracic duct drainage is shown in Figure 8–8. Early patient survival rate was best in the group having contemporaneous thoracic duct drainage, but no advantage was apparent on prolonged follow-up. Pretreatment with thoracic duct drainage had some advantage in patients given their second to fifth transplants.

This and other recent studies support the value of thoracic duct drainage as an immunosuppressive adjunct in patients given cadaver kidneys. Without better maintenance therapy, however, the full value of temporary early lymphoid depletion procedures cannot be fully realized. Although effective and safe recipient conditioning is possible

Fig 8–8.—Actual graft survival in primary cadaveric renal transplants. *TDD*, thoracic duct drainage. (Courtesy of Starzl, T. E., et al.: Surg. Gynecol. Obstet. 153:377–382, September 1981.)

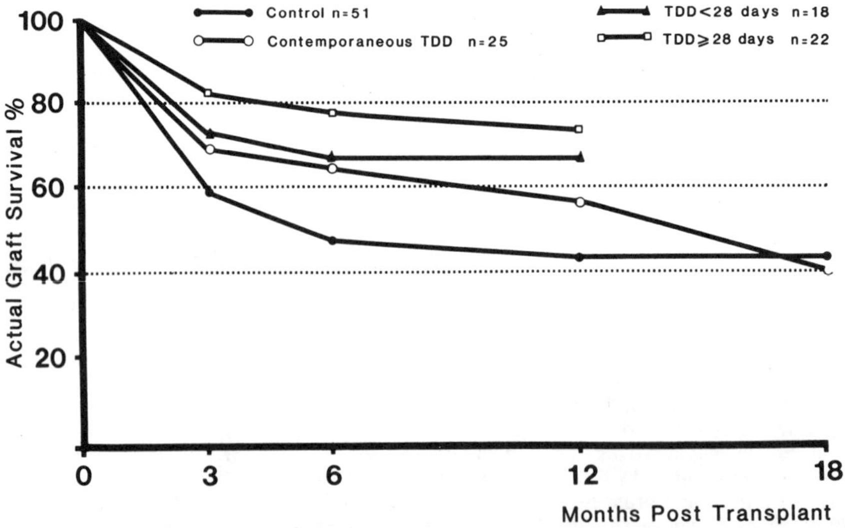

(8–9) Surg. Gynecol. Obstet. 153:377–382, September 1981.

through thoracic duct drainage, the extent to which the procedure will be used in the future is uncertain. The need for a month or more of hospitalization before transplantation involves substantially increased costs. The main use of thoracic duct drainage may prove to be in complicated cases in which patients are undergoing retransplantation or possess widely reactive anti-T warm antibodies.

8–10 **Renal Transplantation After Thoracic Duct Drainage.** Despite documented lymphocyte depletion after thoracic duct drainage (TDD), this technique has been used infrequently for immunosuppression in tissue transplantation. Jay C. Fish, Harry E. Sarles, August Remmers, Jr., Courtney M. Townsend, Jr., John D. Bell, and M. Wayne Flye (Univ. of Texas Med. Branch, Galveston) reviewed experience with TDD in 47 patients undergoing cadaver renal transplantation between 1972 and 1980. Another 63 patients underwent renal transplantation with TDD. All lymph was reinfused after removal of cells by centrifugation. The first available cadaver kidney was transplanted after 28 days of TDD, and TDD was continued for a total of 6 weeks. Both azathioprine and prednisone were given from the day of transplantation. Risk factors and HLA compatibility were similar in

Fig 8–9.—Weekly lymphocyte counts in blood and lymph are plotted during 6 weeks of TDD. Separation of cells into T and B cell components is also graphed. Predominant reduction in circulating lymphocytes occurs in T cell fraction. Solid lines denote peripheral blood lymphocytes; broken lines indicate lymph lymphocytes. (Courtesy of Fish, J. C., et al.: Ann. Surg. 193:752–756, June 1981.)

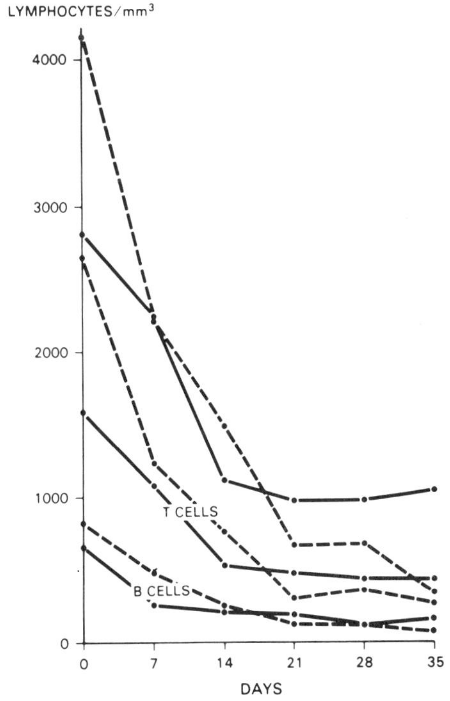

(8–10) Ann. Surg. 193:752–756, June 1981.

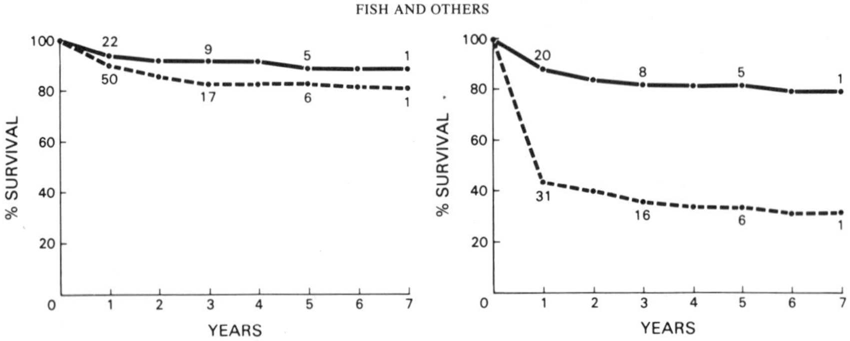

Fig 8–10 (left).—Patient survival after cadaver renal transplantation was not significantly different in the two groups. Solid line indicates TDD (47 patients); broken line denotes non-TDD (63).

Fig 8–11 (right).—Patients prepared with TDD had twice the graft survival as patients treated with standard immunosuppression. Solid line indicates TDD (49 patients); broken line denotes non-TDD (77).

(Courtesy of Fish, J. C., et al.: Ann. Surg. 193:752–756, June 1981.)

the two patient groups. From 1978, all patients received at least 5 units of blood before transplantation.

The single factor that affected graft survival was TDD. Lymph lymphocyte counts fell to 10% to 20% of predepletion values, and blood lymphocyte numbers fell by half in 4 to 6 weeks. Changes in T and B cells are shown in Figure 8–9. The two groups had similar patient survivals, although the TDD group did somewhat better at all intervals (Fig 8–10). Graft survival was twice as good in the TDD group at all intervals (Fig 8–11), despite the use of lower doses of azathioprine and prednisone in this group. Acute rejection occurred in 35% of the TDD group and in 61% of the control group. Two TDD patients lost their grafts, whereas 41 kidneys in the control group were lost from acute rejection. Three grafts in the TDD group were lost and exhibited changes of chronic rejection. Patients treated with TDD were not more susceptible to local or systemic infection. No patient in either group developed cancer.

Several centers now are confirming improved results with TDD, and the present findings indicate significant improvement in the results of cadaver kidney transplantation with TDD. The effect of TDD may be due simply to a reduction in the number of circulating lymphocytes.

8–11 **Cyclosporin A and Steroid Therapy in 66 Cadaver Kidney Recipients.** Thomas E. Starzl, Göran B. G. Klintmalm, Richard Weil III, Kendrick A. Porter, Shunzaburo Iwatsuki, Gerhard P. J. Schroter, Carlos Fernandez-Bueno, and Neil MacHugh reviewed experience with cyclosporin A treatment in 66 consecutive recipients of 67 cadaveric renal homografts, who were followed up for 9–18 months. Mean age was 39 years. Transplants were primary in 57 patients. Average number of Mismatches at the HLA A and B loci was 3.3, and there were no perfect D matches in the 58 recipients studied. Many early

(8–11) Surg. Gynecol. Obstet. 153:486–494, October 1981.

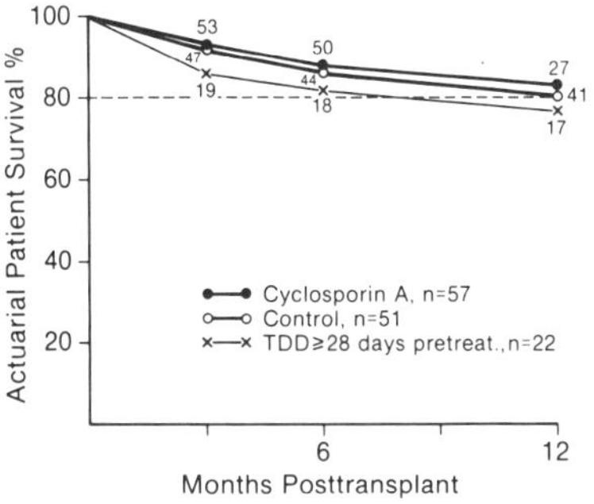

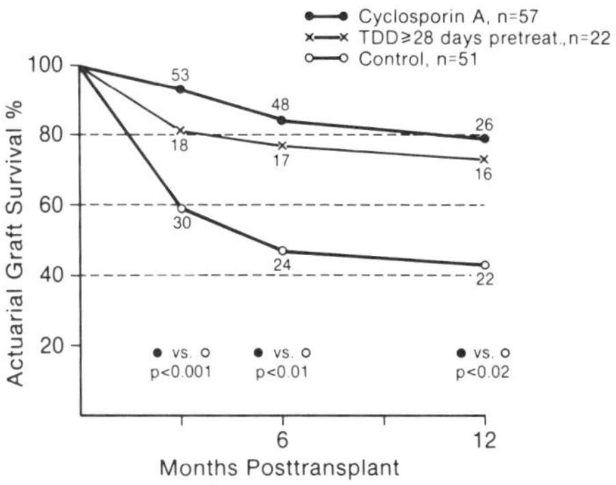

Fig 8–12 (left).—One-year actuarial patient survival of 57 recipients of primary grafts being treated with cyclosporin A and prednisone. Actual follow-up time is 9 to 18 months. Results are compared with actual 1-year patient survival when thoracic duct drainage preoperatively and postoperatively plus conventional immunosuppression and conventional immunosuppression alone were used. TDD = thoracic duct drainage.

Fig 8–13 (right).—One-year actuarial graft survival of 57 primary cadaveric grafts under treatment with cyclosporin A and prednisone are compared with actual 1-year survival of primary cadaveric kidneys under optimal treatment with thoracic duct drainage plus conventional immunosuppression and conventional immunosuppression alone. *P* values were derived with Student's t test.

(Courtesy of Starzl, T. E., et al.: Surg. Gynecol. Obstet. 153:486–494, October 1981.)

patients were pretreated by thoracic duct drainage, lymphapheresis, or cyclosporin A. Cyclosporin A, 17.5 mg/kg, was given daily starting the day of or the day before operation and was continued for 2 months if possible, when the dosage was reduced to 10 mg/kg daily. Prednisone was begun in an adult dose of 200 mg daily on the day of operation and reduced to 20 mg daily within a week after surgery.

Actuarial patient survival is shown in Figure 8–12 and actuarial graft survival, in Figure 8–13. After follow-up for 9–18 months, 80% of the primary grafts were supporting life. Six of 10 retransplants

Indications for Changing Patients From Cyclosporin A to Azathioprine

Patient No.	*Graft function prior to change, creatinine, mgm. per cent*	*Present graft function after change, creatinine, mgm. per cent*	*Time of change after transplant, mos.*	*Indication for therapeutic change*
2	2.3	2.5	13	Hepatotoxicity
3	3.1	1.4	8	Nephrotoxicity plus hepatotoxicity
9	3.6	Graft loss 2½ months later	6	Nephrotoxicity
12	4.6	2.8	4	Nephrotoxicity
14	3.6	2.1	10	Nephrotoxicity
21	3.6	Graft loss 2 weeks later	5	Nephrotoxicity

were functioning after 11–17 months. The results of changing from cyclosporin A to azathioprine in 6 cases are shown in the table. More than half of the surviving recipients have satisfactory and stable renal function. Only one deep wound infection occurred. Nephrotoxicity was suspected in 15 cases, but always decreased when the dose of cyclosporin A was lowered. Two patients had evidence of a lymphoproliferative reaction.

These results confirm the effectiveness and relative safety of cyclosporin A when used with low doses of steroids for immunosuppression in cadaver kidney recipients. Nephrotoxicity and other side effects usually could be managed by adjusting the dose of cyclosporin A. One patient developed a B cell immunoblastic sarcoma, which was not fatal and was associated with a rise in antibody to Epstein-Barr virus. Unless other side effects emerge, cyclosporin A should permit significant advances in whole organ transplantation.

▶ [The present results demonstrate excellent kidney survival when cyclosporin A is combined with steroids for the prevention of renal allograft rejection. These results follow the pioneering efforts by Calne using cyclosporin alone, adding prednisone when rejection episodes occurred. The innovation by Starzl and his group to combine cyclosporin A with prednisone has resulted in less cyclosporin A toxicity and fewer rejection episodes. We have used a similar technique in a randomized prospective study that thus far is incomplete. Nevertheless, cyclosporin A appears to be better than antilymphocyte globulin (ALG) and azathioprine in combination with prednisone because it diminishes hospital days and reduces infectious episodes while achieving excellent graft survival. Of the 50 patients who have received cyclosporin A and prednisone in the University of Minnesota series, only two have lost grafts because of rejection in the past 18 months. Although our results with ALG and azathioprine are almost as good, cyclosporin A appears to be easy to use and relatively nontoxic in the short term. The long-term toxicity, especially the suspicion that lymphoma may be more common in these patients, remains to be assessed. Starzl and his group have found, in the following article, that liver transplantation with prednisone and cyclosporin A is far superior to the use of ALG and azathioprine in these high-risk recipients.—J.S.N.] ◀

8–12 **Liver Transplantation With Use of Cyclosporin A and Prednisone.** Thomas E. Starzl, Göran B. G. Klintmalm, Kendrick A. Porter, Shunzaburo Iwatsuki and Gerhard P. J. Schröter report data on a trial of orthotopic liver transplantation in 14 patients aged 8–41 years; who were scheduled to receive cyclosporin A and prednisone. Ten of the 12 survivors who received the drugs are alive after 8–14½ months. Three survivors had chronic aggressive hepatitis and 3 had Budd-Chiari syndrome. Mismatches at the A and B loci in surviving patients averaged 3.3, and matches averaged 0.6. Treatment with cyclosporin A, 17.5 mg/kg/day intramuscularly or orally, was begun on the day of surgery. After 6–8 weeks the dosage was reduced to 10 mg/kg/day or less. The first few patients did not receive prednisone until rejection occurred; the others received either a low initial dose on the day of operation or, in adults, 200 mg on the day of operation with decreases of 40 mg/day for 4 days and a further decrease of 20 mg/day on day 5.

Improvement in actuarial survival over previous results is striking (Fig 8–14). All 10 surviving patients except 1 with recurrent Budd-

(8–12) N. Engl. J. Med. 305:266–269, July 30, 1981.

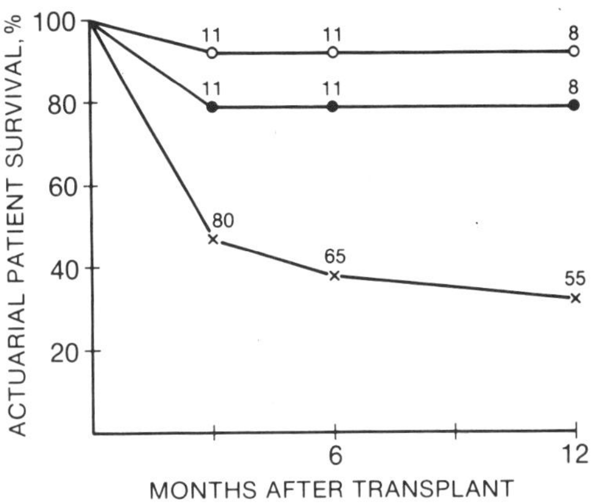

Fig 8–14.—One-year actuarial survival in patients given liver transplants. Follow-up ranged from 8 to 14½ months. Figures above symbols denote numbers of patients alive at different intervals. *Open circles,* survival in 12 patients who survived operation and were treated with cyclosporin A and prednisone; *solid circles,* survival in all 14 patients who underwent transplantation, including 2 who died during operation; *crosses,* survival in 170 patients from previous series who were treated with conventional immunosuppressants. (Courtesy of Starzl, T. E., et al.: N. Engl. J. Med.: 305:266–269, July 30, 1981.)

Chiari syndrome are living outside the hospital. The average postoperative hospital period was 75 days. Most patients have never received more than 20 mg of prednisone daily for longer than 5–6 days. Maintenance doses of cyclosporin A were dependent on abnormalities in renal function. Biopsies most commonly showed acute cellular rejection. Cellular rejection was always responsive to increased steroid administration.

Although the follow-up is short, it is not likely that the striking improvement in early results could be a coincidence. The results appear to be attributable to the use of cyclosporin A in combination with low doses of steroids for immunosuppression. Longer follow-up and more case studies will be needed to establish the safety and effectiveness of this approach to liver transplantation. The toxicity of cyclosporin A has not prevented its long-term use in all surviving patients, and no neoplasms have developed.

–13 **Rejection of Nerve Allografts After Cessation of Immunosuppression With Cyclosporin A.** Host nerve fibers are unable to regenerate through a long nerve allograft because of an immune response that destroys a viral component of the nerve such as the vasculature or the basement membrane of the Schwann cells. Zalewski and Silvers showed that a long nerve isograft could succeed if the recipient was rendered neonatally tolerant to the transplantation antigens of the donor. Andrew A. Zalewski and Adarsh K. Gulati (Natl. Inst. of Health) have now examined the effects of cyclosporin A on regeneration of host axons through a 4-cm nerve allograft in rats. Peroneal nerve grafts were carried out between strains differing at major and multiple minor histocompatibility loci. Study animals received cyclosporin A, 15 mg/kg, subcutaneously daily for 28 days.

(8–13) Transplantation 31:88–89, January 1981.

Six untreated rats had rejected allografts at 28 days, which were infiltrated by mononuclear cells. A large amount of unabsorbed myelin debris was present, and only a few axons were seen in the proximal 5 mm of the grafts. None of the grafts in 6 cyclosporin A-treated animals were rejected at 28 days. Cellular infiltration was absent from surviving grafts, and the perineural sheath was evident. Schwann cells were increased in number and had removed most degenerating myelin. Many host axons were found 2 to 3 cm into the allograft, and some had extended through the entire 4-cm distance. Many regenerated axons in the proximal half were myelinated. All nerve allografts, even those in cyclosporin A-treated animals, were rejected 88 days after surgery.

Cyclosporin A can prevent the rejection of nerve allografts bearing major and minor histocompatibility antigens. Short-term treatment with cyclosporin A did not, however, induce prolonged survival of or tolerance to a nerve allograft.

▶ [This article highlights several facts that have become clear about cyclosporin A immunosuppression. Despite early evidence that cyclosporin A might induce prolonged specific tolerance to the allografted tissue, most evidence now shows that cyclosporin A is a readily reversible immunosuppressive agent. As soon as the drug is stopped, rejection ensues. This has many advantages (i.e., in the treatment of infectious episodes during immunosuppression) but has some disadvantages. For example, the inability to absorb cyclosporin A in the midst of an immunosuppressive course can lead to rejection within days.—J.S.N.] ◀

8–14 **Renal Isotransplantation Without Immunosuppression.** Seventeen of 22 renal transplant recipients of kidneys from presumed identical twins in Boston had probable subacute or chronic glomerulonephritis, and 11 of them developed recurrent glomerulonephritis in their isotransplanted kidneys. Richard Weil, III, Thomas E. Starzl, Kendrick A. Porter, Michael Kershaw, Gerhard P. J. Schröter, and Lawrence J. Koep withheld immunosuppression from 4 recipients of identical twin kidney transplants. Three patients had chronic glomerulonephritis originally, and 1 had chronic pyelonephritis.

All 4 patients currently have good renal function, with serum creatinine values below 1.5 mg/dl, creatinine clearances of at least 60 ml per minute, and no proteinuria. Open biopsies showed normal grafts in 1 patient with chronic glomerulonephritis and the patient with pyelonephritis, but another patient had recurrent glomerulonephritis in the graft. This patient had been operated on 6 years before biopsy. The biopsy findings resembled the initial type 1 mesangiocapillary glomerulonephritis present in the patient's own kidneys. The patient's serum contained low amounts of total hemolytic complement but normal amounts of C3, Clq and C4 and no nephritic factor. The Clq binding assay showed the presence of immune complexes consisting of IgG, IgM and C3. Deoxyribonucleic acid binding was normal. The patient has no clinical evidence of infection. Cytomegalovirus was not found in the urine. The patient has had no proteinuria.

This experience, though limited, suggests that prophylactic immunosuppression is inappropriate for recipients of renal isografts. It seems

(8–14) Ann. Surg. 192:108–110, July 1980.

unlikely that these patients would have had a better clinical course with prophylactic immunosuppression. The possibility that host nephrectomy may reduce recurrences of glomerulonephritis is difficult to assess, as is the possible benefit of antibiotic prophylaxis, which was not used in these patients.

▶ [This is a useful article. Much has been made of the early experience of the Peter Bent Brigham Hospital, Boston, on the recurrence of renal disease in recipients of kidneys from identical twins. For this reason, it has become dogma that such patients require low levels of immunosuppressive agents to prevent the recurrence of glomerulonephritis. This limited experience suggests that this may not be true. The numbers here are small, and further studies are necessary in order finally to determine whether immunosuppression prevents the recurrence of disease in identical twin transplants.—J.S.N.] ◀

–15 **Epstein-Barr Virus-Related Serology in Marrow Transplant Recipients.** Persons with defective cell-mediated immunity can maintain high titers and a broad spectrum of antibodies to Epstein-Barr virus (EBV)-determined antigens, and oropharyngeal excretion of virus is increased in such patients. Beverly Lange, Werner Henle, Joel D. Meyers, Lily C. Yang, Charles August, Penelope Koch, Allan Arbeter, and Gertrude Henle investigated EBV-specific antibody patterns in 50 bone marrow transplant recipients, 34 male and 16 female. Median patient age was 16 years. All patients were given blood products in conjunction with HLA-matched bone marrow transplantation, and all received methotrexate for 100 days after transplantation.

In 28 cases, both the donor and recipient initially had anti-viral capsid antigen (VCA) titers of 1:5 or above. Eight other donors and 7 other recipients were anti-VCA positive with discordance between donor and recipient. All 15 seronegative bone marrow recipients had antibodies to VCA and EBV nuclear antigen (EBNA) in titers of 1:5 or above by the time of transplantation or within a few days afterward. Anti-VCA titers fell to low levels after the cessation of transfusions, and anti-EBNA titers usually became undetectable after 2–4 months. Endogenous antibody production then resumed, with anti-VCA increasing first and gradually reaching elevated titers, as a rule, followed eventually by the emergence of anti-early antigen-R or anti-early antigen-D in low to moderate titers. Finally anti-EBNA appeared in disproportionately low titers. There were no clinical or hematologic signs of EBV infection. Five of 8 patients followed up for over a year showed an exaggerated response to VCA.

Epstein-Barr virus does not cause significant clinical problems in bone marrow transplant recipients. These patients had the same exaggerated immune response to EBV as other immunodeficient patients. The pattern of EBV-specific antibodies may be a more sensitive measure of defective cell-mediated immunity than most conventional measures of immune function. Epstein-Barr virus may be causally related to the development of lymphoma, but only 1 lymphoma has been documented in a bone marrow transplant recipient.

▶ [The Epstein-Barr virus has been little studied after transplantation. Most studies have ruled out significant illness caused by this virus, whereas related viruses, such

(8–15) Int. J. Cancer 26:151–157, August 1980.

as herpes simplex virus, varicella-zoster virus, and cytomegalovirus (herpesviruses all) are responsible for many morbid complications after transplantation. This study is of that ilk, showing that Epstein-Barr virus is of little consequence to recipients of bone marrow transplantation. Unfortunately, considerable evidence is growing that Epstein-Barr virus is the cause of the unfortunately common (0.7% of transplant recipients) posttransplant lymphoma. Posttransplant lymphoma appears to be either a polyclonal or a monoclonal lymphoproliferative disorder, and the Epstein-Barr virus nuclear antigen is present in these cells. In addition, RNA and DNA hybridization studies have shown the Epstein-Barr virus genome to be present in the human tumor cells. Therefore, any declaration of innocence for the Epstein-Barr virus will require long-term follow-up and much more careful study.—J.S.N.] ◀

8–16 **Azathioprine-Induced Leukopenia: Clinical Significance in Renal Transplantation.** A number of factors may promote the development of leukopenia after renal transplantation. Raymond Pollak, Reid A. Nishikawa, Martin F. Mozes, and Olga Jonasson (Univ. of Illinois, Chicago) examined the occurrence of azathioprine-induced leukopenia (AIL) following renal transplantation in a series of 173 consecutive renal allografts performed in 1973–1977. The azathioprine protocol was 5 mg/kg/day for 3 days, 4 mg/kg/day for 4 days, and 2.0–2.5 mg/kg/day thereafter as tolerated. Dosage was reduced by half in patients with a serum creatinine level greater than 3 mg/dl. Methylprednisolone was given for 3 days, and prednisone was given in maintenance doses of about 20 mg/day for 6 months and 15 mg/day thereafter. Azathioprine-induced leukopenia was defined by a white blood cell count of 5,000/cu mm or below in the absence of other factors causing leukopenia and necessitated a reduction in the dose of azathioprine of at least 25%.

Of 154 evaluable patients with 160 renal transplants, 25% developed AIL an average of 3 weeks after transplantation. All episodes occurred within 8 weeks. The disorder was most frequent in cadaver kidney recipients. Poor early renal function commonly was associated with AIL, especially in cadaver kidney recipients. Pretransplant splenectomy significantly reduced the occurrence of AIL. Over half of patients with poor early renal function who did not undergo splenectomy developed AIL. In cadaver kidney recipients, AIL was associated with significantly reduced graft survival at 3 and 6 months. Graft survival also was reduced in related-donor kidney recipients with AIL. Graft survival at 1 year in cadaver kidney recipients who had been splenectomized was not related to AIL.

One fourth of renal transplant recipients in this series developed AIL. Splenectomy reduces the risk of early leukopenia and AIL. Azathioprine-induced leukopenia is associated with decreased allograft survival and patient survival, regardless of the donor source.

▶ [This is an interesting study on two accounts. First, more evidence is presented here that splenectomy decreases the incidence of leukopenia, which, in turn, is associated with a higher incidence of graft loss. It is likely that the leukopenia leads to cessation of immunosuppression so that patients who are not splenectomized develop leukopenia and therefore receive lesser amounts of immunosuppression. The randomized prospective study of splenectomy by Fryd et al. (*Transplant Proc.* 13:48–56, 1981) demonstrate similar phenomena. Second, lymphopenia is much more common in nonsplenectomized patients and is much more commonly associated with

(8–16) J. Surg. Res. 29:258–264, September 1980.

azathioprine toxicity alone. In splenectomized patients, leukopenia is unusual and is most often associated with cytomegalovirus. The problem of a virus-induced leukopenia on the background of bone marrow suppression by azathioprine should certainly be considered here.—J.S.N.] ◀

8–17 **Long-Term Study of Vascularized Free-Draining Intraperitoneal Pancreatic Segmental Allografts in Beagle Dogs.** Heterotopic intraperitoneal implantation of the immediately vascularized, free-draining distal pancreatic segment (FDPS) is technically feasible. George K. Kyriakides, Alexander Rabinovitch, Daniel Mintz, Les Olson, Felix T. Rapaport, and Joshua Miller performed long-term studies of FDPS allografts in beagle dogs with defined histocompatibilities. Donor and recipient dogs were typed for leukocyte antigens (DLA) and tested by mixed lymphocyte culture (MLC). Recipients were made diabetic by total pancreatectomy and were immediately implanted intraperitoneally with an FDPS allograft. Some recipients were immunosuppressed with prednisone and azathioprine. Others were made specifically unresponsive by total body radiation, autologous bone marrow transplantation, and renal transplantation from DLA-MLC-identical donors done a year before FDPS transplantation from the original kidney donors.

Immunosuppressed high-MLC reactors rejected their FDPS grafts in 1–2 weeks, while low-MLC reactors accepted grafts for 25 to over 260 days. Nonimmunosuppressed low-MLC reactors accepted grafts for 9–55 days. Rejection was sudden, permanent, and unpredictable by glucose tolerance testing. Increases in cell-mediated lymphocytotoxicity (CML) were observed before graft rejection in low-MLC reactors. Both CML and MLC responses were reduced before rejection in high-MLC reactors. Graft survival for over 6 months was observed in the dogs made specifically unresponsive, despite low-grade MLC reactivity and CML responses. Biopsy specimens of grafts in normoglycemic dogs showed disappearance of exocrine tissue by 6 months and coalescence of islets. Less fibrosis was seen in immunosuppressed animals.

Immunogenetic disparities remain the chief factors in the outcome of FDPS allograft transplantation. Allograft rejection appears to be an all-or-none phenomenon. Recipients that accept allografts, however, have normal glucose tolerance and insulin secretion several months after transplantation. The use of diabetogenic steroids has not proved deleterious in either dogs or human recipients of FDPS allografts.

▶ [This and the following four articles all relate to the problems of pancreatic transplantation. It is clear from animal studies that careful control of the diabetes can diminish the incidence and severity of secondary diabetic complications such as retinopathy, renal failure, and neuropathy. Pancreatic transplantation, therefore, takes on a new urgency, and the old problems (What do you do with the pancreatic duct?) require a solution. Kyriakides has pioneered in the use of an open intraperitoneal duct technique that is highly successful in pigs and dogs, and his group documents the long-term success in this study. When this technique is attempted in human beings, too often ascites is produced, although a 4-year survivor of pancreatic transplantation that used this technique is currently cured of diabetes. Unfortunately, a fairly high

---

(8–17) J. Clin. Invest. 67:292–303, January 1981.

incidence of graft removal was required to control the ascites in other patients. At least with current techniques, Kyriakides' important work does not seem applicable to most human pancreas transplants.—J.S.N.] ◀

8–18 **Pancreas and Islet Transplantation: II. Clinical Trials** are reviewed by D. E. R. Sutherland (Univ. of Minnesota). Most recipients of pancreas transplants have far-advanced complications of diabetes and are at high risk of complications of transplantation and immunosuppression. An advantage of operating on patients who have, or will require, a kidney transplant is that the risks of immunosuppression are obligatory. The technique of segmental pancreas transplantation is illustrated in Figure 8–15. The use of duct-obliterated segmental grafts has been the most successful method of pancreas transplantation. Intraperitoneal placement or omentoplasty permits residual secretions to be absorbed and is associated with the fewest nonimmunologic graft losses. Of 118 patients having 128 pancreas allotransplants between 1966 and 1980, 15 have functioning grafts and are insulin independent, 4 for over a year. Three others were insulin independent for at least a year. Thirty patients died with functioning grafts, and 30 grafts failed for purely technical reasons. It appears that the procedure may prevent the progress of early lesions and that regression is possible.

Islet transplantation is an attractive alternative, but attempts at clinical application have largely failed. The optimal conditions for digestion of human pancreatic tissue cannot necessarily be extrapo-

Fig 8–15.—Segmental pancreas transplantation. Body and tail are transplanted with anastomoses of splenic vessels of donor pancreas to iliac vessels of recipient. (Courtesy of Sutherland, D. E. R.: Diabetologia 20:435–450, April 1981; Berlin-Heidelberg-New York: Springer.)

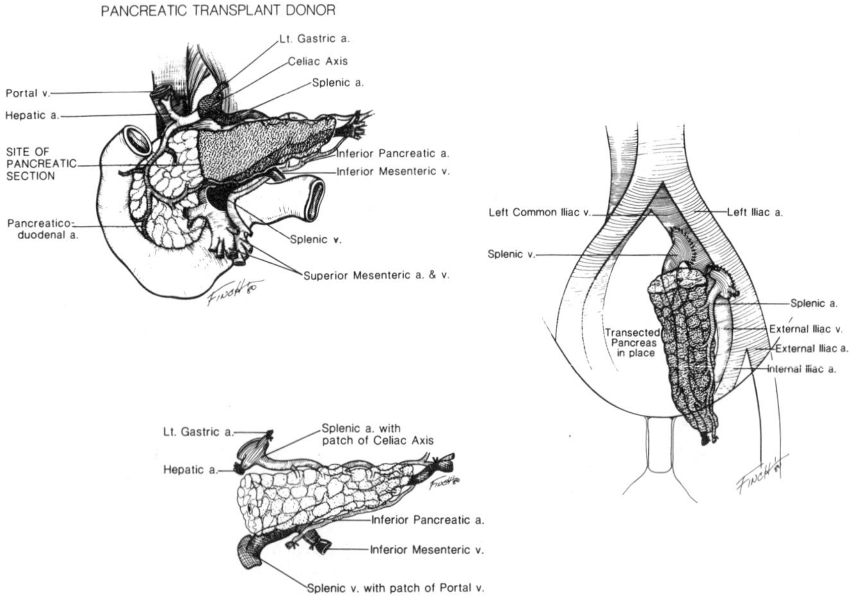

(8–18) Diabetologia 20:435–450, April 1981.

lated from animal studies because of the more fibrous nature of the human pancreas. Only 4 of 74 attempts in the past decade have been followed by long-term withdrawal of exogenous insulin therapy. Islet allografting may fail for immunologic reasons, but failures of islet autografting are clearly technical. The success rates of both islet allotransplantation and islet autotransplantation probably will remain low until more effective means are developed of preparing islets from adult pancreata. For allografting, advances will be required in immunosuppression or in ways of altering islet graft immunogenicity.

Pancreas transplantation could be used at present to treat selected diabetics, who could return to insulin therapy if rejection occurs. This approach should be considered for diabetic renal allograft recipients and for nonuremic patients with advancing retinopathy and neuropathy. Ways are needed of identifying patients early whose diabetes cannot be controlled adequately by insulin and who will develop progressive complications. Enough donor pancreata should be available for treatment of these patients.

▶ [Sutherland here reviews, in the second part of a two-part article, the entire world's literature on pancreatic transplantation. In this article and the following one, he points out two clinical techniques that appear to yield good success. In the first, a segmental graft is drained into a Roux-en-Y jejunal segment. This works best in patients who have not been immunosuppressed previously and whose wound healing, consequently, is not impaired. The second technique is the injection into the duct of silicone rubber, or a related substance, which appears to inhibit pancreatic exocrine function while having lesser effects on pancreatic endocrine function. The institution of cyclosporin A into prophylactic immunosuppression, with a consequent reduction in the need for antilymphocyte globulin, azathioprine, and prednisone, may be an important factor in the pancreatic transplant success currently being observed at the University of Minnesota.—J.S.N.] ◀

8–19 **Segmental Pancreas Transplantation From Living Related and Cadaver Donors: Clinical Experience.** David E. R. Sutherland, Frederick C. Goetz, John J. Rynasiewicz, Dieter Baumgartner, David C. White, Barbara A. Elick, and John S. Najarian (Univ. of Minnesota) performed 20 segmental pancreas transplants from 14 cadaver and 6 related donors in 1978–1981. All 19 recipients had had insulin-dependent diabetes for 12–31 years, and all but 2 had previously received renal allografts for end-stage diabetic nephropathy. Grafts were placed intraperitoneally, 13 with open ducts, 4 with prolamine-injected ducts, and 3 with silicone rubber-injected ducts. Immunosuppression was achieved with azathioprine and prednisone and, in some cases, antilymphocyte globulin and cyclosporin A.

Six patients were normoglycemic at follow-up, with functioning grafts and no need for exogenous insulin. All but 1 of the other patients had a rise in C-peptide levels and normal or nearly normal plasma glucose levels and were insulin independent for up to 4 months after surgery. One patient had the graft removed after 1 day because of venous thrombosis. Three grafts were removed while functioning, while 9 functioned for 1–4 months after transplantation. No symptoms were associated with loss of graft function. Cadaver grafts removed several months after loss of function exhibited thrombosed vessels and fibro-

(8–19) Surgery 90:159–169, August 1981.

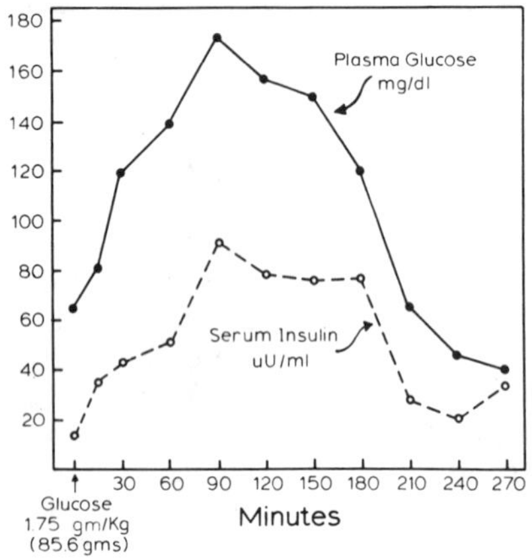

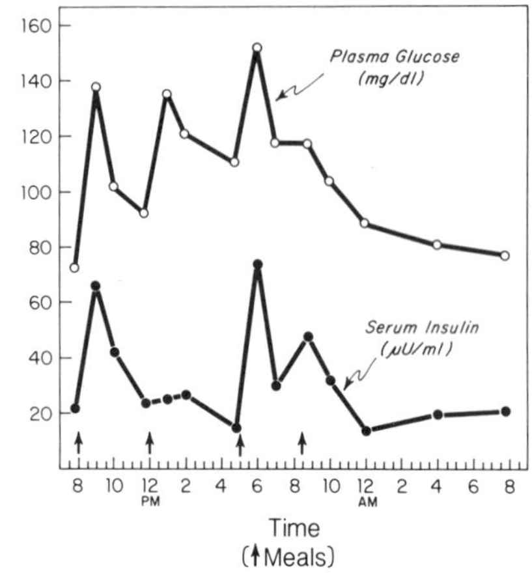

Fig 8–16 (left).—Oral glucose tolerance test results 2 years after pancreas transplantation.
Fig 8–17 (right).—A 24-hour metabolic profile 2 years after pancreas transplantation.
(Courtesy of Sutherland, D. E. R., et al.: Surgery 90:159–169, August 1981.)

sis, with no recognizable endocrine or exocrine tissue present. The metabolic findings in 1 recipient are shown in Figures 8–16 and 8–17. All but 1 of the 6 living related donors had normal glucose tolerance and metabolic profiles; the exception was an obese subject.

Segmental pancreas transplantation is a safe and often very effective treatment for selected diabetics. The limiting factor is allograft rejection. At present, the procedure is indicated only in patients whose diabetic complications are or predictably will be greater than those concomitant upon the immunosuppression required to prevent graft rejection. It would be desirable to perform transplantation early in the course of diabetes, before lesions develop, but this probably is not justified until specific immunosuppression is possible in human beings.

8–20 **Transplantation of Insulin-Producing Tissue.** Paul E. Lacy, Joseph M. Davie, and Edward H. Finke (Washington Univ., St. Louis) report new findings that show the possibility of preventing rejection of thyroid and islet transplants in animals without continued use of immunosuppressive agents in recipients. Thyroid allograft survival has been prolonged by in vitro culture of the thyroid in the presence of 95% oxygen before transplantation. Islet allograft survival was prolonged for more than 100 days by in vitro culture of the islets at 24 C for 7 days before transplantation and using a single injection of rat antilymphocyte serum at transplantation.

Injection of donor peritoneal exudate cells at the time of transplantation induces immune rejection of transplants of cultured thyroids. Rejection of established islet allografts from 100 to 200 days after transplantation can be induced by administration of donor peritoneal exudate cells and donor T lymphocytes. Donor B lymphocytes did not induce rejection of established islet allografts, however.

Apparently the pretreatment regimens used to prolong allograft

(8–20) Am. J. Med. 70:589–594, March 1981.

survival either alter or destroy passenger leukocytes in the grafts. These cells appear to be necessary for induction of immune recognition of the grafts by the recipient. Islet cells in mice express products of the H-2K and H-2D loci, but the cells do not express the I region (Ia) antigens. The presence of H-2K or H-2D antigens would permit recognition of the islet cells as targets after immune rejection was initiated. The lack of Ia antigens may be responsible for the inability of islet cells to induce their own rejection.

The techniques used to prolong thyroid and islet allograft survival also will prolong xenograft survival. Survival of transplants of rat thyroids into mice has been prolonged by in vitro culture of the rat thyroid in 95% oxygen. Survival of rat islets transplanted into diabetic mice has been prolonged more than 100 days by using low-temperature culture of rat islets with a single injection of antiserums to mouse and rat lymphocytes at the time of transplantation. These developments raise questions regarding whether such approaches may be applicable to transplantation of islets into diabetic human beings and also to transplantation of other organs.

▶ [In this study, the St. Louis group has been trying to eliminate alloimmunogeneic tissue from the compound islet allograft. The thinking here is that if various components of the major histocompatibility complex are eliminated, graft rejection will be alleviated. Because the major problem in islet transplantation appears to be the sensitivity of this tissue to minimal amounts of alloimmune function, this work may be of pioneering importance. Both culturing islet tissue and exposing it to anti-Ia antiserum appear to eliminate the blood component of the major histocompatibility complex responsible for the amplification of the immune response (i.e., lymphocyte proliferation) and thereby seems to inhibit the development of immunity to the islet grafts. This appears to be important work and derives directly from basic laboratory research in vitro.—J.S.N.] ◀

8–21 **Prolongation of Murine Islet Allograft Survival by Pretreatment of Islets With Antibody Directed to Ia Determinants.** The survival of islet allografts and xenografts is prolonged by in vitro culture before transplantation, and it has been suggested that organ culture removes the passenger lymphoid cells required for immune rejection. Denise Faustman, Věra Hauptfeld, Paul Lacy, and Joseph Davie (Washington Univ., St. Louis) found that brief treatment of islets with donor-specific Ia antiserums and complement in vitro permits transplantation across major histocompatibility barriers without immunosuppressive therapy of the recipient. Studies with isografts and allografts were performed on mice with streptozotocin-induced diabetes.

Transplantation of isologous islets into the portal vein of diabetic mice resulted in return of the plasma glucose level to normal within a week. Most untreated allografts were acutely rejected, but transplantation of allografts treated with anti-I^k serum and complement resulted in graft survival exceeding 200 days in all animals. The use of an anti-I^k serum produced in different strain combinations also resulted in allograft survival. The nonimmunosuppressed recipients became normoglycemic 10 days after transplantation. Treatment of islets with anti-I^s antiserum and complement did not alter the rapid rejection of 60% of allografts. Animals with established allografts that

(8–21) Proc. Natl. Acad. Sci. USA 78:5156–5159, August 1981.

received lymphoid cells intravenously exhibited prompt rejection of the islets.

Pretreatment of allogeneic mouse islets with donor-specific Ia antiserum and complement prevents their immune rejection in nonimmunosuppressed recipients for at least 200 days. The findings support a possible role for Ia-positive passenger lymphoid cells in the initiation of immune rejection. Immunosuppression of the recipient is not necessary for successful islet transplantation. The prevention of immune rejection by brief pretreatment of grafts with antiserums is an attractive method potentially applicable to a variety of organs.

8–22 **Clinical and Immunologic Effects of Fractionated Total Lymphoid Irradiation in Refractory Rheumatoid Arthritis.** Total lymphoid irradiation has immunosuppressive effects, and there is substantial evidence that sensitized lymphocytes contribute to synovial inflammation in rheumatoid arthritis. David E. Trentham, James A. Belli, Ronald J. Anderson, Judith A. Buckley, Edward J. Goetzl, John R. David, and K. Frank Austen (Boston) evaluated total lymphoid irradiation as a potential alternative to cyclophosphamide therapy in 10 patients with classic rheumatoid arthritis. The 9 women and 1 man had a mean age of 61 years, and had had rheumatoid arthritis for a mean of 11 years. Nine had functional class III involvement and 1, class IV. All patients had persistent involvement of multiple joints and roentgenographic evidence of erosion and progressive joint deformity. All previous treatments had failed to induce remission. A total of 3,000 rad of fractionated total lymphoid irradiation was delivered to each of three regions over 3 to 3½ weeks.

Objective evidence of improvement was obtained in 8 of 10 cases. The response usually began during irradiation of the para-aortic and splenic portal. Decreased joint swelling was noted at 6 months in 7 of 9 patients, but synovitis returned within a year after completion of treatment in all 6 patients followed up for 17 to 21 months. A temporary response of reduction or disappearance of subcutaneous nodules also was observed. Reductions in prednisone dosage were possible for 8 months after the completion of irradiation. Acute reactions were similar to those seen in patients treated for Hodgkin's disease. A marked absolute lymphopenia was induced by irradiation in all patients, with counts returning to normal within a year. In vitro lymphocyte functions were temporarily abrogated in responsive patients. Abnormal antibody responses were not suppressed by lymphoid irradiation.

Eight of 10 patients with refractory rheumatoid arthritis in this study responded objectively to total lymphoid irradiation in conjunction with decreased lymphocyte numbers and reactivities. These preliminary findings suggest that total lymphoid irradiation has an anti-inflammatory effect on rheumatoid arthritis. Most patients had a significant increase in functional capacity. Recurrent active joint disease was substantially less intense than before irradiation. Controlled trials are needed to determine whether total lymphoid irradiation can alter the natural history of rheumatoid arthritis.

(8–22) N. Engl. J. Med. 305:976–982, Oct. 22, 1981.

▶ [The past few years have seen renewed attempts at the clinical manipulation of the immune response with the use of such agents as thoracic duct drainage, cyclosporin A, splenectomy, and total lymphoid irradiation. Total lymphoid irradiation appears to be strongly immunosuppressive and to reduce T cell function. Minimal levels for long periods of time, even without the use of bone marrow transfusion, are highly successful with second transplants to patients who had rejected their first transplant with unusual vigor. Such patients are generally at high risk to reject the second transplant, but in our series at the University of Minnesota, more than 70% of recipients of total lymphoid irradiation who previously rejected their first transplant are currently functioning more than 2 years later with the second transplant. In this study, the usefulness of total lymphoid radiation in the prevention of refractory rheumatoid arthritis is shown, suggesting the important role of continued T cell activity in that disease as well.

Total lymphoid irradiation has, however, many disadvantages in transplantation. The principal one is that the immunosuppression is relatively permanent, so excess immunosuppression can be administered inadvertently. The second problem is of timing the irradiation to coincide with cadaver allograft acquisition, a difficult balancing problem because posttransplant radiation seems not to be well tolerated. Total lymphoid irradiation appears to be associated with a slightly higher incidence of lymphoma, although this is not clear, due to the relatively few patients who have received this treatment and the fact that they had received other immunosuppressive drugs as well.—J.S.N.] ◀

8–23 **Specific Allogeneic Unresponsiveness in Irradiated Dogs Reconstituted With Autologous Bone Marrow** is described by F. T. Rapaport, R. J. Bachvaroff, N. Akiyama, T. Sato, and J. W. Ferrebee (SUNY at Stony Brook). The production of unresponsiveness to transplanted foreign tissues without interference with remaining host immunologic defense mechanisms is a central goal of transplantation. The combined use of total body irradiation and bone marrow transplantation has been shown to induce allogeneic unresponsiveness in adult recipients. Later, transplantation of bone marrow into supralethally irradiated dogs produced long-term individual-specific unresponsiveness to various allografts obtained from the bone marrow donor. The clinical applicability of this observation has been hampered by the high incidence of graft-vs.-host complications associated with bone marrow allotransplantation.

Studies performed with selectively bred dogs uncovered an intriguing exception to the high incidence of such graft-vs.-host complications. Transplantation of allogeneic marrow into irradiated recipients bearing DLA-identical haplotypes derived from the same ancestors as the donors produced long-term chimerism, with no evidence of graft-vs.-host reactions. Further studies suggested the immediate postirradiation and bone marrow replacement period constituted a special, privileged period of immunologic reactivity, during which the host was more likely to react to antigenic challenge by development of unresponsiveness rather than sensitization. A corollary to this hypothesis was the possibility that autologous marrow replacement might be as effective as allogeneic marrow in the induction of unresponsiveness during this privileged period of immunologic ductility.

One hundred consecutive long-term experiments designed to test this possibility showed that hemopoietic reconstitution of supralethally irradiated adult dogs with their own stored bone marrow can

---

(8–23) Transplantation 30:23–30, July 1980.

produce long-term unresponsiveness to DLA-identical kidney allografts with no need for any additional immunosuppression. Eleven of 18 kidneys transplanted 12 hours after replacement of autologous marrow into irradiated recipients have survived with normal function for at least 1,417 days. Eight of 13 organs transplanted 28 hours after marrow replacement, and 8 of 13 organs transplanted 36 hours after marrow injection, have survived at least 502 days, with no further treatment. Alterations in the timing and sequence of each procedure decreased the incidence of unresponsiveness. Implantation of kidney allografts 20 hours before removal of marrow, followed by irradiation and marrow reconstitution, produced unresponsiveness in only 3 of 21 dogs. Kidneys transplanted at the time of marrow replacement were tolerated in 4 of 16 irradiated recipients. When kidneys were placed into irradiated dogs and an interval of 40 hours was provided before marrow reconstitution, only 5 of 19 animals became unresponsive.

Of 12 renal allograft-unresponsive dogs that received skin grafts from the respective kidney donors, 5 were unresponsive to such skin allografts and 7 rejected the skin grafts within 115 days. Second-, third-, and fourth-set skin grafts from the kidney donor were rejected in a progressively more rapid fashion. Survival and function of the kidney allografts were not affected by the rejection of successive skin grafts from the kidney donor. Skin grafts from other DLA-identical donors and DLA-incompatible skin grafts were rejected by the same recipients in uniform fashion.

▶ [Irradiation still may be useful in other ways. Total lymphoid irradiation reduces some of the areas of irradiation and therefore may be more tolerable than total body irradiation. Nevertheless, total body irradiation and reconstitution of the host with bone marrow cells, presumably deficient in T cell precursors, may result in prolongation in grafts between animals who differ at minor histocompatibility loci, as in these pioneering studies. The disadvantage here is that only weak histocompatibility loci can be breached in this way.—J.S.N.] ◀

8–24 **Immunogenicity of Human Amniotic Epithelial Cells After Transplantation Into Volunteers.** Amniotic epithelium has been used successfully as a graft to replace deficient tissue, cover open wounds, and improve the vascularity of ischemic legs, but there is no objective evidence for survival of the implants. C. A. Akle, M. Adinolfi, K. I. Welsh, S. Leibowitz, and I. McColl (Guy's Hosp. and Med. School, London) have examined the survival and immunogenicity of amniotic epithelial membrane implants in 7 volunteer subjects, 6 men and 1 woman aged 28 to 80 years. Implants of amniotic epithelium obtained in elective sections were placed in subcutaneous pockets for periods of 16 to 54 days.

No evidence of acute reaction was obtained in any of the 7 patients. Nodules developed in 2 patients, in 1 of them at the time a rash developed after ampicillin therapy. Amniotic cells were identified by immunofluorescence in all biopsies. Newly formed connective tissue and a granulomatous reaction were observed, as well as an infiltrate of chronic inflammatory cells with small numbers of eosinophils. There

(8–24) Lancet 2:1003–1005, Nov. 7, 1981.

was no evidence of vasculitis or necrosis, and no polymorphonuclear cells were present. None of the 4 subjects tested shared HLA B or HLA DR antigens with the mother; therefore they were incompatible with at least one HLA B and one HLA DR antigen of the child. Three of the 4 were also incompatible with at least one HLA A antigen of the child. None of the 4 had evidence of cytotoxic antibody production. Cytotoxic cells were not formed when amniotic epithelial cells were co-cultured with allogeneic lymphocytes 2 months after implantation. No specific staining occurred when serums from these volunteers were tested by immunofluorescence against the amniotic epithelial cells, but the epithelial cells continued to stain with specific immune serum even after 12 weeks in culture.

The results suggest that acute immune rejection does not occur after transplantation of human amniotic epithelial cells. Further studies are needed to determine whether these cells can be transplanted successfully without immunosuppression to patients with appropriate inborn metabolic errors.

▶ [There has been considerable interest in recent years in varying degrees of tissue immunogenicity. Certain tissues have been found to be deficient in one or another of the components of the major histocompatibility locus, i.e., islet cells seem to be deficient in Ia antigens. This article tends to reinforce this concept. Although the proper selection of tissue to be transplanted may greatly influence the chances of survival by appropriate manipulations, the use of such tissues to correct inborn errors of metabolism can now be considered.—J.S.N.] ◀

9. Oncology and Tumor Immunology

9-1 **Clinical Correlations With Drug Sensitivities in the Clonogenic Assay: Retrospective Study.** Hamburger and Salmon developed an in vitro assay in which human tumor stem cells are cloned in agar, and a high correlation was seen between the in vitro results and clinical responses of ovarian cancer and multiple myeloma. Barry D. Mann, David H. Kern, Armando E. Giuliano, Martyn W. Burk, Mary Ann Campbell, Larry R. Kaiser, and Donald L. Morton correlated the results of colony inhibition in the clonogenic assay (CLAS) with clinical responses to chemotherapy in 32 patients with primary and metastatic cancer. Nineteen patients had melanoma, and 5 had sarcomas. The drugs used in the assay included doxorubicin hydrochloride, bleomycin sulfate, carmustine, decarbazine, fluorouracil, methotrexate sodium, mitomycin, melphalan, cisplatin, and vinblasttine sulfate.

The CLAS predicted tumor sensitivity in 11 of 37 assays, and 9 of these 11 patients had evidence of clinical responsiveness. In 26 assays the CLAS predicted tumor resistance based on less than 75% inhibition of colony growth by the drug concentration tested, and in only 1 of these instances was there evidence of a clinical response to the drug. Of the 9 patients with true positive results, 5 had metastatic melanoma with subcutaneous metastases, 2 had gastric carcinoma, and 1 each had ovarian cancer and a limb sarcoma. The probability of a positive correlation when the CLAS predicted tumor sensitivity was .82, and the probability of a correct correlation when it predicted tumor resistance was .96. The overall association between in vitro and in vivo findings was highly significant.

The CLAS is of value in predicting clinical responses to chemotherapy in patients with multiple myeloma and ovarian cancer, and in patients with a variety of solid tumors. Accurate predictions of chemosensitivity have been obtained in patients with hepatoma and carcinomas of the stomach, breast, and colon. This approach may have great value for individualizing treatment in cancer patients and in avoiding toxicity from ineffective drugs.

▶ [One of the potentially most important findings of the past few years was the finding by Salmon and Hamburger and their associates (*N. Engl. J. Med.* 298:1321–1327, 1978) that clones of tumor cells could be established in soft agar and that such colonies could be the basis for chemotherapeutic assays. In this way, studies similar to sensitivity studies of antibiotics against microbes might be carried out using chemotherapeutic agents acting against cloned tumor cells. Although ovarian tumors and multiple myeloma were studied initially, this is the first study to use the solid tumors seen by surgeons. This report demonstrates that the sensitivity of these assays is great. In particular, the negative correlation is impressive. Tumors that do not respond in vitro tend not to respond in vivo, which permits the selection of appropriate

(9–1) Arch. Surg. 117:33–36, January 1982.

chemotherapeutic agents. Clearly, these results require further confirmation and dissemination so that clonogenic assays can be established within many of the institutions where both surgical and chemotherapeutic modalities are available. There are problems, however, and it is not always possible to establish human tumor stem cells in agar, but the opportunity must be taken.—J.S.N.] ◀

9–2 **Improving the Therapeutic Index in Breast Cancer Treatment** is discussed by Samuel Hellman (Harvard Med. School). A major goal of all cancer therapy is to improve the relationship between the desired and adverse effects of treatment. At the molecular level, an obvious way to gain a therapeutic advantage is by increasing the specificity with which toxic agents are delivered to tumor cells compared with normal cells. Molecular studies have used ^{125}I-tamoxifen as a specific cytotoxic agent for cells containing estrogen receptors, which bind the agent and transport it into the nucleus where its limited-range radiations are cytotoxic. Murine marrow stem cells have varying potential for self-renewal, and chemotherapeutic agents used in the treatment of breast cancer have different effects on these cells. While L-phenylalanine mustard is toxic to the most primitive stem cells and produces a permanent stem cell self-renewal deficit, cyclophosphamide and 5-fluorouracil act chiefly on later stem cells and do not result in proliferative impairment.

The purpose of combining radiotherapy and tumor excision is to eliminate breast cancer while preserving normal structure and function. The results are comparable with those obtained by mastectomy without loss of the breast or chest musculature. The acute effects of irradiation can be minimized by allowing sufficient time between fractions and reducing the size of each fraction to permit adequate proliferation and cellular repair. Selective radiotherapy is enhanced by computer-assisted tomographic scanning. Close cooperation between the surgeon and radiotherapist is necessary to remove gross tumor without distorting the breast, permitting a more moderate dose of radiation to be effective. Adjuvant therapy has improved the relapse-free survival rate and also has enhanced local control in patients with advanced disease. There is little overlapping toxicity with radiotherapy and chemotherapy. Hopefully, both increased survival and preservation of function and structure will result from the combined use of limited surgery, radiotherapy with both external beam and interstitial techniques, and adjuvant chemotherapy when indicated.

▶ [Hellman has made numerous contributions toward the radiotherapeutic treatment of early carcinoma of the breast. As it becomes increasingly apparent that cancer is a systemic as well as a local disease, multimodality control of the primary disease gains rationale. It is becoming clear that limited operation for debulking and staging is approximately as good as radical surgical therapy for disease in the breast. The detailed rationale for this approach is summarized in this article.—J.S.N.] ◀

9–3 **Conservative Surgery and Postoperative Radiotherapy in 300 Adults With Soft Tissue Sarcomas.** Radical surgery was once considered the only effective treatment of soft tissue sarcomas, but conservative surgery and postoperative radiation therapy now are being

---

(9–2) Cancer Res. 40:4335–4342, December 1980.
(9–3) Cancer 47:2391–2397, May 15, 1981.

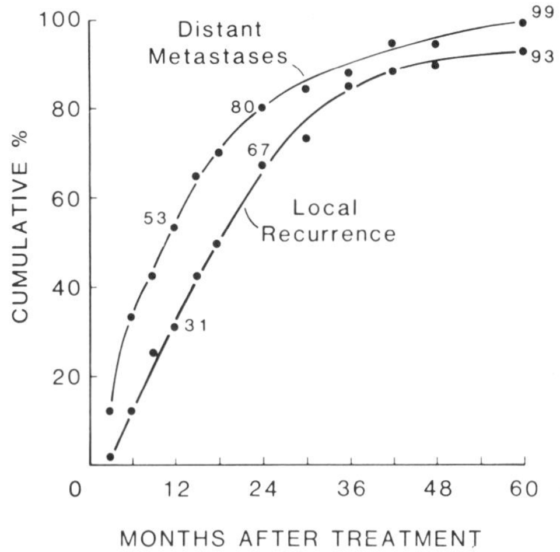

Fig 9–1.—Soft tissue sarcoma, 1963 through 1977; local recurrence versus distant metastases, unlimited follow-up. (Courtesy of Lindberg, R. D., et al.: Cancer 47:2391–2397, May 15, 1981.)

tried in an attempt to preserve limb function. Robert D. Lindberg, Richard G. Martin, Marvin M. Romsdahl, and H. Thomas Barkley, Jr. (Univ. of Texas System Cancer Center, M. D. Anderson Hosp. and Tumor Inst., Houston) reviewed the results of conservative excision and postoperative radiation therapy in 300 adults seen in 1963–1977 with soft tissue sarcoma and no evidence of distant disease at admission. The gross tumor mass usually was simply "shelled out," or removed with a limited amount of normal tissue, and conventional radiation therapy was begun when healing was complete, usually 3–4 weeks after excision. Currently, low-grade lesions are treated with 6,000 rad delivered over 6 weeks, and intermediate- and high-grade lesions are treated with 6,500 rad delivered over 6½ weeks.

The average patient age was 45.2 years. The absolute 2-year disease-free survival rate was 74%. Eighteen of these patients had a recurrence at the primary site but were salvaged by subsequent surgery. Cumulative rates of local and distant disease are shown in Figure 9–1. Eighty-one patients developed distant metastases, the most common initial site being the lungs. Distant disease appeared earlier than local recurrences. Determinate disease-free survival correlated with the stage of disease, and generally with the grade and size of lesions. Most patients had some fibrosis in the irradiated region. Three had soft tissue necrosis, 2 had fractures in the treated area, and 2 had nerve damage. Only 1 patient had a vascular complication.

About 85% of patients in this series with soft tissue sarcoma of the extremity had a functional limb after treatment. The absolute disease-free survival at 5 years exceeded 60%. The low rate of nodal disease at the first evidence of distant spread does not warrant elective treatment of the regional lymphatics. The rate of significant complications in lesions in the extremities is low, and it can be reduced by careful treatment planning.

▶ [This and the following article represent continuing attempts at limb salvage utilizing conservative therapy for sarcoma in conjunction with radiotherapy or chemotherapy, or both. The two articles demonstrate that these modalities are useful alternatives to radical surgical therapy for soft tissue sarcoma. Although it generally is stated that most sarcomas behave alike, one should note carefully the high incidence of recurrence for neurofibrosarcoma or malignant fibrohistiocytoma when compared with liposarcoma, fibrosarcoma, and rhabdomyosarcoma. These differences may or may not prove to be of long-term significance, but local recurrence is a serious problem that is more often than not correlated with distant recurrence as well. The proper selection of the surgical approach with or without radiation is critical.—J.S.N.] ◀

9–4 **Is Amputation Necessary for Sarcomas? Seven-Year Experience With Limb Salvage.** Frederick R. Eilber, Joseph J. Mirra, Todd T. Grant, Thomas Weisenburger, and Donald L. Morton (Univ. of California, Los Angeles) reviewed experience with preoperative multimodal therapy in a prospective series of 105 consecutive patients with soft tissue (65) or skeletal (40) sarcomas. All 40 patients with skeletal sarcomas had grade III tumors, and 52 of the 65 with soft tissue sarcomas had pathologic grade III lesions. Doxorubicin was given intra-arterially before operation in a dose of 30 mg on 3 consecutive days. Radiotherapy from a 6-meV unit was begun the day after completion of chemotherapy. A dose of 3,500 rad was delivered to the midtumor plane over 12 to 14 days. Operation was performed 1 to 10 days after radiotherapy. Most patients received postoperative intravenous doxorubicin therapy, followed by vincristine, high-dose methotrexate and citrovorum treatment.

Over 75% tumor cell necrosis was seen in 80% of resected osteosarcoma specimens in pretreated patients. Over half the grade III soft

Fig 9–2.—Life-table analysis of overall survival for skeletal sarcoma patients comparing those who had limb salvage with those who had amputation. (Courtesy of Eilber, F. R., et al.: Ann. Surg. 192:431–438, October 1980.)

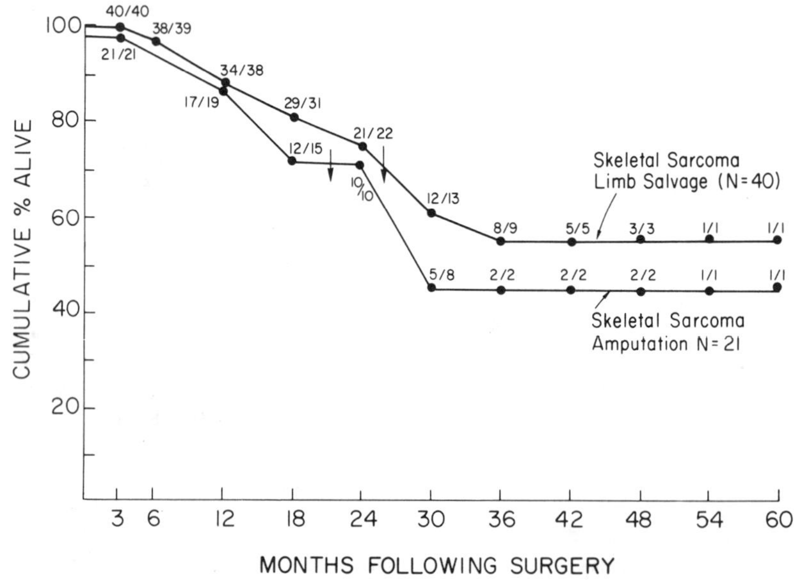

(9–4) Ann. Surg. 192:431–438, October 1980.

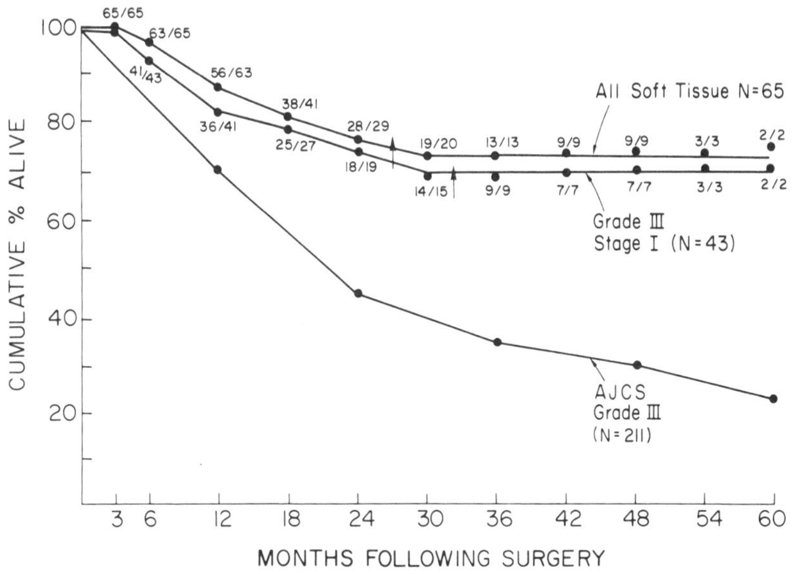

Fig 9–3.—Life-table analysis of overall survival for soft tissue sarcoma patients comparing authors' series with series of American Joint Committee on Staging End Results *(AJCS)*. (Courtesy of Eilber, F. R., et al.: Ann. Surg. 192:431–438, October 1980.)

tissue sarcomas showed greater than 75% necrosis. One of 40 patients with skeletal sarcoma and 2 patients with soft tissue lesions (3%) had local recurrences on follow-up for 3 to 67 months. Four patients with soft tissue lesions required primary amputation. Four patients in the overall series required amputation because of complications. Survival of the patients with skeletal sarcoma is shown in Figure 9–2, and survival of those with soft tissue sarcomas is shown in Figure 9–3.

Local tumor control can be achieved in 90% of patients with skeletal and soft tissue sarcomas without amputation. Excellent function results. The rate of complications from multimodal therapy can be kept below 10%. The results appear to be equal or superior to those achieved by primary amputation. The chief goal of primary tumor treatment is local tumor control rather than limb salvage.

▶ [This is another article in praise of multimodality therapy prior to wide surgical excision. Both Adriamycin (doxorubicin) or methotrexate chemotherapy and radiation therapy were used in these cases. Clearly, limb salvage cannot be achieved in all patients, but it is possible to achieve a high incidence of local tumor control and also preserve the limb. The point here is that the routine use of amputation in the treatment of soft tissue sarcomas is unnecessary and that local control (which is all that can be achieved by amputation) can also be achieved while saving the limb. There is no loss of systemic cure.—J.S.N.] ◀

9–5 **Difficulties Encountered in the Application of Clark Classification and the Breslow Thickness Measurement in Cutaneous Malignant Melanoma.** The histologic classification of Clark and Mihm and the measurement of maximal tumor thickness as described by

(9–5) Int. J. Cancer 26:159–163, August 1980.

CLASSIFICATION FOR HISTOGENESIS AND LEVEL

	Histogenesis
Lentigo malignant melanoma (LMM)	Melanoma, invasive with adjacent intra-epithelial component of Hutchinson's melanotic freckle type.
Superficial spreading Melanoma (SSM)	Melanoma, invasive with adjacent intra-epidermal component of superficial spreading type.
Nodular melanoma	Melanoma, invasive, without adjacent intra-epidermal component.
Unclassifiable melanoma	Melanoma, invasive with intra-epidermal component, impossible to distinguish between LMM type and SSM type.
	Level
Level I	Tumour confined to the epidermis.
Level II	Tumor invading the papillary layer, but not extending to the reticular layer.
Level III	Tumor filling and expanding the papillary layer, but not invading the reticular layer.
Level IV	Tumor Penetrating into the reticular layer.
Level V	Tumor invading the hypodermic fat.

Breslow, shown together in the table, have been used widely to diagnose and classify malignant melanomas of the skin. The EORTC Melanoma Pathologist's Group analyzed the reproducibility of these schemes to determine whether there is general agreement among pathologists regarding the parameters and whether consistent conclusions are reached. Three successive workshops were held by panels of 10 or 11 pathologists, who evaluated about 50 cases of melanoma. Agreement between pathologists regarding histogenesis was markedly improved after discussion, and the same was true for level of involvement. Clark's classification was more difficult to use than the Breslow scheme because it is based on a discontinuous variable, the choice of level of infiltration.

Those who apply the Clark and Breslow methods of diagnosing and classifying malignant melanoma of the skin should consult together in slide readings and projection sessions. In any study utilizing these classification schemes, especially therapeutic trials, all cases should be reviewed and discussed by a panel of pathologists who have agreed on the techniques and interpretations of the classifications. Unclassifiable cases must be excluded. Clark's classification provides better information on the biologic behavior of the tumor, but it is easier to measure tumor thickness, and this method involves less risk of poor interpretation. Variations related to pathologists can be minimized by organizing frequent meetings.

▶ [The discovery by Clark et al. that the prognosis of melanoma is related to the histologic depth of invasion and the quantification of this finding by Breslow have been real advances in the local treatment of malignant melanoma. This article points out that both the Clark classification and the Breslow scheme are useful, but that Breslow's technique is easeir for the pathologist to use. This kind of work has made management of prior malignant malanoma much easier, especially in conjunction with other studies, such as that of Balch et al. (*Ann. Surg.* 188:732, 1978). They pointed out that ultrawide excision is unnecessary on shallow lesions and that prophylactic lymph node dissection is probably unnecessary in extremity lesions of grades I through III and is of questionable value in deeper lesions. In this way, patient morbidity is minimized without loss of ultimate cure.—J.S.N.] ◀

9–6 **Sixty Second-Look Procedures Indicated Primarily by Rise in Serial Carcinoembryonic Antigen.** Carcinoembryonic antigen (CEA) is a sensitive indicator of the efficacy of treatment for carcinoma. Edward W. Martin, Jr., Marc Cooperman, Larry C. Carey, and John P. Minton (Ohio State Univ.) performed second-look operations on 22 patients who were among 300 followed from 1972 through 1975. These patients were reoperated on because of a rise in CEA levels. The mean interval from the rise in CEA to second-look surgery was 4½ months. Of 300 patients followed prospectively from 1976 to the present, 38 (12.6%) were reoperated on solely because of a rise in CEA. The interval from a confirmed increase in CEA level to second-look surgery was 2.6 months in this group. All initial operations involved the removal of all visible tumor with wide resection.

Nineteen of the 22 patients in the retrospective series had recurrent tumor, which was resectable in 6. All 3 patients without recurrence at reoperation later had scan evidence of recurrent disease. Two patients are living after second-look surgery. Of the 38 patients studied prospectively, 23 had resectable tumor. No tumor was found in 1 case. Nineteen patients have no evidence of tumor at present, but the postoperative interval is less than 3 years in most cases. The average CEA level in patients with resectable tumor was 6.5 ng/ml; the interval from the increase to reoperation was only 1.4 months. In patients with unresectable tumor the average CEA was 15.6 ng/ml and the delay before reoperation was 4½ months. In both groups of patients, resectable tumor was found primarily in the liver and pelvis. In all, 24 patients are alive after second-look surgery.

Resectability of recurrent tumor was increased in association with a shorter interval between the finding of an elevated CEA level and second-look surgery. There have been no operative deaths. The rate of major operative morbidity is about 10%. A better tumor marker still is needed.

▶ [The carcinoembryonic antigen (CEA) as an indicator of tumor regrowth has gained routine acceptance. Nevertheless, it is not a panacea, because patients who develop positive CEA levels do not often benefit from resection of the recurrent tumor, even though second-look procedures may be of occasional use. The use of monoclonal antibody against tumor antigens to locate recurrent tumor may be a more sensitive measure of tumor regrowth.—J.S.N.] ◀

9–7 **Cholecystectomy and Carcinoma of the Colon.** Epidemiologic, clinical, and laboratory evidence suggests that bile acids and their byproducts may contribute to the pathogenesis of colonic cancer. If the secondary bile acids are carcinogenic or cocarcinogenic, cholecystectomy, which increases the levels reaching the colon, might predispose to colonic cancer. Dimitrios A. Linos, C. Mary Beard, W. Michael O'Fallon, Malcolm B. Dockerty, Robert W. Beart, Jr., and Leonard T. Kurland (Mayo Clinic) followed up 1,681 residents of Rochester, Minnesota, who underwent cholecystectomy in 1950–1969, 1,221 women and 460 men. Follow-up ranged from 1 to 29 years, the median being

---

(9–6) J. Surg. Res. 28:389–394, May 1980.
(9–7) Lancet 2:379–381, Aug. 22, 1981.

13 years. Patients studied had had colonic cancer diagnosed more than 6 months after cholecystectomy.

Colonic carcinoma was diagnosed in 42 patients after cholecystectomy. The overall relative risk of colorectal cancer was 1.3, not a significant excess. Significantly more women than expected did develop colonic carcinoma; the estimated relative risk for women was 1.7. Women had significantly more cancers of the right colon than expected; the risk was more than double that for the Rochester adult female population. The severity of colonic cancers after cholecystectomy did not differ from that of cancers occurring in the general population.

This study showed a higher than expected number of colonic carcinomas, particularly right-sided colonic cancers, following cholecystectomy in women. Animal studies support an association between cholecystectomy and the subsequent development of colonic cancer. No association has been found between cholelithiasis and colonic carcinoma, which supports the view that cholecystectomy itself may be a predisposing factor. The mechanism of any predisposition is not clear, but the secondary bile acids that predominate in the bile after cholecystectomy may have a carcinogenic or cocarcinogenic effect. The greater number of right-sided colonic cancers could be explained by the more proximal absorption of higher levels of secondary bile acids.

▶ [This epidemiologic relationship between two surgical diseases should be of interest to surgeons, particularly those who advocate routine cholecystectomy for all patients with asymptomatic cholelithiasis. Correlations, however, do not indicate causality.—J.S.N.] ◀

9–8 **Case-Control Study of Diet and Colorectal Cancer** was conducted by M. Jain, G. M. Cook, F. G. Davis, M. G. Grace, G. R. Howe, and A. B. Miller. In all, 348 patients with cancer of the colon and 194 with cancer of the rectum were matched by age and sex with 542 controls living in the same neighborhoods as patients and with 535 controls hospitalized for surgery for nonmalignant gastrointestinal diseases. Postoperatively, each individual completed a personal and medical history questionnaire and a quantitative diet history questionnaire. Data on a number of potential nonnutrient risk factors for bowel cancer and on the consumption of 9 nutrients in the 2-month period immediately prior to interview and in the 2-month period ending 6 months before interview were analyzed. The dietary data thus refer to recent diet consumed in a period antedating the diagnosis of, and in most cases symptoms from, large bowel cancer in the patients, and a corresponding time period in the controls.

The major findings were an elevated risk for the development of colorectal cancer in persons with a history of bowel polyps and in those with an elevated intake of calories, total fat, total protein, saturated fat, oleic acid, and cholesterol. No association was seen with an elevated intake of crude fiber, vitamin C, and linoleic acid. The nutrients for which an increased risk was shown were highly correlated, though multivariate analysis indicated the highest risk for sat-

---

(9–8) Int. J. Cancer 26:757–768, December 1980.

urated fat consumption, with evidence of a dose-response relationship. The findings in both cancer sites, both sexes, and with both sets of controls were quantitatively similar. The population attributable risk for the development of colon and rectal cancer combined was estimated from the neighborhood controls to be 41% in males and 44% in females for saturated fat intake, and 9.8% in males and 6.4% in females with a history of polyps.

These results provide substantial support for the hypothesis that excess consumption of dietary fat is a major risk factor for cancer of the colon and rectum. Attempts to reduce the consumption of dietary fat should now be seriously considered in North American populations. A measurable impact could occur relatively quickly in view of the rapid changes in incidence that occur in migrant populations and the evidence from many sources that dietary fat intake may promote carcinogenesis.

▶ [Colon carcinoma continues to be the most common cause of cancer death in both males and females. This careful epidemiologic study of the relationship of colon cancer to diet may be of some importance to surgeons who are advising their patients at high risk for this disease. The correlation here with consumption of animal fat has been confirmed by many others (e.g., Armstrong, B., and Doll, R.: *Int. J. Cancer* 15:617, 1975).—J.S.N.] ◀

9–9 **Epidemiology of Gallbladder Cancer: Synthesis of Recent Data** is presented by Andrew K. Diehl (Univ. of Texas). Gallbladder cancer accounts for about 2,400 deaths yearly in the United States. There have been no major advances in its treatment in this century; the patients, who are usually untreatable at time of diagnosis, have a median survival of only 5.2 months.

The incidence of gallbladder cancer increases steadily with age in both sexes. The mean age at diagnosis is 60–69 years, with few patients younger than age 50 years. Adenocarcinomas make up 80% or more of most series. Women have an incidence 2–6 times that of men. Since 1968, numbers of total deaths and crude mortality both have fallen consistently in the United States, despite an aging population. This decrease has not occurred in European countries. The improving situation in the United States may reflect an increase over time in cholecystectomies, which reduce the total number of gallbladders at risk and selectively eliminate stone-containing gallbladders, which are at highest risk for cancer.

The incidence of gallbladder cancer shows large (up to a factor of 25) geographic variations. The highest rates are in northeastern Europeans, Israelis, American Indians, and Americans of Mexican origin; the lowest rates are seen in black Rhodesians, black Americans, Spaniards in Spain, and Indians in India. Racial-ethnic heritage has a major impact on incidence; the rates for whites are about 50% higher than those for blacks of both sexes. The incidence in women is 1.4 (per 100,000 per year) in non-Spanish-American Caucasians, 10.5 in Spanish-Americans, and 21.1 in American Indians. These ethnic differences help to explain regional and international variations in incidence.

(9–9) JNCI 65:1209–1214, December 1980.

Gallstones are present in 70%–98% of cases of gallbladder cancer. The epidemiology of cholelithiasis runs parallel to that of gallbladder cancer. Cholelithiasis is a more important risk factor than sex or ethnicity. Drawing a causal inference from the association of gallstones with gallbladder cancer is difficult; cancer develops in fewer than 1% of patients with cholelithiasis, and about 20% of patients with gallbladder cancer have never had stones.

Animal studies suggest that gallstones may facilitate the effects of environmental carcinogens, perhaps by traumatically damaging gallbladder epithelium. Among other carcinogens proposed for the gallbladder is bile itself in altered form. The relation between radiation and gallbladder cancer is uncertain. Bacterial infection associated with gallstones might result in formation from bile of local, highly concentrated carcinogens.

Although cholelithiasis is clearly the strongest risk factor for gallbladder cancer and may be causal with or without cocarcinogens, use of cholecystectomy as prophylaxis for gallbladder cancer cannot be justified. Future epidemiologic research should concentrate on identification of special risk groups; screening for these groups might then be appropriate.

The reasons for the decline in mortality from gallbladder cancer in the United States are far from clear. The best way to continue this trend is to reduce the central risk factor for gallbladder cancer—cholelithiasis. The most productive path for research would be elucidation of why cancers develop in some stone-containing gallbladders but not in others.

9–10 **Recent Concepts of Initiation and Promotion in Carcinogenesis** are reviewed by Frederick F. Becker (Univ. of Texas, Houston). The induction of malignancy by chemical agents has been divided conceptually into phases of initiation and promotion. Current views are that initiation is, or results from, an alteration in DNA and irreversibility is implied. Promotion is the process whereby the initiated cell gains momentum to express the aberrant phenotype in a clinically significant manner.

The finding in viral oncology that a family of highly conserved host genes is central to the transformation process has suggested at least one possible mechanism that might be involved in initiation-promotion sequences. Persistent cell division without further exogenous stimulation is a necessary characteristic of premalignancy for any lesion. Some aggregate perturbation of DNA may have a role in the interaction of carcinogens with DNA. Either a selective alteration in DNA or an aggregate perturbation resulting in DNA instability could activate an appropriate transposable genetic element that would derepress a transforming gene.

The author suggests that in chemical carcinogenesis in parenchymal tissues promotion involves the proliferation of an initiated cell population in which a transforming gene has been activated or a dominant mutation has created responsivity to the action of the promoter.

(9–10) Am. J. Pathol. 105:3–9, October 1981.

A critical mass of altered cells results, which may have a heightened or selective mitotic responsivity to the promoters. The promoter eventually induces an epigenetic programmatic alteration which in some way fixes or impresses the altered cells so as to give them permanence or autonomy. The last increment of progression to true malignancy may involve an inability to communicate or the loss of perception of neighboring cells or finite numbers of cell division. Modulation of the probability of this last occurrence may impose on a given lesion the qualitative character of "degree of premalignancy or risk."

9-11 **Operation-Sequel Carcinoma of the Stomach: Experimental Studies of Surgical Techniques With or Without Resection.** Several pathogenetic factors in carcinogenesis in the stomach after operation have been proposed, but exact proof is lacking. Peter Langhans, Ralph A. Heger, J. Hohenstein, Werner Schlake, and Hermann Bünte have attempted to assess the roles of surgical trauma, duodenogastric reflux, and carcinogen application in rats subjected to Billroth I and Billroth II resections, Billroth II resection plus gastroenterostomy with Roux-en-Y technique, Billroth II resection plus Braun's anastomosis, and gastroenterostomy alone. The carcinogen N-methyl-N′-nitro-N-nitrosoguanidine was given in drinking water. Autopsy was scheduled for surviving animals in week 56 after surgery.

Surgery was performed on 466 rats; 209 (45%) survived for 56 weeks. Weight curves were comparable among animals with and without resection, except for the usual postoperative loss. Carcinomas developed in the stomach of animals that had resection whether or not they were exposed to carcinogen. The rate of carcinoma incidence was influenced strongly by the surgical procedure performed, ranging from zero in animals having gastroenterostomy with Roux-en-Y anastomosis to 70% in animals without carcinogen exposure having gastroenterostomy alone. Carcinomas were present in the immediate vicinity of fistulas in 25 of 29 fistula-bearing animals. The gastric mucosa in these animals exhibited evidence of duodenogastric reflux.

Carcinomas may arise in the stomach with resection whether or not there is application of a chemical carcinogen. Intensified exposure of the gastric mucosa to bile and pancreatic juice is associated with a marked increase in the incidence of tumor, and a direct association with duodenogastric reflux can be postulated. No reflux was noted after Billroth II resection with Roux-en-Y gastroenterostomy in the present study. This supports the interpretation that tumors in this setting are "operation-sequel carcinomas." The findings indicate the advantage of using reflux-preventing techniques in gastric surgery in clinical practice.

▶ [The pathogenesis of cancer of the stomach after operation for peptic ulcer disease has troubled surgeons for years. These experimental studies suggest that exposure of gastric mucosa to refluxed bile after distal gastrectomy or pyloroplasty is associated with an increase in the incidence of the tumor in animals exposed to a known carcinogen, i.e., the bile may be a promoter of carcinogenesis in animals where the carcinogen is the initiator. The preceding article by Becker is important in understanding this process.—J.S.N.] ◀

(9–11) World J. Surg. 5:595–605, July 1981.

9–12 **Cytomegalovirus: Detection in Human Colonic and Circulating Mononuclear Cells in Association With Gastrointestinal Disease.** Cytologic and cultural evidence for the presence of cytomegalovirus (CMV) in the bowel wall has been reported in patients with ulcerative colitis, in which the incidence of colonic cancer is markedly increased, and CMV-DNA has been reported to be present in the bowel in patients with both colitis and colonic carcinoma. J. K. Roche, K.-S. Cheung, I. Boldogh, E.-S. Huang, and D. J. Lang examined the association between epithelial tumors of the colon and CMV in 28 patients having laparotomy for colonic resection at Duke Hospital, Durham, North Carolina, in a 6-month period. Thirteen specimens were examined by a DNA-DNA reassociation kinetics (hybridization) procedure, co-cultivation of fresh tissue with indicator fibroblasts, and immunofluorescence for CMV viral antigens.

Ten of the 13 cancer patients examined by all methods had some evidence of active or previous CMV infection. Four cancer specimens were CMV-DNA positive, and another cancer specimen was culture positive. In 6 instances CMV-DNA was detected in mucosal cells adjacent to adenocarcinoma of the colon. It also was detected in tissue from 1 of 3 patients with ulcerative colitis and from 2 of 7 with other nonneoplastic colonic disease. No fresh colonic tissues had CMV surface or nuclear antigens on immunofluorescence study. Three of 14 cancer patients had peripheral lymphocytes positive for CMV by culture. Most cancer patients had circulating specific antibody to CMV and a normal capacity for CMV-specific antibody-dependent cellular cytotoxicity. All cancer patients except 1 had a capacity for a CMV-specific response. Lymphocytes from cancer patients and other patients had similar responses to stimulation with the mitogen PHA.

Cytomegalovirus frequently can be demonstrated in colonic tissue from patients undergoing intestinal resection, but CMV does not appear to be associated specifically with cancer. The presence of CMV in colonic cells cannot be attributed to preferential replication in damaged tissue or carriage of CMV by peripheral lymphocytes homing to the gut.

▶ [The herpesviruses as a group are known to be oncogenic in animals under some circumstances. There are four herpesviruses that infect human beings: herpes simplex, varicella zoster, cytomegalovirus and Epstein-Barr virus. The Epstein-Barr virus has been implicated in nasopharyngeal carcinoma, Burkitt's lymphoma, and post-transplant lymphoma. Herpes simplex virus has been implicated in carcinomas of the lip, skin, and cervix. This study and the one following suggest that cytomegalovirus may be an initiator or a promoter of tumors in the gastrointestinal mucosa. The following article suggests that immunosuppression associated with cytomegalovirus infection can lead to a variety of other opportunistic infecting agents that may, in turn, be responsible in some way for the high instance of Kaposi's sarcoma in homosexual men. These individuals are prone to opportunistic infections of various types, especially moniliasis and cytomegalovirus infections.—J.S.N.] ◀

9–13 **Kaposi's Sarcoma in Homosexual Men: Report of Eight Cases.** Kaposi's sarcoma is rare in the United States. Most patients are in the seventh decade. Male Ashkenazi Jews and those of Mediterra-

---

(9–12) Int. J. Cancer 27:659–667, May 1981.
(9–13) Lancet 2:598–600, Sept. 19, 1981.

nean origin are most commonly affected. Kenneth B. Hymes, Tony Cheung, Jeffrey B. Greene, Neil S. Prose, Aaron Marcus, Harold Ballard, Daniel C. William, and Linda J. Laubenstein report data on 8 young homosexual men in the New York City area who were seen with Kaposi's sarcoma in 1979 to 1981.

The patients were aged 27 to 45 years. All had multiple sexual partners, and all had sexually transmitted illnesses. Four patients were Jewish, and 1 was Italian. Seven patients presented with skin lesions, and 1 had *Pneumocystis carinii* pneumonia. Seven patients had nodules and papules on the skin, and 1 had plaques. No patient had predominant involvement of the lower extremities; 4 had head and neck lesions. All patients had proved cutaneous and lymph node involvement. The histologic features were typical of Kaposi's sarcoma. Seven patients had clinically detectable generalized lymphadenopathy, and 6 had visceral involvement. Four patients died, 3 of progressive Kaposi's sarcoma despite chemotherapy and 1 of cryptococcosis. Two surviving patients are in clinical remission.

These 8 patients were much younger than typical patients with Kaposi's sarcoma and have an atypical distribution of skin lesions. Sexually transmitted diseases are prevalent in homosexuals, and it has been suggested that cytomegalovirus may be venereally transmitted. The homosexual population apparently may have an increased risk of Kaposi's sarcoma. Further epidemiologic, serologic, and immunologic studies are needed to elucidate this apparent association. Sexually transmissible disease may have a role in the pathogenesis of Kaposi's sarcoma in this population.

▶ [As pointed out in the comment of the preceding article, cytomegalovirus is a common infective agent in immunosuppressed patients and homosexual men. Such men have a high incidence of hepatitis, candidiasis, cytomegalovirus, *Pneumocystis* infection, and other opportunistic infections. Some authors have related this to the use of amyl nitrate by some homosexuals to increase sexual pleasure—that correlation is epidemiologic only. The correlation noted here has been confirmed by others.—J.S.N.] ◀

9–14 **High-Volume Intraperitoneal Chemotherapy With Methotrexate in Patients With Cancer.** Roy B. Jones, Jerry M. Collins, Charles E. Myers, Ada E. Brooks, Susan M. Hubbard, James E. Balow, Murray F. Brennan, Robert L. Dedrick, and Vincent T. DeVita (Natl. Inst. of Health) used methotrexate peritoneal dialysis therapy in 4 patients with stage III or IV ovarian cancer and in 1 with stage IV malignant melanoma. All tumor masses were less than 0.5 cm in diameter and were localized to the peritoneal cavity or liver.

Treatment was begun 1 week after placement of a single-cuff Tenckhoff catheter. Each patient received a 48-hour dialysis weekly for 6 weeks unless otherwise indicated. Dialysis fluid was replaced with fresh solution every 6 hours for a total of 8 exchanges. During the first course, the volume of 1.5% Inpersol (containing methotrexate) was increased progressively from 2,000 ml to patient tolerance and was then held constant for the rest of the 6-week treatment course. The methotrexate concentration in the dialysis fluid was increased

(9–14) Cancer Res. 41:55–59, January 1981.

from 15 to 50 μmoles over the following weeks unless toxicity became prohibitive.

The peritoneal methotrexate level could be maintained 18- to 36-fold higher than corresponding plasma levels using this method; plasma levels remained in the range of 0.2–3.0 μmoles. While local toxicity was generally limited and manageable, mild aseptic peritoneal irritation was common, and 1 episode of bacterial peritonitis occurred. Because of the concentration difference between peritoneum and systemic circulation, systemic toxicity was moderate; only 6 of 29 treatment cycles resulted in myelosuppression. No definite therapeutic benefit was seen, but the tumors of 4 of the 5 patients had shown resistance to a methotrexate-containing chemotherapeutic regimen before the study.

Intraperitoneal treatment with methotrexate is technically feasi-

Fig 9–4 (top).—Implantable infusion pump. Dimensions: 2.82 cm in height, 8.43 cm in diameter. Empty weight is 184 gm.

Fig 9–5 (bottom).—Cross section of implantable infusion pump: *1,* flow restrictor; *2,* silicone rubber coating; *3,* bellows; *4,* charging fluid chamber; *5,* infusate chamber; *6,* charging fluid fill tube (permanently sealed); *7,* filter assembly; *8,* inlet septum; *9,* needle stop.

(Courtesy of Buchwald, H., et al.: Cancer 45:866–869, Mar. 1, 1980.)

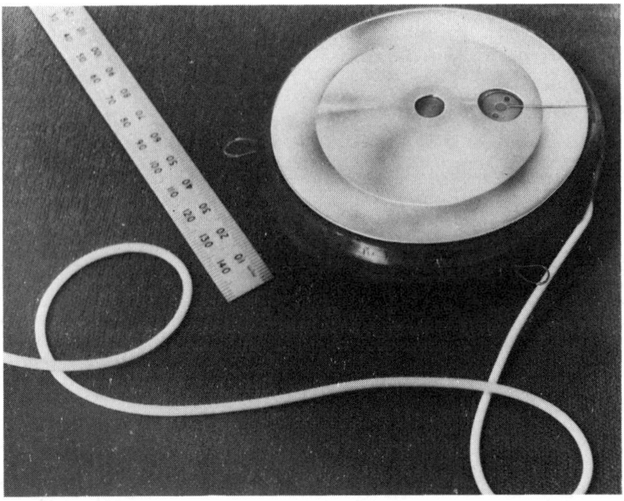

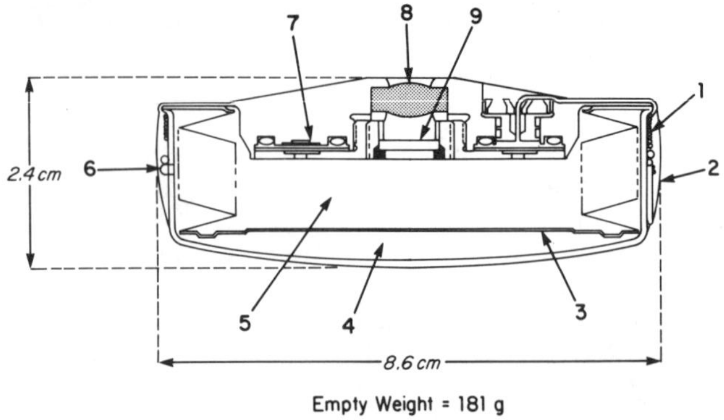

ble, produces manageable toxicity, may be performed with relative safety, and is tolerated adequately. Its therapeutic effectiveness remains to be defined.

▶ [This and the following three articles relate to newer methods of administration of chemotherapeutic agents to deal with special problems. Regional chemotherapy has had a long, and not too productive, history for the treatment of liver metastasis, melanoma of the extremities, and similar disorders. Various infusions have been tried. This method is still under investigation in the hope that it will help relieve a serious problem in selected patients.—J.S.N.] ◀

9–15 **Intra-arterial Infusion Chemotherapy for Hepatic Carcinoma Using a Totally Implantable Infusion Pump.** A high rate of complications has limited the use of intra-arterial chemotherapy for unresectable solid tumors. Henry Buchwald, Theodor B. Grage, Pericles P. Vassilopoulos, Thomas D. Rohde, Richard L. Varco, and Perry J. Blackshear (Univ. of Minnesota) attempted to minimize the problems by using a totally implantable infusion pump. The device is illustrated in Figures 9–4 and 9–5. The delivery cannulas are implanted at laparotomy into the hepatic artery via the gastroduodenal or gastroepiploic artery (Fig 9–6). After several days of infusion of heparin solution, 5-fluorodeoxyuridine (FUDR) is infused at a rate of 0.2–0.5 mg/kg/day, along with heparin. The technique for refilling the pump with medication is shown in Figure 9–7.

Five patients with primary or metastatic carcinoma of the liver were managed with the implantable intra-arterial infusion device; all have

Fig 9–6 (left).—Pump and cannula placement for use in hepatic arterial chemotherapy.

Fig 9–7 (right).—In vivo refilling technique. **A,** pump is being emptied by puncturing the septum with a special needle and allowing pump's pressure to force the remaining infusate into an empty syringe barrel. **B,** fresh infusate is then injected into the pump's reservoir.

(Courtesy of Buchwald, H., et al.: Cancer 45:866–869, Mar. 1, 1980.)

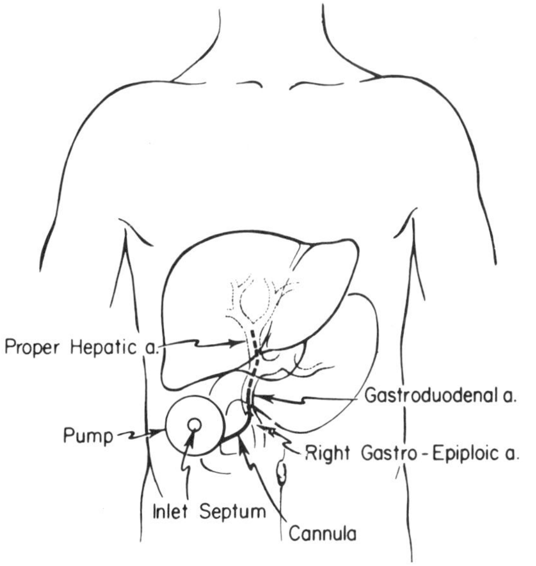

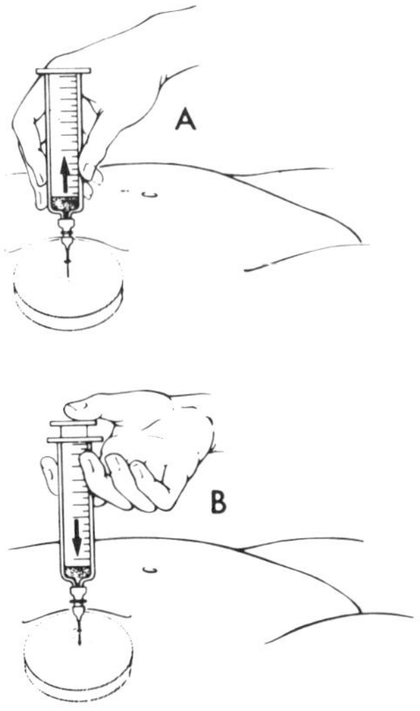

(9–15) Cancer 45:866–869, Mar. 1, 1980.

since died of progressive metastatic disease. The pumps were placed in subcutaneous pockets. In 1 case, a defective pump was removed. The other 4 patients received FUDR for 3 to 29 weeks. Five episodes of presumed FUDR toxicity occurred, resolving rapidly when the FUDR was replaced by sterile water. No complications were specifically related to the implanted pumps or delivery cannulas. Flow through the delivery cannulas was continuous at all times. Three of the 4 functional pumps required refills only about every 30 days.

Continuous long-term intra-arterial infusion chemotherapy is practicable in outpatients with the use of a totally implantable infusion pump. The present patients tolerated the device well and continued their normal daily activities, returning for outpatient visits at about monthly intervals. The device is a versatile mode of access to veins, arteries, or body cavities. A new side port permits bolus injections and angiography through the delivery cannula.

▶ [Buchwald's implantable pump has many potential uses—infusions of heparin, insulin, and cancer chemotherapy are among the most popular at present. The pump is easy to use and to implant and gives highly reproducible and predictable levels of the agent infused. It may prove to be an important advance for the slow infusion of chemotherapeutic agents that are toxic in rapid infusion and whose activity can be prolonged in ambulatory patients in this way.—J.S.N.] ◀

9–16 **Arterial Chemoembolization With Microencapsulated Anticancer Drug: Approach to Selective Cancer Chemotherapy With Sustained Effects.** Mitomycin, a potent anticancer agent, can be prepared in the form of ethylcellulose microcapsules (mitomycin mc) and may in this form be suitable for selective intra-arterial infusion. Tetsuro Kato, Ryosuke Nemoto, Hisashi Mori, Mutsumasa Takahashi, Yoshiharu Tamakawa, and Mosaoki Harada (Akita Univ.) report the use of arterial chemoembolization with mitomycin mc through percutaneous catheterization in 56 patients with invasive or unresectable malignant neoplasms. The most common lesions were renal cell carcinoma, urinary bladder carcinoma, prostatic carcinoma, and primary or metastatic hepatic carcinomas. Thirty-two patients had several metastases or far-advanced disease. Twenty-seven had failed to respond to other treatments. A total of 60 lesions underwent mitomycin mc therapy, followed in 22 instances by radical surgery. The dose of mitomycin mc ranged from 10 to 40 mg. Twenty-six patients received more than one infusion. Twenty renal cell carcinomas received infusions of a mixture of mitomycin mc and gelatin sponge.

Objective tumor reduction was observed in 33 cases, and 13 other tumors showed a moderate response. Improvement in symptoms and such signs as massive hemorrhage and hydronephrosis commonly was observed. Pain was relieved in 80% of 30 cases. Tumor reduction facilitated operation in most instances. Hematologic toxicity occurred in one fourth of patients, but only 7 patients required blood transfusion or corticosteroid administration. Several patients who had hypogastric artery infusions had skin necrosis lasting a few months. Of 22 patients who underwent radical surgery after chemoembolization, 20 with no distant metastasis at the time of operation are doing well.

(9–16) JAMA 245:1123–1127, Mar. 20, 1981.

Early experience indicates that chemoembolization with mitomycin mc is effective as a preoperative and palliative measure in the treatment of locally advanced carcinoma and helpful in controlling hemorrhage and pain in patients with metastases. Survival of the latter might be improved by combining chemoembolization with systemic treatment.

▶ [This is another method for the administration of chemotherapeutic agents for the palliation of advanced solid tumors. Its advantage is that embolization takes place, retaining a high concentration of chemotherapeutic agent within the microvasculature of the tumor. The responses illustrated in the article itself are impressive indeed.—J.S.N.] ◀

9–17 **Tumoricidal Response Induced by Cytosine Arabinoside After Plasma Perfusion Over Protein A.** Spontaneous mammary adenocarcinoma is common in adult female dogs and is considered to be an excellent model of human breast adenocarcinoma. A necrotizing tumoricidal response can be induced by extracorporeal perfusion of plasma over protein A-bearing *Staphylococcus aureus* Cowan 1 (SAC), presumably through the activation of tumor-associated antibodies (TAA). David S. Terman, Tsuyoshi Yamamoto, Richard L. Tillquist, Joseph F. Henry, Gary L. Cook, Abraham Silvers, and William T. Shearer (Baylor College of Medicine, Houston) obtained evidence that a single, nontoxic infusion of cytosine arabinoside (CA), given to dogs after extracorporeal perfusion of plasma over protein A immobilized in collodion charcoal (PACC), results in an enhanced necrotizing tumoricidal response.

Dogs with spontaneous mammary adenocarcinoma underwent extracorporeal PACC. A dose of 10 mg of CA per kg was given intravenously in 4 hours 7 to 12 days before perfusion, and perfusion was repeated 10 to 21 days later with the immediate infusion of CA. The CA-associated procedure led to more rapid and diffuse necrosis. Up to half of the surface area of visible lesions healed in 12 to 18 days, whereas no significant healing was observed after PACC or CA alone in the same dogs. Normal mammary glands showed no morphological changes. The findings in 1 dog are shown in Figure 9–8. Toxic reactions were minimal, except for temperature elevations of 2.5 F in some dogs. Microscopic studies confirmed more extensive necrosis after combined PACC-CA treatment than after perfusion alone.

Tumor necrosis resulting from extracorporeal PACC was augmented by a single, nontoxic dose of CA in this study of dogs with spontaneous mammary adenocarcinoma. This may be an effective chemoimmunotherapeutic approach to breast adenocarcinoma. The effect may be related to observations of a synergistic inhibitory effect of CA on tumor cell replication in tissue culture in the presence of TAA, perhaps due to antibody-enhanced phosphorylation and increased incorporation of the drug into the DNA of cell nuclei.

▶ [Terman, along with Bansal and Ray, has been pursuing a technique of passing human plasma across staphylococcal protein A to induce tumor regression. The rationale originally was to remove "blocking antibodies" in the plasma of patients and permit T cell-mediated destruction of the tumor. Whatever the mechanism, the re-

(9–17) Science 209:1257–1259, Sept. 12, 1980.

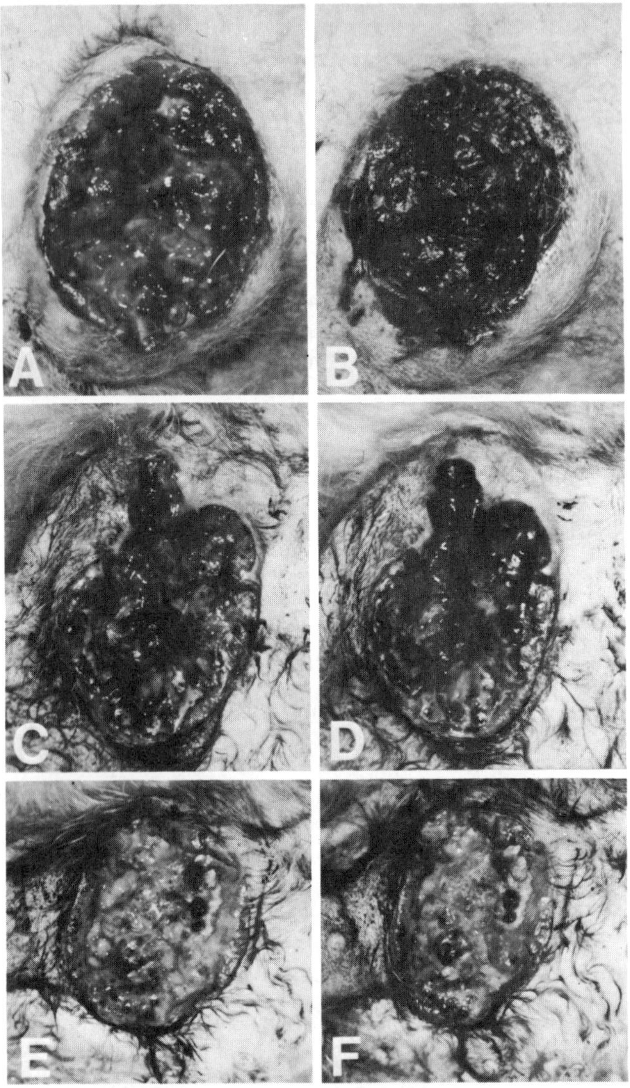

Fig 9–8.—Gross appearance of large, ulcerating mammary adenocarcinoma in dog before (**A, C,** and **E**) and 12 hours after various treatments. **B,** tumoricidal response after PACC plus CA regimen. **D** and **F,** reactions after treatment with PACC and CA, respectively. (Courtesy of Terman, D. S., et al.: Science 209:1257–1259, Sept. 12, 1980. Copyright 1980 by the American Association for the Advancement of Science.)

moval of blocking antibodies does not seem to be it. Nevertheless, impressive tumor regression can be induced both in dogs and occasionally in patients by such extraordinary techniques. More investigators need to be recruited into this field.—J.S.N.] ◀

9–18 **Urine From Patients With Transitional Cell Carcinoma Stimulates Migration of Capillary Endothelial Cells.** Neoplastic cells release a substance that stimulates the migration of capillary endo-

(9–18) N. Engl. J. Med. 305:869–874, Oct. 8, 1981.

thelial cells in vitro, and a similar effect may take place in vivo. Gerald W. Chodak, Cathy J. Scheiner, and Bruce R. Zetter assayed capillary endothelial cell migration-stimulating activity in 125 urine samples from 82 patients with a variety of malignant and nonmalignant diseases and 22 without acute disease. Dialyzed urine samples were analyzed by a phagokinetic-track assay using bovine capillary endothelial cells.

Representative titration curves are shown in Figure 9–9. All 11 matched pairs of samples taken from patients before and after removal of a transitional cell bladder tumor showed a significant reduction in activity after operation. Migration activity increased when new tumor growth was present, but remained low when patients remained free of tumor. Activity in samples from patients with nonmalignant urologic or nonurologic diseases was similar to that in healthy subjects. Low levels of activity were present in urine from patients with prostatic cancer and squamous cell carcinoma of the bladder. Little activity was present in samples from patients with various genitourinary infections.

Fig 9–9.—Capillary endothelial cell migration-stimulating activity in human urine. Five concentrations of dialyzed, concentrated urine from patient with transitional cell carcinoma of the bladder *(solid circles)* and from healthy volunteer *(open circles)* were assayed for migration-stimulating activity. Inset shows tracks made by cells exposed to normal urine *(left)* and tumor urine *(right)*. Data are expressed as mean increase in track size beyond value for cells incubated in medium without urine. Each point represents value for 100 tracks (SEM). (Courtesy of Chodak, G. W., et al.: N. Engl. J. Med. 305:869–874, Oct. 8, 1981.)

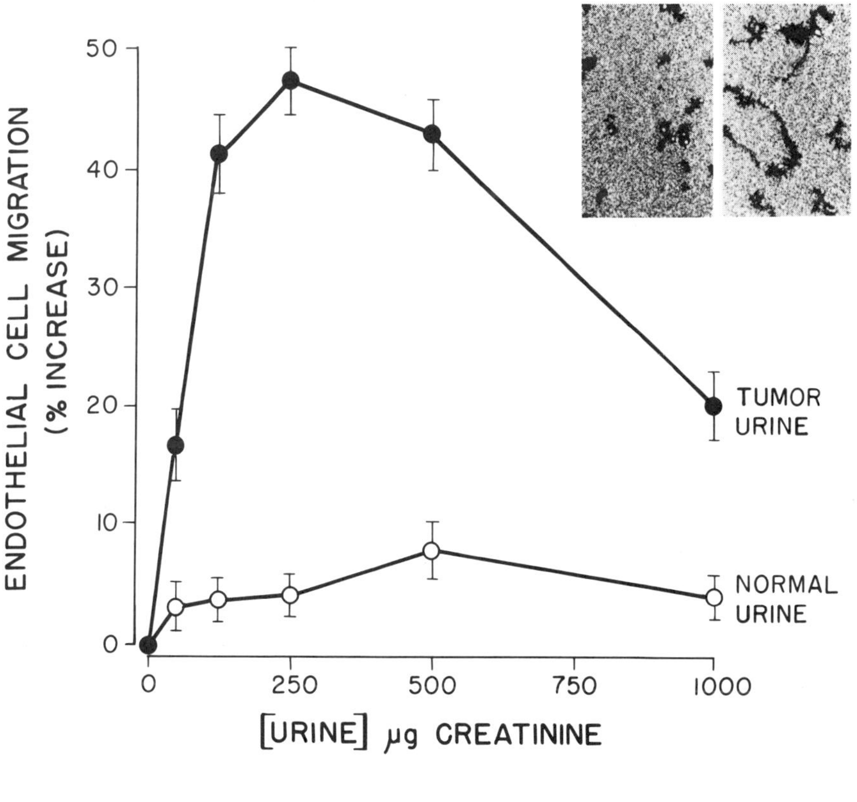

Dialyzed, concentrated urine from patients with transitional cell carcinoma of the bladder can stimulate capillary endothelial cell migration in vitro. The agent responsible for the cell migration-stimulating activity is unknown, and its true biologic function has not been determined. It is possible, however, that it is related to the angiogenic activity produced by solid tumors in vivo. Capillary endothelial cell migration is an essential component of angiogenesis, and studies are underway to determine whether the activity in urine from patients with transitional cell carcinoma is a component of the angiogenic process.

▶ [This article is part of the continuing study by Folkman and his group on tumor angiogenesis factor. These innovative investigators have now been able to perform long-term culture of capillary endothelial cells (*Proc. Natl. Acad. Sci. USA* 76:5217, 1979) and to study the migration of these cells in the presence of tumor angiogenic factors (*Nature* 285:41, 1980). Presumably, the motion of these endothelial cells represents the in vitro correlate of tumor angiogenesis factor on capillary endothelium in vivo. Clearly, this is an important biologic phenomenon. In addition, it becomes an excellent assay for the presence of tumor-associated angiogenesis factors in urine and perhaps in other body fluids.—J.S.N.] ◀

9–19 **Cancer Immunology: Search for Specificity.** In the G. H. A. Clowes Memorial Lecture, Lloyd J. Old (Meml. Sloan-Kettering Cancer Center, New York) states that the major focus of cancer immunology has shifted away from arguments about the validity of the immunosurveillance theory of cancer to the more basic question of tumor-specific antigens. Despite vast effort aimed at demonstrating such antigens, their existence in the generality of cancer remains unproved. Serologic analysis of, mouse leukemia, mouse sarcoma, and human malignant melanoma has received most attention, and a rudimentary classification of the surface antigens expressed by these tumors has begun to emerge.

The prime candidates for antigens that can be considered tumor-specific are the few instances of class 1 antigens that have now been serologically defined on mouse and human tumors. These antigens show an absolute restriction to individual tumors, not being demonstrable on any other normal or malignant cell type. Biochemical and genetic characterization of class 1 antigens represents an essential next step in evaluating the significance of these antigens.

The surprising features of the thymus leukemia (TL) antigens of the mouse provide insight into the genetic origin of another key class of tumor antigens, in this case antigens with characteristic properties of both differentiation antigens and tumor-specific antigens. In normal mice, TL antigens are restricted to cells in the thymus, and strains differ with regard to expression versus nonexpression of TL antigens. Genetic information for TL is universal in the mouse, however, as leukemias developing in mice that normally lack TL are found to express TL.

What is clear from the past 20 years of research in cancer immunology is that a far more detailed knowledge of surface antigens of tumor cells is necessary before the possibility of immunologic control of cancer can be assessed.

(9–19) Cancer Res. 41:361–375, February 1981.

▶ [Although tumor immunotherapy is suffering the effects of clinical disillusionment, the study of tumor cell surface antigens ultimately may permit one to target in on the tumor cell itself. In this important article, Lloyd Old reviews the evidence for specific cell surface antigens on human and animal cancers and the potential for using such antigens as targets. The emergence of monoclonal antibodies to define these antigens has been revolutionary because each cell surface component now can be individually identified and antibody-tailored to its ligand. The following articles review some of the other possibilities for the use of monoclonal antibodies in tumor immunodiagnosis and immunotherapy.—J.S.N.] ◀

9–20 **Monoclonal Antibodies: New Technology for Producing Serologic Reagents** is discussed by Betty A. Diamond, Dale E. Yelton, and Matthew D. Scharff (Albert Einstein College of Medicine, New York). Köhler and Milstein showed that cultured mouse myeloma cells can be fused to normal spleen cells from animals immunized with

Fig 9–10.—Fusion of mouse myeloma cells and immune spleen cells. Mouse myeloma cells that no longer produce their own immunoglobulin *(Ig)* and lack hypoxanthine phosphoribosyl transferase *(HPRT)* activity are fused to spleen cells from an immunized mouse. The hybrid cells are selected in a medium containing hypoxanthine, aminopterin, and thymidine *(HAT)*. The infused myeloma cells are killed by the HAT medium, whereas the unfused spleen cells do not grow in tissue culture. (Courtesy of Diamond, B. A., et al.: N. Engl. J. Med. 304:1344–1349, May 28, 1981.)

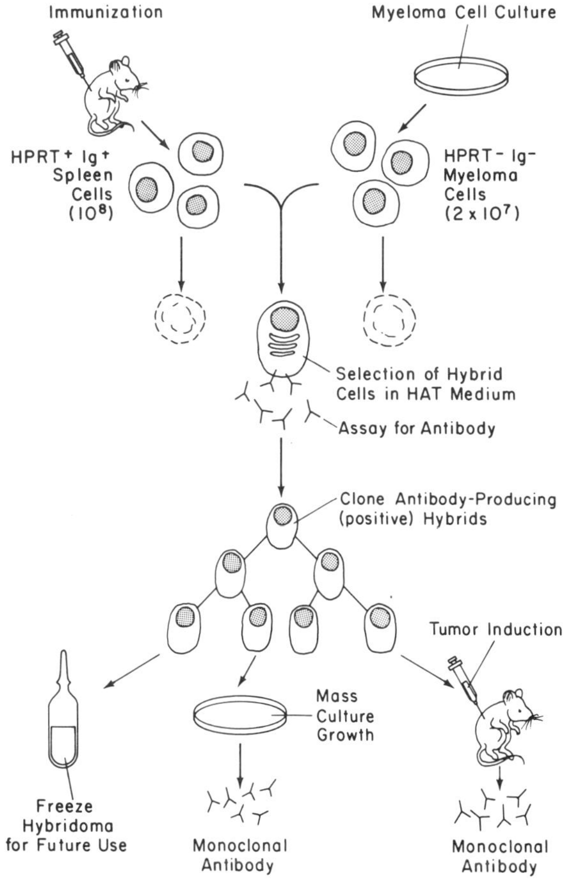

(9–20) N. Engl. J. Med. 304:1344–1349, May 28, 1981.

sheep red blood cells and that some of the hybrids produce large amounts of homogeneous antibody against sheep red cells. The hybrid cell lines grew in culture and could be injected into syngeneic mice to induce an ascites containing large amounts of antibody. The only limit to the amount of antibody available with use of a variety of antigens is the number of animals injected. Impure antigens can be utilized. The hybridoma technique is outlined in Figure 9–10. Antibody-producing clones can be recloned to eliminate nonproducing clones. The likelihood of success depends on the immunogenicity of the antigen, as in traditional immunization.

Problems arise in attempting to use species other than the mouse for immunization; the low frequency of fusion is another continuing problem. The most time-consuming part of the technology is screening hundreds of hybrids for antibody. The screening method is particularly important if an impure antigen has been used for immunization. Not all hybridomas are stable in the expression of antibody or are able to induce large amounts of ascitic fluid in recipient mice. Homogeneous antibodies cannot be used in precipitation assays such as radial immunodiffusion, immunoelectrophoresis, or routine agar diffusion.

It seems certain that most immunoassays eventually will use hybridoma antibodies. Homogeneous antibodies will improve the reliability of tissue typing and lead to the recognition of new specificities that will be useful in organ transplantation and in studies of the role of HLA antigens in various disease states. Radioimmunoassays will become more reproducible. The diagnosis of certain malignant diseases should be improved, and it may become possible to detect small metastases and to deliver cytotoxic drugs to malignant cells. Homogeneous human antibodies against drugs could be used to treat overdosage. Hybrid lines secreting immunoregulatory molecules have been described.

▶ [This article reviews monoclonal antibodies in a language that is clear to the clinician. The benefits of monoclonal antibodies seem obvious. They are highly specific, so that cross-reactivity with normal tissue components would appear to be minimal. Monoclonal antibodies can be tagged with a variety of in vivo or in vitro labels. Radioactive tags then can be used to search out metastases, to analyze body fluids, and to study tissues. Furthermore, therapeutic agents can be attached to the antibody or antibodies that bind complement used as therapeutic vehicles themselves. The biggest current problem is obtaining allomonoclonal antibodies, i.e., human antibodies against human tissue. The major obstruction is finding a human myeloma cell that will fuse with antibody-producing cells to produce stable antibodies. It is likely that this technologic barrier will be breached. Antibodies must be raised that will not generate antibodies against themselves, as do xenomonoclonal antibodies.—J.S.N.] ◀

9–21 **Monoclonal Antibodies to Two Determinants of Melanoma-Antigen p97 Act Synergistically in Complement-Dependent Cytotoxicity.** Ingegerd Hellström, Joseph P. Brown, and Karl Erik Hellström (Univ. of Washington, Seattle) have obtained two hybridomas that produce monoclonal IgG2a antibodies to distinct antigenic determinants of p97, an antigen present at the surface of virtually all normal and neoplastic human cells. Most melanomas express 10 to

(9–21) J. Immunol. 127:157–160, July 1981.

100 times more p97 than normal tissues. Microcytotoxicity tests were used to examine the complement-dependent cytotoxicity of these antibodies, alone and in combination. In 10 of 12 cultured melanoma lines tested by microcytotoxicity technique, complement-dependent cytotoxicity was much greater in the presence of both antibodies than with either antibody alone. Synergism was not noted when the antibodies were tested in combination with an IgG2a antibody to a different cell surface glycoprotein, and it was not detected in tests of 4 nonmelanoma cell lines.

Whether this synergistic cytotoxic effect can be used therapeutically is unknown. The fact that normal cells express some p97 is an obvious difficulty, but observations of killing of melanoma cells under conditions where other cells are not killed are encouraging. The antibodies might be used to remove melanoma cells from a population of normal cells expressing much less p97. The double antibody approach also may be used for other tumor-associated antigens, some of which may have a higher degree of tumor specificity than p97.

▶ [In this article, monoclonal antibodies are used to destroy tumor cells as a consequence of their capacity to fix complement. Monoclonal antibodies can be created with a variety of characteristics and immunoglobulins chosen for immunodiagnostic or immunotherapeutic cells accordingly. This is a similar approach to that taken by Deng et al. in the following article.—J.S.N.] ◀

9-22 **Cytotoxic Monoclonal Antibody to a Human Leiomyosarcoma.** Monoclonal antibodies against tumors have their greatest clinical potential in reacting with tumor antigens while not reacting with antigens of normal tissues. C. Deng, P. I. Terasaki, N. El-Awar, R. Billing, J. Cicciarelli, and L. Lagasse (Univ. of California, Los Angeles) report the production of a highly specific cytotoxic antibody to a human leiomyosarcoma. The tumor, from a woman aged 48, consisted of bundles of spindle-shaped cells, including some large pleomorphic cells with bizarre mitotic figures. Monoclonal antibody was produced by immunizing Balb/c mice with viable tumor cells and boosting them intravenously with tumor cells a week later. After 3 days the spleen cells were fused with myeloma cell 653, a line derived from $P3 \times 63$ AG8. Culture supernatants were screened by the HLA microcytotoxicity test.

The antibody was cytotoxic to the immunizing tumor in dilutions of 1:16,000 to 1:260,000, but not to many other cells including lymphocytes, spleen cells, granulocytes, red blood cells, and leukemia cells. There was no evidence that the antibody is directed against normal smooth muscle antigens. The antibody did not react with cells from 40 patients with leukemia or 8 with other tumors or 7 cultured tumor lines. The only other cell found to react with the antibody, in 1:4000 dilution, was line 8402, a T acute lymphocytic leukemia line. Studies of the monoclonal antibody in a rhesus monkey showed no toxicity.

This monoclonal antibody may prove to be suitable for therapeutic trials. It will be important to determine whether it will react with some or all other leiomyosarcomas. Initially, the antibody will have

---

(9–22) Lancet 1:403–405, Feb. 21, 1981.

to be tested against biopsy material. Monoclonal antibodies may have to be custom produced for each patient.

In an addendum, the authors report that results of recent tests on leiomyosarcoma cells from 2 other patients were negative.

9–23 **Monoclonal Antibodies and Cancer.** Monoclonal antibodies now can be produced to order to recognize a selected antigen. Myelomas of rodent origin can be grown in vitro and in animals and their monoclonal antibody harvested, and Kohler and Milstein developed a way of constructing myelomas, or "hybridomas," which make antibody to an antigen of choice. Stimulated by the antigen, B lymphocytes are fused with cells of a stock myeloma line, and the hybrid cells produce the monoclonal antibody specified by the lymphocyte taking part in the fusion. Antibody to a single component of a mixture of antigens can be produced. An example is the production of interferon by an antibody raised through immunization with partly purified material. Monoclonal antibodies have exceptional specificity, and they can, in principle, be reproduced indefinitely. Hybrid myeloma cells can be stored for years and recloned to eliminate variants. Monoclonal antibodies, however, may have fairly low affinity for their antigens. Disruption of radioimmunoassays is a possibility. The initial production of monoclonal antibodies is expensive.

The most dramatic potential use of monoclonal antibodies is the killing of human tumors and the transport of radioactive labels permitting localization of tumor deposits. Several laboratories have attempted to produce monoclonal antibodies that might bind specifically to the surface of human tumors, but specificity testing is difficult. Tumor cells may be killed in vivo by use of an antibody or mixture of antibodies that is specifically cytotoxic for, or specifically opsonizes, the target cells. In an alternative approach, conjugates are made of toxins with antibodies. Monoclonal antibodies specific for cell types also can be used to separate and manipulate mixed cell populations, such as bone marrow, in vitro. Human myelomas are now available that hybridize satisfactorily with human lymphocytes, and some success has been obtained with interspecies hybrids producing human antibody. Human monoclonal antibodies cannot yet be made to order, however, because human lymphocytes cannot be efficiently immunized in vitro. Further, there may be doubt about injecting products of malignant human cells into patients.

▶ [This article briefly reviews the potentials and problems of monoclonal antibodies in cancer research and is recommended to those wanting a brief review.—J.S.N.] ◀

9–24 **Determination of Incidence and Partial Characterization of Tumor-Associated Antigens Found in the Urine of Patients Bearing Solid Tumors.** Tumor-associated antigens are found in the urine of patients with a wide variety of solid sarcomas, carcinomas, and melanomas, but rarely in normal subjects. N. S. Rote, R. K. Gupta, and D. L. Morton sought tumor-associated antigens in urine samples from 51 patients with sarcomas, 23 with melanomas, 20 with carcinomas, and 37 control subjects. Eighteen of the sarcoma patients had

---

(9–23) Lancet 1:421–423, Feb. 21, 1981.
(9–24) Int. J. Cancer 26:203–210, August 1980.

osteosarcomas. Specimens were tested by complement fixation for antigenic activity against serums from autologous or allogeneic sources. Serums were obtained from patients 4–8 weeks after resection of their tumors.

Antigen was identified in urine samples tested against autologous serum from 84% of sarcoma patients, 91% of melanoma patients, and 89.5% of carcinoma patients. Only 7% of normal subjects were positive. High titers often were present in samples from cancer patients. When allogeneic serum was used, 96% of sarcoma patients, 91% of melanoma patients, and 95% of carcinoma patients had positive findings. Absorption studies indicated that the urinary antigens were tumor-associated. A correlation with tumor burden was observed. The antigenic activity was found to be heat-stable and to consist of molecules of over 1,000,000 daltons, which were dissociated into smaller molecular weight active fractions by treatment with 6M urea.

It appears that tumor-associated antigen is released from solid tumors distal to the urinary tract and somehow find its way into the urine. Passage through the renal glomeruli into the urine would require marked glomerular compromise. It is likelier that smaller antigens are formed into complexes or aggregates after passage of urine or during preparation. Urinary tumor-associated antigens are found in a large proportion of cancer patients. Variations in their excretion may help predict tumor recurrence and may aid the early diagnosis of cancer. Urine provides an excellent source of soluble human tumor-associated antigen for purification and characterization.

▶ [Until recently, tumor-associated antigens could be isolated and identified only by complex chemical techniques, the results of which were never precise and quantitative. These techniques are detailed in this article. The appearance of monoclonal antibodies will permit nice identification of these tumor-associated antigens and, if indeed tumor antigens are filtered and reaggregate in the urine, should permit the immunodiagnosis of cancer by monoclonal urinalysis. The following article by Ueda et al. discusses some of the complexities of this approach in the development of appropriate reagents.—J.S.N.] ◀

9–25 **Cell Surface Antigens of Human Renal Cancer Defined by Mouse Monoclonal Antibodies: Identification of Tissue-Specific Kidney Glycoproteins** is described by Ryuzo Ueda, Shun-Ichiro Ogata, Donna M. Morrissey, Connie L. Finstad, Jerzy Szkudlarek, Willet F. Whitmore, Herbert F. Oettgen, Kenneth Q. Lloyd, and Lloyd J. Old (Meml. Sloan-Kettering Cancer Center, New York). Recently, cell surface antigens of human malignant melanoma were identified by mouse monoclonal antibodies. A comparable analysis of human renal cancer now has been carried out. Mice were immunized with established renal cancer cell lines maintained in supplemented Eagle's medium. Immune spleen cells were fused with mouse myeloma cells. Mouse antibody was detected by the mouse mixed hemadsorption assay.

Seventeen monoclonal antibodies derived from fusions with spleen cells of immunized mice identified 9 cell surface antigenic systems. Six systems are previously undescribed antigens; the other 3 are re-

---

(9–25) Proc. Natl. Acad. Sci. USA 78:5122–5126, August 1981.

lated to HLA A, B, and C heavy-chain and A and B blood group antigens. Three of the new antigens are found only on cells of renal origin, both normal and malignant, and represent differentiation antigens of human kidney. The other new antigens have characteristics of broadly occurring differentiation antigens. They can be distinguished by differences in molecular weight, heat stability, and differential expression on cell types of diverse origin.

The mouse antibodies identified in this study of renal cancer and those identified in the study of melanoma do not recognize antigens that are tumor specific. With regard to human tumor antigens recognized by mouse antibodies, the problem will be to distinguish between tumor-specific reactions and reactions due to highly restricted differentiation antigens. The same problem will arise when human monoclonal antibodies become available for the study of human cancer.

9–26 **On the Mechanism of Tumor "Concomitant Immunity."** Paul Ehrlich described as "concomitant immunity" a situation in which mice bearing a growing tumor suppressed the growth of tumor cells inoculated at a different anatomical site. He attributed the effect to a decrease in essential nutrients for tumor growth caused by the first tumor graft. Bashford et al. later suggested that an antitumor immune response suppressed the second, relatively small tumor inoculum. Eliezer Gorelik, Shraga Segal, and Michael Feldman (Weizmann Inst. of Science, Rehovot, Israel) examined the phenomenon of concomitant immunity in mice bearing Lewis lung carcinoma (3LL), B16 melanoma, EL4 lymphoma, and methylcholanthrene-induced T-10 tumor. Mice were immunosuppressed by irradiation, thymectomy, and splenectomy. Development of metastasis was assayed by inoculating tumor cells into mouse footpads, amputating the extremity when the tumor was 8 to 10 mm in diameter, and evaluating lung metastases 10 days later.

Mice bearing all types of tumor were able to suppress completely the growth of a subsequent intrafootpad inoculum of tumor cells. Inhibitory activity increased with the size of the tumor and reached a maximum during the time the immune response of the host largely was suppressed. Inhibition was as effective in T cell-depleted animals as in normal mice. The effect was seen to be tumor nonspecific, indicating that it is not a result of specific immune responsiveness. Local tumors exerted a strong inhibitory effect on their lung metastases. Removal of local tumor led to an acceleration of metastatic growth in the lungs, even when the local tumor grew in immune-suppressed mice.

It appears that concomitant immunity and suppression of metastatic growth by local tumor are based on similar mechanisms. Concomitant immunity is not a T cell-mediated, tumor-specific immunologic phenomenon. The inhibitory factor may also arrest the replication of normal and of less differentiated, rapidly dividing cells in the tumor-bearing host. Antimitotic factors produced by tumors might suppress the function of bone marrow and the lymphatic system and

---

(9–26) Int. J. Cancer 27:847–856, June 1981.

thus lead to anemia, leukocytopenia, and thrombocytopenia, and subsequently might suppress immune functions.

▶ [The checks and balances that effect tumor growth can be immunologic or nonimmunologic in nature. Unfortunately, the term "concomitant immunity" suggests that tumor specificity is always involved. True concomitant immunity seems to be a phenomenon of tumor-specific concomitant immunity, in which the immunity directed against the tumor borne by the animal depresses specific growth of the self same (but not other) tumors in the same animal. The authors seem to be addressing a different phenomenon or may be expressing a problem in tumor cell heterogeneity. In any case, controlled tumor growth seems at times not to require an immune system. Some tumors appear to inhibit growth of any other cell of the body, malignant or not.—J.S.N.] ◀

9–27 **In Vivo Antitumor Effects of Local Adoptive Transfer of Mouse and Human Cultured Lymphoid Cells.** The possibility of culturing the autochthonous lymphocytes of cancer patients has opened prospects for the application of cytotoxic cells in the immunotherapy of malignant disease. E. Gorelik, E. Kedar, B. Sredni, and R. Herberman (Natl. Inst. of Health) used a radioisotopic assay for in vivo monitoring of natural antitumor immunity, based on serial measurements of elimination of radiolabeled tumor cells from the local site of transplantation, to evaluate the cytotoxic activity of adoptively transferred effector cells. The cytotoxic reactivity of cytotoxic mouse and human cultured T cells (CTC) was assessed and compared with that of effector cells induced by alloimmunization. Studies were done using Madison lung carcinoma, Moloney virus-induced lymphoma, and spontaneous mammary tumor, as well as cell lines from human colonic carcinoma and breast cancer.

Cultured spleen cells of normal mice or mice bearing the lung carcinoma had a high level of cytotoxic activity in vitro against a variety of tumor target cells and had characteristics of natural killer cells. The presence of cells cultured with T cell growth factor in inocula led to a marked reduction in footpad radioactivity within 24 hours. Tumor appearance was delayed but not prevented, and the rate of subsequent tumor growth was not affected. Alloimmune lymphocytes had a more prolonged effect in vivo. Cultured human lymphoid cells initiated from the blood of normal donors had a high level of cytotoxic activity in vitro, and their in vivo cytotoxic activity correlated with their in vitro effects.

Cultured mouse and human effector cells have appreciable in vivo cytotoxic activity against tumor cell lines, but the transient nature of the effect may limit the immunotherapeutic potential. The radioisotopic assay appears to be a more sensitive measure of in vivo cytotoxic activity than parameters of visible tumor growth. It may provide a more sensitive and rapid means of evaluating the potential in vivo efficacy of cytotoxic effector cells or of biologic response modifiers in developing new approaches to immunotherapy.

▶ [The contribution here is a more sensitive assay for demonstrating in vivo cell-mediated cytotoxicity against tumor cells by adoptively transferred immune lymphocytes. These effects are sometimes so subtle they are missed entirely, and chances to pursue this technique further may well help.—J.S.N.] ◀

(9–27) Int. J. Cancer 28:157–164, August 1981.

9–28 **Transfer to Cyclophosphamide-Treated Mice of Natural Killer (NK) Cells and In Vivo Natural Reactivity Against Tumors.** The spontaneous expression of the natural killer (NK) cell response and its ability to be rapidly augmented indicate that it may represent one of the first lines of in vivo defense against tumors. Carlo Riccardi, Teresa Barlozzari, Angela Santoni, Ronald B. Herberman, and Carla Cesarini examined the possibility of adoptively transferring the ability to eliminate tumor cells from the lungs rapidly. Studies were done on mice with YAC, a Moloney-induced lymphoma of A/Sn origin.

Cyclophosphamide led to marked depression of NK activity and of in vivo natural reactivity against intravenous challenge with labeled tumor cells. The adoptive transfer of normal spleen cells restored both activities. Normal spleen cells were particularly active in reconstituting both in vivo and in vitro natural reactivities in mice given cyclophosphamide 4 days earlier, when the greatest depression of natural reactivities was observed. The efficacy of transfer correlated with levels of NK activity of donor cells in a variety of situations. Highly NK-reactive spleen cells from young donors were effective, whereas nonreactive thymus cells were not. Young mice lost their ability to transfer reactivity when their NK activity was depressed by pretreatment with pyran copolymer or carrageenan. The cells responsible for transferring reactivity, like NK cells, were nonadherent, nonphagocytic, and present in nude mice.

These findings support the view that NK cells have a role in the rapid elimination of tumor cells in vivo. The level of NK activity in recipients of transferred cells probably depends on such factors as the number of NK cells transferred and their state of activation, the pattern of donor cell circulation to various organs, and the host environment. It should be possible to restore NK reactivity selectively by transfer of an enriched population of NK cells depleted of macrophages and mature T cells and to determine NK cell effects on the growth and dissemination of primary or transplanted tumors.

▶ [Considerable research continues to be carried out on the natural killer cell, i.e., the cell that mediates cell cytotoxic effects against tumor and other altered cells, rather than against endogenous cells without preexposure. These cells are not cytoxic T cells that have acquired immunity; NK cells are thought of as a surveillance mechanism against the emergence of potential neoplastic cells. The defects in such a hypothesis had previously been the difficulty in demonstrating in vivo elimination of neoplastic cells. Present studies provide strong evidence that certain kinds of NK cells will act to eliminate tumor cells in vivo as well as in vitro.—J.S.N.] ◀

9–29 **Extravascular Natural Cytotoxicity in Man: Anti-K562 Activity of Lymph Node and Tumor-Infiltrating Lymphocytes.** Natural killing (NK) is the functional description of a phenomenon whereby effector cells spontaneously lyse certain syngeneic, allogeneic, and xenogeneic targets. In man, the major NK population probably consists of certain cells of lymphoid origin. M. Moore and B. M. Vose (Manchester, England) investigated whether the low level of NK activity in lymph nodes, a common feature in man and rodents, is attributable to an intrinsic deficit of "mature" NK cells or their precur-

---

(9–28) J. Immunol. 126:1284–1289, April 1981.
(9–29) Int. J. Cancer 27:265–272, 1981.

sors, or both, or to their presence in a suppressed (i.e., functionally inactive) state.

A major distinction was found between the cytolytic activity of peripheral blood lymphocytes and that of lymph node and tumor-infiltrating lymphocytes against targets of the NK-sensitive erythroleukemic cell line K562 in short-term ^{51}Cr release assays. In the peripheral blood lymphocytes of normal donors and lung cancer patients in whom disease was advanced, anti-K562 reactivity, though variable, was consistently detectable; this activity could be augmented to a similar extent in patients and controls by treatment of effectors with exogenous interferon. By contrast, anti-K562 activity in lymph node cells and tumor-infiltrating lymphocytes was virtually absent, and significant levels could not be induced by exposure to interferon. This activity was not attributable to coexistent suppressor cells for NK function, because admixture of lymph node cells and tumor-infiltrating lymphocytes with normal peripheral blood lymphocytes failed to modulate K562 killing by the latter.

The results imply that K562-reactive NK cells and their precursors may frequently be present at subthreshold levels in the lymph nodes of tumor-bearing patients. A similar explanation could account for the inactivity of tumor-infiltrating lymphocytes. However, in the latter situation, actively induced NK dysfunction in situ incapable of regeneration by interferon and attributable to as yet undefined tumor-associated factors also may be involved.

▶ [This is another attempt to clarify the possible role of NK cells in vivo. This and other experiments of this type are necessary in order to help define the role of NK cells in vivo because the prior evidence has been obtained almost exclusively by in vitro studies.—J.S.N.] ◀

9–30 **Randomized Trial of Levamisole Versus Placebo as Adjuvant Therapy in Malignant Melanoma.** The anthelmintic levamisole increases cell-mediated immunity in animals and man and has been reported to result in prolonged disease-free survival in patients with unresectable breast carcinoma. Malignant melanoma seems to be ideal for evaluation of this agent, because the host mounts an immune response to melanoma, and occurrence of halo nevi and vitiligo suggests an immune response involving the pigment-producing cells. Lynn E. Spitler and Richard Sagebiel (Univ. of California, San Francisco) carried out a double-blind, placebo-controlled trial of levamisole as adjuvant therapy in patients with surgically treated malignant melanoma. The patients had Clark level III, IV, or V, mucosal or acral-lentigenous melanoma or cutaneous, subcutaneous, or node recurrence of melanoma. Levamisole was given in a dosage of 150 mg for 3 consecutive days every 2 weeks.

Levamisole was given to 104 patients, and placebo to 99. Median follow-up was 3½ years. No significant differences were found in time to first recurrence, time to first visceral recurrence (Fig 9–11), or survival. Time to visceral recurrence and survival, however, showed trends favoring levamisole-treated patients, particularly those with stage I

(9–30) N. Engl. J. Med. 303:1143–1147, Nov. 13, 1980.

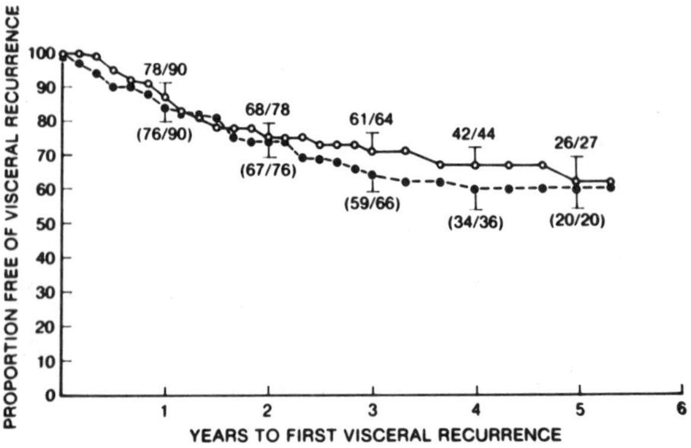

Fig 9–11.—Time to first visceral recurrence in 90 patients with malignant melanoma treated with levamisole *(open circles)* and 90 treated with placebo *(solid circles)*. Numbers represent number of patients free from visceral recurrence during interval per number of patients entering each interval. Vertical bars represent SEM; $P < .48$. (Courtesy of Spitler, L. E., and Sagebiel, R.: N. Engl. J. Med. 303:1143–1147, Nov. 13, 1980.)

disease. No differences were found between levamisole- and placebo-treated patients with stage II melanoma.

This study indicated that levamisole has no benefit over placebo as adjuvant therapy for malignant melanoma. A study appears to be warranted to determine the efficacy of levamisole in patients with stage I melanoma.

▶ [Spitler was once one of the leaders in the optimistic school of immunotherapists. As each and every presumptively immunotherapeutic agent is brought to the test of the randomized prospective blind study, each fails. This is a particularly elegant, well-documented study of such failure. As such, it is an extremely important study.—J.S.N.] ◀

10. Skin, Subcutaneous Tissue, and Hand

10–1 **Arterial Shunting as Adjunct to Major Limb Revascularization.** James A. Nunley, L. Andrew Koman, and James R. Urbaniak (Duke Univ.) used temporary arterial and venous shunting to reduce warm ischemia in major limb replantation and revascularization on 8 occasions since 1979.

METHOD.—In the area from the axilla to the antecubital fossa, the severed ends of the artery are located and freed of soft tissue along 3 cm on both sides of the laceration. The severed proximal end is cut transversely and any clot is removed. A vascular "keeper," made of moistened umbilical tape within a rubber catheter, is inserted over the artery. The distal end is prepared similarly. The Sundt shunt is inserted proximally and the keeper drawn down tight to prevent leakage. The distal end is similarly inserted and the keeper snugged; the tourniquet or clamp is released, thus reestablishing blood flow.

From the antecubital fossa to the wrist crease, the ends of the arteries are dissected free and vascular keepers slipped over the edges. A ventriculoperitoneal shunt is trimmed to the desired length and inserted proximally and distally (Fig 10–1). Before release of the tourniquet, 3,000 units of heparin are given intravenously. (As an alternative, the shunts may be preheparinized by soaking in heparin.)

In all 8 patients, palpable distal pulses with excellent back-bleeding were obtained after shunt insertion. Ischemic muscle, which could not be stimulated prior to reperfusion, contracted after 20 minutes of arterial shunting in all cases. During perfusion of the distal extremity, exploration, efficient and meticulous debridement, and rigid internal or external skeletal fixation were accomplished prior to definitive arterial repair in a controlled environment. There were no complications attributable to the shunt. Sundt shunts were used in 5 repairs of the axillary or brachial arteries and ventriculoperitoneal shunts in 3 radial arteries.

It was unnecessary to shunt both the radial and ulnar arteries in forearm replantation. With the radial artery shunted, good back-bleeding occurred from the ulnar artery. Once the bone was stabilized, the ulnar artery was repaired, the radial artery shunt removed, and this vessel anastomosed. There was no thrombosis within the shunt itself. The only difficulty encountered was bleeding when the vascular keeper slipped off, allowing the vessel to leak.

Temporary arterial shunting is a useful adjunct to major arterial repair associated with massive soft tissue and bony trauma. It is

(10–1) Ann. Surg. 193:271–273, March 1981.

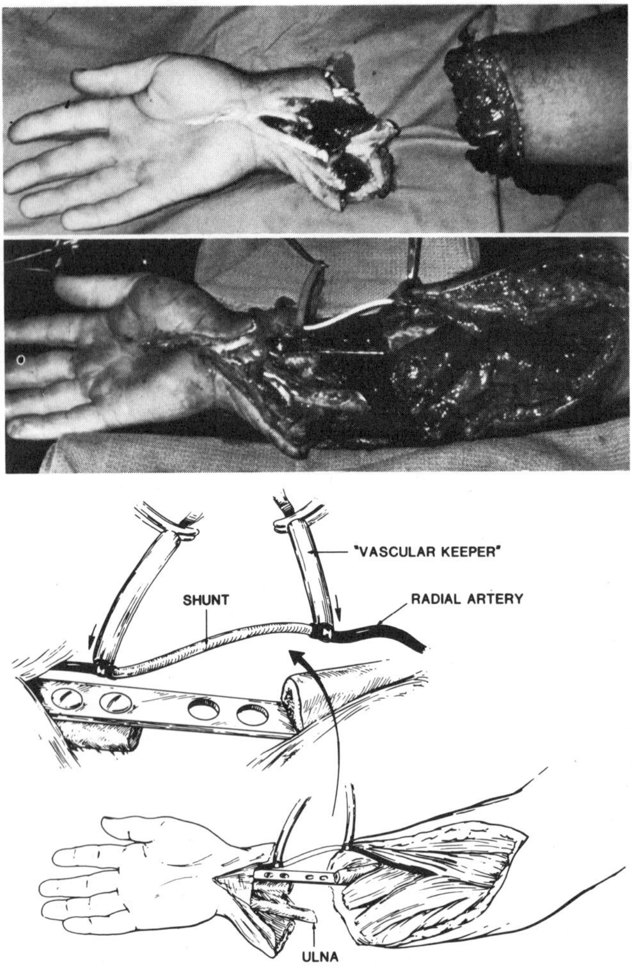

Fig 10–1.—Top, complete amputation of hand proximal to wrist. **Center,** peritoneal shunt within radial artery allowing reperfusion during rigid bony stabilization with dynamic compression plate on radius. **Bottom,** vascular keepers prevent leakage around shunt. (Courtesy of Nunley, J. A., et al.: Ann. Surg. 193:271–273, March 1981.)

probably not necessary for clean sharp amputations treated within 2–3 hours of injury.

▶ [The major importance of this article is its emphasis on rapid revascularization. Whether a shunt is used or the orthopedic aspect of bone stabilization is accelerated, the message is clear: Revascularization must be more rapid than often occurs during major limb replantation.—E.E.P.] ◀

10–2 **Recovery of Function Following Replantation and Revascularization of Amputated Hand Parts.** Frank A. Scott, John W. Howar, and John A. Boswick, Jr. (Univ. of Colorado) reviewed results in 100 patients (two-thirds were aged 10–40 years) who underwent re-

(10–2) J. Trauma 21:204–214, March 1981.

plantation or revascularization of 149 hand units from 1975 to 1979. Replantation of 17 thumbs and 48 fingers was performed in 34 male and 4 female patients. Revascularization of 13 thumbs and 71 fingers was performed in 47 males and 15 female patients. A power saw was the cause of injury in 53% of replantation patients and 24% of revascularization patients. The most common level of injury in both groups was the proximal phalanx of the finger and thumb.

Standard surgical techniques were used. The survival was 79% for replanted units and 97% for revascularized parts. After an average follow-up of 15 months, all replantation patients and 55% of revascularization patients reported cold intolerance. Only 2 patients were not satisfied with the result. The physical appearance of the restored parts was generally satisfactory. Of replanted fingers, 84% had poor (less than 180 degrees) total active motion, and avulsion injuries gave the poorest results. Of revascularized fingers, 28% had poor total active motion, and avulsion injuries responded best. Injuries at the metacarpophalangeal joint, proximal phalanx, and proximal interphalangeal joint produced the poorest results. Grip strength in the replantation group averaged 53% of that of the uninjured hand, and return of pinch strength was 50%; in the revascularized group these figures were 65% and 59%, respectively. Normal two-point sensibility discrimination was regained in 40% of replanted digits and 71% of revascularized digits. Most digits regained two-point discrimination of better than 10 mm. Of replantation patients, 80% underwent secondary operations, usually flexor tendon reconstruction. Of employable replant patients, 88% returned to work (one-third to the same job) within an average of 4.4 months. Of revascularization patients, 97% returned to work within an average of 3.9 months.

Restoration of tendon and joint function was aided by early and aggressive flexor tendon reconstruction, early digital motion, and primary insertion of Silastic rods when a poor result was expected because of tendon or soft tissue damage. Single-digit amputations usually should not be replanted; exceptions include thumb amputations in all age groups and finger amputations in children, who generally obtain better motion and sensibility. Single digits that require revascularization in the presence of fracture and tendon or nerve injuries should also be amputated. The most important digits for power grip are the ring and little fingers, which require good range of motion, whereas the other fingers are used mainly for pinch, making a full range of motion less important. In the thumb, restoration of length and sensibility is more important than range of motion.

▶ [Studies such as this one are needed badly. Recent data suggest that replantation of individual and distal finger tips seldom is indicated. Moreover, in the editor's judgment, replantation of every amputated thumb is not indicated. Even though skin, subcutaneous tissue, nerve, bone, and tendon will heal after repair, the end result of having all of these tissues heal at the same level in a single digit is often functionally inadequate. This basic principle has not permeated the thinking of many microvascular replant enthusiasts.—E.E.P.] ◀

0–3 **Primary Neurovascular Bundle Transfer in the Management of Avulsed Thumbs.** Gary W. Lobay and Gerry L. Moysa (Edmon-

(10–3) J. Hand Surg. 6:31–34, January 1981.

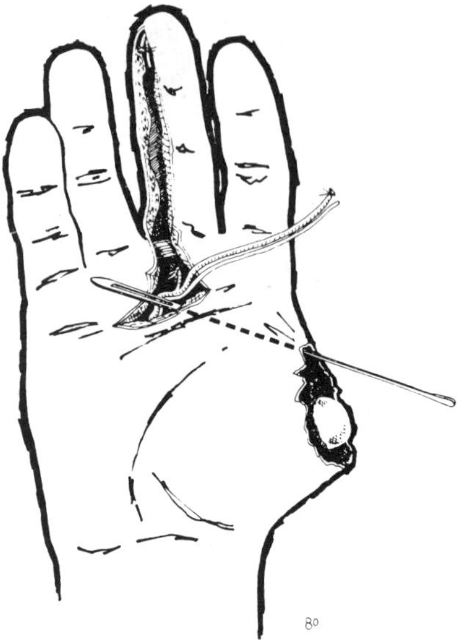

Fig 10–2.—Neurovascular bundle has been divided and is about to be passed through subcutaneous palmar tunnel to lie on ulnar side of thumb. (Courtesy of Lobay, G. W., and Moysa, G. L.: J. Hand Surg. 6:31–34, January 1981.)

ton, Alta.) obtained an initial survival rate of 54% in a series of 13 replantations of avulsed thumbs with the use of conventional microsurgical techniques. The rate for cleanly amputated thumbs approached 75%. The next 10 cases were managed by primary transfer of the neurovascular bundle from the ulnar side of the long finger, and a survival rate of 90% was obtained. Suitable patients with injury proximal to the interphalangeal joint and a warm ischemia time of less than 8 hours are accepted. The neurovascular bundle from the ulnar side of the long finger is mobilized, divided at the level of the distal interphalangeal joint, and passed through a subcutaneous palmar tunnel to the ulnar side of the thumb (Fig. 10–2). Systemic heparinization is used only when there is clinical evidence of arterial or venous insufficiency.

Most patients have been farmers injured in tractor accidents. Most amputations were at the metacarpophalangeal joint and the proximal phalanx. The average time of predominantly "cold" ischemia was 6 to 8 hours. The 5 patients followed up after neurovascular bundle transfer for 9 months to 3 years had sensation confined to the ulnar side of the thumb. Four had less than 10 mm of two-point discrimination, and all 5 perceived pinprick sensation adequately. All patients were satisfied with the outcome. All but 1 have returned to their original work. All have some cold intolerance of the long finger and the thumb.

More recently, 9 additional avulsed thumbs have been replanted or revascularized by using the neurovascular bundle transfer method, and 7 of these thumbs have survived. This procedure has resulted in a dramatic increase in the survival rate and has made primary nerve reconstruction possible. It now is used routinely in cases of avulsion injury of the thumb.

▶ [This is a superb technical maneuver. Avoidance of vein grafts, thus reducing the number of suture lines by half, is well worth the dissection of a vascular bundle from the side of an adjacent finger. When the thumb is being revascularized, the index finger vessels should not be used; transfer of the index finger on a neurovascular bundle may be required if revascularization fails.—E.E.P.] ◀

10–4 **Digital Artery Sympathectomy.** Adrian E. Flatt (Norwalk, Conn.) has developed a very distal sympathectomy at the level of origin of the proper digital arteries and evaluated it in 4 men and 4 women with digital vascular insufficiency due to frostbite, crush injury, scleroderma, or Raynaud's disease. With the aid of magnification, meticulous circumferential excision of the adventitia, which contains sympathetic fibers, is performed beyond the junction of the distal perforating artery with the common digital artery. A palmar approach is used to remove the adventitia over 3 to 4 mm. More extensive clearance of branches arising more distally from the proper digital nerves also can be performed. Postoperative care is minimal.

All 8 patients having this operation benefited, but assessment of the results of surgery has been difficult. Three with sequelae of frostbite have done well. Both patients having sympathectomy of the right long finger for cold sensitivity after crush injury of the digit had a significant rise in skin temperature after operation, but neither had complete relief of symptoms. Three patients had 4 digital sympathectomies for varying presentations of Raynaud-type disease. One of them had scleroderma and 1 had systemic lupus erythematosus. A temperature rise was observed after operation in all patients, and symptomatic improvement was noted.

This very distal digital artery sympathectomy has proved useful in the treatment of patients with sequelae of frostbite or crush injury of the digit and Raynaud-type disease.

▶ [Although the author, a distinguished hand surgeon, has observed beneficial effects from local sympathectomy, I have not been able to confirm such observations. My own experience has been that if a sympathectomy is needed, local measures are not sufficient. A major regional sympathetic block or intravertebral T2, T3, and T4 motor root sections are needed to remove autonomic control of blood vessels in the upper extremity.—E.E.P.] ◀

0–5 **A Randomized Prospective Comparison of Fascicular and Epineural Digital Nerve Repairs.** Although fascicular nerve repair theoretically should allow better function, animal studies have not shown a significant difference from epineural repairs. Leroy Young, R. Chris Wray, and Paul M. Weeks (Washington Univ.) reviewed the results of 34 digital nerve repairs performed in 27 patients in 1977–1979. The 18 male and 9 female patients had a mean age of 29 years. Twenty-four median nerve branches and 10 ulnar nerve branches were repaired. Sharp injuries were present in 27 instances and crushing injuries in 7. Fascicular and epineural repairs were each done in 17 instances. Most of both types of repair were done within a month after injury. Repairs were done at the level of the metacarpals in 12 instances, at the proximal phalangeal level in 15, and at the middle phalangeal level in 7.

The fascicular and epineural repair groups were comparable in age,

(10–4) J. Hand Surg. 5:550–556, November 1980.
(10–5) Plast. Reconstr. Surg. 68:89–92, July 1981.

type of injury, site of injury, and the surgeons performing the operations. No significant difference in the return of two-point discrimination was observed with respect to the type of repair, but age significantly influenced the return of two-point discrimination. No differences in return of light touch or pin-prick sensation were noted.

Digital nerves contain only 3 or 4 fascicles and minimal perineural tissue, facilitating the proper alignment and axial orientation of fascicles at epineural repair. An epineural digital nerve repair is, in a sense, analogous to a group fascicular nerve graft in a larger nerve, and any advantage from aligning the fascicles may be offset by the added trauma and fibrosis resulting from the necessary dissection and suturing. Patients in the present series who were younger than age 20 years had about an 80% chance of achieving useful two-point discrimination. Patients older than age 40 had essentially no chance of obtaining such a result, but protective sensation uniformly returned.

▶ [In my judgment, this is one of the best—if not the only adequate—study comparing fascicular and epineural digital nerve repairs in human beings. Although it is difficult to measure the subjective return of sensation objectively, the authors have done the best that is possible at this time and have presented data that should control some of the unrestrained enthusiasm for fascicular nerve repair. Because fascicular nerve repair has disadvantages, this study is important and should do much to alleviate increased intraneural scarring caused by an excessive number of sutures and intraneural dissection.—E.E.P.] ◀

10–6 **Three Complications of Untreated Partial Laceration of Flexor Tendon: Entrapment, Rupture, and Triggering.** The management of partial laceration of a flexor tendon is controversial. James D. Schlenker, Graham D. Lister, and Harold E. Kleinert have treated 3 patients for complications resulting from unrepaired and untreated partial laceration of flexor tendons.

Man, 29, lacerated the right ring finger when a light bulb burst, and he

Fig 10–3.—Distally based flaps of flexor digitorum superficialis and profundus are demonstrated. With the flexor tendon sheaths open, a retractor has been placed beneath the flexor tendons near the site of partial division. (Courtesy of Schlenker, J. D., et al.: J. Hand Surg. 6:392–398, July 1981.)

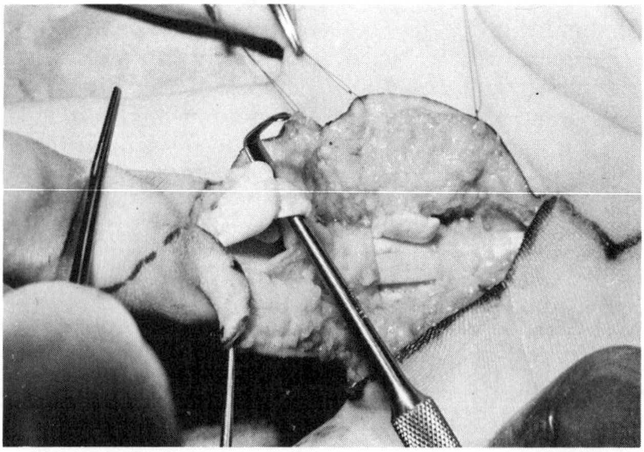

(10–6) J. Hand Surg. 6:392–398, July 1981.

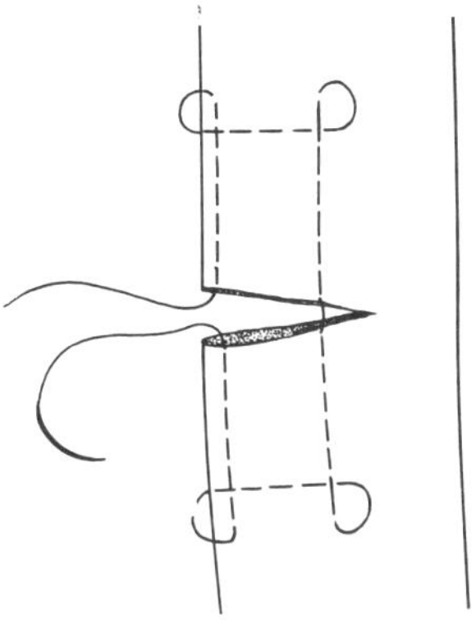

Fig 10–4.—For a 50% or greater laceration of the tendon, a modified Kessler-Mason-Allen suture is placed, followed by a running peripheral suture. (Courtesy of Schlenker, J. D., et al.: J. Hand Surg. 6:392–398, July 1981.)

noted limited flexion after removal of glass fragments and suture of the skin laceration. The proximal interphalangeal joint flexed actively from 0 to 70 degrees at 5 weeks, and the distal interphalangeal joint flexed from 0 to 50 degrees. Passive motion was normal. Exploration showed distally based flaps of the flexor digitorum profundus and superficialis tendons (Fig 10–3). On flexion, the flaps became caught in a rent in the A2 pulley, limiting excursion of the tendons. The flaps were excised, leaving three fourths of the cross-sectional area of the tendons intact. A splint was applied for 3 weeks. The patient eventually regained a full range of function.

A second patient had tendon rupture 2 weeks after injury, and a third experienced triggering 2 months after injury as a result of scar formation on the tendon and pulley. The patient with tendon rupture initially refused treatment, and she subsequently required a tendon graft.

Tendons lacerated less than half of their cross-sectional area may be repaired with a running 6–0 braided synthetic suture, placed only about the lacerated part of the circumference. If more of the tendon is divided, a modified Kessler-Mason-Allen suture of no. 4–0 or 5–0 is utilized (Fig 10–4). The tenorrhaphy is completed by placing the running suture around the periphery of the cut part of the tendon. The suture should be placed more on the palmar than the dorsal aspect of the tendon, and only the ends of the tendon should be approximated. The significant pulleys should be left relatively undisturbed during tendon repair. Immediate mobilization is controlled by use of the rubber band splinting technique.

▶ [Although untreated partial laceration of flexor tendons can result in complications such as are reported in this study, they do not necessarily have to occur if the tendon wound is made "tidy" by adequate debridement and if good judgment is exercised during postoperative care. The work of Weeks showing that it is not necessary to repair all partial lacerations of flexor tendons made a contribution to this field that should not be lost because poor surgical therapy or poor judgment may produce an inferior result.—E.E.P.] ◀

0–7 **Elongation in Profundus Tendon Repair: Clinical and Radiologic Study.** Studies of tendon repair in animals show that separation of the tendon ends sometimes occurs, but no clinical data exist.

(10–7) Scand. J. Plast. Reconstr. Surg. 15:61–68, 1981.

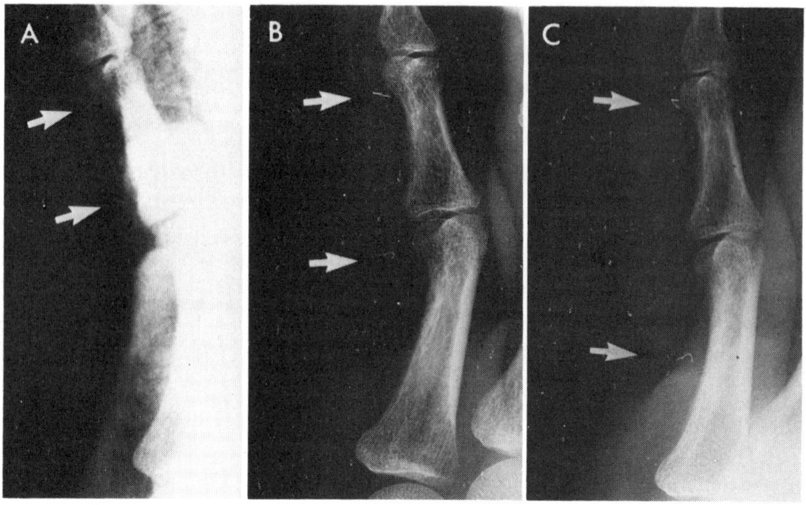

Fig 10–5.—Radiograms showing elongation after primary suture of profundus tendon. **A,** after 1 day; **B,** after 3 weeks; **C,** after 6 weeks. (Courtesy of Ejeskär, A., and Irstam, L.: Scand. J. Plast. Reconstr. Surg. 15:61–68, 1981.)

Arvid Ejeskär and Lars Irstam (Sahlgrenska Hosp., Göteborg, Sweden) repaired severed flexor profundus tendons in 63 digits of 55 patients, aged 8–61 years.

TECHNIQUE.—The tendon was repaired with a crisscross suture using 5–0 stainless steel in 9 cases. A modification of the Kessler method (1963), using 4–0 Silky Polydec, sometimes supplemented by a running circumferential suture of 6–0 Silky Polydec, was used in the other cases. During operation, a small piece of 5–0 steel wire was introduced transversely through each end of the tendon just outside the suture area to serve as a marker. Postoperatively, a cast was applied to hold the wrist and metacarpophalangeal joints in 45 degrees flexion and the interphalangeal joints in the zero position. Graded active movements of the finger were begun 3–4 weeks later.

Radiographic measurement of the distance between markers at operation and postoperatively on three different occasions showed that an increase of the distance by more than 5 mm, considered to indicate elongation in the suture, occurred in 25 (42%) of 59 repaired profundus tendons (Fig 10–5). This usually happened during the period of immobilization. The cause of elongation could be identified in 9 digits: in 5 it was due to rupture of the suture material (5–0 Flexon steel wire) and in 4 to slipping of the knot (4–0 Silky Polydec).

Sixty digits were reexamined 6—36 months (mean, 15 months) after operation. In the distal interphalangeal joint, increased distance between markers and range of active motion showed a strong correlation; only 5 of 17 digits with an increase in intermarker distance exceeding 10 mm had any motion in this joint, whereas all digits with an increase of less than 10 mm had a minumum range of motion of 10 degrees in that joint. Increased intermarker distance and total active motion of the finger also showed a strong correlation; a poor result occurred in 11 of 17 digits with an increased distance of more than 10 mm but in only 4 of 39 with an increased distance of 10 mm or less.

After profundus tendon repair, reoperation should be considered if an increase in the distance between markers exceeding 10 mm is found during the first postoperative week. Tenolysis in digits with small increases in intermarker distance is very successful, but an increase of 10 mm or more indicates extensive adhesions, so that tenolysis is less likely to succeed. In fingers in which elongation did not explain the poor result, long-standing postoperative swelling was present; thus, in cases where resuture is considered, absence of edema preoperatively is mandatory.

▶ [Longitudinal slipping of a crossed suture contributes significantly to the appearance of elongation of the scar between the two ends of a repaired profundus tendon. Inadequate debridement of the tendon ends, inaccurate placement of sutures in the tendon, motion too early, and failure to overcorrect the length of the tendon are factors that produce the appearance of elongation of a profundus tendon. The basic biologic problem is secondary remodeling of the scar tissue between tendon ends to produce an elongated structure. This is one biologic problem that is solvable by expert technique.—E.E.P.] ◀

10–8 **Carpal Tunnel Syndrome: Study of Carpal Canal Pressures.** Richard H. Gelberman, Patrick T. Hergenroeder, Alan R. Hargens, Goran N. Lundborg, and Wayne H. Akeson used a wick catheter to measure intracarpal pressures in 11 men and 4 women, aged 28–70 years (mean, 56 years), who had symptoms of carpal tunnel syndrome for 9 weeks to 10 years (mean, 30 months). The carpal canal pressures of 12 controls were similarly determined.

Mean pressure in the carpal canal was significantly elevated in the patients. Mean pressure with the wrist in neutral position was 32 mm Hg in patients and 2.5 mm Hg in controls ($P < .001$). Mean pressure with the wrist at 90 degrees of flexion was 94 mm Hg in patients and 31 mm Hg in controls ($P < .005$). Mean pressure with 90 degrees of wrist extension was 110 mm Hg in patients and 30 mm Hg in controls ($P < .01$). In the patients, the immediate postoperative carpal canal pressures averaged 5 mm Hg. When measured 2 months later in 7 patients, they averaged 3.5 mm Hg.

Postoperatively, all patients had relief of pain and paresthesias, although 4 had persisting subjective thumb numbness and 1 had persistent mild swelling of the hand. Intracarpal canal pressures were not correlated with age, sex, or duration of symptoms. The symptoms and signs, electric findings. and response to treatment did not correlate with the magnitude of pressure elevations.

Factors other than increases in pressure in the carpal tunnel probably play a significant role in the causation of carpal tunnel syndrome. There may be a use for measurement of tissue pressure in patients with suspected acute carpal tunnel syndrome. Carpal canal pressure measurements may help to differentiate the causes of neural deficits, such as nerve contusion versus acute compression after trauma to the wrist.

▶ [This interesting study confirms the need for opening widely the carpal tunnel.

(10–8) J. Bone Joint Surg. [Am.] 63:380–383, March 1981.

Major problems in carpal tunnel surgery often are missed by inadequate decompression with a small transverse incision performed as an office procedure. Persistence or increasing development of symptoms usually means that the correct diagnosis was missed or that treatment was inadequate. Tumor and significant tenosynovitis are examples of missed diagnoses; inadequate division of the full extent of the carpal ligament is an example of inadequate treatment.—E.E.P.] ◀

10–9 **Wrist Ganglia: Incidence and Recurrence Rate After Operation.** To obtain 5-year follow-up data, Lars Janzon and Igor A. Niechajev (Malmö, Sweden) mailed a questionnaire to 165 consecutive patients (105 female) operated on for primary wrist ganglia during 1970 and 1971. A standard operation was performed under regional intravenous anesthesia. The ganglion, exposed in a bloodless field by a transverse skin incision, was widely excised, in toto, with its base. When it exceeded 1½–2 cm in diameter, it often had to be aspirated to minimize the risk of vessel or tendon damage during dissection. Postoperative immobilization lasted 7–10 days.

The questionnaire was returned by 144 patients. Age distribution showed a peak incidence at 10–30 years. The female to male ratio was 1.7:1. The annual incidence rate was 43 affected individuals per 100,000 for women and 25 per 100,000 for men. Wrist ganglia were 3½ times more common on the dorsal than on the volar side. Nearly 60% of the patients sought medical advice within 1 year of symptom onset; most had a history lasting less than 1 month. The ganglion was 1 cm or less in diameter in 52% of the patients. No correlation was found between sex and ganglion size. The main indication for operation was pain or cosmetic dissatisfaction, or both. Most patients were unable to work for 10–20 days postoperatively. In the 5-year follow-up period, 21 ganglia recurred, for a recurrence rate of 12.7%. Of recurrent ganglia, 60% appeared within 6 months after operation.

In terms of cure rate, convalescence time, and cost, the most important factors to be considered in the surgical treatment of wrist ganglia are gentle technique, bloodless field, wide excision, ample excision of the joint capsule involved, and postoperative immobilization for 7–10 days. Considering the prevalence of preganglionic ducts in the joint capsule, it seems unlikely that the recurrence rate can be further reduced by reconstruction of the joint capsule by transposition of extensor retinaculum or by fascia lata transplant.

▶ [Recurrence of wrist ganglia virtually can be prevented, in my experience, by excising an area rather than a lesion. Ganglia appear to be areas of mucoid degeneration in dense connective tissue. A ganglion, therefore, is not a specific epithelialized cyst that can be excised like other cysts. A procedure not unlike the Sistruck procedure for thyroglossal duct sinus has been most effective in my practice.—E.E.P.] ◀

(10–9) Scand. J. Plast. Reconstr. Surg. 15:53–56, 1981.

11. The Breast

11–1 **Computed Tomographic Mammography: Diagnosis of Mammographically and Clinically Occult Carcinoma of Breast.** If breast cancer can be detected while still localized and nonpalpable, the prognosis for cure is excellent. However, even with conventional mammography, some minimal breast carcinomas are undetectable. Justo L. Sibala, C. H. Joseph Chang, Fritz Lin, and William R. Jewell (Univ. of Kansas) report findings in 2 patients with breast cancer; the lesions, less than 5 mm in diameter, were clinically and mammographically occult, but were correctly diagnosed preoperatively by computed tomographic mammography (CT/M) with use of contrast media enhancement.

Woman, 64, had tenderness in the upper inner quadrant of the left breast for 1 month but no nipple discharge, pain, or lumps. Her mother had had breast carcinoma. Findings on physical examination were normal. Routine mammographs showed a normal fatty left breast. The CT/M study showed a tiny area with a high contrast medium enhancement of 29 CT numbers (5.8% increase in density) in the lower outer quadrant of the left breast compatible with malignancy. Under general anesthesia, the involved quadrant was removed. Frozen-section analysis showed no abnormalities, but study of the permanent sections disclosed a moderately differentiated invasive ductal carcinoma measuring 0.3×0.4 cm. Modified left radical mastectomy was performed. No metastases were found in the left axillary nodes.

The General Electric CT/M system is a prototype CT fan-beam scanner specially designed for breast scanning. Scans are obtained both before and after intravenous infusion of 300 ml of diatrizoate meglumine within 10 minutes. Demonstration of an area of marked contrast medium enhancement, over 25 CT numbers (5% increase in density), is "highly suspicious for malignancy." Normal breast tissue and most benign lesions show only minimal contrast medium enhancement, usually less than 20 CT numbers (4% increase in density).

The CT/M examination appears to be beneficial for the screening of high-risk patients. However, the need for intravenous infusion of iodinated contrast medium, the high cost of the examination, and length of the procedure make CT/M inappropriate as a screening tool for the general population.

▶ [Here is yet another use for CT! It is interesting that CT can be used to diagnose occult breast cancer; in my opinion, there is seldom an indication to do so.—E.E.P.] ◀

11–2 **Scintiscanning of Breast With ^{99m}Tc-Diethylene Triamine Penta-Acetic Acid: Prospective Blind Evaluation** was conducted by A. Cuschieri, F. Hutchinson, G. D. S. Neill, M. L. Wisbey, R. A. B.

(11–1) Arch. Surg. 116:114–117, January 1981.
(11–2) Br. J. Surg. 68:147–149, March 1981.

Wood, P. Preece, and J. Clark (Ninewells Hosp., Dundee, Scotland) in 67 women, aged 22–70 years, with a breast complaint (pain, nipple discharge, lump). An intravenous injection of 8.0 mCi of ^{99m}Tc-diethylene triamine penta-acetic acid (DTPA) was given. Both breasts and axillas were scanned in both lateral and medial modes 30 minutes and 2 hours later. Malignancy was diagnosed when enhanced localized uptake of the isotope, seen at 0.5–1 hour, persisted with the same or increased intensity on the 2-hour image.

The full battery of examinations eventually showed benign disease in 35 patients and malignant disease in 32. The predictive value of positive scans in establishing the presence of breast cancer was 94%, with a false negative rate of 6%. The predictive value of the test when negative in excluding breast cancer was 97%, with a false positive rate of 3%.

Scintigraphic imaging of benign breast disease yielded some useful data. In patients with cyclic pronounced mastalgia, the scans outlined active "hot" breasts with intense uniform uptake of the isotope complex by the entire breast tissue. The DTPA uptake by localized or diffuse benign lesions (fibroadenomas or fibrocystic mastopathy) was sometimes enhanced but was always transient, declining or disappearing in the 2-hour scan. In fibrocystic disease, the cysts were outlined as low-uptake areas surrounded by mottled zones of increased uptake in adjacent breast parenchyma.

The technique of DTPA scintiscanning has a high diagnostic accuracy in differentiating benign from malignant lesions of the breast. It may also be useful in differentiation of the various clinical forms of mastalgia and in objective assessment of the results of specific therapy.

▶ [The data in this report seem encouraging in regard to the diagnosis of a primary lesion in the breast. Remember, however, that lymphoscintigraphy has not been proved successful in diagnosing breast cancer in axillary lymph nodes.—E.E.P.] ◀

11–3 **Clinical Benign Disorders of Breast and Carcinoma of Breast.** Studies of the relationship between benign and malignant breast disorders have involved microscopic examination of cancerous breast tissue for the concurrent presence of benign disorders; also, findings in women who had breast biopsies have been reviewed retrospectively to determine the number in whom breast carcinoma develops. Both types of studies usually showed that women with benign breast disorders are at greater risk for the development of breast carcinoma. However, there are inconsistencies and contradictions in these studies; physicians usually have to deal with gross physical signs rather than with microscopic findings, and data on the incidence of benign breast disorders in the general population are limited.

James E. Devitt (Univ. of Ottawa) studied the relation between preexisting clinical, rather than microscopic, benign breast disorders, and breast carcinoma. Of 2,506 consecutive women aged 15 years and older seen between 1970 and 1979 for a mammary problem, 345 had carcinoma and 2,161 had clinical benign disorders. Thus, clinical be-

---

(11–3) Surg. Gynecol. Obstet. 152:437–440, April 1981.

nign breast disorders occurred 6.3 times more often than carcinoma of the breast. The lifetime risk of clinical benign breast disorder was calculated to be more than 50%. Clinical benign breast disorders occurred chiefly in young women, reached a peak at age 45–49 years, and declined rapidly thereafter. The incidence of breast carcinoma began to increase in women aged 45–49 and became more common thereafter. Thus, clinical benign breast disorders precede carcinoma because of the age at which the disorders occur.

A total of 390 women had a history of benign findings on a previous breast biopsy or cyst aspiration. The incidence of a previous benign biopsy in women with carcinoma was 10.4%; it was estimated to be at least 8.2% in the general population. Only 36 women with carcinoma had a previous benign biopsy. The likelihood of finding carcinoma was 9.2% in women with a previous benign biopsy and 14.6% in those without a previous benign biopsy. Of the 36 women with breast carcinoma and a previous benign biopsy, 31 were older than age 50 and 18 were older than age 60.

Women with clinical benign breast disorders do not have an increased risk for the development of breast carcinoma.

▶ [Such studies as this are important to place in proper perspective the plethora of reports that claim that there is an increased incidence of carcinoma of the breast in patients with benign breast disease. The fact is that we do not know. If there is an increased incidence of breast cancer associated with benign disease, it seems doubtful that the incidence is high enough to justify routine use of subcutaneous mastectomy to prevent cancer.—E.E.P.] ◀

11–4 **Multifocal Breast Carcinoma.** In considering local excision of breast cancer, the risk of multiple foci of tumor growth must be taken into account. Sighild Westman-Naeser, Evert Bengtsson, Olle Eriksson, Torsten Jarkrans, Bo Nordin, and Björn Stenkvist (Uppsala, Sweden) examined the problem of multifocality of breast cancer in 173 women having a mean age of 63 years who had a diagnosis of operable breast cancer in a 5-month period. Simple mastectomy, radical mastectomy, or mastectomy with exploration was carried out, with exeresis of the axilla where necessary. Controls included age-matched women without breast cancer.

Fifteen of the breast cancers (8.7%) had grossly visible multiple tumors that were clearly separate from one another. Study of tissue sections showed unrelated foci of invasive cancer in another 26 (15%) cases. Epithelial proliferation combined with severe atypia or carcinoma in situ was present in 11 (6.4%) cases. In all, 52 (30%) patients had multifocal tumor growth. Thirteen (7.5%) had bilateral breast cancer. Ten patients had already had one breast removed because of cancer, and 3 had cancer diagnosed on the other side within 3 years postoperatively. These patients did not have an increased incidence of multifocal tumors. The size of the primary tumor and the presence of axillary or distant metastases did not correlate with multifocality, nor was death from breast cancer so related. Multifocal growth did not correlate with age or with a previous diagnosis of benign breast

(11–4) Am. J. Surg. 142:255–257, August 1981.

disease. Abnormality of the cell nucleus also appeared to be unrelated to multifocal growth of breast cancer.

Nearly one third of patients in this series had multifocal growth of cancer in the same breast as the dominant breast cancer. This high rate must be considered when planning treatment by less than radical operation. A biologic experiment such as tylectomy or partial removal of the breast appears to be associated with considerable risks for patients.

▶ [There is little doubt that cancer is multifocal in many patients. This fact cannot be used at this time, however, as a reason to stop investigation of conservative therapy, including "lumpectomy." The biologic significance of microscopic multifocal breast carcinoma has not been determined. Untold numbers of patients were taken back to the operating room for an unnecessary total thyroidectomy when carcinoma was found after lobectomy or subtotal thyroidectomy—before it was realized that multifocal microscopic thyroid cancer was not the same as clinically discernible gross cancer. The biologic significance may or may not be the same in breast cancer.—E.E.P.] ◀

11-5 **Comparing Radical Mastectomy With Quadrantectomy, Axillary Dissection, and Radiotherapy in Patients With Small Cancers of the Breast.** Few advances have been made in conservative surgical procedures that would save a major part of the breast in patients with small cancers. Umberto Veronesi, Roberto Saccozzi, Marcella Del Vecchio, Alberto Banfi, Claudio Clemente, Mario De Lena, Giuseppe Gallus, Marco Greco, Alberto Luini, Ettore Marubini, Giuseppe Muscolino, Franco Rilke, Bruno Salvadori, Annamaria Zecchini, and Roberto Zucali (Milan) conducted a controlled study comparing the classic Halsted mastectomy with a conservative procedure

Fig 11–1.—Actuarial overall survival in patients treated with Halsted mastectomy or with quadrantectomy, axillary dissection, and radiotherapy (log-rank test: overall χ^2, .02 with 1 degree of freedom; P = .88). (Courtesy of Veronesi, U., et al.: N. Engl. J. Med. 305:6–11, July 2, 1981.)

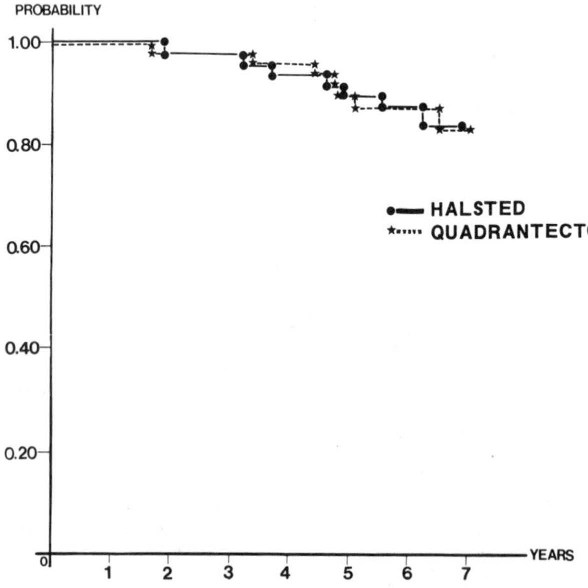

(11–5) N. Engl. J. Med. 305:6–11, July 2, 1981.

in patients with breast cancers up to 2 cm in maximum diameter. Cases of in situ lobular carcinoma and noninfiltrating ductal carcinoma were excluded. The conservative operation involved the resection of a breast quadrant and dissection of axillary nodes, followed by irradiation with 5,000 rad within 6 weeks. In recent years, patients with positive nodes have received 12 cycles of CMF chemotherapy.

Of 701 evaluable patients, 349 underwent the Halsted mastectomy and 352 had the conservative procedure. The groups were clinically comparable; about 45% of patients had primary cancers less than 1 cm in diameter. About one fourth of both groups had microscopic evidence of axillary metastases. Survival did not differ in the two groups after 7 years of follow-up (Fig 11–1). Analysis of survival taking axillary metastasis into account failed to show any differences between the treatments. Five patients had late fibrosis in the breast after conservative treatment, and 11 had mild lymphedema of the upper arm. Lymphedema of varying degrees was present in 23 patients having the Halsted operation.

Patients with early breast cancer have survived as well after quadrantectomy and axillary dissection plus radiotherapy as after the Halsted mastectomy and have had the same rates of local and distant recurrences. Radical mastectomy appears to be unnecessary in patients with breast cancers measuring less than 2 cm and no palpable axillary nodes.

▶ [These data support earlier predictions that the treatment of choice for small carcinomas of the breast would become lumpectomy or quadrantectomy with axillary dissection and radiotherapy. Leading radiation centers are beginning to assimilate data that suggest that even this approach will entail more surgery than is necessary.—E.E.P.] ◀

11–6 **The Accuracy of Clinical Nodal Staging and of Limited Axillary Dissection as a Determinant of Histologic Nodal Status in Carcinoma of the Breast.** Despite convincing evidence that a Halsted axillary dissection does not influence the rate of distant disease or the ultimate survival of patients with breast cancer, the true axillary nodal status provides the best index of prognosis and identifies those patients who should be considered for systemic adjuvant therapy. Bernard Fisher, Norman Wolmark, Madeline Bauer, Carol Redmond, and Mark Gebhardt (Pittsburgh) assessed the value of careful clinical nodal assessment and of axillary sampling to determine the true axillary nodal status in a series of patients in a prospective trial of radical mastectomy and total mastectomy, with and without postoperative radiotherapy. Of 641 women having conventional radical mastectomy, 286 were clinically node positive, as were 99 of 296 patients undergoing total mastectomy with removal of 1–10 axillary nodes.

The overall error rate in clinical assessment of the axillary node status in the radical mastectomy group was 33.5%. More than one third of patients who were clinically node negative had positive nodes on pathologic examination, and no tumor was found in about one fourth of patients who were clinically node positive. The results did not appear related to the number of nodes examined, but the number of

(11–6) Surg. Gynecol. Obstet. 152:765–772, June 1981.

patients with 4 or more positive nodes increased with the number of nodes examined. The number of nodes examined could not be related to recurrence rates or survival 5 years after radical mastectomy. There was little difference in treatment failure rates between clinically negative and pathologically positive patients and clinically and pathologically positive patients.

These findings support the view that the regional nodes are primarily indicators, not instigators, of distant disease in patients with breast cancer. Palpable nodes that are pathologically negative do not appear to represent a favorable host response to tumor. Removal of the lower two levels of axillary nodes appears to be more than adequate in preventing subsequent axillary node involvement.

► [These data are important because there seems to be continued emphasis on developing techniques for performing a complete axillary dissection at the time of mastectomy. Technical exercises such as dividing the insertion of the sternal portion of the pectoralis major muscle and reconstructing the pectoralis major and pectoralis minor muscles after a Halsted type of axillary dissection are not warranted to provide nodal staging.—E.E.P.] ◄

11–7 **The Effect of Pregnancy on the Prognosis of Carcinoma of the Breast Following Radical Mastectomy.** It remains unclear whether or not pregnancy influences the lives of patients treated for breast cancer. Many have suggested that such patients avoid pregnancy completely or for some stated interval. James C. Harvey, P. P. Rosen, Roy Ashikari, Guy F. Robbins, and David W. Kinne (Meml. Sloan-Kettering Cancer Center, New York) reviewed data on 41 patients who conceived after treatment for primary operable breast carcinoma from 1940 to 1970. Median age at mastectomy was 34 years. No patient had evidence of metastasis at the time of pregnancy. Treatment consisted of radical mastectomy, with radiation therapy in 14 cases with positive axillary nodes.

The overall 10-year disease-free survival rate of 27 patients with negative axillary nodes was 80%. Four patients who conceived within 2 years after mastectomy died; 1 had a second episode of breast carcinoma after the pregnancy. Three patients had recurrent disease after more than 10 years; they had become pregnant within 2 years after mastectomy. All patients with noninfiltrating tumors survived and were free of disease from 15 to 22 years. The 14 patients with positive axillary nodes had an overall 10-year disease-free survival rate of 79%. The disease-free survival rate for patients who conceived within 2 years after mastectomy was 71%.

No detrimental effect of subsequent pregnancy on the course of these patients with breast cancer was apparent, even in those with positive axillary nodes or those who became pregnant within 2 years after mastectomy. Abortion does not appear to improve patient survival. Pregnancy need not be avoided or terminated in patients who are apparently free of recurrent disease after being treated for carcinoma of the breast.

► [The patients described in this study almost assuredly did not have estrogen-sensitive neoplastic cells remaining somewhere. The data are reassuring, as they proba-

(11–7) Surg. Gynecol. Obstet. 153:723–725, November 1981.

bly apply to most patients; pregnancy should not be considered a no-risk factor, however, in patients who have remaining estrogen-sensitive neoplastic cells.—E.E.P.] ◀

11-8 **Postmastectomy Breast Reconstruction Using a Rectus Abdominis Musculocutaneous Island Flap** is described by Thomas H. Robbins (Melbourne). Breast reconstruction should not be withheld from any mastectomy patient with a reasonable prognosis. Such methods as the multistaged migration of tubed pedicles and subcutaneous prosthetic implants have not given optimal esthetic results. The latissimus dorsi musculocutaneous island flap technique is better, but a prosthetic implant usually is necessary because of the thinness of this muscle. Improved results have been obtained in a one-stage procedure with use of a musculocutaneous island flap on the rectus abdominis muscle. The operating time is shorter, and the scar at the donor site is acceptable.

The flap consists of the upper part of the ipsilateral rectus abdominis with the overlying skin and subcutaneous tissue. It is marked preoperatively with the patient standing (Fig 11–2).

METHOD.—The upper part of the muscle with the flap is freed from the thoracic cage, the flap is transposed through 90 degrees over the recipient site as a "trial run" before the recipient bed is prepared, and the donor site is closed with 000 nylon sutures in one layer. The distal and medial ends of the flap are deepithelialized and buried under the extremities of the wound on the chest wall to create an anterior axillary fold and increase cleavage medially. A dog-ear on the upper flap edge is deepithelialized and buried.

Patients usually are discharged 3 days postoperatively. The sutures are removed 2 weeks later.

The esthetic results have been better than those obtained by other methods of reconstruction, and the operating time is considerably less.

Fig 11–2.—Preoperative markings with the patient standing. (Courtesy of Robbins, T. H.: Br. J. Plast. Surg. 34:286–290, July 1981.)

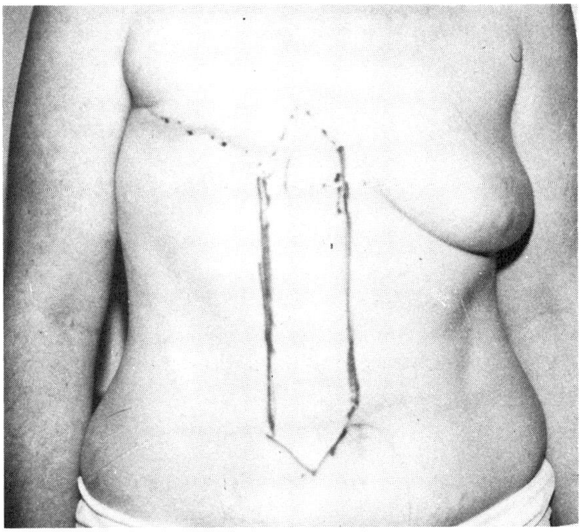

(11–8) Br. J. Plast. Surg. 34:286–290, July 1981.

No prosthetic implant is necessary. Should muscle atrophy occur, it may well be masked by normal involutional atrophy of the other breast. A transverse mastectomy scar gives the best results with this procedure. The neurovascular bundle is deep to the thoracic cage and is well protected. Delayed primary or early secondary reconstruction is the best approach.

▶ [This method of breast reconstruction is superior to most other. Transplanting a local composite tissue graft from an area where soft tissue is redundant and constructing a breast without a prosthesis meet some of the most demanding standards in reconstructive surgery. Contrary to popular practice, it is not necessary to repair or replace the anterior rectus sheath superior to the semilunar line; the posterior rectus sheath is adequate to prevent hernia.—E.E.P.] ◀

11–9 **Early Versus Delayed Shoulder Motion Following Axillary Dissection: Randomized Prospective Study** of the role and timing of physical therapy following axillary dissection for melanoma, or in conjunction with modified radical mastectomy, was conducted by Michael T. Lotze, Mary A. Duncan, Lynn H. Gerber, Eugene A. Woltering, and Steven A. Rosenberg (Natl. Inst. of Health). A total of 36 patients, aged 20–69 years (mean, 47 years), with 40 axillary dissections, 19 for melanoma (15 men and 4 women) and 21 for breast cancer (all women), received graduated increases in allowed range of motion beginning either on postoperative day 1 or day 7. All patients were advanced to full pain-free range of motion when the suction catheters were removed.

Patients starting motion on day 1 had more total wound drainage (805 vs. 420 cc, $P < .01$), more days of drainage (10.3 vs. 6.2 days, $P < .01$), and later postoperative day of discharge (12.8 vs. 9.2 days, $P < .02$) than did patients who began motion on day 7. Wound complications (e.g., infection and small areas of skin breakdown) occurred more often in the early motion group (7 vs. 1 patient, $P < .02$). Almost all patients achieved excellent shoulder function. No significant differences in number of patients achieving functional range of motion were found between the two groups 1, 3, or 6 months after operation. Transient serratus anterior palsy (12 patients) and latissimus dorsi palsy (2 patients) occurred in approximately 30% of all patients regardless of group (breast or melanoma, early or delayed), but returned to normal in all patients.

Early institution of flexion and abduction exercises following axillary dissection thus appears to have a deleterious effect on wound healing and drainage and no beneficial effect on time to attainment of full range of motion. Shoulder flexion beyond 40 degrees and abduction beyond 40 degrees should be delayed until the seventh postoperative day, or until after the suction catheters are removed. After the initial postoperative period, a physical therapist should guide the advancement of range of motion until the patient can continue appropriate home exercises without assistance.

▶ [No more fundamental principle has ever been established in surgery than "injured tissue needs rest." Shoulder and arm motion at a time when skin flaps are held in place only by fibrin always results in collection of serum and sometimes in develop-

(11–9) Ann. Surg. 193:288–295, March 1981.

ment of a bursa beneath the skin flap. Adequate immobilization by external air pressure (suction drainage) or external compression produced by dressings must be maintained long enough to prevent shearing forces from detaching the skin flap from the chest wall and axillary fascia before collagen synthesis and deposition occur. This objective can be attained without producing pulmonary complications or a permanently stiff shoulder.—E.E.P.] ◀

11–10 **Social, Emotional, and Financial Implications of Adjuvant Chemotherapy in Breast Cancer.** C. S. McArdle, K. C. Calman, A. F. Cooper, A. V. M. Hughson, A. R. Russell, and D. C. Smith (Glasgow) studied the incidence and severity of toxicity, extent of emotional disturbance, and cost of adjuvant chemotherapy in 107 women with stage II breast cancer; the patients were randomized to receive radiotherapy, chemotherapy, or both. The chemotherapy regimen included cyclophosphamide, methotrexate, and 5-fluorouracil administered intravenously on an outpatient basis on days 1 and 8 of 28-day cycles. Chemotherapy was begun 4–6 weeks after mastectomy and continued until recurrence or for 1 year. Patients allocated to receive both treatments had radiotherapy 4–6 weeks after mastectomy and chemotherapy 4–6 weeks after completion of radiotherapy.

Nausea and vomiting, which occurred in 85% of patients receiving chemotherapy, contributed significantly to distress. More than one third of the patients required a wig for hair loss or had mucosal ulceration. Nevertheless, most were able to return to work during treatment. Leukopenia was more common in patients who received radiotherapy prior to chemotherapy.

One year after mastectomy, psychiatric morbidity was present in 13 of 34 patients receiving chemotherapy with or without radiotherapy and in only 1 of 18 receiving radiotherapy alone ($P < .05$). Depression occurred in 7 patients receiving chemotherapy and 1 receiving radiotherapy. Anxiety was common in both groups. This trend was still present 6 months after completion of chemotherapy (18 months after mastectomy).

Chemotherapy was expensive but, like radiotherapy, could be administered on an outpatient basis. A 1-year course of chemotherapy cost about £400 in 1980. This does not include the costs of antiemetics, wigs, laboratory time, and similar expenses. The overall costs of chemotherapy recently have been compared favorably with forms of treatment for other chronic diseases and with conventional forms of cancer therapy.

▶ [At a time when increasing numbers of patients are being subjected to chemotherapy (including patients with no evidence of lymphatic spread of carcinonia), it is time to review some of the implications of adjuvant chemotherapy and to rethink the use of chemotherapy for breast cancer.—E.E.P.] ◀

(11–10) Br. J. Surg. 68:261–264, April 1981.

12. Head and Neck

12–1 **Is Aggressive Surgical Treatment Indicated for Recurrent Benign Mixed Tumors of the Parotid Gland?** Benign mixed tumors, or pleomorphic adenomas, are the most common parotid neoplasm and management of local recurrence remains a common clinical problem. Robert J. Piorkowski and Oscar M. Guillamondegui (Univ. of Texas, Houston) reviewed data on 58 patients with benign mixed tumors of the parotid gland, seen in 1955–1974, who had received primary surgical treatment elsewhere. Forty-five had obvious tumor recurrence, and 13 others had had a recent incomplete excision. Mean follow-up was 10 years.

Thirteen patients had superficial parotidectomy with preservation of the facial nerve. Eleven remained free of recurrent disease, the other 2 had further treatment without sacrifice of any branch of the facial nerve. Seven patients had total parotidectomy with preservation of the facial nerve, and 5 have been free of disease for 7–10 years. One had further treatment with the facial nerve preserved. Twelve patients had superficial or total parotidectomy with partial resection of the facial nerve. Eight have been free of disease, and 2 died of intercurrent disease. Eight of 9 patients having total parotidectomy with complete resection of the facial nerve have been free of disease. All 4 patients having local resection of recurrent tumor nodules have been free of disease for 8–13 years. Five of the 13 patients seen shortly after incomplete excision or biopsy had residual tumor present. One patient without residual cancer had a recurrence next to the parotid duct at 7 years and was treated successfully.

No particular operative procedure proved to be superior in this series of patients with residual or recurrent benign mixed parotid tumors. Surgery must be individualized in these cases. Patients without residual tumor after biopsy or recent incomplete excision should have superficial parotidectomy and excision of the cutaneous scar. Radiation therapy has been used after operation in some of these cases. In general, aggressive but selective surgical treatment is indicated for patients with recurrent mixed tumors of the parotid gland.

▶ [The answer to the question in the title of this article depends on the measurement used. Histologically, it is seldom necessary to be surgically aggressive in the treatment of a recurrent benign mixed tumor. Significant change in cell types can be found in less than 5% of patients. The old adage that once a benign tumor is excised inadequately it becomes a malignant tumor is not completely false, however. Although cells may appear histologically benign, benign mixed tumor cells (spread through the face by repeated inadequate surgery) present a formidable problem. I have seen a patient die with mixed tumor producing cavernous sinus thrombosis while the tumor was still being reported by pathologists as benign mixed tumor. Really, any tumor is benign, "only if you get it all out."—E.E.P.] ◀

(12–1) Am. J. Surg. 142:434–436, October 1981.

12–2 **Conservative Parotidectomy by Peripheral Approach.** Steven Chan and Alastair Gunn (Ashington Hosp., Northumberland, England) reviewed the results of 30 consecutive conservative parotidectomies performed by the peripheral approach between 1975 and 1980. The 16 women and 14 men had a mean age of 51 years. Using Patey's incision, a skin flap is dissected anteriorly superficial to the parotid with a scalpel. The cervical branch of the facial nerve is dissected carefully proximal to the main facial trunk, as shown in Figure 12–1. The superficial lobe of the parotid is removed by tracing the facial nerve branches distally, constantly reorienting the gland with respect to the proximal and distal aspects of the nerve. The entire superficial

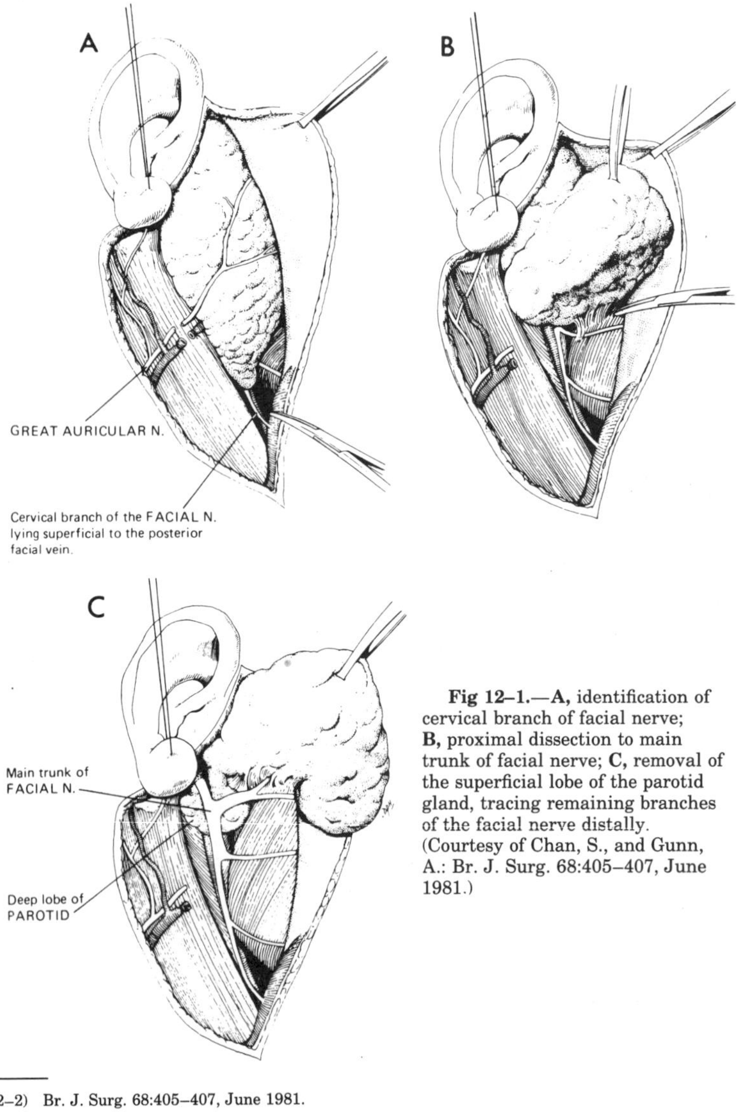

Fig 12–1.—**A,** identification of cervical branch of facial nerve; **B,** proximal dissection to main trunk of facial nerve; **C,** removal of the superficial lobe of the parotid gland, tracing remaining branches of the facial nerve distally. (Courtesy of Chan, S., and Gunn, A.: Br. J. Surg. 68:405–407, June 1981.)

(12–2) Br. J. Surg. 68:405–407, June 1981.

lobe need not be removed if the tumor is located in the lower pole. The superficial temporal vessels are not routinely ligated. Tumors of the deep lobe are removed after superficial parotidectomy by gentle dissection deep to the nerve.

The lesions treated included 20 pleomorphic adenomas, 4 involving the deep lobe of the parotid. Ten patients received radiotherapy postoperatively. One patient had severe temporary paralysis, and 11 had temporary paralysis affecting the lower lip. The recovery time ranged from 6 weeks to 6 months. No patient had permanent paralysis. Two wound hematomas had to be evacuated. Other complications included neuromas of the great auricular nerve in 3 patients and the development of Frey's syndrome in 4. No recurrences have been recognized to date, but a patient with Hodgkin's disease died of widespread involvement.

The peripheral approach to removal of parotid tumors appears to be safe. Severe temporary paralysis occurred in 1 patient, but no permanent paralysis developed in any.

▶ [For many years, I have practiced peripheral identification of the facial nerve and retrograde simultaneous nerve-tumor section. The disadvantage is that continual stimulation of peripheral nerve branches makes the distal ramifications less responsive at the end of the procedure than at the beginning. The advantage, however, is that identification of a peripheral branch is safer than searching for the major track of the facial nerve, particularly when the tumor is a large one in the preauricular or infra-auricular area. If a mistake is made during proximal dissection and the nerve is damaged, the deformity is much more severe than during peripheral dissection.—E.E.P.] ◀

12–3 **Head and Neck Cancer: Early Detection.** Harry W. Southwick (Rush-Presbyterian-St. Luke's Med. Center, Chicago) states that early detection is very important in cases of head and neck cancer because the overall survival rate is 60% for patients with localized oral cancer, compared with only 25% for those in whom the disease has spread.

Tumors of the head and neck have a wide variety of presentations. The probable existence of a neoplastic rather than an inflammatory process is suggested by a sore or soreness that persists; a lump that persists, particularly if nontender, or evidence of nerve dysfunction such as hoarseness, facial weakness, or dysphagia. The probability is enhanced if a careful history shows high risk factors such as heavy smoking, poor oral hygiene, or prior irradiation. Careful inspection and palpation may reveal the probable diagnosis.

A skillful biopsy is essential. Both aspiration needle biopsy and large-gauge needle biopsy are often useful. Biochemical studies are important, particularly for the detection of thyroid cancers. Ultrasound techniques give much improved delineation of lesion consistency. Xerography (Fig 12–2) is sometimes superior to radiography. Nuclear scanning remains integral in the evaluation of thyroid nodules. Computerized axial tomography can often delineate the extent of disease. Arteriography remains essential in the diagnosis of carotid body tumors.

▶ [Advanced techniques such as ultrasonography and computerized tomography may

---

(12–3) Cancer 47(Suppl.):1188–1192, Mar. 1, 1981.

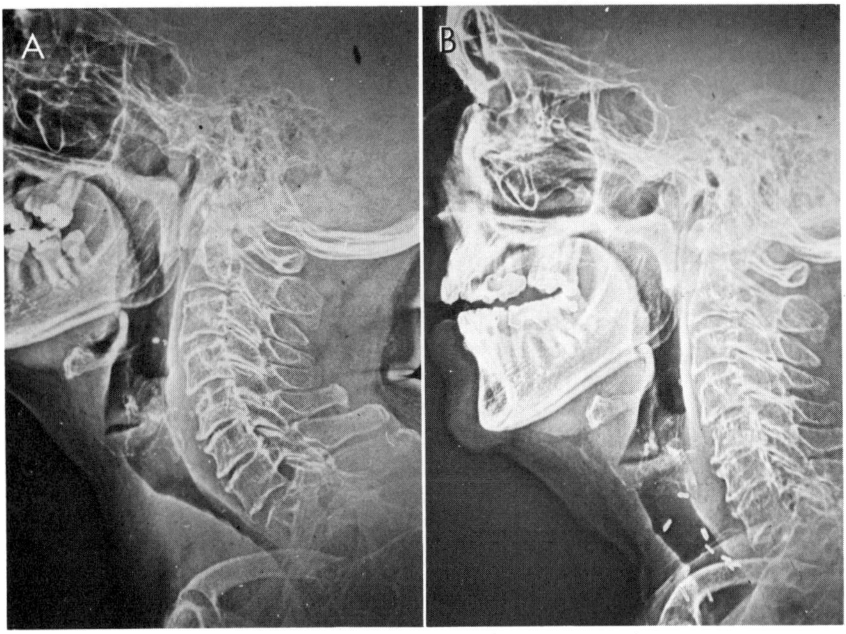

Fig 12–2.—A, lateral xeroradiogram of patient with thyroid cancer, showing marked tracheal compression. **B,** postoperative study of same patient; normal tracheal dimensions are restored. (Courtesy of Southwick, H. W.: Cancer 47(Suppl.):1188–1192, Mar. 1, 1981.)

make it possible to define operative control of head and neck cancer preoperatively, but the data available at this time do not support such a claim. Inoperability occurs with the spread of the tumor into the base of the skull and along deep fascial plains adjacent to the internal carotid artery. Surgical exploration is necessary in most patients to be certain whether neck metastases can or cannot be removed.—E.E.P.] ◀

12–4 **Evolution of Clinically Negative Neck.** There is controversy concerning the benefits of elective neck dissection in patients with head and neck cancer and clinically negative findings in the neck. E. M. Skolnik, A. H. Katz, R. Mantravadi, S. P. Becker, and S. Stal (Univ. of Illinois, Chicago) retrospectively studied the results (minimum follow-up, 3 years) in 615 patients with squamous cell cancer of the upper aerodigestive tract and clinically negative neck findings at the time of presentation between 1960 and 1976 when there was no uniform policy as to treatment of N_0 necks. Overall, 213 patients had radiation therapy alone as the initial treatment modality, 149 had surgery for the primary tumor and no radical neck dissection, and 253 had surgery for the primary tumor and concomitant radical neck dissection.

Ipsilateral or contralateral metastases developed in 12.9% of the 149 patients receiving surgery for the primary tumor only. Palpable nodal disease developed in 22% of the 253 receiving both surgery for the primary tumor and neck dissection. Only 3% of patients had development of positive lymph nodes when the primary tumor was con-

(12–4) Ann. Otol. Rhinol. Laryngol. 89(Pt. 1):551–555, Nov.–Dec. 1980.

trolled. The recurrence rate of neck lesions was 23% when the specimens were histologically positive and 21% when they were negative. The number of positive nodes did not seem to affect the recurrence rate.

The rate of evolution of nodal disease when primary neck tumors are controlled is not close to that predicted by the percentage of positive neck specimens. Microscopic ipsilateral neck histopathology is not a reliable guide for predicting future contralateral neck conversion. The number of neck recurrences when the primary lesion is controlled is very low with elective radical neck dissection or elective radiation therapy. In a series with predominantly T_1 and T_2 lesions, the recurrence rate in the neck is low with no neck therapy. Radiation therapy is as effective as surgery in controlling microscopic neck disease when the primary tumor is controlled. The number of microscopically positive nodes found in elective radical neck dissections does not correlate with subsequent neck recurrences. The most important factor affecting subsequent lesion recurrence in the neck is primary tumor control. Radiation therapy is effective in controlling in-field occult metastasis when the primary tumor is controlled. Low cervical or supraclavicular tumor recurrence, or both, occur rarely when the primary lesion is controlled, making elective treatment of these areas unwarranted. These conclusions are not applicable to patients with a primary tumor in the head and neck, a palpable ipsilateral node, and negative findings in the contralateral neck.

▶ [Anatomical location of the primary tumor is the most valuable factor in evaluating a clinically negative neck. Biologic predisposition of the tumor to metastasize is another important factor. Better radiation therapy is making the decision about prophylactic neck dissection somewhat easier. Generally speaking, a statistical approach such as that described in this article, is the third best way to approach the problem of a potentially dangerous primary lesion in the absence of palpable lymph nodes.—E.E.P.] ◀

12–5 **Bilateral Radical Neck Dissection.** Until recently, the presence of bilateral cervical metastases in patients with head and neck cancer was regarded as a sign of inoperability, and ligation of both internal jugular veins was thought to be fatal. Upon demonstration of adequate collateral formation after division of the internal jugular veins, it was shown that bilateral cervical metastases could be managed safely and effectively in either one or two stages. Mohamed S. Razack, Raul Baffi, and Kumao Sako (Roswell Park Meml. Inst, Buffalo) retrospectively studied data concerning 61 patients who had a simultaneous bilateral (one-stage) neck dissection and 63 who underwent therapeutic second (two-stage) neck dissection between 1960 and 1977. Median patient age was 60 years, 80% being between 51 and 70 years.

Of the 61 patients undergoing one-stage procedures, 51 had a classic bilateral neck dissection and 10 had preservation of either 1 or both internal jugular veins, or spinal accessory nerve, or both. Of the staged second neck dissections, 58% were done 6–12 months after the first. In both the one- and two-stage procedures, the most common postoperative complication was facial swelling and edema (table).

(12–5) Cancer 47:197–199, Jan. 1, 1981.

POSTOPERATIVE COMPLICATIONS*

	No. of patients (simultaneous neck)	No. of patients (nonsimultaneous)
Facial edema and swelling	39 (63)	19 (30)
Wound infection	39 (63)	9 (14)
Orocutaneous fistula	22 (36)	4 (6)
Carotid artery blowout	7 (11)	—
Pulmonary infection	10 (16)	—
Cyanosis	5 (8)	—
Major flap loss	3 (4.9)	—
Unconsciousness	3 (4.9)	—
Mortality	6 (9.8)	2 (3.2)

*Numbers in parentheses indicate percent.

In patients undergoing simultaneous bilateral neck dissection, the 30-day postoperative mortality was 9.8%; the incidence of life-threatening postoperative complications was 11% (carotid artery hemorrhage), and 3- and 5-year survival was 20% and 12.5%, respectively. Staged second neck dissections showed histologically positive nodes in 57 (91%) of the 63 patients. In these 63 patients, the postoperative mortality was 3.2%, postoperative complication rate was 54%, and 3- and 5-year survival was 60% and 38%, respectively.

Bilateral cervical node metastases arising from oropharyngeal and laryngeal carcinomas may not indicate inoperability and incurability. Bilateral neck dissection can be done in either one or two stages. Patients treated for an "early" stage of disease, and who subsequently have contralateral cervical metastases, have the same 5-year salvage rates as those treated initially for stage IV disease. Little can be done to prevent postoperative facial swelling and edema; these conditions are best managed by elevation of the head postoperatively to facilitate lymphatic and venous drainage. Although only 10 patients were treated with preservation of one or both jugular veins, they experienced minimal complications and no postoperative deaths. Thus, preserving one jugular vein, if and when possible, may be helpful in preventing facial edema.

▶ [Although it has been known for some time that it is possible to perform a bilateral radical neck dissection in one stage, complications are significant and there is usually no valid reason why the procedure cannot be done in stages. Also, it is usually possible to retain one internal jugular vein without compromising the chances for cure. Although surgeons have been taught almost routinely that the internal jugular vein must be removed in a complete neck dissection, persistence of metastatic cancer along the internal jugular vein when it has been preserved does not support such a view.—E.E.P.] ◀

12–6 **Preoperative Irradiation for Head and Neck Cancer: Results of a Prospective Study.** Preoperative radiotherapy often is recommended as an adjuvant to surgery for head and neck cancer despite lack of convincing objective evidence of benefit. Jose J. Terz, E. R.

(12–6) Surgery 89:449–453, April 1981.

King, and Walter Lawrence, Jr., undertook a prospective trial of preoperative radiotherapy in 248 previously untreated patients with primary epidermoid carcinoma of the oral cavity, oropharynx, and hypopharynx of stages II to IV. Irradiated patients received a midline total dose of 1,400 rad delivered in two equal fractions 24 and 48 hours before operation. Cobalt teletherapy was used. The two patient groups were similar in age, stage of disease, primary sites, and incidence of node metastasis. Follow-up ranged from 4 to 9 years.

Local wound complications were comparable in the study and control groups, but irradiated patients more often had postoperative exposure of the mandible or mandibular prosthesis. Operative mortalities were 7% in the irradiated group and 8% in the control group. Carcinoma recurred in 22% of irradiated and 36% of control patients. Patients in both groups with involved nodes in the surgical specimen more often had recurrences. Distant disease was comparably frequent in the two groups. The 5-year disease-free survival rates were 32% for irradiated patients and 26% for control patients, not a significant difference. Among patients with node involvement, those given radiotherapy had better survival and the difference approached significance. Benefit was apparent in patients with oral cavity lesions, but not in those with pharyngeal primary sites.

No improvement in overall survival resulted from radiotherapy in this study, but local recurrences may be less frequent in patients with involved cervical nodes who receive radiotherapy. A trial with 5,000 to 6,000 rad might be worthwhile, although a higher rate of postoperative complications might preclude such an approach. Postoperative radiotherapy is a reasonable alternative.

▶ [In my judgment, this is the best of the few real prospective studies evaluating preoperative evaluation for head and neck neoplasms. The results should put to rest the often-repeated claim that a combination of radiation and surgery is superior to the best of radiation or the best of surgery alone.—E.E.P.] ◀

12–7 **Practical Palliative Care for Patient With Terminal Head and Neck Cancer.** In patients with incurable tumors of the head and neck, the dying process is slow and painful, and the anatomical areas involved tend to be visible. Thus, these patients present problems that differ from those of patients with cancer of other areas. Nigel R. T. Pashley (Univ. of Michigan) offers guidelines for the palliative management of patients with head and neck cancer.

In changing the approach from that of aggressive cure-dominated treatment to that of making a patient comfortable for the rest of his life, absolute frankness can be disarming; however, the "ignorance is bliss" policy can later backfire into resentment at not being told the truth. It is basically a personal attitude and interaction problem for the physician and patient to discuss together, with or without involving the family. Because colleagues often have differing interests in regard to the terminally ill, a team approach including members of the oncology group, social services, nursing staff, and pastoral service is useful.

(12–7) J. Otolaryngol. 9:405–411, October 1980.

Many therapeutic modalities can be used for palliation of local factors (e.g., to control pain, odor, physical deformity, drooling) and systemic factors (e.g., nutrition, mood or confusion, dyspnea, pain), but they should avoid long-term morbidity or unpleasant side effects and allow the patient to function as normally as possible; even unorthodox modes of application are acceptable. To relieve the pain and fear of pain that are usually present in patients with recurrent head and neck cancer, simple analgesics should be tried first. The anti-inflammatory effects of aspirin may be useful in the combined narcotic-aspirin medications. Narcotics are the mainstay of pain relief, with oral morphine or diamorphine preferred over methadone or heroin. Rather than using these drugs "as needed," a scheduled dose every 4 hours should be used, titrating up to the normal plateau, which commonly appears with about 10–15 mg of morphine. A parenteral route may allow faster onset of action and more potency, thus giving patients periods of pain-free mobility. Pharmacologic adjunctive therapy may assist in pain control. For example, indomethacin, an antagonist of prostaglandin synthetase for the E and F prostaglandins, may alleviate metastatic bone resorption pain.

Extirpative surgical procedures (e.g., debulking the primary tumor) should generally not be used as palliation in head and neck cancers, due to the high morbidity, but cryotherapy may be successful. Local nerve block, stereotactic thalamotomy, and percutaneous tractotomy control pain poorly because of the multiple neural supply to the head and neck area; however, retrolabyrinthine nerve section using an extradural approach may be useful. Regional radiation even after full-course conventional radiotherapy can aid in pain control. Short high-dose bursts of radiotherapy are better for the dying patient than a daily lower dose. A lowered maximum dose, or even cessation of therapy as soon as symptoms are controlled, is applicable in palliation and effective for pain and bulk reduction. Tumoricidal chemotherapeutic drugs generally cause too many side effects to be applied to the terminally ill, but these are used actively as palliation once widespread disease is identified. Prednisone induces a sense of well-being and stimulates appetite.

Anorexia of terminal disease may be hypothalamic in origin. In patients with head and neck cancer, alcohol-based appetite stimulants may cause confusion, but judicious use of alcohol may help. Nasogastric tubes are uncomfortable and difficult to self-insert. A long-term feeding gastrostomy may be satisfactory, but a cervical hypopharyngostomy may be preferred as it can be done with the use of local anesthesia and the patient may change the tube himself. To control nausea or vomiting, the phenothiazines are the most useful group of medications.

Mood swings and pain control are managed more easily and predictably if insomnia can be avoided. Nonbarbiturate sedatives (e.g., chloral hydrate or methyprylon) should be tried before using barbiturate combinations. Small doses of antidepressants (e.g., imipramine) may be useful, but larger doses may precipitate confusion and agitation.

Disfigurement and discomfort can be improved by the judicious use of antibiotics to reduce superficial infection and thus reduce malodorous discharge. Superficial cleansing with a water jet device, benzalconium, or topical antibiotic spray may be useful. A soda and salt mouthwash may be of comfort to a patient with lack of saliva or with a prosthesis.

▶ [In my experience, the single most important principle in the palliative care of a patient with terminal head and neck cancer is, "Always have something else to offer the patient." The worst mistake in palliative care is abandonment. It is always possible to clean out an ulcer, apply a local anesthetic, or just give the patient believable assurance that whatever lies ahead, he or she will not be alone. Fear of suffocation makes such reassurance especially timely.—E.E.P.] ◀

12–8 **Application of Biologic Principle of Induced Osteogenesis for Craniofacial Defects.** Demineralized, devitalized bone matrix induces mesenchymal cells in nonskeletal tissue to transform into chondroblasts with subsequent bone formation. This transformation has been used in rats with both isogeneic and xenogeneic material to repair large, nonhealing defects of the skull and mandible. Julie Glowacki, Joseph E. Murray, Leonard B. Kaban, Judah Folkman, and John B. Mulliken (Harvard Med. School) show that this principle of induced osteogenesis is applicable in man.

Demineralized bone implants, in the form of chips, blocks, and powders, were used in 34 patients aged 1¼–59 years (mean, 18 years) to augment bony contours, fill intraosseous defects, and construct new bone. Six patients had acquired defects, and 28 had congenital deformities. The implants were obtained from cadaver femurs in 33 cases and from the skull of the patient in 1. In defects that could be palpated or stressed, solid healing was demonstrable by 2–3 months. The 3 patients who could be assessed radiologically had signs of osseous healing as early as 6 weeks after implantation (Fig 12–3). Biopsy specimens from 4 patients, obtained during secondary procedures, showed that the induced bone was united to the unresorbed deminer-

Fig 12–3.—**A,** roentgenogram before implantation of demineralized bone powder in mandibular defect. **B,** roentgenogram 10 weeks after operation. (Courtesy of Glowacki, J., et al.: Lancet 1:959–963, May 2, 1981.)

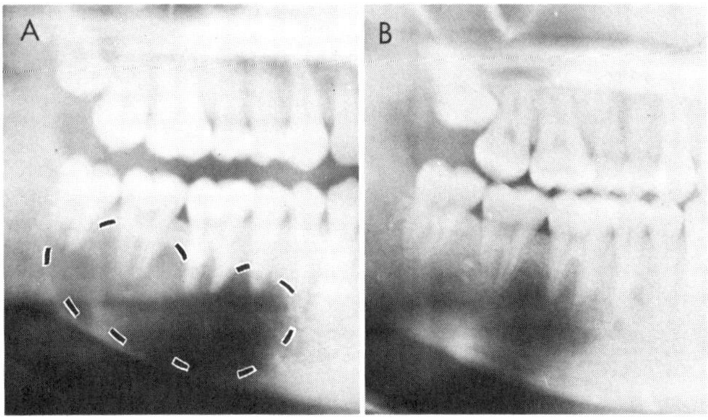

(12–8) Lancet 1:959–963, May 2, 1981.

alized implants. Complications included 2 instances of postoperative wound infection necessitating removal of the implants.

The clinical advantages of demineralized implants are rapid healing of skeletal defects, ability to induce large quantities of new bone, avoidance of harvesting procedures, and the potentially unlimited supply of banked material, which increases treatment options. Because the inductive process is not species specific, xenogeneic bone matrix may be useful clinically. Longer follow-up will be required to determine whether resorption has been avoided.

▶ [This report—highly publicized in lay publications—of using demineralized bone implants to stimulate osteogenesis is interesting. It should be remembered that similar principles were established many years ago by Marshal Urist and others. Even plaster of Paris has been used successfully as a substitute for bone and as a substrate for ultimate bone replacement by natural osteogenesis.—E.E.P.] ◀

12-9 **Surgical Treatment of Exophthalmos and Enophthalmos** is outlined by S. Anthony Wolfe (Univ. of Miami). Exophthalmos may be a result of Graves' disease, soft tissue tumors of the orbit, mucoceles, or hamartomas (Fig 12–4). The exorbitism associated with shallow orbits in the craniofacial stenoses usually is associated with a generalized retardation of maxillary growth and is corrected by the Le Fort III osteotomy with midface advancement. When retromaxillism is not present, a Le Fort III osteotomy can be combined with a Le Fort I osteotomy to permit forward movement of the upper part of

Fig 12–4.—Previous exploration of the right orbit elsewhere had failed to disclose a cause for unilateral exophthalmos, but CT scan showed a large mass in the posterior part of the orbit. Removal of the entire lateral orbital wall through a coronal incision made possible subtotal removal of the benign hemartoma. A small amount of persistent exophthalmos probably could have been corrected completely if the lateral orbital wall had been repositioned in a slightly more lateral position. Visual acuity was unchanged after the operation. (Courtesy of Wolfe, S. A.: Ann. Ophthalmol. 13:995–1002, August 1981.)

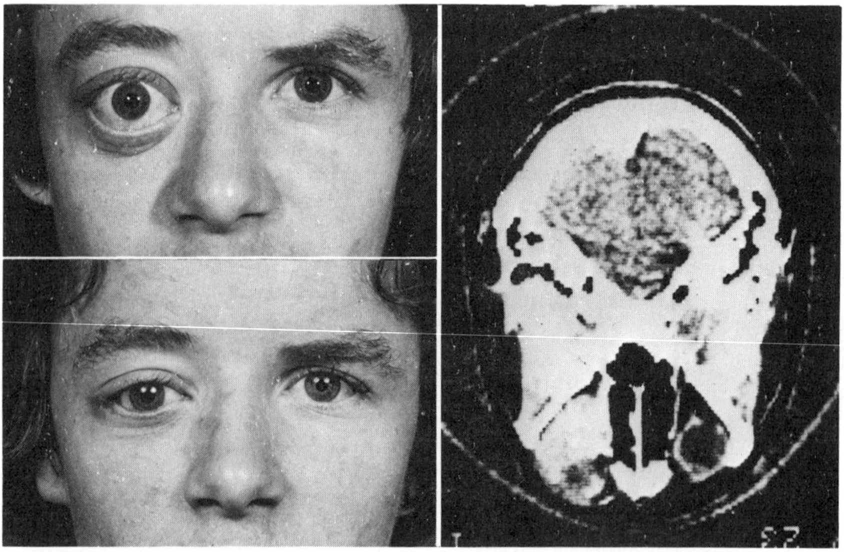

(12–9) Ann. Ophthalmol. 13:995–1002, August 1981.

the maxilla only. Any of the orbital walls can be removed in approaching an orbital tumor. Exophthalmic Graves' disease can be managed by lowering the orbital floors and infracturing the medial walls into the ethmoid sinuses, or by a three-wall expansion including a valgus step osteotomy of the lateral orbital wall. Exophthalmos of more than 8 mm is managed by Le Fort III and I osteotomies.

Attempts to treat enophthalmos with the use of glass beads or silicone injections have generally failed. Even severe late enophthalmos can nearly always be greatly improved, or even totally corrected through circumferential orbital dissection back to the orbital apex, reintegration of the orbital contents into the orbital cavity, and restoration of the orbital walls with autogenous bone grafts. An inferior marginotomy aids in retrieval of orbital contents from the maxillary sinus. Cancellous bone from the ilium can be shaped exactly as required and inserted under direct vision to restore completely the orbital floor. Where outward and downward displacement of the malar bone is present in cases of old orbital fracture, an osteotomy following the old fracture lines is very effective in reducing the orbital volume, but care must be taken not to overcorrect and cause exophthalmos.

► [Many simple procedures have been designed to decompress the orbit in extreme exophthalmos. Recent advances in radical craniofacial surgery have provided the only uniformly successful way of relieving exophthalmos. Decompressing the roof of the orbit, removing the lateral wall of the orbit, or making a window in the roof of the maxillary antrum have not been uniformly successful. At least three of the four orbital walls must be expanded to provide significant decompression of severe exophthalmos.—E.E.P.] ◄

13. Thorax

13–1 **Tracheostomy in Neonates and Small Infants: Problems and Pitfalls.** The number of tracheostomies done in infants and neonates is increasing with the wider use of ventilatory support in small infants and the increase in complications of prolonged endotracheal ventilation. J. J. Tepas III, James H. Heroy, Dennis W. Shermeta, and J. Alex Haller, Jr. reviewed the results of tracheostomy in 74 infants younger than age 2 years who were treated in a 13-year period. Tracheostomy was required in 48 neonates the first days or weeks of life. The other 26 infants had an average age of 14.9 months.

Neonates were tracheostomized with a soft siliconized polymer tube, without technical difficulties in any case. Two of 14 neonates without hyaline membrane disease required long-term tracheostomy. Half the 34 neonates with hyaline membrane disease died of continued respiratory failure. Five others have required prolonged tracheostomy and have remained cannulated for at least 6 months. Two of these infants have significant tracheomalacia. Sixteen older infants were treated for acute respiratory distress, whereas 10 had congenital cardiac lesions. Significant morbidity from tracheostomy occurred in 12 of the 16 infants with croup. Postmortem findings in 2 infants were related to tracheostomy, although the procedure was not the primary cause of death. The infants treated in conjunction with congenital heart disease had no significant complications directly related to tracheostomy.

Tracheostomy can be done safely and precisely in young infants if an endotracheal tube or bronchoscope is in place. Decannulation over 48 hours usually is possible after short-term tracheostomy by progressive reduction of the size of the tube. Before decannulation is begun, infants who have had prolonged tracheostomy should undergo endoscopy in order to treat any obstructing lesion adequately.

▶ [A familiar problem to all thoracic surgeons is the hazard of tracheostomy in infants. This experience reviews 74 tracheostomies performed during a period of 13 years. Forty-eight of the 74 patients were newborns. It is particularly significant that no complications occurred in this group.

This report is especially gratifying to me, as I well remember the erroneous dictum repeated again and again 30 years ago: "Tracheostomy performed in an infant will have to remain until the child's first birthday!" The exact origin of this myth will probably never be known. As I have written several times, my observations in the neonatal unit in South Africa with the use of tracheostomy and mechanical ventilation for 6 weeks for neonatal tetanus in a series exceeding 300 patients, with excellent results, well refuted this erroneous concept. These data fully support the fact that tracheostomy, with proper care and a silicone rubber tracheostomy tube, can be performed with confidence and safety, even in the newborn.—F.C.S.] ◀

(13–1) Surgery 89:635–639, May 1981.

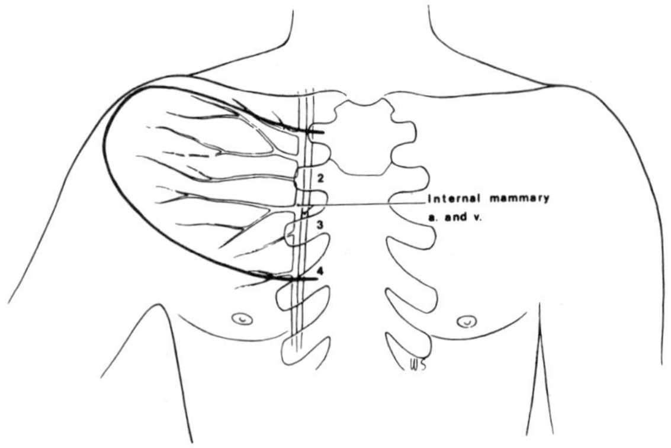

Fig 13–1.—An axial pattern flap is a single pedicle flap of skin and subcutaneous tissue with an intrinsic vascular supply paralleling its long axis. It can be used without the need for prior surgical delays. (Courtesy of Boyd, A. D., et al.: Ann. Thorac. Surg. 32:337–346, October 1981.

Fig 13–2 (top).—Latissimus dorsi myocutaneous flap based on the thoracoabdominal vessels, branches of which extend through the muscle to supply overlying skin; *a.v.n.*, artery, vein, nerve.

Fig 13–3 (bottom).—Pectoralis major myocutaneous flap based on pectoral branches of thoracoabdominal vessels.

(Courtesy of Boyd, A. D., et al.: Ann. Thorac. Surg. 32:337–346, October 1981.)

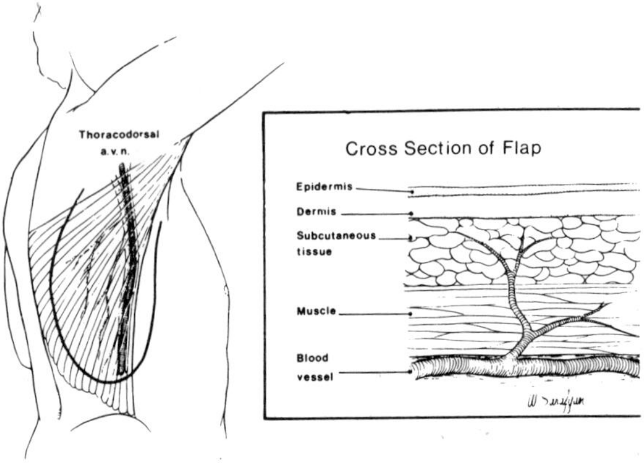

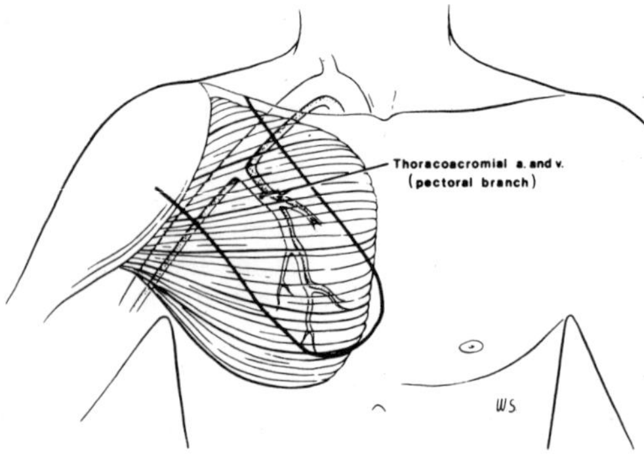

13–2 **Immediate Reconstruction of Full-Thickness Chest Wall Defects.** Full-thickness chest wall defects secondary to resection of malignancy or radiation necrosis require prompt, secure repair. Arthur D. Boyd, William W. Shaw, Joseph G. McCarthy, Daniel C. Baker, Naresh K. Trehan, Anthony J. Acinapura, and Frank C. Spencer (New York Univ. Med. Center) performed full-thickness chest wall resections on 21 patients during the past 10 years. Eleven patients had a necrotic radiation ulcer excised, 4 had a primary chest wall tumor resected, and 6 had recurrent tumor removed. Wide, full-thickness resections were performed. Marlex mesh was used to stabilize the defect in patients who were not given radiotherapy and in whom more than 2 ribs were resected. Local tissue in the form of a broad-based rotation or advancement random pattern flap was used in 6 patients to resurface the defect immediately. Distant normal tissue was used in 5 other cases. An axial pattern flap was used in 1 patient. Six patients had reconstruction with a myocutaneous flap and 3, with a myocutaneous free flap. Figures 13–1 to 13–4 show the types of flaps used.

All but 1 of the 21 patients gained satisfactory chest wall stability. One patient with a total sternectomy without the use of Marlex mesh

Fig 13–4.—Tensor fascia lata myocutaneous free flap based on lateral circumflex femoral vessels provides excellent functional and cosmetic repair for full-thickness chest wall defects. (Courtesy of Boyd, A. D., et al.: Ann. Thorac. Surg. 32:337–346, October 1981.)

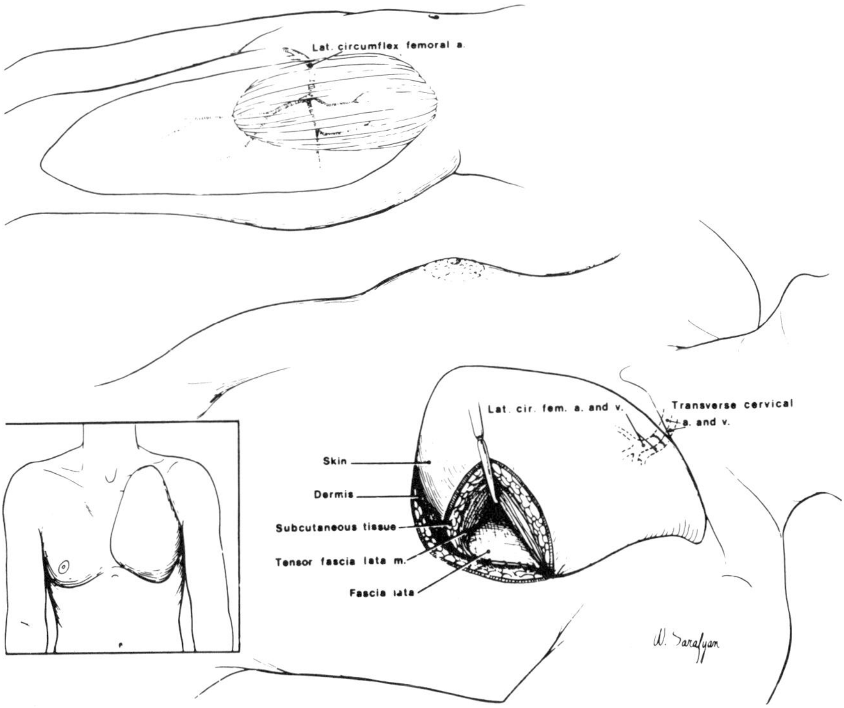

(13–2) Ann. Thorac. Surg. 32:337–346, October 1981.

had severe ventilatory insufficiency postoperatively. Extensive necrosis developed in 2 of 6 random pattern flaps of local tissue and in 2 of 6 distant-tissue flaps. Two patients required more than 1 myocutaneous flap for closure. The 3 patients given tensor fascia lata myocutaneous free flaps had primary healing and excellent esthetic results.

Full-thickness chest wall defects can be reconstructed immediately in nearly all cases using myocutaneous, myocutaneous free, and axial pattern flaps and Marlex mesh or viable fascia lata for stability. Excellent functional and esthetic results can be expected. A tensor fascia lata myocutaneous free flap is apparently the best means of providing chest wall stability and coverage of large, potentially contaminated defects. The use of a foreign body such as Marlex mesh is questionable.

▶ [This report by Boyd and his colleagues on the reconstruction of chest wall defects in 21 patients operated on at New York University indicates well the substantial progress made in the field, especially with the availability of myocutaneous flaps, either rotated or free. With their availability, immediate reconstruction is feasible in the vast majority of patients. Reinforcement with Marlex mesh and methyl methacrylate has been satisfactory in the experience of Nael Martini in a series of 48 patients, as reported in his discussion of this paper. With myocutaneous flaps, Marlex may be unnecessary.—F.C.S.] ◀

13–3 **New Trends in Skeletal Reconstruction After Resection of Chest Wall Tumors.** Patricia McCormack, Manjit S. Bains, Edward J. Beattie, Jr., and Nael Martini (Meml. Center for Cancer, New York) reviewed the results of chest wall resection performed in continuity with tumor in 155 patients between 1963 and 1978. The 96 males and 59 females had a median age of 54 years. A total of 159 thoracotomies were done. Eighty-five patients had carcinomas and 70, sarcomas. Three fourths of the carcinomas were primary lung tumors. A large majority of the sarcomas arose from the chest wall; osteogenic sarcoma and chondrosarcoma were most common. Most patients had a mass, with or without pain. Hemoptysis was present in fewer than one third of patients with carcinoma, and 20% had no symptoms.

Since 1973, 12 patients have had chest wall reconstruction with a composite of Marlex mesh and methylmethacrylate. Pulmonary resections were performed in 72 patients. One fourth of patients required only muscle and skin closure over a small defect. Marlex mesh was used in 94. Twenty patients required respiratory support. Most pulmonary complications occurred in the earlier cases. Operative mortality was 4.5%; 5 of 7 operative deaths occurred earlier in the series. Operative mortality in the past 5 years was 2%.

Immediate reconstruction and preservation of adequate function and cosmetic appearance make wide excision with adequate surgical margins achievable in most instances. Excellent palliation can be achieved even in patients who are not curable. Reconstruction of chest wall defects with Marlex mesh and methylmethacrylate provides excellent functional and esthetic results in patients requiring resection of chest wall tumors.

▶ [Reports are becoming more frequent about reconstruction of the chest wall after

---

(13–3) Ann. Thorac. Surg. 31:45–52, January 1981.

treatment for trauma, radiation necrosis, malignancy, or sternal infections. This experience, describing the use of the composite of Marlex mesh and methyl methacrylate in 12 patients since 1973, indicates the reliability of the technique. Might it perhaps be applicable to patients with extensive flail chest after trauma, who may require prolonged therapy with a respirator before the chest wall stabilizes?—F.C.S.] ◀

13–4 **The Outcome of Patients With Pleural Effusion of Indeterminate Cause at Thoracotomy.** Thoracotomy is not uncommonly done to determine the cause of pleural effusion, although in some cases it does not provide a cause. Casey J. Ryan, Rosemary F. Rodgers, Krishnan K. Unni, and Norman G. G. Hepper (Mayo Grad. School, Rochester, Minn.) reviewed the course of 51 patients in whom the cause of pleural effusion was indeterminate immediately after thoracotomy in 1962–1972. The 37 men and 14 women had a median age of 56 years. The mean known duration of pleural effusion before thoracotomy was 15.7 weeks. One patient had a bilateral effusion.

In 18 cases the cause of effusion became apparent after thoracotomy. In 31 cases the effusion did not recur and no cause became known. Two patients died relatively soon after thoracotomy with the cause of effusion still uncertain. Thirteen patients had malignancy, including 6 with lymphoma. The effusion was or became chylous in 3 of these patients. Four patients ultimately had a diagnosis of malignant pleural mesothelioma. Two patients had intra-abdominal adenocarcinoma, and 1 had anaplastic carcinoma. Two patients had systemic lupus erythematosus, and 1 had rheumatoid arthritis. There was 1 case each of yellow-nail syndrome and rheumatic mitral stenosis. None of the 8 deaths of undiagnosed patients that occurred 1½–8 years after thoracotomy could be related to the previous effusion. In no case did tuberculosis become evident.

An entirely benign course with no recurrence of effusion can be expected in about 60% of patients after diagnostic thoracotomy for effusion that shows only nonspecific pleuritis. Pleural effusions due to malignancy may go undiagnosed despite careful examination of the pleura, lung, and mediastinum at thoracotomy. Pleural effusion is a frequent presenting manifestation of malignant mesothelioma. Tuberculosis was not observed in the present series.

▶ [A puzzling problem to the thoracic surgeon is the recurrent pleural effusion of unknown etiology. The prevailing concept is that such effusions are almost always due to malignant disease, which will become apparent sooner or later. The editor has long been puzzled by this, as he has seen an occasional patient with an effusion of unknown cause cured by decortication. Hence, this report is of particular significance. Sixty-one percent of the 51 patients had no recurrence of the effusion. No cause was found in a follow-up of from 1 to 15 years in 31 cases. Malignant disease was found in 13 patients and other causes in the remainder.

It seems clear that patients with a pleural effusion of unknown etiology should not be subjected to repeated tests that are not diagnostic. However, a thoracotomy should be done after a reasonable length of time, which will correct the effusion, establish the diagnosis, if possible, and probably cure the patient in over 50% of the instances in which the diagnosis remains uncertain.—F.C.S.] ◀

13–5 **Survival of Patients Surgically Treated For Stage I Lung Cancer.** David E. Williams, Peter C. Pairolero, Charles S. Davis, Philip

(13–4) Mayo Clin. Proc. 56:145–149, March 1981.
(13–5) J. Thorac. Cardiovasc. Surg. 82:70–76, July 1981.

E. Bernatz, W. Spencer Payne, William F. Taylor, Mary A. Uhlenhopp, and Robert S. Fontana (Mayo Clinic) examined the survival of patients with postsurgical stage I non-small cell bronchogenic carcinoma who underwent curative pulmonary resection as the sole treatment. The 624 patients represented 16% of all those seen in 1972–1978 with bronchogenic carcinoma. The operative mortality was 2.4%. A total of 495 patients were followed up for a mean of 37 months, including 350 patients enrolled in a prospective 4-monthly follow-up program and 145 patients enrolled later or followed up less frequently. Survival rates were comparable in these two groups.

An actuarial analysis showed 84% of the patients alive at 2 years, and 69% at 5 years. The 2- and 5-year survival rates of T1N0M0 patients were 91% and 80%, respectively. Survival was poorer for patients who were aged 70 or older at the time of surgery and was poorer for men than for women. Patients with bronchioloalveolar cell carcinoma had the best 5-year survival. Patients with wedge or lobectomy resections survived better than those with more extensive operations. Multivariate analysis showed that the effects of age and cell type on survival, when adjusted for sex, tumor node metastasis classification, and extent of resection were not significant.

Of patients in this series with T1N0M0 disease, 80% survived for 5 years or longer, compared with an expected survival of 84% (deaths from all causes) when adjusted for age and sex. The American Joint Committee Cancer staging method is helpful in assessing risks preoperatively, especially in patients with stage I cancer, for whom resection may provide long-term control.

▶ [As with many series, reports from the Mayo Clinic are invaluable because of their extensive clinical experience and careful follow-up. This article analyzes 3,900 patients, selecting a group of 624 with stage I lung cancer of whom 495 were suitable for analysis. The most encouraging finding is that the 5-year actuarial survival was 69%, emphasizing the importance of early diagnosis as well as the fact that adjuvant chemotherapy would theoretically add little to this excellent survival rate.—F.C.S.] ◀

13–6 **Bronchogenic Carcinoma and Postoperative Empyema: Is Survival Really Enhanced?** There are conflicting reports about the effect of postoperative empyema on survival after pulmonary resection for bronchogenic carcinoma; some workers have reported improved survival, and others, decreased survival in patients in whom empyema followed resection. Alan Peterson, Marvin Kirsh, and Herbert Sloan (Univ. of Michigan) reviewed experience with 542 patients who underwent curative resection of bronchogenic carcinoma between 1959 and 1974. Postoperative empyema developed in 17 patients (3.1%), in 10 after pneumonectomy and in 7 after lobectomy. Survival at 5 years was 18% in these patients, compared with 27% for patients who did not develop empyema. All 3 5-year survivors had stage I disease. All but 1 of 14 patients who died did so of recurrent carcinoma. Treatment of empyema was with open or closed tube thoracostomy and antibiotics. A variety of organisms was cultured from the empyema cavity in each patient.

The findings fail to show enhanced survival of patients with em-

(13–6) Ann. Thorac. Surg. 31:240–243, March 1981.

pyema after resection of bronchogenic carcinoma. Patient selection did not contribute to the poor prognosis. No patient died of septicemia or other complications of empyema. Reports in the literature do not show conclusively that postoperative empyema favorably influences survival in patients who have had pulmonary resection for bronchogenic carcinoma.

▶ [To explore the hypothesis that empyema after resection for bronchogenic carcinoma enhances survival, experiences with 542 patients treated in Ann Arbor, Michigan, between 1959 and 1974 were reviewed. Empyema occurred in 17, but no beneficial effect on long-term cure rates could be found. This report indicates well the problem of determining whether chance observations about neoplasm are statistically important or are simply associated factors that do not influence the results of therapy significantly.—F.C.S.] ◀

13–7 **Superior Sulcus Tumors: Results of Irradiation of 36 Patients.** Proper management of superior sulcus (apical) tumors has been controversial. Ritsuko Komaki, James Roh, James D. Cox, and Alberto Lopes da Conceicao (Med. College of Wisconsin, Milwaukee) encountered 36 patients with superior sulcus tumors confined to the thorax during 1963–1977, representing 2.7% of all patients with lung carcinoma. Two patients had stage II and 34 patients had stage III disease. All but 5 patients received megavoltage photon or gamma irradiation of 1–25 megavolts. The average field size was 13.5 sq cm. The median tumor dose was 5,800 rad over 6 weeks. The spinal cord was spared after 4,000 rad were delivered. The median patient age was 55 years. Fourteen patients had squamous cell carcinoma.

Symptomatic relief was obtained by 86% of the patients; median duration of palliation was 1 year. Local control of tumor was achieved in 47% of the patients, and this was the chief determinant of survival. The median survival of patients with local control was 26.5 months, compared to 6.5 months for the others. Performance status also was an important prognostic factor, but age was not. Mediastinal involvement did not indicate a poor prognosis, and rib and/or vertebral involvement did not preclude local control. Distant disease developed in 9 patients; it initially was most common in the brain. The actuarial survival at 5 years was 23%; 11 patients have lived more than 2 years without evidence of disease. There were no major complications. One patient had temporary findings of subclavian vein obstruction.

Intensive external irradiation of carcinomas of the superior pulmonary sulcus can give results equivalent to those of resection with or without preoperative irradiation. The primary tumor, upper and middle level of the mediastinum, and lower cervical and upper thoracic vertebrae must be included in the treatment field. A megavoltage dose of 6,000 rad in 6–6½ weeks is recommended. Prophylactic whole brain irradiation should be considered for patients with undifferentiated or poorly differentiated tumors.

▶ [Nearly 15 years ago, Paulson and associates reported significant improvement in the treatment of superior sulcus tumors by the combination of preoperative irradiation and surgery. For reasons puzzling to the editor, no group has been able to demonstrate comparable good results in a large series of patients.

This report challenges the role of operation, describing 36 patients treated with

---

(13–7) Cancer 48:1563–1568, Oct. 1, 1981.

high-dose irradiation who had a 5-year actuarial survival of 23%. The authors' thesis is that the previous concept of radiation alone being ineffective was due to the use of small doses applied to a small field. In general, their approach was to irradiate a field 13 cm wide with 6,000 or more rad over 6 to 6½ weeks. The best approach for this serious neoplasm remains uncertain.—F.C.S.] ◀

13–8 **Small Cell Carcinoma of the Lung** is discussed by John A. Meyer and Frederick B. Parker, Jr. (SUNY, Upstate Med. Center). Like bronchial carcinoid tumors, small cell carcinomas arise from the argentaffin cells in the bronchial mucosa and are members of the APUD (amine precursor uptake and decarboxylation) group. Small cell carcinomas appear to have the highest labeling indices and shortest volume-doubling times among lung tumors. Surgical resection alone has done nothing to alter the rapidly lethal course of these tumors. A great majority of patients with small cell carcinoma have stage III disease at diagnosis. A histologic biopsy specimen is generally necessary, besides thorough studies to determine the extent of disease.

Small cell carcinoma responds better to combinations of effective drugs than to a single effective agent given to maximum tolerance. An optimal regimen has not been found, and treatment to the absolute limit of patient tolerance is not necessarily desirable. Nearly all patients without distant metastases respond to treatment, and complete remission rates of 70% to 90% have been reported. In the presence of distant disease, complete remission rates may average 25% to 30%. Radiotherapy does not prolong survival in this group, but it can be of considerable palliative value in patients with severe local symptoms. Limited small cell carcinoma is clearly responsive to radiotherapy, and eradication of disease has been described in a few instances. Prophylactic irradiation of the CNS is a consideration.

Radiotherapy and chemotherapy do not necessarily control disease at the primary site, but incomplete excision is not helpful. Radiotherapy must not be used to facilitate the initial response. Immunotherapy has not shown promise in small cell carcinoma, but Cohen et al. reported increased survival in patients given thymosin fraction V besides chemotherapy. Further study of immune support or repletion is warranted.

▶ [Recent developments in the therapy of small cell carcinoma of the lung, a combined approach with chemotherapy, radiation, and operation in selected cases, have been reviewed in this article. This is important in regard to both the disease and evolving concepts in the treatment of neoplasms. Although results are still scanty, there clearly has been substantial improvement in the grim prognosis formerly associated with such neoplasms, which resulted in death for most patients within 6 to 12 months.—F.C.S.] ◀

13–9 **Small Cell Lung Cancer: Analysis of Treatment Factors Contributing to Prolonged Survival.** Combination chemotherapy has improved the results of radiotherapy for treatment of small cell lung cancer (SCLC), but the optimal combination of treatment remains poorly defined. R. Catane, A. Lichter, Y. J. Lee, H. D. Brereton, J. G. Schwade, and E. Glatstein (Natl. Inst. of Health) reviewed the results of treatment in 71 consecutive patients with biopsy-proved SCLC, who

---

(13–8) Ann. Thorac. Surg. 30:602–610, December 1980.
(13–9) Cancer 48:1936–1943, Nov. 1, 1981.

were seen during 1974 to 1977. Forty-two patients had limited disease, defined as tumor confined to the chest, and 29 had extensive disease. The 50 men and 21 women had a median age of 55 years. Chemotherapy consisted of cyclophosphamide, vincristine, and doxorubicin. Both local-field irradiation and prophylactic cranial irradiation were delivered with a 6-meV linear accelerator, and six different radiation regimens were used. The dose of cranial irradiation was 2,000 rad per 10 fractions.

A complete response was seen in 72% of the patients, in 81% with limited disease and 59% with extensive disease. Twelve patients who obtained a complete response died of acute treatment-related toxicity, most often sepsis associated with leukopenia or radiation pneumonitis. Nine of the 12 were disease free at autopsy. Eight patients remain alive without disease 33 to 57 months after treatment. All the long-term survivors had limited disease. Toxicity from treatment was substantial. Three patients had an esophageal stricture. Radiation pneumonitis and infection, with or without esophagitis, resulted in 17 deaths. The overall results appeared to favor concurrent combined modality treatment over sequential treatment.

Ultimate local control of SCLC may be enhanced by concurrent combined-modality treatment. Three weeks of concurrent therapy appears to be optimal for obtaining a maximal antitumor effect with acceptable toxicity. Controlled clinical trials are needed to define the optimal timing of chemotherapy and radiotherapy and to determine the optimal dose of radiotherapy for use in SCLC.

▶ [A dramatic development in the field of oncology in recent years has been the finding that certain types of neoplasms, especially sarcomas of the extremities and small cell carcinomas of the lung, can respond to a combined approach with x-ray, chemotherapy, and operation. Long-term data are not yet available, but the previous outlook with small cell tumor was so dismal, approaching 100% mortality within 1 to 2 years, that the results currently being obtained clearly represent an advance. This report describes six different patterns used at the National Cancer Institute in 71 consecutive patients.

A complete response was achieved in 51 patients (72%), although 12 died from the toxicity of the treatment. Nine of the 12 were free of disease at autopsy. Twenty-nine patients subsequently relapsed, but 8 remain alive and free of disease between 33 and 57 months after operation, a most encouraging finding.—F.C.S.] ◀

14. Congenital Heart Disease

14–1 **Atrial Septal Defect in Patients Aged 60 Years or Older: Operative Results and Long-Term Postoperative Follow-up.** Martin G. St. John Sutton, Abdul J. Tajik, and Dwight C. McGoon (Mayo Clinic) report the first long-term follow-up study of a large number of elderly patients who underwent operative closure of atrial septal defect. Seventy-two patients aged 60 and older were treated during 1955–1977. Sixty-four had a secundum atrial septal defect, and 8 had a sinus venosus defect associated with partial anomalous pulmonary venous connections. Sixty-six patients with a mean age of 64.5 years underwent surgical repair of atrial septal defect. Forty-four were in New York Heart Association functional classes III and IV preoperatively. Eighteen of the 56 patients studied had a pulmonary artery pressure greater than 60 mm Hg, but all except 6 had a pulmonary arteriolar resistance below 7 units/sq m.

Direct suture was used in 47 cases and a Dacron patch graft in 19. The hospital mortality was 6%. All 4 patients who died had undergone additional surgical procedures. There were 14 late deaths among the 47 patients with follow-up for 2 years or longer. Six of 8 patients who died of stroke had long-standing systemic hypertension. Three deaths were due to congestive heart failure. The surgical patients lived significantly longer than medically managed patients, the difference becoming apparent 4–5 years after operation. All but 6 of 47 patients were improved by at least one functional class at follow-up, the rest being unchanged; no patient deteriorated. Patients with significant pulmonary hypertension improved as often as the others.

Atrial septal defect is not rare in the elderly. Most patients are symptomatically improved on a long-term basis after operative repair, and the mortality risk is low. Surgery significantly increases life expectancy and restores subsequent survival of the patients to normal. Surgery can be recommended for all patients except those with the most severe pulmonary vascular obstructive disease and those with associated debilitating medical illness that results in shortened survival.

▶ [At the Mayo Clinic between 1955 and 1977, 66 patients older than age 60 years had an atrial septal defect closed. Four deaths occurred, all unrelated to pulmonary vascular resistance. Symptomatic benefit occurred in all groups.

Quite important is the fact that no patient was seen in whom increased pulmonary vascular resistance made the risk of operation prohibitive. However, only 10% of the group had pulmonary arteriolar resistance greater than 8 units/sq m. Benefit from operation was significant. An important unsolved problem is that 8 of 14 late deaths were from cerebrovascular accidents. Six of these deaths occurred in patients who had had atrial fibrillation; 3 had hypertension. Autopsies performed on 4 patients

---

(14–1) Circulation 64:402–409, August 1981.

found that the cause of death was intracranial hemorrhage in 3, not thromboembolism. Hence, the best treatment for postoperative hypertension remains unknown. The data did not show any difference in patch versus suture closure, and the authors did not mention obliterating the left atrial appendage.—F.C.S.] ◀

14–2 **Long-Term Results of Repair of Incomplete Persistent Atrioventricular Canal.** Daniel M. Goldfaden, Michael Jones, and Andrew G. Morrow (Natl. Inst. of Health) reviewed the records of 44 patients who had operative repair of uncomplicated incomplete persistent atrioventricular canal during 1956–1976. None had other major cardiac anomalies. The median age at operation was 12 years. The 39 consecutive operative survivors had follow-up for an average of 10.8 years.

All patients had a typical low-lying atrial septal defect of the ostium primum type and 37 had a cleft of the anterior mitral leaflet. Repair involved patch closure of the septal defect and direct suture closure of the mitral cleft. Three patients also had annuloplasty or suture closure of a cleft in the tricuspid valve. An anomalous left superior vena cava was ligated in 3 patients, and a small membranous ventricular septal defect was sutured closed in 3.

Five operative deaths occurred. Three patients had significant arrhythmias at discharge. Five of 35 patients catheterized an average of 11 months postoperatively had signs of mild mitral regurgitation, and 2 appeared to have serious regurgitation. The findings correlated well with residual symptoms; 5 of 6 patients with symptoms had abnormal catheterization findings. There were 3 late deaths, 2 of cardiac causes. Three patients have required late reoperation.

The predicted survival without reoperation at 13 years is 82%. Four patients had significant arrhythmias or conduction disturbances late after operation. Of 30 late survivors who were not reoperated on and were followed for an average of 13 years, 25 are currently asymptomatic and have no evidence of significant mitral regurgitation. The other 5 have mild cardiac symptoms and are thought to have mild to moderate mitral regurgitation.

Continued follow-up of patients operated on for incomplete persistent atrioventricular canal is necessary. However, with appropriate management of late complications, most late survivors have been free of cardiac symptoms.

▶ [This report is a valuable source of data, as it includes an average long-term follow-up of 12 years for 39 patients operated on before 1976. Thirty-five of the 39 patients had repeat catheterization. It is encouraging that only 20% had some mitral regurgitation, which was severe in 2%. Two of the patients required mitral valve replacement for mitral insufficiency. Long-term survival is excellent, but the need for continued medical surveillance is clearly indicated by the fact that only about one half of the patients were free of any serious cardiac problems 13 years after operation.—F.C.S.] ◀

14–3 **Results of Aortic Valve Replacement in Patients With a Narrow Aortic Annulus: Effects of Enlargement of the Aortic Annulus.** A narrow aortic annulus that will not accept a prosthesis of adequate size may be encountered at aortic valve replacement. Nicks

(14–2) J. Thorac. Cardiovasc. Surg. 82:669–673, November 1981.
(14–3) Ann. Thorac. Surg. 31:111–116, February 1981.

et al. devised a method of enlarging the aortic annulus at the noncoronary cusp. Tohru Mori, Yasunaru Kawashima, Soichiro Kitamura, Susumu Nakano, Kanji Kawachi, and Takeshi Nakata (Osaka Univ.) used this procedure in 10 male and 3 female patients with a narrow aortic annulus who were among 71 consecutive patients who underwent aortic valve replacement between 1975 and 1979. The average age of the patients at operation was 34.4 years. Eight patients had dominant aortic regurgitation, and 5 had dominant stenosis. Nine patients were in New York Heart Association functional class III or class IV preoperatively. Nine patients also had mitral stenosis. When the annulus did not accept a Björk-Shiley prosthesis greater than 23 mm in tissue diameter, the incision was extended about 8 mm toward the intervalvar fibrous trigone under the noncoronary cusp, and teardrop-shaped Teflon patches with pericardium were sutured to the edges of the subannular incisions.

One patient died of low-output syndrome and another of recurrent endocarditis with dehiscence of the suture line on the aortic wall of the patch used to enlarge the annulus. Leakage had resulted in a large pseudoaneurysm outside the ascending aortic wall. The other 11 patients are leading normal lives; 7 are in functional class I and 4 are in class II. The average postoperative cardiothoracic ratio was 55%. The aortic annulus was increased by an average of 3.3 mm in diameter. The enlarged annulus accepted a prosthesis at least one size larger than it could initially. The average pressure gradient across the prosthesis was 9.3 mm Hg.

Enlargement of a narrow aortic annulus by the method of Nicks et al. gave good results in these patients. The operation permitted placement of a prosthesis at least one size larger than was accepted by the annulus at first. Such enlargement is necessary if better postoperative prosthetic hemodynamics are to be expected.

▶ [Experiences with 13 patients with enlargement of the aortic annulus a bit over 3 mm to permit insertion of an adequate Björk-Shiley aortic prosthesis are described. The technique used was the one originally reported from Australia by Cartmill and associates, which is simpler and is associated with less morbidity than the procedure by Konno. This would seem to be the method of choice for enlarging the aortic annulus in most patients, because, except with extreme hypoplasia, enlarging the annulus 3 to 4 mm should be sufficient. A 19-mm Björk-Shiley prosthesis is almost never needed in adults, whereas a 23-mm prosthesis is ordinarily used only with patients weighing more than 200 lb.—F.C.S.] ◀

14–4 **Operation for Aortic Arch Anomalies.** James V. Richardson, Donald B. Doty, Nicholas P. Rossi, and J. L. Ehrenhaft (Univ. of Iowa) reviewed the results of operation in 42 patients seen between 1948 and 1978 with various forms of aortic arch anomaly resulting in tracheoesophageal compression. The 25 males and 17 females were aged 3 days to 71 years at operation; 27 were under age 2 years. Ninety percent of patients had symptoms of tracheal compression, and 86% had dysphagia, aspiration, or feeding difficulties. Esophagograms clearly showed esophageal compression in 90%. Nineteen patients had a right-sided aortic arch with a left-sided ligamentum arteriosum, and

---

(14–4) Ann. Thorac. Surg. 31:426–432, May 1981.

17 had a double aortic arch. Six patients had aberrant right subclavian arteries. Fifteen patients had associated defects.

All patients but 1 underwent surgical repair. In all other patients with a right-sided aortic arch, obstruction was relieved by division of the ligamentum arteriosum (Fig 14–1). Two patients with double aortic arch underwent division of the posterior arch, and the rest underwent division of the anterior arch, either distal to the left subclavian artery or between the left common carotid and left subclavian arteries (Fig 14–2). Five patients with aberrant right subclavian artery

Fig 14–1 (top).—Anatomy and surgical treatment of right-sided aortic arch and left-sided ligamentum arteriosum. Esophagus and trachea are compressed by ligamentum. After complete mobilization of aorta and left subclavian artery, ligamentum arteriosum is divided. *PA,* pulmonary artery.

Fig 14–2 (middle).—Anatomy and surgical treatment of double aortic arch. Here compression of trachea and esophagus occurred from left-sided arch. Obstruction can be relieved by dividing narrowest area of left-sided or anterior arch either between left common carotid and left subclavian anterior *(a)* or distal to left subclavian artery *(b)*. Ligamentum arteriosum is also divided. *PA,* pulmonary artery.

Fig 14–3 (bottom).—Anatomy and surgical treatment of aberrant right subclavian artery. This artery takes abnormal origin from upper descending thoracic aorta and has course posterior to esophagus to right axilla, causing posterior obstruction of esophagus. Division of anomalous subclavian artery after mobilization allows retraction of artery from behind esophagus. In older patients, revascularization of subclavian artery may be necessary. *PA,* pulmonary artery.

(Courtesy of Richardson, J. V., et al.: Ann. Thorac. Surg. 31:426–432, May 1981.)

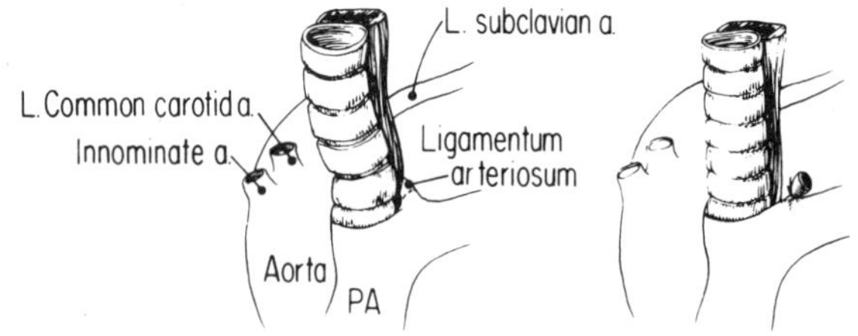

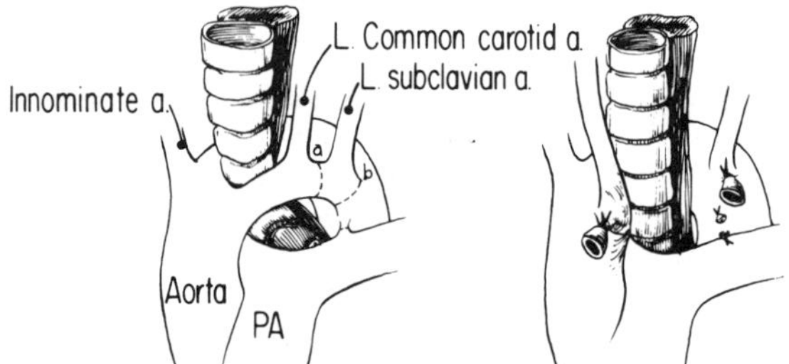

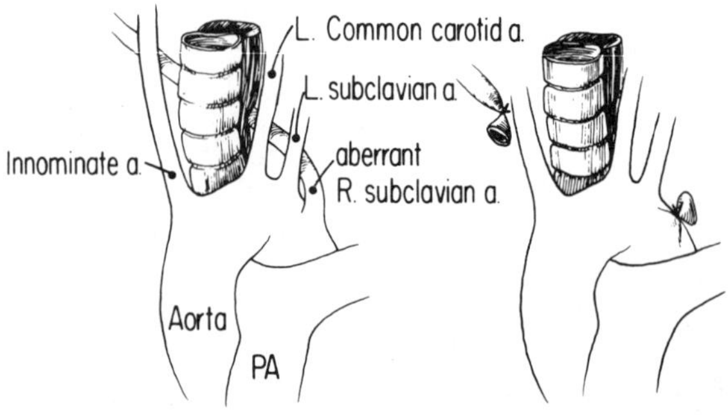

underwent ligation and division of the vessel (Fig 14–3). One had a subclavian-common carotid artery anastomosis as well. Two patients (5%) died after operation. Respiratory complications were common, and over half the patients required prolonged ventilatory support. There was 1 late death. All other patients were greatly improved or completely relieved from symptoms on follow-up for a mean of 94 months. Esophagograms showed complete resolution of esophageal obstruction in all 25 patients so examined. Five patients have severe mental retardation, and 4 others are ill with or disabled by associated congenital anomalies.

Aortic arch anomalies are a relatively common cause of respiratory distress and dysphagia in infants and small children. Barium esophagography is an accurate diagnostic method. Surgical repair is safe and has generally given quite good results.

▶ [This report provides significant data about the unusual condition of aortic arch anomalies, describing experiences with 42 patients treated during a 32-year period. Although Gross described the varieties of aortic arch anomalies decades ago, there is a paucity of data in the surgical literature about this condition. Hence, this article should be quite helpful. Most anomalies are of three types: a right aortic arch with a ligamentum arteriosum, a double aortic arch, or an aberrant right subclavian artery. With well-defined surgical principles, results of operation are excellent.—F.C.S.] ◀

14–5 **Appraisal of the Mustard Procedure for the Physiologic Correction of "Simple" Transposition of the Great Arteries: 80 Consecutive Cases, 1970–1980.** Gian Piero Piccoli, James L. Wilkinson, Robert Arnold, Francesco Musumeci, and David I. Hamilton (Liverpool, England) reviewed the findings in 80 consecutive patients who underwent the Mustard operation for so-called simple transposition of the great arteries during a 10-year period. The patients had atrioventricular concordance and ventriculoarterial discordance, an intact ventricular septum or a small septal defect, and absence of left ventricular outflow tract obstruction or, if present, a systolic pressure gradient of not more than 40 mm Hg. The average age was 14.7 months (Fig 14–4). Balloon atrial septostomy had been done in all but 2 patients, in 72 of them before age 3 weeks. The best palliation was obtained with the use of larger balloons. The Mustard operation was done with deep hypothermia and circulatory arrest with the use of a 7.5×2.5-cm pericardial baffle.

The early mortality was 2.5%. Six patients required intensive care for persistent low cardiac output postoperatively. On follow-up of 76 patients at an average of 4½ years, 59 were symptom free and leading normal lives. Six of 13 symptomatic children had pulmonary venous obstruction; 4 underwent successful plastic enlargement of the pulmonary atrium, whereas 1 died at reoperation and 1 at home. Seven patients had superior vena cava obstruction; 2 underwent plastic enlargement of the upper part of the interatrial baffle and closure of a residual interatrial communication. Several patients with arrhythmias were well at follow-up.

These findings compare favorably with those reported for other types of physiologic or anatomical correction in patients with simple trans-

---

(14–5) J. Thorac. Cardiovasc. Surg. 82:436–446, September 1981.

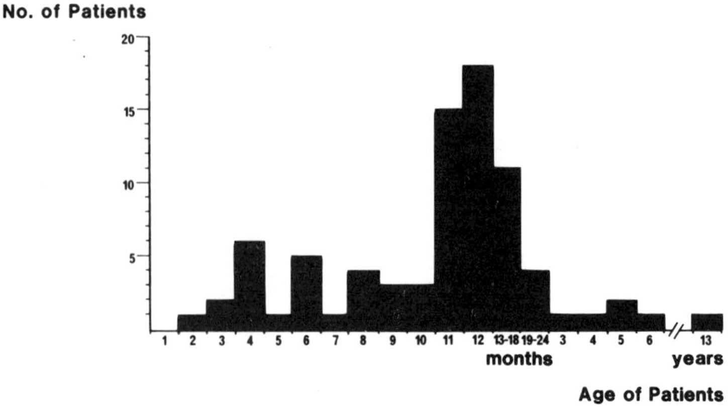

Fig 14–4.—Age of patients at operation. (Courtesy of Piccoli, G. P., et al.: J. Thorac. Cardiovasc. Surg. 82:436–446, September 1981.)

position of the great arteries. The present results warrant the continued use of the Mustard operation in this setting, although many more years of follow-up are needed before a final judgment can be made regarding the best means of correcting simple transposition. Elective repair is done at age 10 to 12 months or earlier if the patient's condition deteriorates.

▶ [At present, there are inadequate data to indicate which type of operation is superior for correction of "simple" transposition, the Mustard and the Senning procedures being those most commonly used. This report from England describes experiences with 80 cases during a 10-year period and concludes that the results compared favorably to those with other techniques. The data did not show any reason to alter surgical policy. A significant point regarding this series is that most patients were operated on before age 24 months (Fig 14–4).—F.C.S.] ◀

14–6 **Two-Dimensional Echocardiographic Evaluation of Mustard Operation for d-Transposition of the Great Arteries.** After the Mustard operation for transposition, the intra-atrial baffle can be detected by M mode echocardiography, but only limited segments of the atria are visualized, and abnormalities such as vena caval or pulmonary venous-atrial stenosis cannot be diagnosed. Kalim U. Aziz, Milton H. Paul, Saroja Bharati, Roger B. Cole, Alexander J. Muster, Maurice Lev, and Farouk S. Idriss (Northwestern Univ.) used two-dimensional sector scan echocardiography to evaluate the revised atria in 17 patients with d-transposition of the great arteries who underwent the Mustard operation. Seven were thought to have an ideal repair, 1 had superior vena caval and pulmonary venous-atrial obstruction, 3 had stenosis of the pulmonary venous atrium, and 6 had tricuspid regurgitation. Images were recorded from several planar projections (Fig 14–5).

In patients with an ideal repair, the dimension of the superior vena caval-isthmic segment of the systemic venous atrium was narrower than that of the superior vena caval segment. The anterior segments

---

(14–6) Am. J. Cardiol. 47:654–664, March 1981.

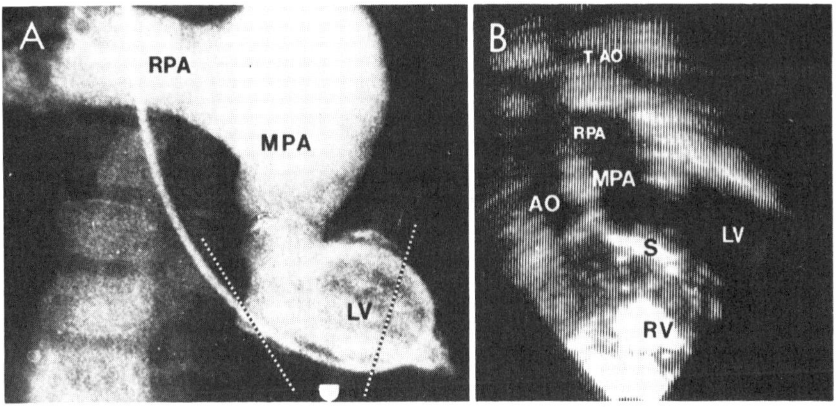

Fig 14–5.—Left ventricular angiogram (**A**) and subxiphoid view sector scan (**B**). Imaging of superior vena cava segment of systemic venous atrium is begun by obtaining four-chamber image and orienting sector beam in horizontal plane. With superior and anterior tilting of echographic beam, origin of pulmonary artery *(MPA)* from left ventricle *(LV)* and its branches can be defined. In this patient, origin of aorta *(AO)* from right ventricle *(RV)* is unusually well visualized. Further anterior and rightward beam angulation from this position shows superior vena cava segments and systemic venous atrium. *RPA,* right pulmonary artery; *S,* interventricular septum; and *TAO,* transverse aorta. (Courtesy of Aziz, K. U., et al.: Am. J. Cardiol. 47:654–664, March 1981.)

of the pulmonary venous atrium were slightly larger than those of the posterior or isthmic segments. Three patients had mild to moderate abnormal narrowing of the isthmic part of the pulmonary venous atrium. One had evidence of stenosis of the superior vena caval-isthmic segment, with a pressure gradient of 9 mm Hg across the isthmus. Patients with tricuspid regurgitation had increased sector scan dimensions of all segments of the pulmonary venous atrium. The mild isthmic narrowing seen in patients with ideal repairs was not present. The angiographic and echocardiographic findings correlated well.

Qualitative and quantitative two-dimensional sector echocardiography can reliably detect structural abnormalities of the surgically revised atria after the Mustard operation for transposition of the great arteries.

▶ [Periodic cardiac evaluation after the Mustard operation is most important because of the complications of caval or pulmonary vein obstruction that may occur. This technique apparently has significant potential in permitting periodic evaluation of the patient noninvasively. Hopefully, others can duplicate these findings.—F.C.S.] ◀

14–7 **Current Status of the Septation Procedure For Univentricular Heart.** Robert H. Feldt, Douglas D. Mair, Gordon K. Danielson, Robert B. Wallace, and Dwight C. McGoon (Mayo Clinic) reviewed the results of surgery in 45 patients with univentricular heart and 2 atrioventricular valves who, since 1973, underwent an operation in which an intraventricular patch was used to divide the ventricular chamber into two functional ventricles. Of the 24 patients who were discharged, 8 died during a 2½- to 62-month follow-up. The 16 surviving patients have been followed up for an average of 38½ months. Ten have undergone cardiac catheterization at least once.

(14–7) J. Thorac. Cardiovasc. Surg. 82:93–97, July 1981.

Most patients had levomalposition with a subaortic chamber. None of the 5 patients with univentricular heart and no outlet chamber have survived. Three of the 10 surviving patients who had catheterization had no residual shunt and good myocardial function. Seven survivors have required further surgery. Seven of the 16 survivors are currently free of symptoms without cardiac medications or diuretics, while 3 others are significantly disabled. Long-term survival could not be related to age, and only 2 of 15 patients with a documented history of congestive heart failure have survived. Patients with previous palliative surgery did not do as well as the others. The need for valve repair or replacement at septation had an adverse influence on the outcome. The patients with the best results were 5–15 years old at surgery for levomalposition with a subaortic outlet chamber. They had no history of heart failure or previous palliative surgery, and had preoperative hemoglobin values below 20 gm/100 ml.

The septation operation has not so far favorably altered the outcome compared with the natural history of univentricular heart, but conclusions are not yet possible. Currently, a modified Fontan procedure is performed in surgical candidates. Palliative surgery may improve the quality of life in other cases. Septation apparently is appropriate for selected patients, especially those with modestly elevated pulmonary vascular resistance.

▶ [With the rapid progress in the development of operations for congenital heart disease, the concept of creating a ventricular septum to treat the "single ventricle" is mechanically very attractive. This report from the Mayo Clinic of 45 operations during a period of more than 5 years is sobering, for the hospital mortality was 47%, and 18% of the patients died subsequently. Of the 16 survivors, 12 have a fairly good result—a small yield, about 25% of the original 45 patients. As detailed in the manuscript, several major problems await future solution.—F.C.S.] ◀

15. Valvular Heart Disease

15-1 **Tricuspid Valvulectomy Without Prosthetic Replacement: Ten Years of Clinical Experience.** Agustin Arbulu and Ingida Asfaw (Wayne State Univ.) reviewed the results of tricuspid valvulectomy without prosthetic replacement in 61 patients operated on since 1970 for intractable infective endocarditis. Gram-negative bacteria were responsible in 37 cases and gram-positive bacteria in 19. The most common bacterium involved was *Pseudomonas aeruginosa,* followed next by *Staphylococcus aureus.* Three patients had *Candida albicans* infection, and 1 each had traumatic endocarditis and cancerous invasion of the tricupsid valve. Fifty-two patients were addicted to intravenous drugs, usually heroin. The average time of intensive antibiotic therapy before operation was 4½ months. The tricuspid valve was totally excised with cold potassium cardioplegia and aortic cross-clamping. Intravenous antibiotic therapy was administered for 2 to 6 weeks postoperatively. Two patients also had pulmonic valvulectomy without prosthetic replacement.

There were 6 hospital deaths, whereas 55 patients survived and were cured of endocarditis. No hemodynamic problems were present in 46 survivors, and no patient had a poor outcome. There were 5 late deaths, 2 from recurrent endocarditis. Ten patients subsequently had insertion of a tricuspid prosthesis; 1 died with an infected, thrombosed prosthesis, and 9 are well. One other patient among those who did not have prosthetic replacement died of recurrent infective endocarditis. The actuarial survival at 1 year was 88.7% and at 2 years, 86.3%, subsequently remaining unchanged through 10 years.

Surgery is indicated for tricuspid endocarditis when intensive antibiotic therapy has failed. Insertion of a prosthesis may be necessary in some patients with ventricular failure unresponsive to medical treatment who are cured of their addiction. Tricuspid valvulectomy without prosthetic replacement is, however, the procedure of choice for intractable right-sided endocarditis in drug-addicted patients. It also is of value in this setting in nonaddicted patients. A valve prosthesis can be inserted later in this group of patients with minimal risk after the infection has been eradicated.

▶ [This surely is the largest experience with tricuspid valvulectomy in the world, 61 patients operated on since 1970. Fifty-two of the 61 were addicted to drugs. The mortality is reasonably low with such a serious illness, 6 hospital deaths and 5 late deaths, 3 unrelated to operation. Eleven of the surviving patients had a prosthetic valve inserted. Comparison of these patients with the larger group without a prosthetic valve showed no significant difference. Hence, the authors make the interesting point that subsequent insertion of a prosthetic valve is an elective decision. Certainly, it should probably not be done unless the patient has been cured of his drug addic-

(15–1) J. Thorac. Cardiovasc. Surg. 82:684–691, November 1981.

tion. Otherwise, there is a high probability of subsequent infection of the prosthesis. The contributions of Arbulu and his associates in Detroit in the past decade have been substantial and of great benefit to everyone.—F.C.S.] ◀

15–2 **Safe Technique for Removal of Massive Left Atrial Thrombus** is described by J. I. Gallo, B. Ruiz, and C. M. G. Duran (Santander, Spain). A large, intracavitary atrial thrombus creates a risk of intraoperative embolization at attempted removal.

Procedure.—The heart should be handled particularly carefully at bypass. With aortic cross-clamping and cardioplegia, a 2 to 3-cm incision is made in the left atrial wall, close to the atrial septum and paralleling it, and the atriotomy is widened after introduction of a sucker. A blunt subendocardial dissection is carried out to separate the thrombus from the septal wall. The mitral orifice is closed with an inflated 24 F Foley catheter (Fig 15–1). Gentle wall suction is used when the atrial cavity is aspirated. The cavity is washed out thoroughly, and Valsalva maneuvers are performed to aspirate the left pulmonary veins. Appropriate mitral surgery then is carried out.

Thirty of 968 patients undergoing open mitral operations between 1974 and 1979 were found to have massive left atrial thrombus. Seven of 8 early patients died of irreversible cerebral damage. This problem was avoided in the next 22 patients by use of the foregoing approach. The goal is to avoid fragmenting the thrombus during atriotomy and when retractors are introduced. Subendocardial removal of the thrombus reduces the number of fragments, and blocking of the mitral orifice avoids their passage into the left ventricular cavity. Wall suction is used when the atrial cavity is aspirated. Use of these measures can make removal of massive left atrial thrombus a safe procedure.

▶ [The unexpected finding of a massive left atrial thrombus is a significant complication at operation for mitral valve disease. Massive embolization of clot or air can occur. Ischemia time is prolonged, and others have reported a significant hazard of thromboembolism afterward.

For several years, I and my associates have used a technique like the authors describe, excising the clot with a plane of the diseased endocardium, taking care not to weaken the atrial wall and cause a perforation. It has not been necessary to occlude the mitral orifice as long as this is exposed, usually with the placement of a

Fig 15–1.—Foley catheter is placed through mitral orifice, and plane of cleavage is created between thrombus and atrial wall both anteriorly and posteriorly by blunt dissection. (Courtesy of Gallo, J. I., et al.: Ann. Thorac. Surg. 31:283–284, March 1981.)

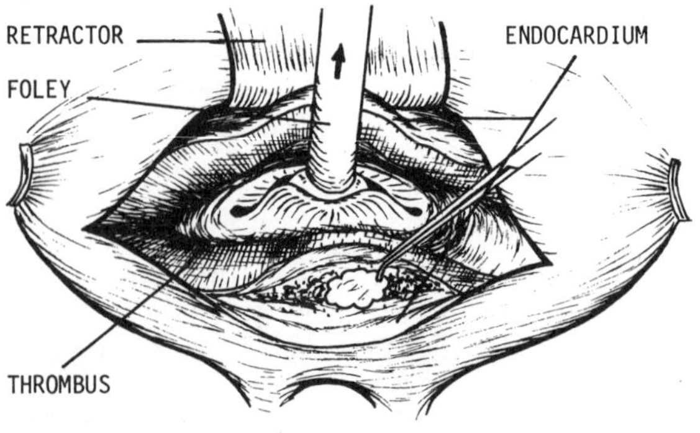

(15–2) Ann. Thorac. Surg. 31:283–284, March 1981.

sponge in the opening as additional protection. Finding the proper plane can be awkward, but, when done, the plane readily can be developed, usually with the finger, essentially removing all of the endocardium from the left atrium. The technique is not only a simple and effective way to remove the thrombus, but, to date, has been associated with negligible postoperative risk of embolization. Such patients have been managed similarly to those without left atrial thrombi, without any increased hazards, contrasting with reports by other authors of the need for anticoagulation. It would seem reasonable that removal of disease in the cardium is probably the technique that prevents recurrence of the thrombus.—F.C.S.] ◀

15–3 **Open Mitral Commissurotomy: Modern Reevaluation.** The anticoagulation necessary after valve replacement with mechanical prostheses is an added risk, and the long-term durability of porcine heterografts is in question. William L. Halseth, Donald P. Elliott, E. L. Walker, and E. A. Smith (Denver) reviewed the results of open surgery in 222 patients operated on for mitral stenosis between 1969 and 1978. The 161 female and 61 male patients were aged 15 to 72 years. Thirty-two patients had previously had closed mitral commissurotomy. Open commissurotomy was done in 197 patients; the other 25 patients had initial mitral valve replacement. Commissurotomy was done under bypass with moderate systemic hypothermia and aortic cross-clamping. Cold cardioplegia solution has been injected into the aortic root in recent operations. Anticoagulants were not used routinely after valve repair. Twelve patients who underwent open commissurotomy had other cardiac procedures also.

Of the 32 patients who had had previous closed mitral commissurotomy, 8 required initial mitral valve replacement, and 2 of the others later required mitral valve replacement. Hospital mortality was 1.5%. Two moribund patients who underwent emergency operations died. Fourteen of 191 open commissurotomy patients followed for a mean of 53 months died of heart-related causes, 2 after mitral valve replacement and 2 of thromboembolism. Three patients, all in atrial fibrillation, had cerebral embolism postoperatively. Seven other patients had nonfatal postoperative complications. No patient has required further surgery for restenosis after open commissurotomy. Fourteen patients (7.2%) required mitral valve replacement. The actuarial survival for patients who did not require reoperation for mitral valve replacement was 86% at 10 years.

All patients requiring surgery for mitral stenosis should have an open operation. Fused subvalvular structures should be released to provide adequate mitral leaflet motion and prevent restenosis. Patients with a large left atrium and those in chronic fibrillation should have the atrial appendage oversewn and should be considered for long-term anticoagulant therapy.

▶ [This experience with 222 patients undergoing open mitral valvulotomy over a 10-year period is significant and emphasizes that open mitral commissurotomy is reliable and durable in selected patients. During this time, mitral valve replacement was performed in only 25 patients, 11% of the group. These data indicate that most patients with mitral disease in some series can be treated by commissurotomy, rather than by replacement.

In the discussion, I describe experiences at New York University and report results very similar to those from Denver. To achieve an effective valvulotomy, division of

---

(15–3) J. Thorac. Cardiovasc. Surg. 80:842–848, December 1980.

fused chordae and papillary muscles is often required, the ideal being an orifice area as near as possible to normal to minimize turbulent flow and subsequent fibrosis. For example, a normal mitral valve is usually greater than 3 sq cm, and symptoms usually appear when the orifice is narrowed to between 1 and 2 sq cm. Improvement can result by enlarging the orifice to about 2 cm, far less than normal, but it is probable that recurrences within 3 to 5 years are common in this group because of recurrent stenosis.—F.C.S.] ◀

15–4 **Mitral Valve Replacement With the Hancock Bioprosthesis: Five- to Ten-Year Follow-up.** A. Michael Borkon, Charles L. McIntosh, Thomas J. Von Rueden, and Andrew G. Morrow (Natl. Inst. of Health) reviewed the results of implantation of a Hancock, glutaraldehyde-preserved, porcine mitral valve prosthesis in 111 patients in 1970–1974. Aortic or tricuspid valve replacement, or both, was also performed in 55 patients. Twenty-four bioprostheses were used in the aortic or tricuspid position. The average age at operation was 51 years. The operative mortality was 10%, with most deaths due to low cardiac output. The mean follow-up of hospital survivors was 5.4 years. Anticoagulant therapy was not used routinely in patients with bioprostheses except when there were documented emboli.

Of 70 patients who had follow-up for 5–10 years after surgery, 59 are alive. Actuarial survival rates were 76% at 5 years and 60% at 10 years. Patients with mitral valve replacement only had 5- and 10-year survival rates of 82% and 65%, respectively. The incidence of thromboembolism in this group was 2.4% per patient-year. Five episodes were fatal. The incidence of fatal thromboembolism in patients with bioprostheses was 0.8% per patient-year. A mitral bioprosthesis failed in 16% of 94 hospital survivors. Ten patients have had intrinsic failure of 11 bioprostheses due to leaflet calcification or disruption, thrombosis, or deformity of the stent post. Valve failures occurred an average of 86 months after operation. Reoperation was done in 9 cases, with 1 hospital death; 1 patient died before reoperation.

The Hancock bioprosthesis is a valuable cardiac valve substitute primarily because of a low rate of embolic complications and the lack of a need for anticoagulation. Whether these factors will outweigh the long-term risks of late intrinsic valve failure and reoperation remains unclear. Currently, the Hancock valve is used for mitral replacement only in patients older than age 60 and those with contraindications to anticoagulant therapy.

▶ [The group at the National Institutes of Health, led by Andrew Morrow, has investigated the Hancock porcine prosthesis carefully for several years. Hence, their experience with 111 patients is particularly significant. Analysis of their data has led them to conclude that the prosthesis should be used only in patients older than 60 years of age. At New York University, we have followed a contrary approach, using the porcine prosthesis in about 90% of patients operated on in the past 3 years, with the principal objective being to avoid anticoagulants. Knowing the danger of anticoagulant administration, with the worst ultimate result—having to reoperate on all patients within 8 to 10 years, with a reoperative risk of 4% to 5%—one may have more surviving patients at 15 years, including those reoperated on, than would be achieved if all patients had had a metallic prosthesis and permanent anticoagulation at the first operation. Only time and the accumulation of data will tell which approach is correct.—F.C.S.] ◀

(15–4) Ann. Thorac. Surg. 32:127–137, August 1981.

15–5 **Aortic Valve Replacement Without Myocardial Revascularization in Patients With Combined Aortic Valvular and Coronary Artery Disease.** Myocardial revascularization at valve replacement has been suggested for symptomatic patients with both aortic valve disease and coronary artery disease, but it is not clear that long-term survival is significantly impaired when only aortic valve replacement is performed. Robert O. Bonow, Kenneth M. Kent, Douglas R. Rosing, Lewis C. Lipson, Jeffrey S. Borer, Charles L. McIntosh, Andrew G. Morrow, and Stephen E. Epstein (Natl. Inst. of Health) compared the results of aortic valve replacement in 55 consecutive, symptomatic patients who had coronary artery disease with those in 142 patients without coronary disease also operated on between 1972 and 1978. Forty-three patients had 70% or greater stenosis of at least one major coronary artery, and 10 had a history of myocardial infarction. Starr-Edwards and Björk-Shiley prostheses and porcine heterografts were used.

Mean follow-up after operation was 3.7 years. Patients with coronary disease were significantly older than the others. Operative mortality and infarction were comparably frequent in the two patient groups. Late survivals did not differ significantly. Eight patients with coronary disease (15%) had recurrent angina after aortic valve replacement, but only 3 required coronary bypass grafting. The results in patients with coronary disease were similar to those reported from other centers after aortic valve replacement plus coronary bypass grafting.

The detection of coronary artery disease before aortic valve replacement does not necessitate myocardial revascularization in all patients at the time of replacement. Coronary disease did not affect survival adversely in this series, and the outcome of operation was as good as that reported for patients undergoing both aortic valve replacement and coronary bypass grafting.

▶ [The necessity for routinely grafting the coronary arteries at the time of aortic valve replacement was studied in this report. It was found that results in the first 2 to 3 years after operation were similar in the two groups, indicating that coronary bypass grafting is not mandatory at the time of aortic valve replacement. Survival at up to 4 years after operation was similar between the two groups.—F.C.S.] ◀

15–6 **Clinical Durability of the Hancock Porcine Bioprosthetic Valve.** The function of the glutaraldehyde-fixed xenograft bioprosthetic valve is generally satisfactory, but its clinical durability is uncertain. Philip E. Oyer, D. Craig Miller, Edward B. Stinson, Bruce A. Reitz, Ricardo J. Moreno-Cabral, and Norman E. Shumway (Stanford Univ.) reviewed data on 1,407 patients who received Hancock xenobioprosthetic valves between 1971 and 1979, 707 in the aortic and 700 in the mitral position. Cumulative follow-ups were 1,732 patient-years for aortic and 1,843 for mitral prostheses. Currently patients undergoing aortic valve replacement receive warfarin for 6 weeks after operation, and those undergoing mitral valve replacement receive it for 12 weeks.

The overall rate of valve failure was 1.1% per patient-year in both

(15–5) Circulation 63:243–251, February 1981.
(15–6) J. Thorac. Cardiovasc. Surg. 80:824–833, December 1980.

groups of patients. The probabilities of freedom from valve failure were 95.4% for adult aortic valve patients 5 years after operation and 90.9% for adult mitral valve patients 6 years after operation. Valve failure was more frequent in children than in adults; the risk decreased after age 15 years. Primary tissue failure was slightly more frequent in mitral valve cases. No primary tissue failure has occurred in adults given modified-orifice aortic bioprostheses. Endocarditis occurred at respective rates of 1.2% and 0.4% per patient-year in the aortic and mitral groups. Seventeen of 28 patients with endocarditis diagnosed before death have survived their infection with no valve dysfunction. Eight patients developed a new regurgitant murmur of unknown origin within 5 years after operation. Three bioprosthetic valve thromboses have occurred. Thirteen patients underwent reoperation for valve failure due to endocarditis, with 8 operative deaths. All 13 patients reoperated on for bioprosthetic tissue failure in the absence of infection survived the operation.

Close surveillance of patients with xenograft bioprostheses is necessary to assure timely reoperation if necessary, but the available data support the continued use of these valves in adult patients. The long-term risk for young patients remains to be clarified.

▶ [The total Stanford University experience with porcine prostheses, 1,407 patients operated on between 1971 and 1979, is reviewed. The probability of freedom from tissue failure in adults was 99% at 5 years in those with aortic valve replacement, and 94% at 6 years in those with mitral replacement. Data beyond 6 or 7 years are too few to permit conclusions.

This report is a good data base for evaluating long-term results with porcine prostheses. Findings between 8 and 10 years after operation are urgently needed, because several reports indicate that failure occurs much more commonly after 7 or 8 years. Whether this may be altered by better techniques of preservation is a leading question in the years ahead.—F.C.S.] ◀

15–7 **Year of Operation as a Risk Factor in the Late Results of Valve Replacement.** Quentin Macmanus, Gary L. Grunkemeier, Louis E. Lambert, Joseph F. Teply, Bradley J. Harlan, and Albert Starr (Univ. of Oregon) reviewed the results of valve replacement with silicone ball-valve prostheses with respect to time of operation. A total of 158 Model 6120 Starr-Edwards mitral prostheses and 363 Model 1200/60 aortic prostheses were implanted between 1965 and 1979 at the authors' institution. All patients had replacement of a single valve, but concomitant procedures were commonly performed. All patients received warfarin postoperatively, but warfarin often was temporarily interrupted, usually for trauma or unrelated surgery.

There were 39 late deaths in the mitral replacement group. Eight patients required removal of the prosthesis. A total of 44 thromboembolic events occurred, 6 of them fatal and 14 causing residual disability, in patients operated on before 1973. Subsequently 1 transient thromboembolic event occurred. In the aortic replacement group there were 65 late deaths. There were 39 deaths from events causally or temporally related to valve replacement, compared with 19 in the mitral replacement group. Sixty-eight embolic events occurred, 7 fatal and 22 causing residual disability. Three deaths resulted from bleed-

---

(15–7) J. Thorac. Cardiovasc. Surg. 80:834–841, December 1980.

ing complications. In both groups, rates of thromboembolism were significantly lower in the more recent part of the review period than in the initial years.

The standard silicone ball-valve prostheses currently has a thromboembolic risk as low as that reported for other presently used valve substitutes. The time frame of valve replacement must be considered when results are evaluated. Improved late results may not necessarily reflect improved prosthesis design or material. Selection of a prosthesis in a given case is based chiefly on considerations of durability and the relative risk of anticoagulation.

▶ [There is a striking difference in the frequency of thromboembolism in ball valves implanted after 1973 as compared with those implanted earlier. The embolus-free rates were 96% for mitral prostheses implanted after 1973, compared with 68% for the earlier implants. With aortic prostheses, the corresponding figures were 87% as compared with 77%. Reasons for this difference are unclear, but this is a finding of great significance.—F.C.S.] ◀

15–8 **Isolated Mitral Valve Replacement and Ventricular Rupture: Presentation of Six Patients.** F. Gosalbez, F. A. de Linera, J. L. Cofiño, J. L. Naya, J. Rodríguez and A. Ortuña (Oviedo, Spain) encountered 2 cases of intraoperative left ventricular rupture during mitral valve replacement before 1977 and subsequently 4 cases in less than 2 years among 55 isolated mitral prosthetic procedures. The 3 operative deaths represented three fourths of total early mortality for mitral valve replacement. Myocardial protection with aortic root cardioplegic solutions was used routinely at the time of the last 4 cases. All 4 patients had slight or minimal valve fibrosis and no calcium. Mitral insufficiency was the dominant lesion. There was little fibrous ring in which to place sutures in these patients. Björk-Shiley prostheses were used in all procedures.

The posterior leaflets were excised almost completely, and sutures were placed in the muscle next to the annulus. It was assumed that, apart from perforations due to mechanical trauma from the procedure itself, the patients most at risk were those with mitral insufficiency and soft, pliable leaflets, with little fibrosis and smaller fibrous rings. In patients with noncalcified valves, excision of the posterior mitral leaflet is now avoided, or merely the edge is removed with the chordae. Sutures are placed through the leaflet and annulus only, not through muscle. If muscle is entered, sutures buttressed with Teflon pledgets on the ventricular side should be used. Postoperative hypertension is avoided by using vasodilators, and left ventricular volume overloading is avoided postoperatively. No ruptures have occurred in 23 subsequent operations, 15 on patients with no calcium present.

The authors have had little success with the repair of ruptures, but others have reported better results. Delayed rupture is a hopeless situation.

▶ [This report describes experiences with 6 patients with rupture of the left ventricle after mitral valve replacement, 5 of whom died. This article was selected because it focuses attention on a grave problem that has appeared with mitral valve replacement, probably increasing in frequency with the use of potassium cardioplegia, which relaxes the left ventricle more than ischemic arrest. The conclusions of the authors

(15–8) Ann. Thorc. Surg. 31:105–110, February 1981.

are not significant in that they are sequential observations without controls, and, like many areas in medicine, once attention becomes focused on a problem, the problem diminishes, although the exact reason for the improved results is unclear.

At New York University, I and my associates have studied this problem in considerable detail. Observations are principally hypotheses because there is virtually no way of either performing a controlled experiment or evaluating the problem in the laboratory. There seem to be three types of ventricular rupture, rupture beneath the annulus, rupture in the free wall of the left ventricle from strut perforation of a porcine valve, and transverse rupture of the left ventricular wall beneath the annulus of the mural leaflet.

Subannular rupture results from any maneuver that applies excessive traction to the mitral valve annulus, tearing it away from the underlying ventricular muscle. This injury results from two factors, the amount of force applied and the tensile strength of the heart. It can occur many ways, from traction during removal of the valve, insertion of sutures, tying down of the sutures, anchoring of the prosthesis, or tilting of the heart after the prosthesis has been inserted.

The strut perforation of the ventricle results from inserting a prosthesis too large for the ventricular cavity, which is relaxed with potassium arrest in diastole. If the posterior strut is near the ventricular muscle, resumption of cardiac contractions results in the muscle being gradually perforated by the strut. This can be avoided by both careful selection of the size of the prosthesis and inspection of the position of the posterior strut before insertion.

The third type of rupture, described in detail in a report by Cobbs from Emory University in 1980, is the most lethal and is of unknown origin. It is probably the result of increased friability of the potassium-arrested heart and weakening of the ventricular wall from removal of chordae tendoneae. Preservation of chordae to the mural leaflet may be the best protection. Another method used at Emory University has been carefully to prevent forceful contraction of the left ventricle for 20 to 30 minutes after the aortic clamp is removed.—F.C.S.] ◀

16. Coronary Heart Disease

16–1 **Clinical and Angiographic Predictors of Operative Mortality From the Collaborative Study in Coronary Artery Surgery (CASS)** were analyzed by J. Ward Kennedy, George C. Kaiser, Lloyd D. Fisher, James K. Fritz, William Myers, J. Gerard Mudd, and Thomas J. Ryan (Univ. of Washington). Isolated coronary artery bypass surgery was performed on 6,630 patients with coronary artery disease at 15 centers participating in the CASS between 1975 and 1978. All patients had 70% or greater stenosis of at least one major coronary artery segment or 50% or greater stenosis of the left main coronary artery. Overall operative mortality was 2.3%.

Mortality was 4.5% in women and 1.9% in men. It tended to be higher with advancing age in men, but not significantly so in women. Risk factors for coronary disease could not be related to operative mortality, and previous myocardial infarction did not increase the risk of bypass surgery. Operative mortality was higher in patients with more severe angina and in those with more marked congestive heart failure. Mortality was increased insignificantly in patients with lower ejection fractions. It increased significantly with left ventricular wall motion scores and with increasing left ventricular end-diastolic pressure. Severe left main coronary disease increased operative mortality significantly, especially in patients with a left-dominant system. Operative mortalities were 1.7% for elective surgery, 3.5% for urgent surgery, and 10.8% for emergency surgery. Thirty patients with severe left main coronary stenosis who had emergency surgery had an operative mortality of 40%.

Operative mortality after coronary bypass surgery is influenced by advanced age, female sex, symptoms of heart failure, left main coronary artery stenosis, left ventricular dysfunction, and nonelective surgery. These factors should be taken into account in selecting patients for operation.

▶ [Data from experiences with over 6,600 patients from 15 institutions are described here. Operative mortality was slightly more than 2%. It increased with age, female sex, heart failure, left main coronary stenosis, impaired left ventricular function, and emergency operations. This cooperative study, a landmark in this area of investigation, should produce much valuable information because of the size of the data sample and the number of institutions participating.—F.C.S.] ◀

16–2 **A Rationale For the Use of Sequential Coronary Artery Bypass Grafts.** Sequential coronary artery bypass grafts have been increasingly used for coronary revascularization. Martin J. O'Neill, Jr., Patrick D. Wolf, Thomas K. O'Neill, Ralph M. Montesano, and John A. Waldhausen (Pennsylvania State Univ., Hershey) analyzed intra-

---

(16–1) Circulation 63:793–802, April 1981.
(16–2) J. Thorac. Cardiovasc. Surg. 81:686–690, May 1981.

operative measurements of saphenous vein graft dimension, coronary perfusion pressure, and coronary bypass graft flow to determine whether sequential grafting creates favorable hemodynamic conditions. Studies were made of 106 single grafts and 35 double sequential grafts, both after aortic anastomosis and after completion of the coronary anastomosis. Proximal sequential anastomoses were done in a diamond or parallel manner. Anastomoses were made with a running 6–0 Prolene suture under hypothermic potassium cardioplegia.

The diameters of single and sequential grafts were comparable, but the single grafts were significantly shorter. The resistance of the venous conduit was 15.5 resistance units (RU) in single grafts and 16.5 RU in sequential grafts, which was not a significant difference. However, total resistance was significantly greater in single graft cases (190.1 vs. 116.5 RU). Coronary resistance was 100 RU for sequential grafts and 174.6 RU for single grafts. Velocity of blood flow was 11.1 cm/second in the proximal segment of sequential vein grafts and 7.5 cm/second in single grafts, which was a significant difference. Arterial pressures were equal in the 2 groups of patients.

Double sequential coronary artery bypass grafts have nearly half the coronary vascular resistance of single bypass grafts. Coronary vascular resistance is the chief determinant of blood flow through the grafts, and therefore of the velocity of blood flow. Sequential bypass grafting creates favorable hemodynamics. Every effort is now made to attach the smaller coronary system proximally on a sequential graft with the larger coronary vessel used for the distal anastomosis. The more frequent use of sequential grafts provides the best opportunity to obtain complete revascularization of the ischemic heart with small coronary arteries.

▶ [For unclear reasons, sequential grafts have been proved neither superior nor inferior to single grafts, although the concept was introduced several years ago. Sequential grafts have the attraction of a higher rate of blood flow through the parent graft, but a thrombus occurring in one segment may extend into the lumen and embolize to the other segment, causing failure of several anastomoses. This article analyzes different hemodynamic variables, indicating that in a sequential graft the velocity of blood flow through the proximal segment is significantly higher. The maximum advantage occurs if the smaller coronary artery is used for the proximal sequential anastomosis.

Although it is only a hypothesis, the editor would judge that the failures in the past have resulted from inadequate myocardial preservation. With present techniques, sequential grafts will probably be used more and more frequently, both for simplicity and for hemodynamic advantages, permitting the bypass of all significantly occluded coronary arteries greater than 1.5 mm in diameter.—F.C.S.] ◀

16–3 **Life Expectancy After Coronary Artery Surgery** was reviewed by Floyd D. Loop, Delos M. Cosgrove, Bruce W. Lytle, and Leonard R. Golding (Cleveland Clinic). Operative experience and technical advancements in the 1970s are responsible for a documented reduction in operative mortality after coronary artery surgery. The 15-center Collaborative Study in Coronary Artery Surgery confirmed a reduced operative risk from bypass graft surgery. Ten-year survival rates compare favorably with the 50% survival achieved with conservative

---

(16–3) Am. J. Surg. 141:665–671, June 1981.

management of patients eligible for surgery. Five-year survival rates with surgery have exceeded significantly those for solely medical management in controlled studies of patients with multivessel coronary atherosclerosis. Revascularization is indicated whenever possible for left main coronary artery disease because of the grim prognosis with medical treatment alone. The results of surgery in patients with poor left ventricular function are improving, and are superior to those of medical management. Significant palliation has been obtained in reoperation with respect to both relief of symptoms and longevity.

The operative risk from coronary artery surgery has declined in the face of an increasing incidence of multi-vessel disease and worse preoperative left ventricular function. Improvements in mortality and morbidity are attributed to improved methods of myocardial protection. Survival rates at 5 and 10 years in patients with chronic stable angina are 92.3% and 77.3%, respectively. Ejection fraction is apparently the best indicator of late survival. Controlled studies have shown significantly better 5-year survival rates with surgery than with medical management. Coronary artery surgery has improved medium-term survival in patients with poor left ventricular function. The surgery appears to alter favorably the annual rates of fatal myocardial infarction and sudden death. The number of candidates for reoperation has increased gradually; the 5-year survival after reoperation now is about 90%.

▶ [This article summarizes data on the principal question regarding coronary bypass: What is its influence on longevity? Data from several sources indicate that bypass surgery significantly improves longevity in patients with triple-vessel disease and those with left main artery disease, and probably those with significant impairment of ventricular function. Data are less convincing for single- and double-vessel disease. This report describes a survival between 88% and 93%.—F.C.S.] ◀

16–4 **Long-Term Results of Myocardial Revascularization in Early-Onset Arteriosclerosis.** Although it generally is supposed that early-onset coronary arteriosclerosis is accelerated and operation may be less beneficial, observations of the natural history do not support an overly pessimistic view. James W. Jones, John L. Ochsner, Noel L. Mills, and Larry Hughes (Ochsner Med. Inst.) compared the outcome of coronary bypass in 116 patients younger than age 40, operated on between 1971 and 1978, with that of 2,090 older patients treated in the same period. Follow-up ranged from 1 to 9 years and was complete in 98% of cases. The only risk factor that was significantly more frequent in the younger patients was an elevated serum cholesterol concentration. Hypertension was significantly more common in the older patients. The extent and pattern of anatomical disease and ventricular function were comparable in the two groups.

There were no operative deaths in the younger group, compared with a 2.4% operative mortality in patients over age 40 years. Only 2 young patients (1.7%) had perioperative myocardial infarction. Failure of angina to improve and other adverse, nonfatal consequences were comparably frequent in the two groups. Survival curves

---

(16–4) Surgery 88:760–765, December 1980.

at 5 years did not differ significantly. Cumulative 5-year survival for early-onset patients who were operated on was greater than that for an early-onset group treated medically.

The findings do not warrant concern that the clinical course of early-onset coronary artery disease is accelerated. Younger patients with coronary artery disease are effectively managed by coronary bypass grafting.

▶ [A comparison was made of results after coronary bypass in patients younger than age 40 and those operated on later in life; 116 patients younger than age 40 were compared with more than 2,000 older patients. Results were excellent, with no evidence that the disease process was accelerated, supporting the application of bypass in symptomatic patients younger than age 40.—F.C.S.] ◀

16–5 **Influence of Aspirin and Dipyridamole on Patency of Coronary Artery Bypass Grafts.** Up to 25% of coronary bypass grafts are occluded within the first year after operation, and graft occlusion continues to occur for several years. Aspirin and dipyridamole have enhanced arterial patency after intimal injury in animals. J. E. Mayer, Jr., W. G. Lindsay, W. Castaneda, and D. M. Nicoloff (Univ. of Minnesota) evaluated these agents in a prospective, randomized trial in 174 patients undergoing coronary bypass grafting for refractory angina between 1973 and 1975. Study patients received 650 mg of aspirin and 50 mg of dipyridamole twice daily by mouth, starting after transfer from the intensive care unit after operation. Forty-seven drug-treated and 66 control patients were satisfactorily evaluated after operation. The groups were roughly comparable. Each group had an average of 1.9 grafts per patient.

Graft patency was significantly greater in study patients than in controls, with respective overall patency rates of 94% and 82%. The patency rates for saphenous vein grafts were 92% in the study group and 78% in the control group 3 to 6 months after operation. Differences in patency between grafts in drug-treated and those in control patients were greater for females than for males.

Administration of aspirin and dipyridamole can improve the early patency rate of saphenous vein-coronary artery bypass grafts in patients by 15%. The authors are continuing to administer these drugs to patients after coronary bypass grafting in the hope of improving graft patency rates. The decreased platelet aggregation observed after aspirin ingestion is attributed to decreased production of thromboxane A_2, secondary to inhibition of cyclo-oxygenase. Dipyridamole inhibits phosphodiesterase within platelets, leading to a rise in intraplatelet cyclic adenosine monophosphate and decreased ability of the platelets to aggregate.

▶ [The beneficial effects of antiplatelet agents on coronary bypass grafts after operation have been unknown. This report, a well-designed prospective randomized trial, fully supports the use of antiplatelet agents, finding a 15% difference in patency between the treated group and the control group.—F.C.S.] ◀

16–6 **Surgical Treatment of Ventricular Arrhythmias in Coronary Artery Disease** is discussed by Leonard N. Horowitz, Alden H. Harken, Mark E. Josephson, and John A. Kastor (Philadelphia). Serious

(16–5) Ann. Thorac. Surg. 31:204–210, March 1981.
(16–6) Ann. Intern. Med. 95:88–97, July 1981.

ventricular arrhythmias are a common complication of organic, especially ischemic, heart disease and have an important impact on patient welfare. Some patients in whom tachyarrhythmias do not respond to pharmacotherapy will respond to pacing, but pacing is not effective when recurrent ventricular fibrillation or tachycardia produces immediate hemodynamic collapse. The implanted automatic defibrillator offers promise in the future in this setting.

Coronary bypass surgery may actually worsen ventricular premature depolarizations. Revascularization appears promising, however, for recurrent ventricular fibrillation caused by discrete acute episodes of reversible myocardial ischemia, especially when medical treatment has failed. Experience with sympathectomy is limited. Sympathectomy may help certain patients with recurrent sustained ventricular tachycardia but typically fails as a sole method of treatment. Large series have shown less benefit than hoped from routine aneurysmectomy, but newer procedures have been developed, including encircling endocardial ventriculotomy and simple ventriculotomy guided by epicardial mapping. The latter procedure has given extremely encouraging results in patients without coronary artery disease. Endocardial excision guided by endocardial mapping may be a better approach. Some have recommended the use of activation mapping during sinus rhythm to identify areas responsible for ventricular arrhythmias.

More sophisticated means of acquiring and analyzing activation mapping of extremely rapid, transient, or multiform tachycardias are anticipated. Standardization of preoperative and postoperative clinical data is needed to assess accurately the efficacy of various surgical procedures for the treatment of ventricular arrhythmias.

▶ [Over two thirds of the 600,000 annual deaths from coronary artery disease occur outside the hospital. The dramatic data from Seattle, accumulated over a period of 10 years, clearly indicate that arrhythmias—rather than massive infarctions—are responsible for well over half these deaths. Bypass has been ineffective for abolishing arrhythmias. This paper reviews the background of the treatment of arrhythmias, defining the currently most effective method. The group in Philadelphia, led by Alden Harken, have used endocardial mapping successfully to find the trigger zone, followed by local excision. Their experiences include 39 patients, 31 of whom have been totally relieved of the arrhythmias without any antiarrhythmic agent whatever. Undoubtedly, this is an area of surgical therapy whose horizons should expand greatly in the next 2 to 3 years.—F.C.S.] ◀

16–7 **Improved Long-Term Survival Following Myocardial Revascularization in Patients With Severe Left Ventricular Dysfunction.** Conflicting results from revascularization have been reported in patients with symptomatic coronary artery disease associated with left ventricular dysfunction. J. G. Coles, C. Del Campo, S. N. Ahmed, R. Corpus, A. C. MacDonald, M. M. Goldbach, and J. C. Coles (Univ. of Western Ontario) reviewed the results obtained in 59 consecutive patients with severe left ventricular dysfunction operated on during a time when the policy was to accept all such patients with severe angina as the predominant symptom. The 54 men and 5 women had a mean age of 54 years. The mean left ventricular ejection fraction in

(16–7) J. Thorac. Cardiovasc. Surg. 81:846–850, June 1981.

55 cases was 0.28%; it was 0.35% or under in 76% of patients. The mean left ventricular end-diastolic pressure was 18 mm Hg. All patients had evidence of severe coronary obstructive disease. An average of 2.8 grafts was placed. Right coronary artery endarterectomy was necessary in 19% of cases.

The mean follow-up was 37 months. The single operative death resulted from low cardiac output and sepsis. Seven of 9 late deaths were cardiac in origin; 5 were associated with myocardial infarction. The 5-year actuarial survival rate was 80%. All but 1 of 44 long-term survivors report improvement in angina, and two thirds are completely asymptomatic. Nine of 12 patients with congestive heart failure preoperatively are significantly improved. Of long-term survivors under age 65 years, 80% are currently employed.

These encouraging long-term results warrant the continued use of an aggressive surgical approach in patients with angina complicated by severe left ventricular dysfunction. Operative mortality in the present series approached that of bypass grafting in patients with normal left ventricular function. Survival depends on the selection of patients with severe angina as the predominant symptom, and exclusion of patients solely with heart failure secondary to irreversible myocardial fibrosis.

▶ [The role of bypass for patients with severe left ventricular dysfunction has been controversial for a decade. At one time, the American Heart Association officially stated that this should not be done. Experience proved that this was an incorrect statement, because such patients not only can be operated on safely with relief of angina, but actually may be in more urgent need of operation than a patient with a normal ventricle. Everything depends on how well the myocardium is preserved during operation.

The data in this paper fully support operation in these patients. Operative mortality in the 59 patients was 1.7%, and 9 late deaths occurred; the 5-year actuarial survival rate was 80% ± 6%. Angina was relieved in most. Hence, the results were very satisfactory in terms of both relief of angina and longevity. Evolving data from 25,000 patients undergoing catheterization in the CASS study have shown thus far that the prognosis for medically treated patients with triple-vessel disease and severe impairment of left ventricular function is dismal, approaching only 45% survival within 4 years.—F.C.S.] ◀

16–8 **Immediate Coronary Artery Bypass For Acute Evolving Myocardial Infarction.** Ralph Berg, Jr., Samuel L. Selinger, Jack J. Leonard, Ronald P. Grunwald, and William P. O'Grady (Spokane, Wash.) reviewed the results of coronary bypass grafting for acute evolving myocardial infarction in 227 consecutive patients operated on in 1971–1979. Patients too far into infarction were excluded, as were those with small coronary branch occlusions and patients with small infarctions as the result of obstructions of nondominant right or circumflex arteries. Under hypothermic cardioplegic protection, vessels with proximal stenoses of 50% or more were grafted, starting with the vessel to the dyskinetic area of myocardium. Probing of the coronary arteries was minimized.

More than 80% of patients were men; the age range was 28–79 years. The left anterior descending artery was most often involved. An average of 2.2 grafts was placed in an average of about 3¼ hours.

(16–8) J. Thorac. Cardiovasc. Surg. 81:493–497, April 1981.

Significant preoperative complications occurred in 41% of patients; the most common was arrhythmia. Cardiogenic shock was present in 8% of cases. The operative mortality was 1.8%. Nine patients required intra-aortic balloon pumping postoperatively. Four patients required reoperation for bleeding. Seven patients had pulmonary embolism, 7 had pneumothorax, and 7 had typical postpericardiotomy syndrome. Two patients had permanent pacing for complete heart block. The patency rate for grafts to ischemic areas a year postoperatively was 94%. There were 3 late deaths. All but 2% of patients had the same or an improved quality of life at follow-up.

Cineangiography should be done if possible in patients with acute evolving myocardial infarction, and appropriate patients should be offered prompt coronary bypass graft surgery. Perisistent angina is much less frequent in operative patients than in those treated conventionally.

▶ [Since 1971, the group led by Ralph Berg in Spokane, Washington, has pursued an aggressive policy of prompt operation on acute infarction, a method of therapy contrasting sharply to that followed by the vast majority of cardiologists worldwide. Hence, their data are of particular significance. Their logistical arrangement is impressive, attempting to have a bypass graft functioning within 6 hours after the onset of symptoms, which includes admission to the hospital, catheterization, and operation. This report with 227 patients indicates a low operative risk—less than 2%—an even more impressive figure of mortality in the first year of less than 2%, no impairment in the ejection fraction in 86% (which indicated that the evolving infarction was not harmed), and a graft patency of 94% in 102 patients. These data are most impressive. The principal question is the severity of the infarction and how many of the patients would have recovered with conventional medical therapy. Further experiences will be of particular significance.—F.C.S.] ◀

16–9 **False Aneurysm and Pseudofalse Aneurysm of the Left Ventricle: Etiology, Pathology, Diagnosis, and Operative Management.** S. Stewart, R. Huddle, I. Stuard, B. F. Schreiner, and J. A. DeWeese (Univ. of Rochester) report 4 cases of false or pseudofalse aneurysm of the left ventricle that followed myocardial infarction.

Woman, 50, experienced burning substernal pain radiating into the neck and became progressively disabled over the next year. The right coronary artery was totally obstructed, and there was an inferior false aneurysm that expanded in systole and emptied in diastole. It communicated with the ventricular cavity through a relatively small orifice. A large posterior aneurysm was found at operation. It contained a large amount of old thrombus and communicated with the left ventricle through a 2 × 4-cm orifice in the posterobasal wall of the ventricle (Fig 16–1). The fibrotic edge of the orifice was sutured closed. The postoperative course was satisfactory.

The findings in another patient are shown in Figure 16–2. A false aneurysm follows hemorrhagic dissection into an area of transmural myocardial infarction. Most often the process ends in free intrapericardial rupture of the heart, cardiac tamponade, and death, but adherent overlying pericardium can contain a hematoma. In this instance a false aneurysm is formed by the transmission of left ventricular pressure through the hematoma tract to the fused pericardium-epicardium. Occasionally the hematoma is contained within the area

---

(16–9) Ann. Thorac. Surg. 31:259–265, March 1981.

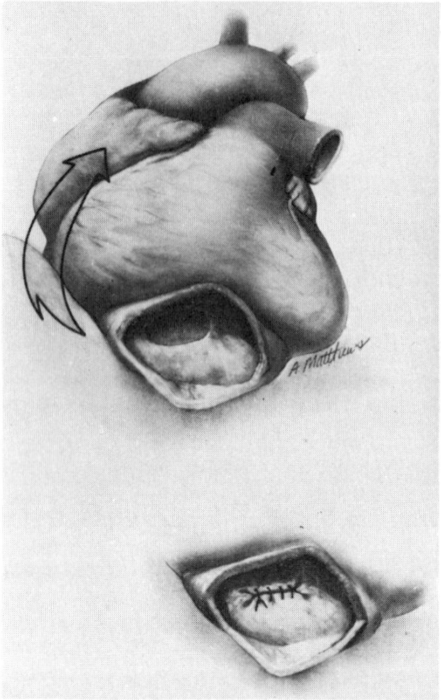

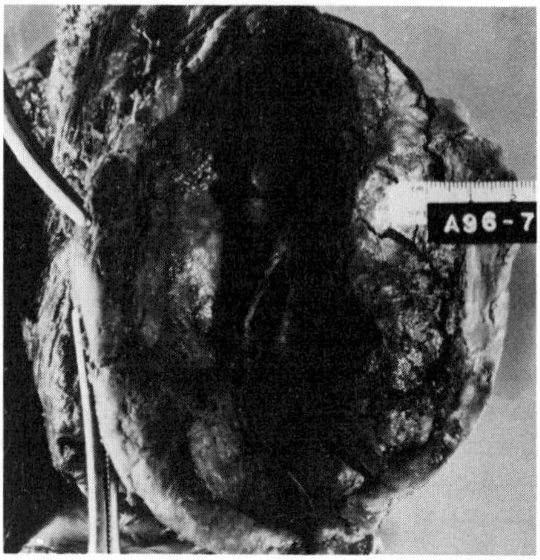

Fig 16–1 (left).—Patient 1. Small opening into cavity of left ventricle was identified and closed. Aneurysm sac was not resected.

Fig 16–2 (above).—Patient 2. Postmortem external view of posterior aspect of left ventricle. Wall of unroofed false aneurysm was composed of pericardium and organized mural thrombus. Here it is retracted by clamps to expose small central orifice leading into left ventricle from which Teflon felt and sutures have been removed.

(Courtesy of Stewart, S., et al.: Ann. Thorac. Surg. 31:259–265, March 1981.)

of the infarct, and this segment expands to form a pseudofalse aneurysm, as seemed likely in 2 of these 4 patients.

Both true and false aneurysms can affect ventricular performance adversely, false aneurysms by unloading the ventricle during systole, reducing cardiac output, and indirectly resulting in left ventricular dilation. The false aneurysm need not be excised, but only opened, with removal of thrombotic debris and direct closure of the communication with the left ventricular cavity. There is no need to dissect the aneurysm from surrounding tissue. False aneurysms should be repaired, even in asymptomatic patients, to prevent rupture.

▶ [The importance of recognizing a false aneurysm of the left ventricle from a true aneurysm is emphasized in this report of experiences with 4 patients. A true aneurysm of the left ventricle almost never ruptures; hence, operation is not urgent and is related to the size of the aneurysm and its influence on ventricular function. By contrast, a false aneurysm represents a hematoma that is formed after actual rupture of the left ventricle and, like posttraumatic aneurysms in peripheral arteries, is apt to both expand and rupture. Hence, operation is urgent.—F.C.S.] ◀

16–10 **Early and Late Patency of Expanded Polytetrafluoroethylene Vascular Grafts in Aorta-Coronary Bypass.** R. N. Sapsford, G. D. Oakley, and S. Talbot (London) examined the fate of 27 expanded polytetrafluoroethylene (PTFE) grafts and 19 saphenous vein grafts inserted in 16 patients with coronary artery disease during 1974–1978. The PTFE grafts were used only when a sufficiently suitable

(16–10) J. Thorac. Cardiovasc. Surg. 81:860–864, June 1981.

vein was unavailable. The 12 men and 4 women had a mean age of 59 years. All bypasses were constructed with 4-mm expanded PTFE grafts and were inserted in the same way as the saphenous vein grafts. Cold cardioplegia was used in the more recent cases. The material proved to be easy to use, although the anastomoses were technically more difficult to perform. Eleven patients were restudied within 3 months of surgery and 6 after 12–30 months. Nine patients received both expanded PTFE and vein grafts.

There were 3 postoperative deaths, 1 perioperative death, 1 perioperative infarction, and 1 late infarction. Eleven of 14 expanded PTFE grafts and 7 of 12 saphenous vein grafts were patent within 3 months of surgery. Ten of the 11 patients restudied were improved symptomatically. In patients given both types of graft, occlusion was related to the quality of the grafted vessel rather than to the material used. Six of 9 expanded PTFE grafts and 4 of 7 vein grafts were patent 12–30 months after operation. Late graft occlusion occurred when poor vessels had been grafted and was unrelated to the material used. Four patients remained symptomatically improved 2–3 years after operation. One had mild angina, and 1 has had another infarction.

Although these results seem disappointing, extremely high-risk patients were treated. Under favorable circumstances, expanded PTFE grafts can remain patent and functional for more than 2 years and provide good relief of symptoms. They are a suitable alternative to vein grafts, and their use is practicable when no vein is available.

▶ [A satisfactory prosthetic graft has never been developed for vessels smaller than 4 or 5 mm. This is especially true for coronary arteries with a diameter between 1.5 and 3 mm. The problem, of course, exists in the patient in whom the saphenous veins are inadequate, smaller than 3 to 4 mm.

This group reports experiences with 27 grafts in 16 patients. Angiography of 18 grafts within 3 months after operation found 11 patent and 7 occluded. Subsequently, 9 grafts were studied between 12 and 29 months, and 6 were found to be patent. Hence, the occlusion rate is 30% or greater.

At New York University, we have preferred to use the cephalic vein when the saphenous vein was unsatisfactory. The long-term results are not available in terms of late dilatation of the graft, but the clinical results for at least 2 to 3 years are excellent and would seem superior to either the use of prosthetic grafts or homograft veins.—F.C.S.] ◀

16–11 **Patency and Flow Response in Endarterectomized Coronary Arteries.** Conventional coronary bypass grafting may be difficult or impossible if diffuse coronary disease is present, and endarterectomy may be indicated in such instances before vein grafting. M. Laxman Kamath, Donald H. Schmidt, Pablo M. Pedraza, Fred M. Blau, A. Sampathkumar, Linda L. Grzelak, and W. Dudley Johnson (Univ. of Wisconsin, Milwaukee) reviewed the results of coronary endarterectomy in 90 patients operated on in 1978 and 1979 for coronary artery disease who survived operation and were recatheterized. Twenty-five other patients refused recatheterization, and 7 died postoperatively. Where more than one difficult endarterectomy had to be done besides conventional bypass grafting, intermittent ischemic arrest with total

(16–11) Ann. Thorac. Surg. 31:28–35, January 1981.

body hypothermia was used. Total clamp time averaged 100 minutes.

Of 118 grafts to endarterectomized arteries, 87.3% were patent, compared with 93.1% of 233 conventional vein grafts in the same patients. Myocardial blood flow on isoproterenol-induced stress in 33 vein grafts to endarterectomized arteries was comparable with that in 28 conventional saphenous vein grafts and 7 normal coronary arteries. Endarterectomized patients without heavy scarring or residual disease had flow responses identical with those of patients who had conventional vein grafts. Three endarterectomized patients (2.6%) had perioperative infarction. Abnormal pyrophosphate scans were obtained in 12.4% of 105 patients.

The early patency of saphenous vein grafts to endarterectomized coronary arteries is comparable with that of conventional vein grafts. The flow response of grafts to endarterectomized vessels is normal, provided that there is no residual distal disease and the myocardium is not heavily scarred. Endarterectomy did not increase the rate of perioperative infarction in this series. Coronary endarterectomy appears to be an effective treatment for diffuse coronary artery disease.

▶ [Experiences with coronary endarterectomy in 90 patients operated on over a period slightly greater than a year are described, with a patency of 88% in 103 of 118 arteries, only slightly lower than that of vein grafts.

The operative technique was a difficult one, with an arteriotomy as long as 18 cm in some patients and a clamp time with ischemic arrest that totaled between 100 minutes and 3 hours. This series represents very complex operations in patients with diffuse disease. The fact that such patients can be operated on successfully, with a good early patency, is encouraging. The long-term patency is unknown, because in the lower extremities endarterectomized arteries function well for a few months, but a high percentage close within 1 to 2 years due to progressive stenosis.—F.C.S.] ◀

16–12 **Long-Term Clinical Assessment of the Efficacy of Adjunctive Coronary Endarterectomy.** D. Craig Miller, Edward B. Stinson, Philip E. Oyer, Bruce A. Reitz, Stuart W. Jamieson, Ricardo J. Moreno-Cabral, and Norman E. Shumway (Stanford Univ.) examined the impact of adjunctive distal right coronary endarterectomy on the outcome of myocardial revascularization in 80 patients who had both procedures and in 592 patients who had right coronary artery bypass surgery plus 1 or more other bypass grafts but not endarterectomy. The former patients had more left ventricular dyssynergy and higher pulmonary wedge pressures. Currently, antiplatelet agents are given for 2–3 months to patients with coronary endarterectomy. Follow-up was 98% complete and averaged 4.8 years.

Perioperative infarction was twice as frequent in the endarterectomy group. Operative mortality did not differ significantly in the two groups. Recurrence of angina was comparable in the two groups, and no significant difference in the incidence of postoperative infarction was evident. Repeat revascularization was comparably frequent in the two groups. Overall late survival was similar in the two groups. Highly symptomatic patients in both groups had low right coronary bypass graft rates, and also low rates of patency for all the grafts restudied.

The findings in this review support the continued use of adjunctive right coronary endarterectomy in carefully selected patients. More late

---

(16–12) J. Thorac. Cardiovasc. Surg. 81:21–29, January 1981.

postoperative angiographic studies are needed to determine to what degree right coronary thromboendarterectomy influences the results of myocardial revascularization. The only contraindication to adjunctive coronary endarterectomy is a nondominant right coronary artery.

▶ [The role of endarterectomy in association with bypass grafting remains debatable; it is used frequently in some groups and rarely or not at all in others. At New York University, endarterectomy rarely has been done in the past 4 to 5 years.

These data compare results in two groups at 5 years. The operative infarction rate was twice as high in the group undergoing endarterectomy, but the 5-year results regarding angina and survival were virtually the same. Therefore, endarterectomy demonstrated neither a benefit nor a harm. The crucial question, as the authors indicate, concerns the long-term patency of the endarterectomized vessel. This can only be determined by angiography performed a year or more after operation. Endarterectomized vessels of similar caliber in the lower extremity have shown a prohibitive rate of occlusion between 6 and 24 months after operation.—F.C.S.] ◀

16–13 **Late Clinical and Arteriographic Results in 500 Coronary Artery Reoperations.** Floyd D. Loop, Delos M. Cosgrove, John R. Kramer, Bruce W. Lytle, Paul C. Taylor, Leonard A. R. Golding, and Laurence K. Groves (Cleveland Clinic) report experience with 500 coronary artery reoperations performed in 12 years, most of them during 1972–1979. These represented 2.7% of the isolated myocardial revascularization experience. About 90% of the patients were men. The median age was 49 years at initial operation and 54 years at reoperation. All patients but 6 had angina; 5 of the 6 were reoperated on for progression to three-vessel disease without angina. About half of the patients were reoperated on for atherosclerosis progressive in previously ungrafted vessels or progressing beyond the graft anastomosis. Graft closure was the indication in about 30% of the patients.

Operation was performed with normothermic arrest in 387 patients and with systemic hypothermia and cold cardioplegia in 113. The 324 patients having bypass graft surgery only at initial operation received an average of 1.6 grafts. Complete revascularization was achieved in 56.6% of the reoperations.

The operative mortality was 4%. The incidence of perioperative infarction was 7.8% with anoxic arrest and 2.7% with cardioplegia. Definite or probable infarction occurred in 6.6% of the patients. Of the 451 survivors followed up for a mean of 42 months, about 60% had no angina, whereas about 11% were in New York Heart Association classes III and IV. The patency rate of saphenous vein grafts was 78.8%. The 5-year actuarial survival rate was 89.2%. Survival was better with more than 1 graft at reoperation, and with bypass grafting rather than a Vineberg implant initially. Only 1.8% of late survivors were completely disabled at follow-up. All 6 patients having more than 1 reoperation are still alive, and 4 are employed.

Most patients reoperated on for angina exhibit clinical improvement and relief of angina. Selected patients with recurrent angina after revascularization may gain further effective palliation when reoperated on by experienced surgeons.

▶ [With the combination of two known factors—the slow rate of occlusion of coronary bypass grafts, about 3% per year after the first year after operation, and the

(16–13) J. Thorac. Cardiovasc. Surg. 81:675–685, May 1981.

progression of atherosclerosis—it is inevitable that some patients will require repeat operation after a few years. This summary by Floyd Loop of the Cleveland Clinic is probably the largest such experience published in the English literature. The operative death rate of only 4% is most encouraging. Equally encouraging is the fact that angina was relieved or improved in 86% of the group after an average follow-up of 42 months. With reoperation, the internal mammary is clearly superior to the vein if it is suitable for use.—F.C.S.] ◀

17. Miscellaneous Cardiac Disease

17-1 **Fulminating Noncardiogenic Pulmonary Edema: Newly Recognized Hazard During Cardiac Operations.** Alfred T. Culliford, Stephen Thomas, and Frank C. Spencer (New York Univ.) report 3 cases of pulmonary edema that occurred during or within 6 hours after uneventful coronary bypass in conjunction with successful cardiac operations. The patients, seen in an 18-month period, suddenly passed copious secretions via the tracheal tube and then experienced circulatory collapse, severe hypoxia, and respiratory acidosis. None had signs of left ventricular dysfunction. All 3 patients recovered completely within 72 to 96 hours of the start of aggressive therapy. The course in 1 patient is shown in Figure 17–1. All patients had a low left atrial mean or pulmonary wedge pressure, excluding cardiac causes of pulmonary edema. The protein concentrations of edema fluid were 3.0 and 3.5 gm/dl in the 2 patients in whom they were measured.

Fulminating noncardiogenic pulmonary edema in cardiac surgery patients is virtually indistinguishable clinically from pulmonary edema secondary to acute left ventricular failure. A low or normal left atrial

Fig 17–1.—Serial roentgenograms of 1 patient taken over 72 hours after he had received 50 gm of albumin, showing progressive resolution of pulmonary congestion. **A,** chest film on admission to recovery room; **B,** 8 hours later; **C,** 16 hours later; **D,** 24 hours later; **E,** 36 hours later; and **F,** 72 hours later. (Courtesy of Culliford, A. T., et al.: J. Thorac. Cardiovasc. Surg. 80:868–875, December 1980.)

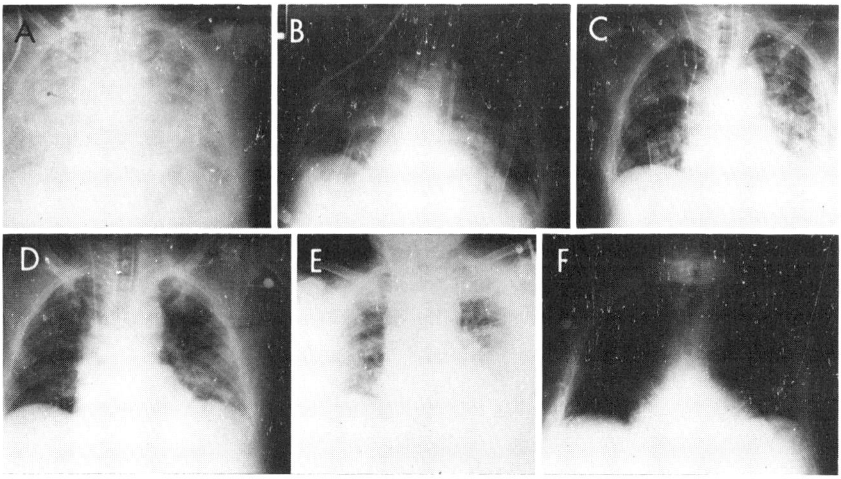

(17–1) J. Thorac. Cardiovasc. Surg. 80:868–875, December 1980.

or pulmonary wedge pressure is recorded, in conjunction with high protein content of the pulmonary edema fluid. The condition probably is caused by an unknown type of allergic reaction to blood or blood products. The pulmonary capillary membranes are the first to be exposed to intravenously administered fluids. Treatment includes infusion of corticosteroids and antihistamines, positive-pressure ventilation, diuretic therapy, and subsequently albumin administration. Inotropic agents and balloon counterpulsation were helpful in 2 of the present cases. Both patients given albumin showed a dramatic shrinkage of the lungs, indicating reversal of the membrane injury. Sternal closure in the presence of stiff, distended lungs can be fatal, but it is safe and effective simply to stabilize the sternum, completing the closure 2 to 4 days later.

▶ [This report from New York University defines an unusual syndrome related to the administration of plasma or a plasma product. In all probability, this syndrome has been present for many years, closely resembling left heart failure unless pulmonary wedge or left atrial pressure can be measured. The therapeutic importance of the diagnosis is great, for the condition may be rapidly fatal unless treated. With appropriate treatment with steroids, albumin, and ventilation, the condition may resolve completely within 2 to 3 days. Since this report has been submitted, additional experiences with other patients have confirmed these conclusions. Vulnerability to the injury probably is related to the dose of the unknown antigen and to the permeability of the pulmonary capillaries and the capacity of the pulmonary lymphatics to transport excess fluid.—F.C.S.] ◀

17–2 **Emergency Thoracotomy in the Surgical Intensive Care Unit After Open Cardiac Operation.** Ronald M. Fairman and L. Henry Edmunds, Jr. (Univ. of Pennsylvania) reviewed the records of 64 patients who had 74 emergency thoracotomies in the intensive care unit after cardiac surgery during a 42-month period. They represented 3% of all cardiac surgical patients. In all instances, thoracotomies were done because of inadequate circulation. Most patients already were intubated. A Swan-Ganz catheter was in place in all except 3 patients. Forty-four patients (group 1) had sudden profound hypotension because of arrhythmia (13 patients), sudden massive bleeding (15), suspected tamponade (6), or unexplained reasons (10). Twenty patients (group 2) had progressive circulatory insufficiency while receiving maximal cardiac support, including intra-aortic balloon pumping.

More than two thirds of the thoracotomies were done within 12 hours of surgery. The 37 men and 27 women had a mean age of 60 years. Twenty-five patients in group 1 were resuscitated, and 19 were ultimately discharged. Seven patients in group 2 were resuscitated, but none survived hospitalization. Half of all the thoracotomies were initially successful. Survivors in group 1 included only 2 of 13 patients having 16 thoracotomies for refractory arrhythmias, 9 of 15 patients with hypotension caused by sudden massive bleeding, 3 of 10 patients with unexplained hypotension, and 5 of 6 patients treated for suspected pericardial tamponade. Two patients, both in group 2, had wound infections, but in neither was this the cause of death.

Thirty percent of these patients survived after emergency postoperative thoracotomy in the surgical intensive care unit. Overall, 43%

(17–2) Ann. Thorac. Surg. 32:386–391, October 1981.

of the patients in group 1 survived. The results justify the procedure as possibly lifesaving if performed promptly in patients with sudden, unexpected hypotension. The incidence of wound infection was equivalent to that in the operating room.

▶ [This paper reports experiences with 64 patients undergoing emergency reopening of the sternum in the recovery room, 44 for acute hypotension, and 20 for progressive circulatory insufficiency. None of the patients in the second group ultimately survived, but 19 of 44 in the first group did. The wound was prepared with povidone-iodine and irrigated in the operating room with the same material before closure. The infection rate was only 5%.

I consider it crucial in any unit performing open heart surgery to have the equipment, experience, and personnel to reopen the sternum promptly in urgent circumstances. Clearly, the fear of infection should not be a deterrent in a life-threatening situation. At New York University, we have had one dramatic instance of a patient who recovered after *2 hours* of open cardiac massage before satisfactory cardiac function was obtained and the wound sutured in the operating room. Infection did not occur.—F.C.S.] ◀

17–3 **Delayed Sternal Closure Following Open Heart Operation.** Isaac Gielchinsky, Victor Parsonnet, Bhaktan Krishnan, Mark Silidker, and Ronald M. Abel (Newark, N. J.) reviewed the results of delayed sternal closure in 29 patients having open heart surgery during 1976–1980, representing 1.5% of all patients having cardiac surgery in this period. The 14 men and 15 women had a mean age of 55.5 years. The indications included an enlarged heart with tamponade when the mediastinum was closed, poor lung compliance, hemodynamic instability from intractable arrhythmia or coagulopathy, and the presence of a mediastinal assist device. Sixteen patients required insertion of an intra-aortic balloon pump. Eleven patients had a cardiac tamponade-like syndrome. Only the skin was closed, or when even this produced hemodynamic difficulty, the wound was simply covered with adhesive plastic material. Closure was achieved when the clinical condition was stabilized, usually after 24–96 hours.

Nineteen of the 29 patients are long-term survivors at 3–42 months. The only wound complication was a superficial infection that cleared with local care. All surviving patients now are in New York Heart Association functional class I or II. None of the 10 patients who died had evidence of sepsis or wound infection at the time of death. Six died of low cardiac output secondary to left ventricular dysfunction, 2 of perioperative myocardial infarction, and 2 of hemorrhage.

Delayed sternal closure was not complicated by early or late major wound infections in these patients. The procedure provides hemodynamic stability and permits rapid access to the heart for massage or evacuation of clots. An intra-aortic balloon can be removed without leaving a large Dacron tube in place. Although the procedure should not be used routinely, its selective use will make the management of difficult cases more flexible.

▶ [This report of 29 patients undergoing delayed sternal closure over a period of nearly 5 years indicates the value of this technique in extreme circumstances. The absence of significant infection in any of these patients is most impressive, indicating that fear of infection should not prevent the surgeon from using the procedure. Equally

---

(17–3) Ann. Thorac. Surg. 32:273–277, September 1981.

important is that certain pathologic conditions, usually edema of the myocardium, and occasionally edema of the lungs, can lead to fatal tamponade if the sternum is closed. Ordinarily, such problems are rare if myocardial preservation is effective. If patients with acute infarction are operated on, however, significant cardiac edema may be present. Hence, such a technique should be considered in planning the operative procedure. Our preference at New York University is partly to approximate the sternum with wires, leaving the edges of the sternum about 2 in. apart, which provides stability but still permits free drainage.—F.C.S.] ◀

17–4 **Embolization of Bone Wax From Sternotomy Incisions** was investigated by Francis Robicsek, Thomas N. Masters, Laszlo Littman, and Gustav V. R. Born. It is usual to employ bone wax to control bleeding from the sternotomy incision at cardiac surgery. The authors discontinued use of bone wax when an outbreak of *Mycobacterium fortuitum* sternal infections developed. Blood loss did not increase appreciably as a result, and there was a considerable reduction in postoperative pulmonary complications, suggesting that bone wax squeezed into the sternal marrow may embolize in the lesser circulation. The sternal marrow has been used as an entry for blood transfusions in patients with unsuitable peripheral veins.

Hypaque-M was injected under pressure into the midportion of the sternum of dogs in conjunction with cineangiography and serial roentgenography. Other dogs underwent median sternotomy, and tritium-labeled bone wax was pressed into the marrow in a dose of about 5 gm per dog; lung tissue was sampled up to an hour later. In the roentgenographic study, contrast medium appeared in the azygos and hemiazygos system and then in the superior vena cava, right side of the heart, and pulmonary circulation. Significant radioactivity was found in the lungs after sternal placement of tritium-labeled bone wax. Activity in the liver, kidneys, and spleen was unchanged from control values; the increase in activity appeared to be limited to the lungs.

Discontinuance of the use of bone wax for sternotomy at open heart surgery has not increased the risk of postoperative bleeding, and animal studies have given evidence of bone wax embolization. Such embolization probably also occurs under clinical conditions and may have a role in the development of postoperative pulmonary complications.

▶ [This report is an interesting one for two reasons, the fact that not using bone wax did not result in increased hemorrhage and the fact that emboli could be produced in the lung, presumably from liquefied wax. These observations, though not conclusive, are of considerable potential significance and should be evaluated carefully by others.—F.C.S.] ◀

17–5 **Lack of Correlation Between Activated Clotting Time and Plasma Heparin During Cardiopulmonary Bypass.** Large doses of heparin are used during cardiopulmonary bypass. The activated clotting time (ACT) has been recommended as a means to determine the proper dosage and to indicate the amount of protamine needed for heparin neutralization. Alfred T. Culliford, Sanford N. Gitel, Norman Starr, Stephen T. Thomas, Francis G. Baumann, Stanford Wessler,

---

(17–4) Ann. Thorac. Surg. 31:357–359, April 1981.
(17–5) Ann. Surg. 193:105–111, January 1981.

and Frank C. Spencer (New York Univ.) used the ACT with a Hemochron system to determine heparin requirements during bypass with hemodilution and hypothermia in 28 patients undergoing coronary bypass graft surgery for refractory angina. The 23 men and 5 women had an average age of 58 and received an average of 2.7 grafts per patient. Patients received 300 USP units of heparin per kg intravenously before bypass, and 8000 units of beef lung heparin were added to the pump prime solution. Heparin was given in a dose of 100 units/kg every hour starting an hour after the institution of bypass. Protamine was given in a dose of 1 mg/100 units of heparin given at the time of initial heparinization.

The mean pre-bypass plasma heparin level was 4 units/ml, and the ACT was 493 seconds. During bypass the plasma heparin level fell significantly to 3.1 units/ml, while the mean ACT increased significantly to 674 seconds. The mean protamine requirement predicted from the ACT was 43% higher than that predicted from plasma heparin levels. In the presence of heparin, cooling and hemodilution significantly prolonged the ACT in vitro. Scanning electron microscopic study of arterial line filters in 6 cases showed few microthrombi or microemboli trapped on the fibers.

The ACT did not reflect plasma heparin levels accurately during bypass in this study, or predict protamine requirements accurately. A fixed-dose regimen of heparin can prevent intraoperative thrombosis and clotting on arterial line filters, and does not require anticoagulant monitoring during surgery. Studies are under way to simplify the unmonitored fixed-dose schedule.

▶ [One of the significant developments with measurement of coagulation factors during open heart surgery is the technology for rapid determination of activated clotting time. Exactly what this represents—simultaneously measuring a large number of factors in the clotting process and those in the coagulation cascade, platelets, and other factors—is still uncertain. The data in this paper clearly indicate that activated clotting time does not correspond with plasma heparin levels.

What is uncertain at present is whether activated clotting time or plasma heparin level is the best measurement of proper anticoagulation. At New York University, though data are inadequate for a final conclusion, an activated clotting time above 400 seconds is obtained in most cases, often requiring 4 mg of heparin per kg, and sometimes as much as 6 or 7 mg/kg. We have not found a level of activated clotting time so high that it is dangerous, such as 800 or 900 seconds.—F.C.S.] ◀

17-6 **Myocardial Preservation With Nifedipine: Comparative Study at Normothermia.** Prevention of increased intracellular calcium associated with ischemia and reperfusion might result in less myocardial stiffness and loss of contractility after cardiac surgery with cardiopulmonary bypass. Richard E. Clark, Ignacio Y. Christlieb, John A. Spratt, Philip D. Henry, Albert E. Fischer, Joseph R. Williamson, and Burton E. Sobel (Washington Univ.) evaluated the effects of a cardioplegic solution containing the calcium antagonist nifedipine on the consequences of ischemia and reperfusion in dogs subjected to normothermic global ischemia and cardiopulmonary bypass. Ischemia was induced for 1 hour, in conjunction with infusion or bolus injections of normal saline, normal saline plus potassium chloride, Nor-

(17–6) Ann. Thorac. Surg. 31:3–20, January 1981.

mosol-R at pH 7.4, or cardioplegic solution with and without 0.17 to 0.2 μg of nifedipine per ml.

Measurements of left ventricular performance indicated consistent superiority of nifedipine-treated dogs after bypass, compared with the cardioplegic and control groups. Nifedipine-treated dogs had normal preischemic stroke work indices and Sarnoff curves 2 hours after bypass. Cardioplegic solution gave modest protection when injected as a bolus, but it was ineffective when given by continuous infusion. Morphological changes were much less marked in nifedipine-treated dogs than in the hearts of dogs given cardioplegic solution alone.

Nifedipine appears to be useful as a calcium-blocking agent to enhance myocardial preservation during operative myocardial ischemia and the initial reperfusion period. The use of calcium antagonists to alter abnormal transmembrane fluxes during ischemia may extend the "safe" ischemic interval in the clinical setting. The light sensitivity of nifedipine minimizes its systemic accumulation. The effects of the drug are reversed readily by administering calcium chloride.

▶ [The use of nifedipine as a cardioplegic agent, lowering calcium concentration, has been studied extensively by Clark and associates, and the first clinical trial was reported this year. Results to date appear good, though clear superiority over techniques using potassium cardioplegia has not yet been demonstrated. The physiologic importance of these studies is that they evaluate both the beneficial and the possible harmful effects of calcium blockade during cardioplegia.—F.C.S.] ◀

17–7 **Multiprogrammable Pacemakers** provide an opportunity to alter the rate, output energy, sensitivity, and mode of pacemakers. G. Frank O. Tyers, Edward H. Williams, Alberto J. Larrieu, W. R. Eric Jamieson, Richard Calfee, and Michael Hardage reviewed experience gained over 3 years with a multiprogrammable pacemaker, the CyberLith, in 164 patients. This pacemaker offers over 3,000 combinations of mode, rate, pulse width, sensitivity, and telemetry.

Over three fourths of the patients have undergone permanent therapeutic programming, and multiple variables were programmed in several units. Over 40% required multiple programming of a single variable. Rate, pulse width, and mode were the most frequently programmed therapeutic variables. Rate usually was reduced to maximize the time in sinus rhythm, and pulse width usually was decreased to extend pacemaker cell life. Mode programming was undertaken so that an electrocautery could be used safely during unrelated operations. Eight patients with arrhythmias, congestive failure, or both were programmed to the atrioventricular sequential mode. All patients have been programmed to the telemetry transmission setting for multivariable follow-up. No cell failures or lead breaks have occurred, and no unit has even begun to approach the end of life. Initial telemetry transmissions have closely confirmed electrode impedance data obtained at pacemaker implantation.

The CyberLith, Spectrax, and Programalith are the most frequently used multiprogrammable pacemakers. There is little doubt that most patients given standard demand pacemakers are at a higher risk of reoperation than if they had received multiprogrammable

---

(17–7) Can. J. Surg. 24:252–256, May 1981.

pacemakers. New programmable units will include both local and transtelephonic digital telemetry of multiple variables. "Physiologic" pacing modes will be available in most units. Future pacemakers will have the potential for automatic programming to appropriate frequency and duration settings for the treatment of most troublesome arrhythmias.

▶ [Experiences with pacemakers since 1962 are described here by Dr. Tyers, a leading investigator in this field, and his co-workers. The multiprogrammable pacemakers were introduced in 1977 and 1978. The beneficial effects, as opposed to the limitations from the complex electric circuits, are evaluated in this report. At present, data suggest that the multiprogrammable pacemaker is preferable, despite the increased expense.—F.C.S.] ◀

17–8 **Pacemaker Implantation in Infants and Children: Simplified Approach** is described by Serafin Y. DeLeon, Michel N. Ilbawi, and Farouk S. Idriss (Northwestern Univ.). Limited space for the power pack and lead and scanty subcutaneous tissue are problems in pacemaker implantation in infants and children, as is providing for growth. A new approach has been used in 12 patients aged 4 months to 14 years. A midline subxiphoid incision is made or, in patients who have been operated on, the lower end of the midsternotomy scar is reopened and extended downward. The epicardial electrode is implanted, usually over the diaphragmatic surface of the right ventricle, and a pocket is made under the posterior rectus sheath for the power pack. If necessary, the lower end of the sternum may be split to gain better exposure.

No problems have occurred with skin erosions, and the results are cosmetically acceptable. There are no unnecessary scars. Reoperation for electrode and power pack replacement is relatively simple. This approach obviates the need for extra incisions and provides a good cosmetic outcome of pacemaker implantation in infants and children.

▶ [A technique for insertion of an epicardial pacemaker in infants and small children, which has been used in 12 patients over the past 4 years, is described. The cosmetic effects are significant in the infant. Placing the pacemaker between the rectus muscle and the posterior rectus sheath avoids the problems associated with subcutaneous implantations.—F.C.S.] ◀

17–9 **Approaches to the Artificial Heart** are reviewed by William S. Pierce, John L. Myers, James H. Donachy, Gerson Rosenberg, Donald L. Landis, G. Allen Prophet, and Alan J. Snyder (Pennsylvania State Univ., Hershey). Some severe forms of heart disease never will be amenable to operative repair. The mechanical heart eventually may offer a better approach to these cases than cardiac transplantation, with its problems of donor heart availability and host rejection. The optimal blood pump design currently involves a flexible, ultrasmooth elastomer bladder in a relatively rigid housing. Blood-contacting properties have been improved by incorporating a polydimethyl siloxane moiety in the polyurethane solution. The pneumatic power unit provides timed pulses of gas to compress the pump bladder and a vacuum to aid prompt filling. Automatic control systems that interact with the power unit to achieve a wide range of cardiac output while

---

(17–8) Ann. Thorac. Surg. 30:599–601, December 1980.
(17–9) Surgery 90:137–148, August 1981.

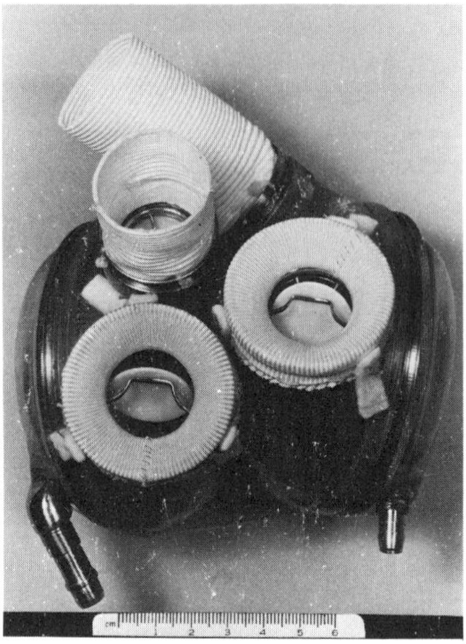

Fig 17–2.—Pneumatically powered artificial heart being developed by Hershey group includes separate right and left ventricles, smooth polyurethane blood-contacting surfaces, and tilting disk valves. (Courtesy of Pierce, W. S., et al.: Surgery 90:137–148, August 1981.)

Fig 17–3.—This Holstein calf has had an artificial heart for 60 days. The cabinet contains separate right and left air power units. A spare unit and battery inverter are included for use in the event of a mechanical or electric failure. On top of the cabinet are the automatic control unit *(left)* and oscilloscope *(right)* for displaying the air line pressure wave contours. (Courtesy of Pierce, W. S., et al.: Surgery 90:137–148, August 1981.)

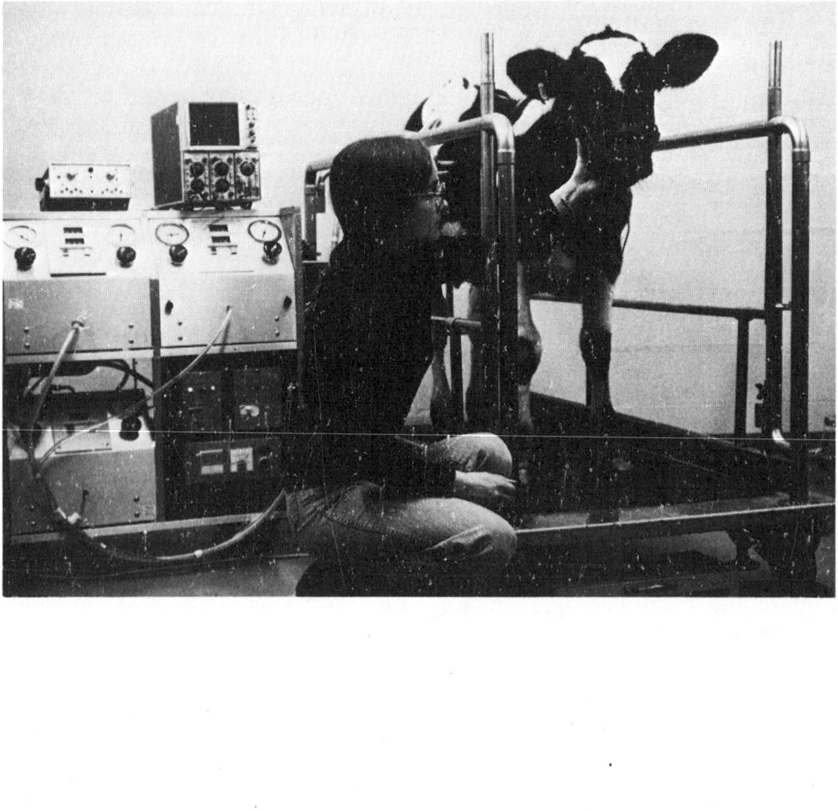

maintaining balance between the outputs of the two ventricles have been developed (Fig 17–2).

Calves now survive for several months after artificial heart implantation, and apparently do well (Fig 17–3). Problems include blood stream infection, tissue overgrowth or pannus formation at the junction of the atrial sewing cuff and inlet valve, and elastomer bladder calcification. Increasing attention is centering on the development of an implantable artificial heart that does not require a bulky external pneumatic power unit or large percutaneous tubes. The most logical designs utilize electric energy transmitted to an electric motor within the thorax. The motor may be mechanically linked to pusher plates, or may pressurize a hydraulic fluid that activates the blood pumps. An energy converter similar to that being developed by the National Heart, Lung, and Blood Institute for use in an implanted left ventricular assist pump will be used in the artificial heart. Atrial collapse must be prevented in the event that inadequate blood is present for ventricular refilling. A pack of rechargeable batteries and the electronics required for recharging will be necessary. Motor-driven left ventricular assist devices probably will be available for clinical use in this decade, with total artificial hearts to follow.

▶ [This is an excellent summary by one of the leading investigators in the field of the artificial heart, William Pierce, and his colleagues. It details well the mechanical problems associated with the device, the progress to date, and the goals for the future. Doctor Pierce's emphasis on polyurethane as being the best available type of tubing for the artificial heart is particularly significant. At present calves may live for 4 to 6 months with the device.—F.C.S.] ◀

17–10 **Long-Term Survival and Function After Cardiac Transplantation.** Incomplete control of allograft rejection has limited the use of biologic cardiac replacement in treatment of irreversible heart disease, but some patients have gained prolonged and useful survival.

Vincent A. Gaudiani, Edward B. Stinson, Edwin Alderman, Sharon A. Hunt, John S. Schroeder, Mark G. Perlroth, Charles P. Bieber, Philip E. Oyer, Bruce A. Reitz, Stuart W. Jamieson, Lois Christopherson, and Norman E. Shumway (Stanford Univ.) reviewed the records of 92 patients who underwent cardiac transplantation during 1968–1975 and report on 25 who lived 5 years or longer with the same graft. The average age at the time of transplantation was 40 years. All but 2 of the 25 study patients were men. All had irreversible myocardial failure as the indication for transplantation; 7 patients had dilated cardiomyopathy, and 18 had severe coronary disease. The average time from the first annual postoperative study to the most recent follow-up evaluation was 4.4 years.

The average survival is 6½ years. Six patients died 5–8 years after transplantation, 4 with severe graft coronary artery disease. Sixteen study patients (64%) were gainfully employed throughout their postoperative course, and 7 others were more than 50% rehabilitated. There were fewer than 0.1 hospitalizations per patient-year for late graft rejection. The average ECG sum voltage declined 14% throughout the study period; 12 patients had reductions of over 20% of first year

---

(17–10) Ann. Surg. 194:381–385, October 1981.

baseline values. No significant change in LV ejection fraction was observed. Eight patients had reductions in the function of one or more segments below the accepted norm. Four of 21 patients developed graft coronary artery disease.

Extended survival is possible after cardiac transplantation in some patients with otherwise fatal heart disease, and the quality of survival is acceptable. Cardiac graft function may remain intact for prolonged periods. Better methods of immunosuppression are needed, however. Complications of current immunosuppression and graft coronary atherosclerosis are the chief remaining problems in cardiac transplantation.

▶ [As everyone recognizes, Shumway's group at Stanford University has been the world leader in cardiac transplantation for a long time. Hence, the data from this group are probably the most significant in the field. This report describing 25 patients surviving more than 5 years is most encouraging. At least 1 patient has survived more than 10 years. Equally encouraging is the fact that the left ventricular ejection fraction remains constant (0.60) after the first postoperative year. Since 1975, the 5-year actuarial survival has been about 40%.—F.C.S.] ◀

17–11 **Sequential Orthotopic Heart Transplantation in Man.** Donald C. Watson, Bruce A. Reitz, Philip E. Oyer, Edward B. Stinson, and Norman E. Shumway (Stanford Univ.) reviewed the results of sequential orthotopic cardiac transplantation in 16 patients who had two procedures between 1968 and 1980. They were among 185 patients given a total of 202 hearts in this period. Immunosuppression was with azathioprine, prednisone, and antithymocyte globulin. Treatment of rejection was with methylprednisolone and occasionally actinomycin D also. Secondary transplants were necessary because of initial allograft dysfunction. One patient required a tertiary allograft.

Overall survival rates at 1 and 2 years were 56% and 50%, respectively; the rates improved to 63% and 59% after 1973. Patients requiring secondary transplants had 1- and 2-year survival rates of 60% and 57%, respectively. The secondary allograft survival rates at 1 and 2 years were 31% and 29%, respectively. The patient given 3 hearts was alive 1.4 years after the most recent implant. Four patients are still alive. Seven patients died of infection. Of 114 patients in the overall series who died, 52% died of infection, and 24% had acute or chronic rejection. The secondary and primary transplant groups did not differ in number of rejection episodes, number or type of infections, occurrence of malignancy, or hemodynamic and pathologic findings.

Secondary and tertiary cardiac transplantation can be performed with an expectation of success. Replacement of the orthotopically transplanted heart appears to offer a reasonable chance of survival. Infection of the secondary transplant patient appears to play a more significant role in mortality, but the number and type of infections have not differed substantially from those in patients given primary cardiac transplants.

▶ [Two hundred and two transplantations were done in 185 patients at Stanford University in the 12-year period from January 1968 to March 1980. In 16 patients, a sec-

---

(17–11) Transplantation 30:401–403, December 1980.

ond transplant was done, the results of which are described in this brief report. Although the technique of heart transplantation is at the stage of clinical investigation and is limited, as it should be, to a few experienced centers, this article indicates that in the unusual patient a second transplant may be beneficial.—F.C.S.] ◀

17–12 **Surgical Treatment of Constrictive Fibrous Endocarditis.** Constrictive fibrous endocarditis is characterized by a trend toward cardiac insufficiency that may be chiefly right-sided or left-sided and rapidly leads to death. The cause is obscure. Charles Dubost, Claude Prigent, Alain Gerbaux, Pierre Maurice, Jacqueline Passelecq, Roger Rulliere, Alain Carpentier, and Alain Deloche (Paris) treated 20 patients with fibrous endocarditis seen during 1971–1979 by resection of ventricular endocardium and replacement of the atrioventricular (AV) valve. The 13 male and 7 female patients were aged 12–58 years. The mean duration of symptoms was 4.2 years. All patients but 1 were in New York Heart Association (NYHA) classes III and IV. Patients generally presented with signs of severe combined right and left heart failure. Resection was carried out from the side of the fibrosis to remove the entire fibrous shell from the AV orifice to the apex (Figs 17–4 to 17–7).

Three postoperative deaths resulted from intractable heart failure and renal insufficiency or from cerebral hemorrhage. Three other patients had low cardiac output, 2 had functional renal insufficiency, and 1 had hemopericardium. Complete AV block necessitated per-

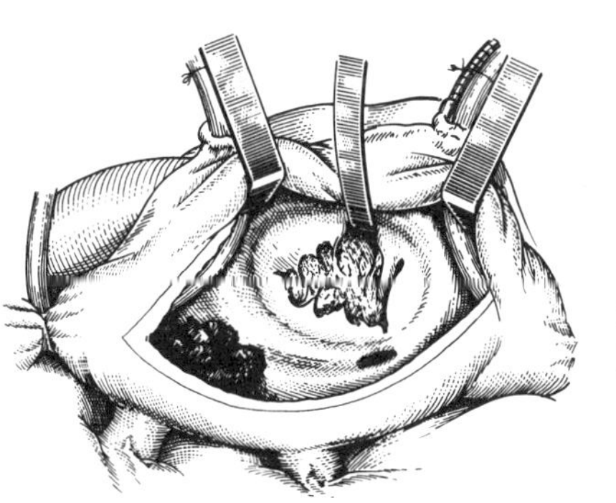

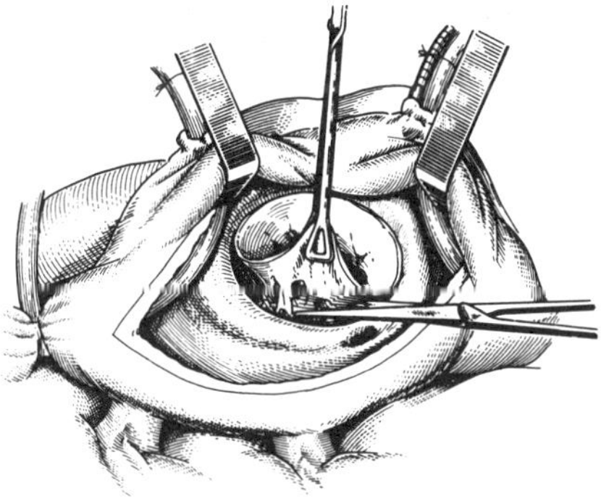

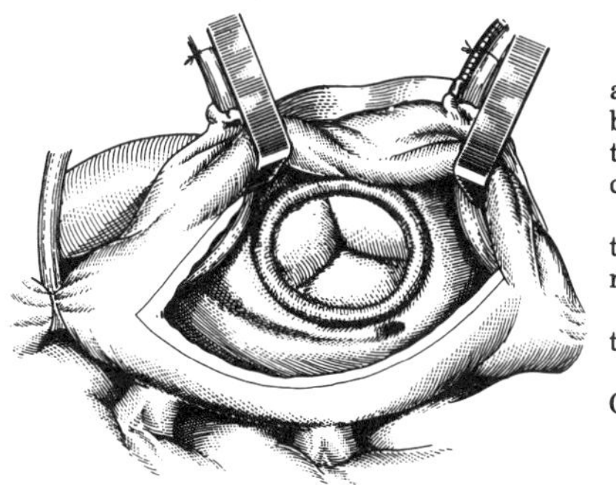

Fig 17–4 (above left).—Opening of the right atrium. The fibrous ventricular endocardium can be seen below the retracted leaflets of the tricuspid valve, whose papillary muscles and chordae tendineae are involved.

Fig 17–5 (above).—After resection of the tricuspid valve, the thick endocardium is resected from the inner ventricular wall.

Fig 17–6 (left).—Replacement of the tricuspid valve with a bioprosthesis.

(Courtesy of Dubost, C., et al.: J. Thorac. Cardiovasc. Surg. 82:585–591, October 1981.)

(17–12) J. Thorac. Cardiovasc. Surg. 82:585–591, October 1981.

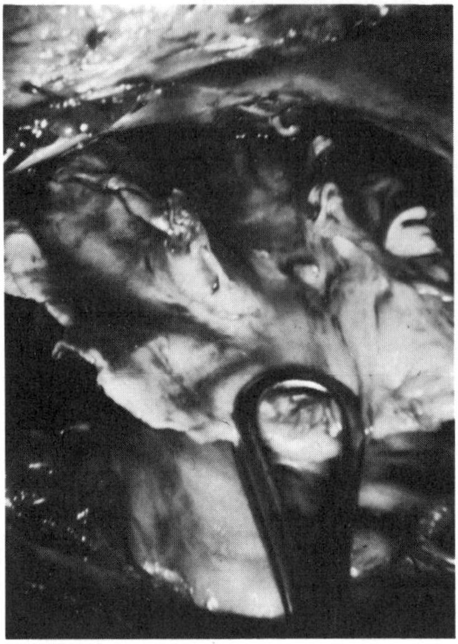

Fig 17–7.—Intraoperative photograph showing technique of resection of ventricular fibrosis. (Courtesy of Dubost, C., et al.: J. Thorac. Cardiovasc. Surg. 82:585–591, October 1981.)

Fig 17–8.—Chest roentgenogram taken before **(A)** and 6 months after **(B)** operation. (Courtesy of Dubost, C., et al.: J. Thorac. Cardiovasc. Surg. 82:585–591, October 1981.)

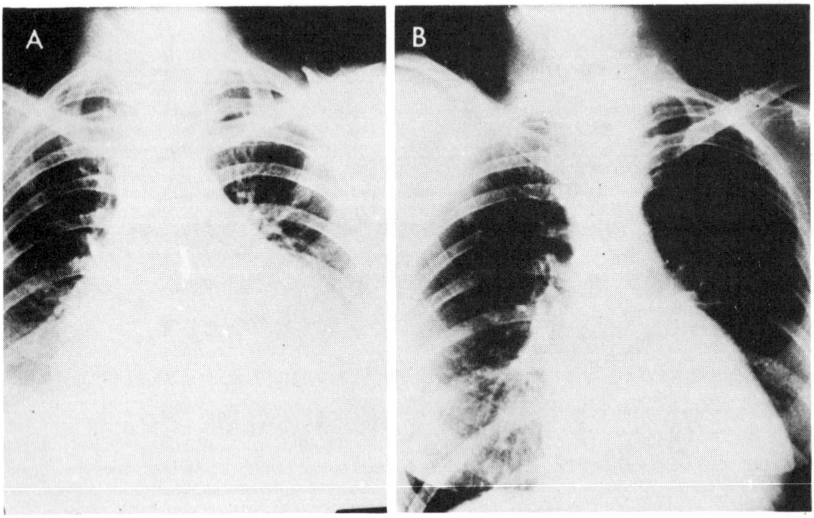

manent pacemaker implantation in 7 patients. One of 4 late deaths was due to arrhythmia, and 1 to thrombosis of the prosthesis. All patients were improved (Fig 17–8); 11 of 13 were in NYHA classes I and II at follow-up. Follow-up hemodynamic and angiographic studies showed normal atrial and ventricular pressure curves and a return to normal of the configuration of the left ventricle.

Endocardiectomy appears to be the treatment of choice for even the most advanced cases of constrictive fibrous endocarditis. The late functional results have been satisfactory, with most patients returning to full employment. A better understanding of the role of hypereosinophilia in the origin of this disease might permit medical treatment or even prevention of the disease.

▶ [This report by the group headed by Dubost, a world-recognized pioneer in cardiac surgery, of experiences with 20 patients with fibrous endocarditis over a period of 9 years is of particular significance because, to date, this disease has rarely been recognized in the United States. The disease seems to be mainly from central Africa, northeastern Brazil, and southern India.

Although this disease virtually is unknown in the United States, the concept that cardiac function may be improved significantly by extensive excision of endocardial scar may be applicable with other diseases, such as extensive fibrosis after subendocardial infarction from coronary artery disease.

The operative technique may require excision of both the mitral and tricuspid valves, as the disease is limited primarily to the ventricular endocardium, not the atrium. Hence, the operative procedure is somewhat analogous to that of pericardiectomy.—F.C.S.] ◀

7–13 **Etiologic Considerations in Superior Vena Cava Syndrome.** James M. Parish, Robert F. Marschke, Jr., David E. Dines, and Robert E. Lee reviewed experience with 86 cases of superior vena cava obstruction seen at the Mayo Clinic during 1960 to 1979; 67 (78%) were due to malignancy and 19 (22%) to benign causes. The 61 male and 25 female patients had an average age of 53.4 years. The most common symptoms were fullness in the head, dyspnea, and cough. Only 20% of the patients reported pain. The most common findings were dilatated neck veins, a prominent venous pattern over the chest wall, edema of the face and arms, and cyanosis. Mediastinal widening was found in about two thirds of the cases. The diagnosis was evident clinically in all patients but 1. The most productive studies were bronchoscopy, open lung biopsy, and biopsy of a superficial lymph node. The most common benign causes of superior vena cava obstruction were mediastinal fibrosis and thrombosis. Most of the tumors were primary lung cancers.

Patients with a rapid onset of obstruction because of malignancy were managed primarily by radiotherapy; chemotherapy, alone or combined with radiotherapy was also used. Patients with nonmalignant disease received steroids, diuretics, or a low-salt diet and conservative management. Fifty-five patients, including 50 with malignant disease, died. The average intervals from onset of symptoms to diagnosis were 42 months in patients with benign disease and 3.2 weeks in those with malignant disease; average survivals from diagnosis until death were 16.9 months and 7.7 months, respectively. Of the 67 patients with malignant obstruction, 60 had metastatic disease at the time of diagnosis. The most common site of metastasis was the mediastinum.

Radiotherapy remains the standard treatment for superior vena cava obstruction from malignant disease. Benign cases caused by superior vena cava thrombosis may result from the use of central venous cath-

---

(17–13) Mayo Clin. Proc. 56:407–413, July 1981.

eters. Radiation fibrosis is unusual. The role of surgical decompression of the vena cava remains unsettled.

▶ [This report of 20 years' experience at the Mayo Clinic with superior vena cava obstruction totaling 86 cases, is a valuable source of data. It confirms that 4 of 5 cases (78%) are caused by malignancy. The vast majority of patients live less than 1 year. Radiotherapy is the palliative treatment of choice.

Of equal significance, 1 case in 5 is caused by benign disease. Conservative management suffices in most of these, as collaterals will develop in time, usually 6 to 12 months. The role of the composite autogenous vein grafts for benign obstruction remains unproved, although it certainly can be performed effectively. Finally, the fact that 3 of the authors' cases resulted from the use of central venous catheters is an alarming statement, indicating the hazard of these catheters when left in situ for a long time.—F.C.S.] ◀

17–14 **Pulmonary Embolectomy.** Pulmonary embolism remains a major clinical problem, and pulmonary embolectomy may be indicated for patients with life-threatening embolism for whom anticoagulation alone is inadequate or contraindicated. David M. Glassford, Jr., William C. Alford, Jr., George R. Burrus, William S. Stoney, and Clarence S. Thomas, Jr. (Nashville, Tenn.) reviewed the results of pulmonary embolectomy in 20 patients operated on during 1969 to 1979, 12 of whom survived. The 12 women and 8 men were aged 22 to 77 years. Age appeared not to influence the outcome. All 5 patients who had lung scanning and pulmonary arteriography before operation survived, as did 3 of 5 having pulmonary arteriography alone. Of 10 patients undergoing active cardiopulmonary resuscitation at the time of operation, 5 survived.

Patients with pulmonary embolism tend to deteriorate dramatically. Embolectomy should be considered when arteriography shows more than half the pulmonary arterial tree to be obstructed. The pulmonary artery pressure also is a reasonably good guide to the severity of obstruction. Embolectomy also should be considered in patients who have had cardiac arrest caused by pulmonary embolism and in whom initial resuscitative efforts have failed. In patients who are responding poorly or not at all to cardiopulmonary resuscitation, surgery should not be delayed in order to perform diagnostic studies. The results of surgery will not be statistically impressive in this setting, but immediate pulmonary embolectomy offers the only hope of salvage.

▶ [This article summarizes experiences with pulmonary embolectomy performed on 20 patients during 10 years, with 12 survivors. Of 10 patients who had a pulmonary arteriogram before operation, 7 survived. Of 10 operated on without an arteriogram, 5 survived. I could not find in this article how many of this second group were found to have a pulmonary embolus at operation. This remains a difficult question. In desperate circumstances, pulmonary arteriography may not be possible, but in a significant number of patients, no pulmonary embolus will be found.

As the authors indicate, if arteriography demonstrates that more than 50% of the pulmonary arterial tree is obstructed, embolectomy should be performed regardless of the clinical status of the patient. Such patients are at serious risk for sudden decompensation and death.—F.C.S.] ◀

17–15 **Perforation of the Pulmonary Artery With Swan-Ganz Catheters: Diagnosis and Surgical Management** are reviewed by Thomas

(17–14) Ann. Thorac. Surg. 32:28–32, July 1981.
(17–15) Ann. Surg. 193:686–692, June 1981.

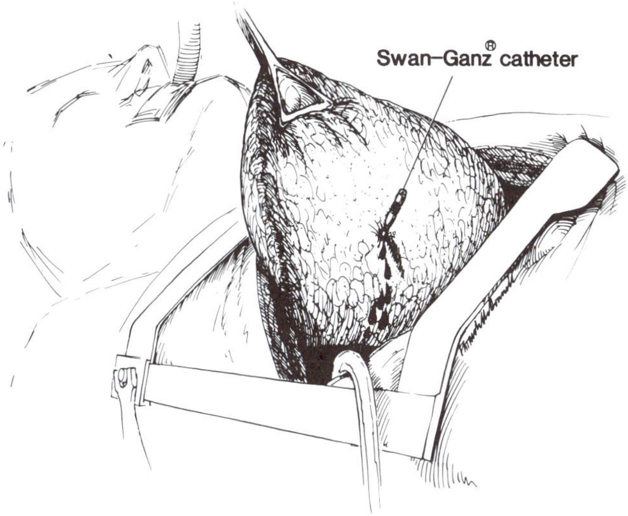

Fig 17–9.—Artist's concept of free perforation. (Courtesy of Kelly, T. F., Jr., et al.: Ann. Surg. 193:686–692, June, 1981.)

F. Kelly, Jr., George C. Morris, Jr., E. Stanley Crawford, Raphael Espada, and Jimmy F. Howell (Baylor College of Medicine). Swan-Ganz catheter placement has been used increasingly for hemodynamic monitoring. Pulmonary artery rupture is a rare complication that can range from a small amount of parenchymal bleeding to free rupture with massive bleeding into the pleural space (Fig 17–9). Three cases of pulmonary artery rupture are presented, including one nearly fatal exsanguination into the pleural space. Fifteen cases, including the present ones, have been reported. All patients but 2 were older than age 60. Most of the patients had cardiac or vascular disease, and all but 1 of the evaluable patients had elevated pulmonary artery pressures. The mortality was 53%. Several patients received anticoagulants.

Balloon inflation should be done under constant pressure monitoring and stopped instantly when a wedged or a damp tracing is observed. If possible, the catheter tip should be refloated each time. Wedge time should be minimized, especially in patients with pulmonary hypertension. Chest roentgenograms should be freely used to check catheter position and identify migration. Fluids should not be used for balloon inflation. Pulmonary artery perforation should be suspected in any patient with a catheter in place who exhibits hemodynamic changes, respiratory embarrassment, or hemoptysis. The catheter should be removed immediately if a complication is suspected. Airway maintenance and appropriate surgery are indicated in patients with hemoptysis. Free rupture into the pleural space calls for resection or ligation, or both as indicated.

▶ [This article is one of two selected this year to emphasize the rare but lethal complication of perforation of the pulmonary artery. The Swan-Ganz catheter has been a very valuable diagnostic advance for monitoring seriously ill patients in a variety of conditions, including any operation associated with heart disease, septic shock, hemorrhagic shock, and other problems. However, there are many pitfalls with a Swan-Ganz catheter, almost all of which can be avoided by careful teaching and training.

The use of the Swan-Ganz catheter to measure wedge pressure while a patient is heparinized during cardiopulmonary bypass probably should be abandoned. An alternate approach with the chest open is to measure left atrial pressure directly or to use the pulmonary artery diastolic pressure. Rupture of the pulmonary artery in a heparinized patient, in our experience, almost always has been fatal. The 3 patients in this report who survived were not heparinized. Although only 15 cases were found by the authors in the literature review, our institution knows of more than 8 such instances in the past 2 years. Undoubtedly, there are far more cases than are reported.—F.C.S.] ◀

17–16 **Catheter-Induced Pulmonary Artery Perforation: Mechanisms, Management, and Modifications.** Pulmonary artery perforation is a rare but usually lethal complication of use of the Swan-Ganz catheter. P. G. Barash, D. Nardi, G. Hammond, G. Walker-Smith, D. Capuano, H. Laks, C. J. Kopriva, A. E. Baue, and A. S. Geha (Yale Univ.) review 6 cases of pulmonary artery perforation associated with use of Swan-Ganz catheters. The 7 F Swan-Ganz catheter was introduced into the right atrium by a standard method, the balloon was inflated with 1.5 cc of air, and the catheter was allowed to float into the wedge position.

Balloon inflation preceded perforation in all 6 cases. At least one risk factor, such as anticoagulation, hypothermia, and pulmonary hypertension, was present in the 4 patients who died. The 2 survivors had not received anticoagulation therapy, nor were they hypothermic. An autopsy study showed that balloon inflation can result in an eccentric configuration. The balloon can disrupt the pulmonary artery, the tip can be propelled through the vessel wall on balloon inflation, or the catheter tip can be advanced too far distally and perforate the vessel.

At present, the catheter is floated to a position 4–5 cm above the pulmonary valve. Care is taken not to fill the balloon with more than 1.5 ml of air. Wedge pressure measurements are obtained only when absolutely necessary, with the catheter advanced through an external sheath. If an "overwedge" pattern is seen, the catheter is immediately withdrawn 2–3 cm. Further study is needed of possible changes in the catheter body, the balloon, and the balloon pressure-release valve. The catheter tip should be made of softer material than is presently available. Observation is necessary if a small amount of hemoptysis occurs. If it exceeds 15–30 cc, a "wedge" angiogram should be considered. With massive hemoptysis, a double-lumen endotracheal tube is passed to facilitate ventilation and prevent aspiration of blood into the unaffected lung. Emergency pneumonectomy or lobectomy may be necessary.

▶ [Reports of rupture of the pulmonary artery by a Swan-Ganz catheter are appearing with increasing frequency. These probably can be avoided in most instances by proper technique, although rupture may be inevitable in a small group of patients. The Swan-Ganz catheter is invaluable in the management of critically ill patients, so the technique of its use must be studied carefully and precisely, not delegated to someone inexperienced.

(17–16) J. Thorac. Cardiovasc. Surg. 82:5–12, July 1981.

Perforation is especially dangerous, probably lethal, when it occurs during open heart surgery in the heparinized patient. We have had only one such patient survive at New York University. Hence, the measurement of wedge pressure rarely should be used in the heparinized patient. During operation, left atrial pressure can be measured directly or, alternately, the pulmonary artery diastolic pressure can be compared with the left atrial pressure, making determinations of wedge pressure unnecessary.—F.C.S.] ◀

17–17 **Repair of Dissection of the Thoracic Aorta: Evaluation of False Lumen Utilizing Computed Tomography.** Thoracic aortic dissection has a persistently high risk of late rupture. Recent angiographic studies have questioned whether obliteration of the false lumen commonly is achieved and whether attempted obliteration contributes substantially to altering the course of the process. Kevin Turley, Daniel J. Ullyot, J. David Godwin, James M. Wilson, Martin Lipton, Erik Carlsson, and Paul A. Ebert (Univ. of California, San Francisco) used computed tomography (CT) to examine the fate of the false lumen in 21 patients with thoracic aortic dissections who were operated on in 1975–1980. The 14 men and 7 women had a mean age of 52 years. There were 11 acute and 10 chronic dissections. The ascending aorta or transverse arch was involved in 11 dissections, and in 10 only the descending aorta was involved. Surgery involved resection of the site of intimal tearing and prosthetic graft interposition. Obliteration of the false lumen was attempted in 10 cases by directing flow to the distal true lumen only.

Eighteen of the 20 survivors, including 8 in whom obliteration had been attempted, were followed up for a mean of 32 months. No late ruptures have occurred. A postmortem examination of a patient who died of amyloidosis showed both true and false lumens; both lumens had been anastomosed in this case. The false lumen persisted on CT study in 7 of the 8 patients in whom obliteration had been attempted. The false lumen persisted in both type A and type B lesions. Preoperative angiographic studies showed major branches were perfused by the false lumen in all 5 patients with persistence of the false lumen on CT. The patient with documented obliteration had no false-lumen perfusion of major vessels preoperatively. In this case, the dissection ended above the diaphragm, and both the intimal tear and reentry site, if any, probably were resected.

False luminal perfusion persists in patients with thoracic aorta dissections in whom obliteration is attempted, presumably because of major vessel runoff. Long-term survival apparently is a result of resecting the segment of aorta containing the entry site, which often is the site of subsequent enlargement and rupture, rather than of obliterating the false channel. Computed tomography is safe for postoperative follow-up of asymptomatic patients.

▶ [This report from San Francisco, and the department headed by Paul Ebert, is particularly significant, detailing experiences with 21 patients over a period of about 5 years. The occurrence of only 1 operative death is one of the lowest operative mortalities ever reported with acute dissection. The authors clearly emphasize that the object at operation should be to excise the entry site as well as any area of gross dissection of the aorta, but one should not attempt to excise the entire area of dis-

(17–17) J. Thorac. Cardiovasc. Surg. 81:61–68, January 1981.

sected aorta, anatomically impossible in many patients in whom the dissection may involve both the thoracic and abdominal aorta.—F.C.S.] ◀

17–18 **Aortic Dissection: Anatomy, Consequences, and Causes** are discussed by William C. Roberts (Natl. Inst. of Health). All aortic dissections are characterized by separation of the media in a course paralleling blood flow. In addition, a continuous, more or less transverse intimal and medial tear occurs in all but a few cases and usually is located in the ascending aorta. The dissecting, or false channel is in the outer half of the aortic media, leaving a thin outer wall that is prone to rupture. Most commonly, about half the circumference of the aorta is dissected at a given level. The most common cause of interruption of the longitudinal dissection is apparently atherosclerotic plaquing. Aortic isthmic coarctation is another cause. The most common cause of death is through-and-through rupture of the aorta, usually near the site of the initial intimal-medial aortic tear. Extension of medial dissection or hematoma into a major artery can lead to ischemia or necrosis of the perfused tissue. Healing of a dissection results in a double-barrel aorta; the large false channel may contain saccular aneurysms.

The cause of spontaneous aortic dissection usually is unknown, but about two thirds of patients have or have had systemic hypertension. Hypertension can increase plaquing in major arteries and cause luminal narrowing, and it can weaken the media of some arteries to cause aneurysms or tears. If systemic hypertension were eliminated, spontaneous aortic dissection virtually would disappear. Pregnancy is not a well documented "cause" of aortic dissection. Dissection may be associated with the Marfan syndrome and its variations, and also with congenitally bicuspid aortic valves, with or without associated aortic valve stenosis. Aortic isthmic coarctation is clearly associated with a high rate of aortic dissection. Trauma is a rare cause of aortic dissection. Both cannulation and aortic incision can cause traumatic aortic dissections. Atherosclerosis and syphilis are not likely "etiologies" of aortic dissection.

▶ [This survey paper of aortic dissection should be studied carefully by everyone encountering this problem, because Roberts is one of the most experienced cardiac pathologists in the world. With the increasing ability of prompt operation to correct the condition, wide familiarity with the variations in this remarkable disease is essential. In all likelihood, such problems increasingly will be treated as a surgical emergency, similar to a perforated ulcer or a ruptured abdominal aneurysm.—F.C.S.] ◀

17–19 **Transverse Aortic Arch Aneurysm: Improved Results of Treatment Employing New Modifications of Aortic Reconstruction and Hypothermic Cerebral Circulatory Arrest.** Problems of cardiac and cerebral protection complicate the management of patients with transverse aortic arch aneurysms that involve the segment from which both the innominate and left common carotid arteries arise. E. Stanley Crawford and Salwa A. Saleh (Houston) operated on 8 such patients, 5 men and 3 women aged 51–72 years. Seven had fusiform arteriosclerotic aneurysms, and 1 had a sacciform my-

(17–18) Am. Heart J. 101:195–214, February 1981.
(17–19) Ann. Surg. 194:180–188, August 1981.

cotic aneurysm. The ascending, transverse, and descending thoracic aorta was involved in 4 cases (Fig 17–10). Two patients had annular involvement with severe aortic insufficiency. Two patients had symptomatic coronary artery disease. The left pulmonary artery was occluded in 1 patient (Fig 17–11).

The mycotic aneurysm was replaced with a patch graft. In 3 patients the distal half or two thirds of the ascending aorta and entire transverse arch were replaced with a graft. Resection of the descend-

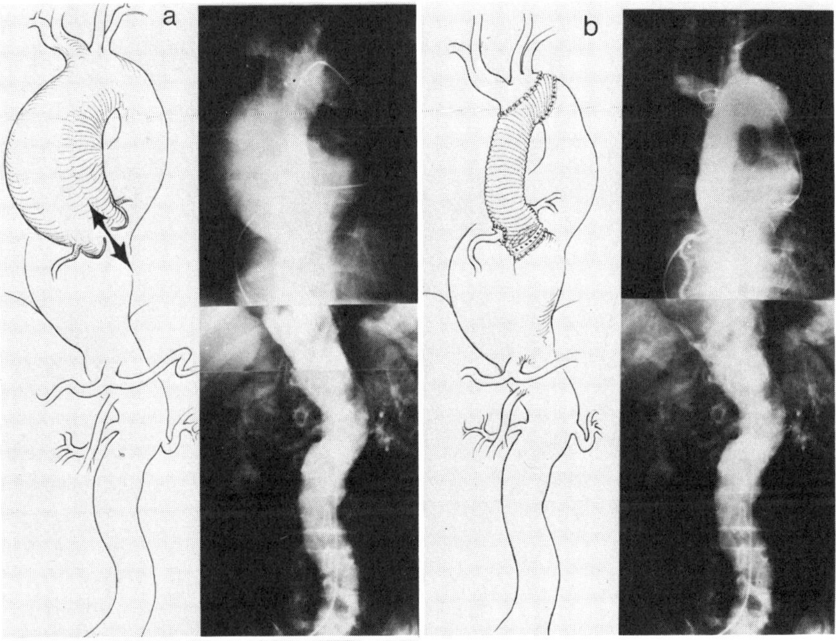

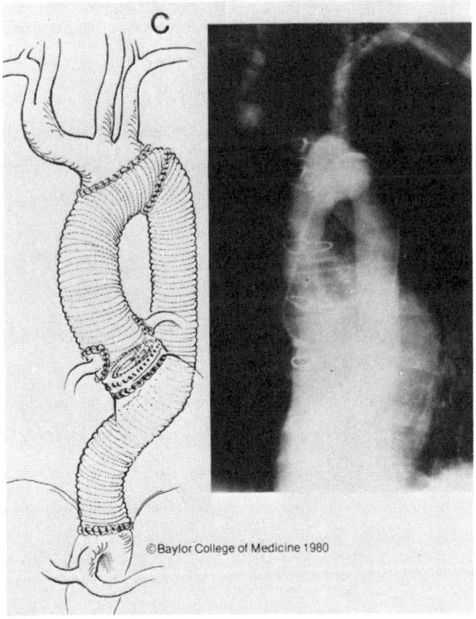

Fig 17–10.—Diagrams of patient with aortic aneurysm extending from aortic annulus to celiac axis treated by graft-valve composite graft replacement of ascending aortic arch at one operation and graft replacement of extensive aneurysm of descending thoracic aorta at second operation. Preoperatively **(a)**, extent of aneurysm and aortic insufficiency is shown. After first operation, proximal graft and aortic valve were in place and functioning **(b)**. After second operation **(c)**, diagram shows total replacement of thoracic aorta and aortic valve with reattachment of coronary and brachiocephalic arteries. (Courtesy of Crawford, E. S., and Saleh, S. A.: Ann. Surg. 194:180–188, August 1981.)

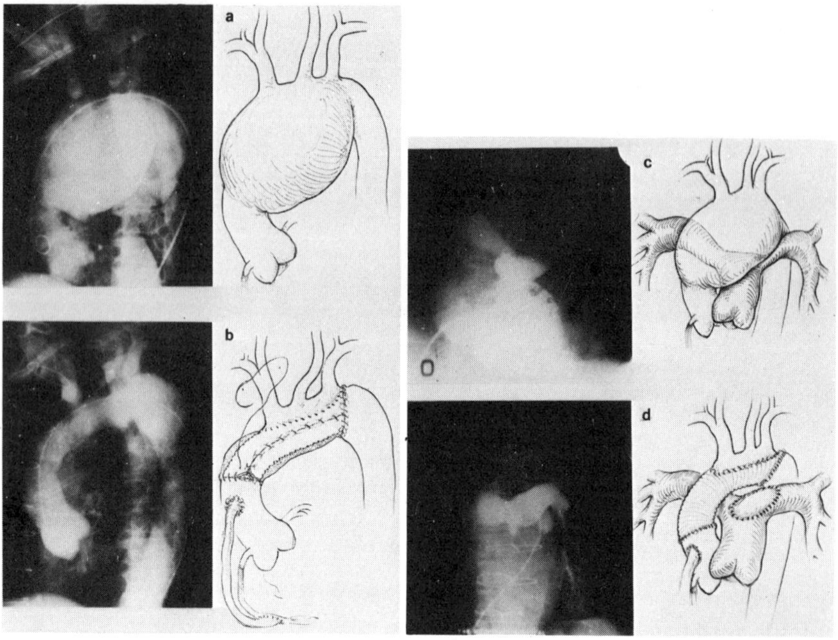

Fig 17–11.—Diagrams showing treatment of patient with coronary artery disease and aneurysm of the transverse aortic arch producing obstruction of the left pulmonary artery. Extent of the aneurysm (**a**). Postoperatively (**b**), aortic graft and coronary artery bypass were in place and functioning. Compression of the left pulmonary artery by the aneurysm (**c**). Method of repair (**d**) using pericardial patch. (Courtesy of Crawford, E. S., and Saleh, S. A.: Ann. Surg. 194:180–188, August 1981.)

ing aortic segment was deferred in all 4 patients with this form of involvement, and has subsequently been achieved in 3 of them. Profound hypothermia was used for cerebral protection. Graft inclusion and direct brachiocephalic arterial reattachment were used to prevent bleeding. All patients survived surgery without complications. Heart failure, angina, aortic insufficiency, and respiratory failure were relieved. All patients had patent anastomoses and competent aortic valves shown angiographically before discharge. No vascular complications resulted from subsequent surgery in patients with descending thoracic aortic involvement.

This approach has proved successful in a small series of extensive, complicated arch aneurysms. Bleeding is well controlled by combining techniques of proximal reconstruction with a composite valve-graft with the method of graft inclusion and major vessel reattachment. Innominate, common carotid, and subclavian artery attachment of the proximal end of a coronary artery bypass graft permits easy bypass without losing the effects of aortic graft inclusion. Patients with extensive lesions that involve the entire thoracic aorta should be managed by staged surgery.

▶ [This is a most significant article because data regarding operations on the transverse aortic arch are meager, usually describing a high mortality, exceeding 50% to 75%. Profound hypothermia and circulatory arrest, with the technique of intralumenal insertion of the graft described in this report, seem to represent a significant advance, although the article describes only 8 cases. The uncertain feature, of course, is how long the cerebral blood flow safely can be decreased. The enigma for years has been whether cerebral injury after such operations is due to ischemia or to emboli from particulate matter in the aneurysm.—F.C.S.] ◀

17-20 **Acute Traumatic Disruption of the Thoracic Aorta: Ten-Year Experience.** Although disruption of the thoracic aorta from nonpenetrating trauma usually is rapidly fatal, 10% to 15% of patients live to reach medical treatment. Urgent operation is the accepted approach, but the best means of protecting the distal circulation is uncertain. Cary W. Akins, Mortimer J. Buckley, Willard Daggett, Joseph B. McIlduff, and W. Gerald Austen reviewed information on 44 patients treated between 1970 and 1979 for proved acute thoracic aortic injury secondary to nonpenetrating trauma. The 32 male and 12 female patients had a mean age of 33 years. Most were involved in automobile accidents. Associated injuries were frequent. In 2 cases, mediastinal widening was not observed until several weeks after injury. Three patients had subcutaneous emphysema, and 9 had evidence of left-sided pleural effusion. Two had abdominal viscera in the left side of the chest.

All injuries but 2 involved the proximal descending thoracic aorta. Twenty-one patients were operated on within 48 hours of injury. One patient died during angiography, and 1 refused operation. Operation was electively delayed in 19 cases. Modified left heart bypass was used in most surgical patients. A Dacron graft was used in most instances. Overall hospital survival was 75%. Twelve of 14 patients in whom operation was electively delayed for healing or stabilization of concomitant injuries survived. All 5 patients in whom operation was deferred indefinitely because of extensive concomitant injuries survived hospitalization. Four patients died in the operating room. Several survivors of operation had significant postoperative complications.

Immediate operation is not necessary in all cases of traumatic disruption of the aorta, but prompt diagnosis is essential. Currently, all patients with suspected thoracic aortic trauma receive antihypertensive therapy and β-blockade, if they are hemodynamically stable, until the diagnosis can be confirmed by urgent aortography.

▶ [Experiences with 44 patients treated during 10 years at the Massachusetts General Hospital are reported. The gravity of the injury is indicated by a mortality of 24% in a group operated on within 48 hours of injury. The mortality was related to both the aortic injury and associated injury with sepsis. A Dacron graft was needed in 33 patients. The preferred technique includes the use of the Gott heparin shunt, avoiding systemic heparinization.—F.C.S.] ◀

-21 **Incremental Risk Factors For Spinal Cord Injury Following Operation For Acute Traumatic Aortic Transection.** Emergency surgery for acute traumatic transection of the descending thoracic aorta requires temporary interruption of the blood supply to the spinal cord and lower body. The need for a shunt procedure to avoid cord injury is unclear. Nevin M. Katz, Eugene H. Blackstone, John W. Kirklin,

(17-20) Ann. Thorac. Surg. 31:305–309, April 1981.
(17-21) J. Thorac. Cardiovasc. Surg. 81:669–674, May 1981.

and Robert B. Karp (Univ. of Alabama, Birmingham) reviewed 35 cases of surgery for acute traumatic descending thoracic aortic transection in 1967–1980. Eight of the 33 evaluable patients had postoperative paraplegia or paresis; all had had normal cord function preoperatively. Four patients were paraplegic, and 4 had bilateral lower limb paresis.

No single factor was significantly associated with cord injury, but preoperative shock and use of a shunt procedure were possibly associated with less frequent spinal cord injury. When no shunt procedure was used, aortic cross-clamp times were longer in patients who incurred cord injury; these patients were younger and had longer operations. Multivariate analysis indicated that only a long cross-clamp time and no shunt procedure were associated with a higher risk of cord injury, with an apparently possible significant interaction of these factors. The risk of cord injury in patients in whom a shunt procedure was not used increased as the aortic cross-clamp time increased beyond 33 minutes. More interposition grafts were inserted in patients in whom a shunt procedure was used.

Spinal cord injury after surgery for acute aortic transection is related to a long or aortic cross-clamp time. When a shunt was used, the risk of cord injury did not increase with the cross-clamp time in the present study. Repair without shunting should be limited to cases where surgery can be completed within 30 minutes of aortic cross-clamping. When a shunt procedure is to be used, aortoaortic shunting has no apparent advantage over femorofemoral bypass with a pump oxygenator.

▶ [This report reviews experiences with 35 patients operated on for acute traumatic rupture of the aorta during 1967 to 1980. Some spinal cord injury occurred in 8 of 33 patients in whom sufficient data were available for analysis, an alarming frequency exceeding 25%. Our preference at New York University is that unless associated injuries make the risk of heparinization prohibitive, all such injuries should be repaired with partial bypass, preferably between the femoral artery and the femoral vein. The associated heparinization of the patient does not add significantly to the risk of bleeding, provided proper precautions are taken. Spinal cord injury is virtually unknown. Admittedly, some patients recover promptly in whom expeditious clamping and reconstruction of the aorta is necessary, but this can not be anticipated in advance, especially as most of these patients will require a graft for reconstruction.—F.C.S.] ◀

18. Arteries

18–1 **Antithrombin Deficiency: A Cause of Unexplained Thrombosis in Vascular Surgery.** Antithrombin III is a potent plasma inactivator of thrombin and other serine proteases such as activated factor X. It also functions as a heparin cofactor. Antithrombin deficiencies may be the cause of otherwise unexplained thrombotic episodes. Jonathan B. Towne, Victor M. Bernhard, Clara Hussey, and John C. Garancis (Med. College of Wisconsin, Milwaukee) encountered 5 men and 4 women, aged 31–65, with antithrombin deficiencies as a cause of hemorrhage in 1978–1980 (table). Three patients presented with early thrombosis of distal femoral grafts, 2 had spontaneous arterial thrombosis, 1 had ileofemoral venous thrombosis, and 1 had spontaneous thrombosis of the tibial outflow vessels during extended profundoplasty.

PATIENTS WITH ANTITHROMBIN DEFICIENCY

Patient No.	*Age (yr)*	*Sex*	*Complication*	*Antithrombin II level*	*Antithrombin III level*	*Results*
1	63	F	Intraoperative thrombosis of femoral-anterior tibial graft	11 sec	7 sec	Graft patent at 1 yr
2	50	M	Thrombosis of femoral-peroneal bypass; persistance of clotting noted in operative field despite heparinization	18.5 sec	Normal	Graft occluded, but limb salvaged
3	65	M	Thrombosis of tibial-peroneal trunk as well as runoff vessels into foot during performance of common femoral endarterectomy and extended profundaplasty for mild rest pain	18.5 sec	9.5 sec	Below-knee amputation
4	56	M	Thrombosis of tibial vessels and femoral-popliteal graft done for isolated superficial femoral block	17.5 sec	10.5 sec	Below-knee amputation
5	62	M	Spontaneous thrombosis of distal superficial femoral, popliteal, and tibial arteries; past history of multiple episodes of thrombosis and pulmonary embolism	Normal	10.5 sec	Successful femoral anterior tibial graft
6	52	M	Spontaneous thrombosis of left brachial and femoral, popliteal, and tibial vessels of both legs	14.5 sec*	Normal*	Patient required femoral distal posterior tibial bypass because of residual ischemia following thrombectomy of left leg
7	30	F	Ileofermoral venous thrombosis while hospitalized for treatment of viral encephalitis	Normal	8.5 sec	Resolved without sequelae

*Values obtained after administration of fresh frozen plasma. True values are probably lower.

(18–1) Surgery 89:735–742, June 1981.

Two patients required below-knee amputation. Another had successful thrombectomy with long-term graft patency when the coagulation defect was identified the day after surgery and corrected with fresh frozen plasma. Both patients with spontaneous arterial thrombosis had correct diagnoses shortly after admission. Both required bypass procedures. The patient with ileofemoral thrombophlebitis was treated, with sequelae. The patient with multiple thrombi noted during surgery had extension of the graft. Antithrombin II assay gave abnormal results in 5 patients. The antithrombin III assay time was abnormally shortened in 5 cases. Three patients had both antithrombin II and III deficiencies. In 2 cases, heparin failed to prevent clotting in the operative field until fresh frozen plasma was given.

Venous thrombosis of the legs and mesenteric circulation has been attributed to antithrombin III deficiency, but no well-documented cases of arterial thrombosis have been reported. The cause of antithrombin deficiency in the present cases is unknown. A platelet count is made and blood taken for antithrombin measurements. If the platelet count is normal, fresh frozen plasma is given until the results are available. Patients with antithrombin deficiency continue to receive the plasma for 5 days. Warfarin therapy is given indefinitely, because it has been shown to increase antithrombin III levels in some patients.

▶ [This is a relatively new concept that merits emphasis. Karl et al. (*Surgery* 89:429, 1981) described a patient with congenital antithrombin deficiency in whom superior mesenteric vein thrombosis developed after cessation of warfarin therapy, resulting in gangrene of the small intestine. Initial treatment of the deficiency with fresh frozen plasma and long-term management with warfarin were effective in avoiding further thrombotic events. The presence of antithrombin deficiency in both Scandinavian and New England populations has been estimated to be 1 in 2,000, and it is felt that these deficiencies may account for as much as 2% of cases of venous thromboembolism. In families with inherited deficiencies, the incidence of thromboembolic events in patients with abnormally low levels of antithrombin III is approximately 50%. These have been reported to include iliofemoral thrombosis, superficial calf vein thrombosis, pulmonary embolism, caval thrombosis, mesenteric vein thrombosis, and thrombosis of the sinuses. Heparin resistance is common in these patients, and the administration of warfarin has been demonstrated to increase the antithrombin III levels in deficient patients.—S.I.S.] ◀

18–2 **Preliminary Experience With Prostaglandins E_1 and I_2 in Peripheral Vascular Disease.** The management of ischemic extremity pain and focal tissue necrosis in patients in whom sympathectomy or reconstructive surgery is not indicated, or has failed, remains an important problem. Bruce J. Pardy, John D. Lewis, and H. H. G. Eastcott evaluated intravascular infusions of prostaglandin E_1 (PGE_1) and prostacyclin (PGI_2) in 19 patients with limb ischemia and 1 with vasculitic leg ulceration. They were treated on 25 occasions for 72–96 hours. The mean patient age was 48 years. The most common underlying conditions were arteriosclerosis and Buerger's disease. Focal tissue necrosis was present in 13 patients. Prostaglandin E_1 was given by intermittent or continuous infusion at a rate of 10 ng/kg/minute. PGI_2 was given intravenously in a final dose of 8–15 ng/kg/minute.

(18–2) Surgery 88:826–832, December 1980.

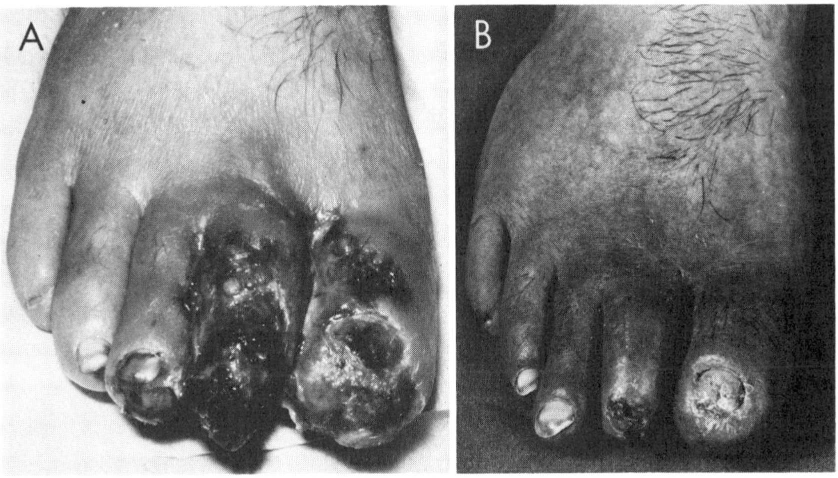

Fig 18–1.—A, gangrene and sepsis in right foot of 31-year-old white man with Buerger's disease diagnosed in 1972. Left lumbar sympathectomy was performed in 1973, and left hallux amputation was performed the following year. Amputation of the right first and second toes was considered necessary after failure of conservative management for 7 weeks (right lumbar sympathectomy was not performed because of possible sexual complications). Prostaglandin E_1 was given via the femoral artery, with immediate healing response. **B,** 2 months after PGE_1 treatment, the patient was pain-free and working. (Courtesy of Pardy, B. J., et al.: Surgery 88:826–832, December 1980.)

Four patients with foot ischemia responded poorly or not at all to low-dose PGE_1 given intravenously, but pain was relieved after 10 of 20 intra-arterial or intravenous high-dose infusions of either agent. Healing of tissue necrosis followed 7 of 14 infusions, either spontaneously or after debridement (Fig 18–1). Arterial patency was associated with a high success rate, and occlusion was associated with a low success rate. Arm pain from high-dose intravenous PGE_1 therapy was avoided by advancing the cannula tip beyond the shoulder. Administration of PGI_2 often led to facial flushing and headache.

If the proximal axial artery is patent, intravascular infusion of PGE_1 or PGI_2 for 72–96 hours is likely to relieve severe ischemic extremity pain and promote tissue healing. Continuous intravenous infusion of PGE_1 causes few side effects when the cannula tip is proximal to the shoulder. Prostaglandins may be of value in carrying patients with distal arteriopathy over acute episodes of sever pain, gangrene, and sepsis. Healing of the ischemic extremity after local surgery may be aided by initial prostaglandin infusion. The significance of the platelet inhibitory effects of PGE_1 and PGI_2 is difficult to assess.

▶ [This represents an interesting and innovative approach to the management of peripheral vascular disease. The antiplatelet effects of prostaglandin have been shown in other experimental models in which platelet trapping in the lung associated with endotoxin has been obviated by a combination of acetylsalicylic acid and the prostaglandins. It is pointed out in the discussion that the prostaglandin also has an important vasodilating effect that probably accounts for the results described in this clinical study. Salzman makes a particularly appropriate suggestion regarding the use of prostaglandin D_2 in naturally occurring prostaglandin, which has the same antiplatelet effect as prostaglandin E_1 but is active when administered orally.—S.I.S.] ◀

18-3 **The Extended Retroperitoneal Approach for Treatment of Extensive Atherosclerosis of the Aorta and Renal Vessels.** A retroperitoneal approach has been suggested in place of the traditional transperitoneal approach for the correction of aortic and renal vascular disease, to reduce ileus and respiratory complications. G. Melville Williams, John Rocotta, Michael Zinner, and James Burdick (Johns Hopkins Hosp., Baltimore) evaluated this approach in 53 consecutive patients having abdominal aortic surgery. Access to the retroperitoneum was gained through a long flank incision. Aortic endarterectomy and treatment of orifice lesions of the renal or visceral arteries were accomplished by clamping the aorta above the celiac axis and below the renal arteries. The distal aorta was replaced in all cases but 1. The technique for incorporating the right renal arteries into a Dacron graft is shown in Figure 18–2.

Two of 28 patients with severe atherosclerosis or occlusive disease died postoperatively. None of 25 patients having the aorta occluded above the celiac axis required hemodialysis. One patient had disseminated intravascular coagulation. One patient with occlusion of a graft limb underwent thrombectomy and femoropopliteal saphenous vein grafting. One renal artery has experienced thrombosis. The blood pressure response to renal artery reconstruction was good in 15 of 18

Fig 18–2.—The technique for incorporating the right renal arteries into the Dacron graft utilizing the posterior flank approach. It was not unusual to find normal-appearing intima extending from the upper abdominal aorta to include renal arteries even when they were part of the aneurysm. In such cases, a slot was cut into the graft (**A**) and the area of normal endothelium was incorporated into the suture line (B, C, and D). (Courtesy of Williams, G. M., et al.: Surgery 88:846–855, December 1980.)

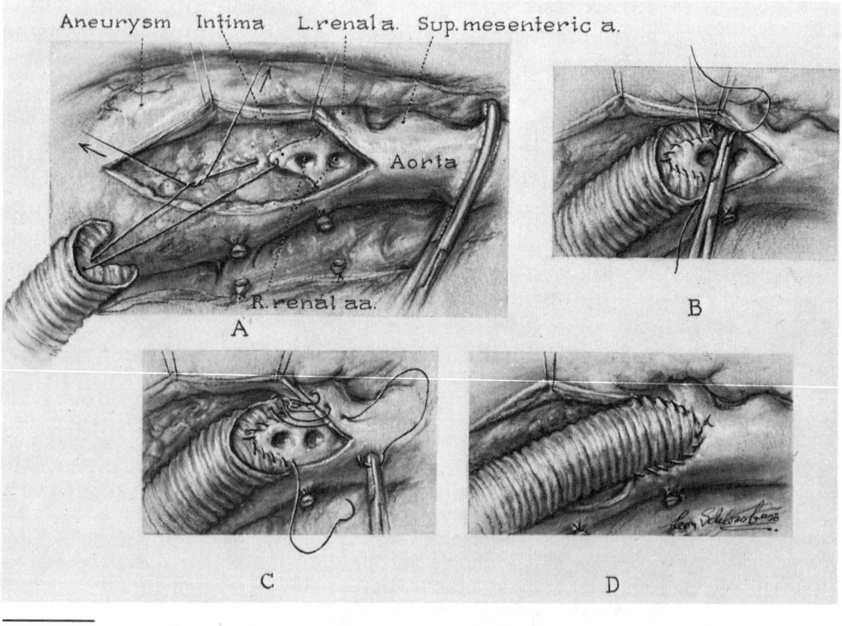

(18–3) Surgery 88:846–855, December 1980.

patients followed up for 1 month to 3 years postoperatively. The overall operative mortality was 8%.

The retroperitoneal approach is recommended for reoperations on the aorta and for patients with extensive aneurysmal and/or occlusive disease of the aorta, renal, or visceral arteries. The approach is ideal for the repair of contained abdominal aortic rupture, especially in the area of renal arteries. The posterior exposure is superior for some bilateral renal artery orifice endarterectomies. It is more difficult to assess the results of right renal reconstruction than with the standard transperitoneal approach.

▶ [This extension of Charles Rob's retroperitoneal approach for lower lesions of the aorta is a significant addition to the vascular surgeon's technical armamentarium. The technique for incorporating the renal arteries with a Dacron graft is particularly attractive. There is little question that the retroperitoneal approach offers a distinct advantage as far as the postoperative course is concerned, because the extent of ileus is reduced markedly and the patients are significantly more comfortable.—S.I.S.] ◀

18–4 **Infrarenal Abdominal Aortic Aneurysm: Factors Influencing Survival After Operation Performed Over a 25-Year Period.** E. Stanley Crawford, Salwa A. Saleh, Julius W. Babb III, Donald H. Glaeser, Patrick S. Vaccaro, and Abraham Silvers (Houston) reviewed survival factors in a series of 920 consecutive patients operated on for infrarenal abdominal aortic aneurysm in the past 25 years. Sixty patients were operated on for rupture, with a survival of 77% that did not vary much with the time of treatment. The patients without rupture were predominantly men; the median age was 65.5 years. No aneurysm-related symptoms occurred in 390 of the 860 cases. Associated disease was frequent; more than half the patients had arteriosclerotic heart disease. The graft inclusion technique was used increasingly after the late 1950s.

The 30-day mortality was 4.7% in patients without rupture. Cardiac causes were responsible for more than half of the early deaths. Both overall mortality and death from heart disease declined steadily over the review period. Forty percent of the operative survivors followed up died after discharge. The mean follow-up was 4.5 years. Overall survival rates at 5, 10, and 15 years were 63%, 38%, and 18%, respectively. Survival was highest in patients without associated disease and lowest in those with arteriosclerotic heart disease. The most important single factor that influenced long-term survival was the age at the time of operation. False aneurysm occurred in 23 patients, and 3 had graft erosion into the gastrointestinal tract. No patient in whom the aortic bifurcation had been spared required iliac artery aneurysm surgery.

The results of graft replacement of infrarenal abdominal aortic aneurysms have improved steadily since the early 1950s. Operative mortality is now less than 2%, although the proportion of patients with risk factors has increased. The surgery effectively controls the disease, extends life expectancy, and can be performed safely in nearly all cases. Aneurysm size should not be a major factor in selecting

(18–4) Ann. Surg. 193:699–709, June 1981.

patients for surgery. The only factors that severely limit life expectancy are advanced age and associated disease.

▶ [This article is an excellent survey of experiences with 920 patients operated on by one group during 25 years. A survival of 77% in cases of ruptured aneurysm is significantly better than that for many groups. More important is the progressive decline in elective operative mortality, decreasing to less than 2% in recent years. Separately, the 5-year survival of 84% if heart disease is not present is impressive. Equally impressive is the fact that it is 54% with heart disease, emphasizing the fact that the major cause of death after resection of abdominal aneurysm is coronary artery disease, which, hopefully, can be treated better in the future with careful monitoring and treatment.—F.C.S.] ◀

18–5 **Aortic Graft-Enteric Fistula.** Aortic-enteric fistula has been described after reconstructive aortic surgery in 0.4% to 2.4% of patients. Paul D. Kiernan, Peter C. Pairolero, John P. Hubert, Jr., Peter Mucha, Jr., and Robert B. Wallace (Mayo Clinic) reviewed the records of 20 patients who underwent 24 operations for intestinal bleeding from aortic graft-enteric fistula between 1964 and 1978. The 16 men and 4 women were aged 45 to 86 years. Duodenal ulcer was documented in 8 patients before development of the fistula. Ten patients were initially operated on for aneurysms and 10 for arteriosclerosis obliterans. Eleven patients underwent resection of the abdominal aorta with graft interposition, and the other 9 had aortofemoral or aortoiliac bypass surgery. Dacron prostheses were used in 15 patients, Teflon prostheses in 2, and a nylon prosthesis in 1. In 4 cases the graft and proximal anastomosis were inadequately covered by autogenous tissue.

The mean interval between initial operation and onset of gastrointestinal bleeding was 37 months, and the mean time from onset of bleeding to operation for repair of the fistula was 15 days. Melena occurred in 70% of patients, hematemesis in 40%, and hematochezia in 35%. Fifteen patients had abdominal pain, usually with lumbosacral radiation. Arteriography failed to confirm the diagnosis in the 8 patients so examined. A fistula was present at the proximal anastomosis in 13 patients and at the distal anastomosis in 1. Three patients had blood loss through intact but bile-stained defibrinated grafts. In 16 patients the enteric component of the fistula was oversewn. Four patients had intestinal resection with primary anastomoses. Three of the 6 patients who had complete excision of the aortic prosthesis and extra-anatomical arterial bypass grafting died postoperatively, and 1 died later of abscess formation and a fistula that developed after further surgery. Two of 5 patients who had complete excision of the prosthesis and immediate retroperitoneal anatomical graft replacement died postoperatively, and a third died at reoperation for a recurrent fistula. In all, 11 patients died postoperatively, 4 after repair of a recurrent aortoenteric fistula and 2 of apparently unrelated causes. Only 3 patients (15%) are well.

Adequate coverage of both the graft and the proximal anastomosis with retroperitoneal tissue and peritoneum is necessary to avoid development of an aortoenteric fistula. Graft infection is best controlled

---

(18–5) Mayo Clin. Proc. 55:731–738, December 1980.

by complete excision of the fistulous tract, with or without extra-anatomical arterial bypass. If the diagnosis is made at exploration, the abdomen may be closed after excision of the graft and extra-anatomical bypass carried out with new instruments after repeat preparation.

▶ [This report from the Mayo Clinic summarizes experiences with 20 patients with aortoenteric fistulas treated during a 15-year period. Mortality remains at a grim level, around 50%, similar to that reported by others. The suggestion by the authors that the major factor was the soft tissue coverage of the graft and the proximal anastomosis, generally using retroperitoneal tissue, but using omentum if this were inadequate, seems to be most important.

The authors emphasize that the diagnosis may not be made before surgical exploration is done. Endoscopy was the most useful measure, but if this were not diagnostic, additional studies with x-rays and arteriography were not helpful. At operation, excision of the graft with axillary femoral bypass seems to be the best approach, though the aortic stump remains a hazardous problem, with fatal rupture in 2 of the authors' 6 patients and in 3 of 10 previously described in the literature.—F.C.S.] ◀

18–6 **Secondary Aortoenteric Fistula: A 20-Year Experience.** Charles S. O'Mara, G. Melville Williams, and Calvin B. Ernst (Johns Hopkins Med. Inst.) reviewed the findings in 17 patients operated on during 1960 to 1980 for secondary aortoenteric fistula. All but 1 were male, and the average age was 66 years. Twelve patients had had synthetic graft replacement of an abdominal aortic aneurysm, 3 on an emergency basis for rupture. Five patients had had synthetic bypass grafting for aortoiliac occlusive disease. Fifteen Dacron and two Teflon grafts had been used. The average interval from initial surgery to onset of fistula symptoms was 2.8 years. All patients had evidence of gastrointestinal (GI) hemorrhage, which in 13 was acute. Seven patients required urgent surgery for exsanguinating hemorrhage. Five had sepsis. Ten had significant abdominal or back pain. The diagnosis was made by upper GI endoscopy in 2 of 8 patients. Aortography showed a false aneurysm at the aortic-graft anastomosis in 3.

The distal duodenum was involved in 14 patients, the jejunum in 1, and the ileum in 2. Five patients had bowel erosion by the prosthesis, and 12 had a fistulous communication between the bowel and aortic lumen. A false aneurysm of the aortic-graft anastomosis was seen in 8 of the latter patients. Purulence was seen in 5 patients, and 5 others had organisms isolated from the graft. Two moribund patients died shortly after aortic control was obtained. Three patients had local repair by suture or patch grafting, but 2 died of recurrent fistula and massive bleeding. Graft excision combined with axillobifemoral or bilateral axillofemoral bypass was performed in 8 patients, with 5 hospital deaths. The overall hospital mortality was 59%, and only 2 patients survived longer than 6 months. Only graft excision and extra-anatomical reconstruction were compatible with survival and absence of recurrent fistula formation.

Esophagogastroduodenoscopy followed by aortography and barium contrast GI series should be performed when secondary aortoenteric fistula is suspected in a patient with sepsis, abdominal pain, or GI bleeding after aortic reconstruction. Gentle dissection around the

---

(18–6) Am. J. Surg. 142:203–209, August 1981.

duodenum during the initial operation is essential to avoid this complication, as may the prevention of direct contact between a synthetic graft and the bowel wall. Successful repair requires graft excision and axillofemoral bypass.

▶ [The data in this report are quite valuable for determining management of this highly lethal complication. Of 17 patients treated over a period of 20 years, 12 had their initial operation performed elsewhere. The aortoenteric fistula appeared as late as 8 years after operation. Significantly, diagnostic studies were accurate in only about 50% of patients, the more important being gastroduodenoscopy, aortography, and barium contrast studies.

A separate important point is that all such patients should be considered contaminated, even though no signs of infection are present. The involvement of the intestine will lead almost surely to contamination of the graft. Hence, in the vast majority of cases any operation short of graft removal is doomed to failure.

Some initial survivors die later from dehiscence of the aortic stump, an unsolved problem at present. The grim nature of the complication is indicated by the fact that of the 7 patients who left the hospital after treatment, only 2 survived longer than 6 months. The ideal management at present is prompt excision of the graft, combined with bilateral axillary-femoral bypass, followed by a long course of appropriate antibiotic therapy.—F.C.S.] ◀

18–7 **Aneurysms of the Splanchnic Arteries.** Aneurysms of the splanchnic arteries, though usually asymptomatic, can cause catastrophic exsanguinating hemorrhage. Joseph M. Graham, Charles H. McCollum, and Michael E. DeBakey (Baylor College of Medicine) reviewed the findings in 18 patients with 19 splanchnic artery aneurysms (table). The 10 women and 8 men had an average age of 52 years. Ten patients were asymptomatic at the time of diagnosis. In only 1 case did the aneurysm rupture acutely. A calcified ring was noted on roentgenography in 8 cases. Angiography demonstrated the aneurysm in 13 patients, while in 4 cases it was found at surgery for other intra-abdominal disease. Thirteen fusiform and 6 saccular aneurysms were observed.

Six patients had resection of the aneurysm and ligation of the involved artery. Four patients with splenic artery aneurysms had sple-

DATA ON 18 PATIENTS WITH ANEURYSMS OF THE SPLANCHNIC ARTERIES

	Type of Aneurysm				
	Celiac	Splenic	Hepatic	Superior Mesenteric	Total
No. of Aneurysms	2	5	6*	6	19
Type					
Saccular	1	4	0	1	6
Fusiform	1	1	6	5	13
Men	1	1	5†	2†	8
Women	1	4	1	4	10
Age					
Average	51	47	63	49	
Range	49–52	44–67	55–73	27–72	

*Two aneurysms involved the origin and proximal portion of the gastroduodenal artery.
†One patient had 2 aneurysms.

(18–7) Am. J. Surg. 140:797–801, December 1980.

nectomy as well. Six patients had resection with primary arterial reconstruction. Seven patients had replacement of the resected aneurysm with a Dacron graft. Five patients had resection of a concomitant abdominal aortic aneurysm. One operative death occurred. None of the 4 late deaths were caused by aneurysmal disease. The surviving patients were asymptomatic 12–217 months after operation. Survival rates at 3, 5, and 10 years were 87.5%, 78.6%, and 55.6%, respectively.

Splenic artery aneurysms are the most common aneurysms of the splanchinic vessels. The risk of rupture of these aneurysms is about 10%. Hepatic artery aneurysms carry a high risk of rupture. Superior mesenteric artery and celiac trunk aneurysms are less frequent. Several of the present patients were asymptomatic before admission. In only 1 case did the aneurysm rupture acutely, resulting in the only death in the series. Long-term follow-up has shown continuing good results. One patient subsequently had a visceral artery aneurysm at another site.

▶ [This article focuses on the most unusual of aneurysmal lesions. Although the number of patients who spontaneously ruptured splenic artery aneurysms is admittedly small (the highest was in the third trimester in pregnancy), the risk of the operation is such that intervention in this age group is indicated. In other circumstances, particularly in patients who live in an area where medical care is available, the presence of a splenic artery aneurysm does not mandate removal. In an age of appreciation of the importance of the preservation of the spleen, it would be appropriate in the younger patient to resect the splenic artery with its aneurysm, leaving the spleen to be supplied by collaterals and avoiding the issue of an asplenic state. Our experience with hepatic artery aneurysms is such that they are usually fusiform and have reached significant size. In two instances in which ligation was carried out, there was no evidence of hepatic dysfunction.—S.I.S.] ◀

18–8 **Mycotic Emboli of the Peripheral Vessels: Analysis of 44 Cases.** Nghia M. Vo, John C. Russell and Donald R. Becker (Univ. of Connecticut) report 2 cases of peripheral mycotic embolization and review 42 other cases reported in the English literature since 1950.

Man, 22, underwent an above-knee amputation, as well as several other operations, after a severe motorcycle accident and received multiple courses of antibiotic therapy. After a focal seizure, a saddle embolus of the terminal aorta was diagnosed and an embolectomy was performed, showing *Aspergillus fumigatus*. Mitral vegetations were found, and valve replacement was carried out. Emboli recurred despite therapy with amphotericin and 5-flucytosine, and the patient died 11 months after injury.

Man, 64, developed a femoral embolus 5 months after aortic valve replacement, and *Aspergillus* was found in association with aortic valve vegetations. The patient died during aortic valve replacement.

Fungal endocarditis may be indolent at its outset. Patients with peripheral embolization have had a mortality of 84%. Predisposing factors include open heart surgery, antibiotic therapy, concomitant infection, drug therapy, and intravenous hyperalimentation. Both aortic and mitral involvement are seen. Peripheral embolization generally has preceded clinical involvement of the brain or mesenteric organs. Femoral emboli are most common, followed by distal aortic, brachial,

---

(18–8) Surgery 90:541–545, September 1981.

iliac, popliteal, and axillary artery emboli. *Candida* and *Aspergillus* are the most common fungi involved. Only 43% of patients had positive blood cultures, usually in association with candidal infection. Mycotic embolization after open heart surgery is particularly lethal. More than half of the patients subsequently experienced generalized embolization. Two patients had mycotic aneurysms.

Embolectomy is necessary in these cases. It was performed in 81% of patients, with a 19% survival rate; no patient not having embolectomy survived. The role of valve replacement is not defined fully, but early valve replacement combined with prolonged antifungal drug treatment probably will give optimal results.

▶ [This important review focuses on an entity that undoubtedly will increase in the future. We recently have had experience with patients in whom mycotic emboli of Candida developed after insertion of a lifeline for massive chemotherapy as treatment for leukemia. In our patients, the mycotic emboli developed in the spleen and liver, and in one case the emboli were responsible for spontaneous rupture of the spleen and intraperitoneal bleeding. In all circumstances, aggressive therapy should consist of removing the site of embolization and the site of implantation, if at all possible, followed by aggressive chemotherapy.—S.I.S.] ◀

18–9 **Local Antibiotic Irrigation in the Treatment of Arterial Graft Infections.** Infection of an anastomotic line or synthetic prosthesis is one of the most serious complications of reconstructive vascular surgery. Debridement with drainage and local antibiotic irrigation is an alternative to removal of the infected graft. B. Almgren and I. Eriksson (Univ. of Uppsala) reviewed the management of 12 infected arterial reconstructions, representing 1.25% of the operations done in 1972–1978. Eight infections followed synthetic grafting; 3, autologous vein grafting; and 1, thromboendarterectomy. Two patients died of hemorrhage from a ruptured aortic anastomosis. Three had an infected false aneurysm and required ligation of the artery and excision of the graft. The other 7 patients were managed by continuous local antibiotic irrigation and drainage after removal of necrotic tissue. Where possible, the graft was covered with healthy tissue. A solution of cloxacillin in saline was instilled for 7–13 days, and systemic cloxacillin was given in a daily dose of 8 gm. Subsequently, cloxacillin was given orally in a dose of 4 gm daily for 3–6 months.

The clinical data are summarized in the table. Four infections involved synthetic grafts but not the anastomoses; 3 occurred in patients with Dacron bifurcation grafts. Three patients had infected vein-artery anastomoses and local hemorrhage caused by disruption of an anastomotic suture line. *Staphylococcus aureus* was isolated in all cases but 1, in which *Escherichia coli* was present. One patient died of cerebral hemorrhage more than a year after treatment with a patent graft. In another patient, a false aneurysm of an anastomosis later developed without infection. The other 5 patients were well on follow-up 34–59 months after treatment and had well-functioning grafts with no signs of late infection.

Arterial graft infections can be eradicated by local antibiotic irrigation and systemic antibiotic therapy without removal of the graft.

(18–9) Acta Chir. Scand. 147:33–36, 1981.

CLINICAL DATA ON SEVEN PATIENTS TREATED BY LOCAL CONTINUOUS ANTIBIOTIC IRRIGATION

Patient no.	Site and type of graft	Part of graft involved	Time after operation (weeks)	Organism	Result	Follow-up (months)
1	Aortofemoral bifurcation graft (Dacron)	Shaft and limbs	3	*E. coli*	Recovered Non-infected false aneurysm of right distal anastomosis 47 months postop.	59
2	Aortofemoral bifurcation graft (Dacron)	Right limb	19	*Staph. aureus*	Recovered	39
3	Aortofemoral bifurcation graft (Dacron)	Shaft and limbs	8	*Staph. aureus*	Recovered	14
4	Iliofemoral (Dacron)	Shaft	3	*Staph. aureus*	Recovered	34
5	Femoropopliteal (vein)	Proximal anastomosis	2	*Staph. aureus*	Recovered	56
6	Femoropopliteal (vein)	Distal anastomosis	4	*Staph. aureus*	Recovered	56
7	Saphenofemoral dialysis shunt (vein)	Anastomosis	1	*Staph. aureus*	Bleeding from anastomosis Removal of graft	–

Graft excision is indicated for infection involving an anastomosis of a synthetic graft, but infection along a synthetic graft without involvement of anastomoses should be treated by local antibiotic irrigation initially. Infection of a saphenous vein-artery anastomosis is treated by ligation or, alternately, by resuturing and local antibiotic irrigation.

▶ [Although the series is small, the message is large. It does run counter to consensus opinion indicating that the presence of an infection surrounding a graft necessitates removal of the entire graft. A sense of insecurity relates to the question of whether or not the suture line is involved. Because we are dealing with a single space in continuity, it is difficult to imagine the infection being confined to the midportion of the prosthetic material and not tracking up to the suture line. Even more interesting than the success achieved with infections of the prosthetic material is the ability to manage leakage at the suture line in patients with an infected saphenous vein artery anastomosis.—S.I.S.] ◀

8-10 **Percutaneous Angiographic Embolization—A Procedure of Increasing Usefulness: Review of a Decade of Experience.** Frederick S. Keller, Josef Rösch, Gerald M. Baur, Lloyd M. Taylor, C. T. Dotter, and John M. Porter (Univ. of Oregon) reviewed 152 selective transcatheter embolizations performed in 124 patients for a wide range of problems. The most commonly used embolic materials were Gelfoam, bucrylate, and Ginaturco steel coils. Diagnostic angiography always preceded vaso-occlusion. Where possible, the therapeutic procedure was separated from the diagnostic study. All but 5 of the 120 arterial embolizations were done from the femoral approach.

Twenty-five patients had 26 embolizations for acute upper gastrointestinal arterial bleeding; usually the left gastric artery was embolized. Bleeding was controlled in all but 2 patients. There were no procedure-related deaths. Thirty-two patients had transhepatic occlu-

(18–10) Am. J. Surg. 142:5–13, July 1981.

sion of the left gastric and short gastric veins and gastroesophageal varices for variceal bleeding, and the procedure succeeded in 94% of cases. Active variceal bleeding was initially controlled in all but 3 of 18 cases of emergency embolization. Thirty-one infarctions were done for renal carcinoma. Eight patients with congenital arteriovenous malformations had 21 vaso-occlusive procedures. One patient had pulmonary embolization as a complication. Four patients had cutaneous and large subcutaneous hemangiomas embolized. Eleven had embolization of the pelvic arteries without significant procedure-related complications. Three patients with iatrogenic arteriovenous fistulas had fistula closure by the transcatheter technique. Two patients with recurrent massive hemoptysis had therapeutic bronchial artery embolization.

Transcatheter embolization is a safe and effective measure in selected cases. Its indications will be extended in the future, and its use will be common wherever angiographic facilities exist.

▶ [This presentation of the panoramic indications for selective embolization, coming from the center that initiated much of the work, is an expression of increasing interest in the subject. Lang (*Diagn. Radiol.* 140:331–339, 1981) reported on an experience in 46 patients with transcatheter embolization for intractable hemorrhage from pelvic organs. Autologous blood was advocated if later restitution of vascular continuity was desired, such as hemorrhage attributed to trauma or iatrogenic causes; Gelfoam was favored if permanent or semipermanent occlusion was desired, such as in hemorrhage caused by neoplasm. Excellent results were obtained. Palmaz et al. (*AJR* 137:117–122, 1981) used particulate intra-arterial embolization in the management of pelvic arteriovenous malformation to provide symptomatic relief, but recurrence of these lesions is expected.—S.I.S.] ◀

18–11 **Arterial Embolization: Problems of Source, Multiplicity, Recurrence, and Delayed Treatment.** Joseph P. Elliott, Jr., John H. Hageman, D. Emerick Szilagyi, Vellore Ramakrishnan, Jose J. Bravo, and Roger F. Smith (Henry Ford Hosp., Detroit) reviewed the course of 225 patients having 309 episodes of arterial embolism in 1950 to 1979. The prevalence increased in the latter part of the review period. Of the 337 individual emboli, 95 represented recurrences. Multiple simultaneous emboli constituted 11.6% of initial emboli and 23.2% of recurrent emboli. Cardiac abnormality was present in 86.3% of cases, and atherosclerotic heart disease was seen in 60.4%. Rheumatic heart disease was present in 20.9% of instances. More than 80% of emboli were in peripheral arterial trunks, particularly in the legs. Angiography was performed before embolectomy in 134 cases.

Mortality in nonoperative cases was 34.4%. Use of the Fogarty balloon catheter markedly improved the results of arterial embolectomy, especially in patients with aortoiliac embolization. The results of surgery for carotid and visceral embolism were relatively disappointing. Unfavorable results also were obtained in cases of simultaneous multiple emboli. Anticoagulation was the chief management of the site of origin of emboli in most cases. The recurrence rate was reduced markedly in permanently anticoagulated patients (Fig 18–3). Limbs that did not become obviously nonviable within 1 week did well with or without surgical treatment. Mean postoperative survival was 3.1

(18–11) Surgery 88:833–845, December 1980.

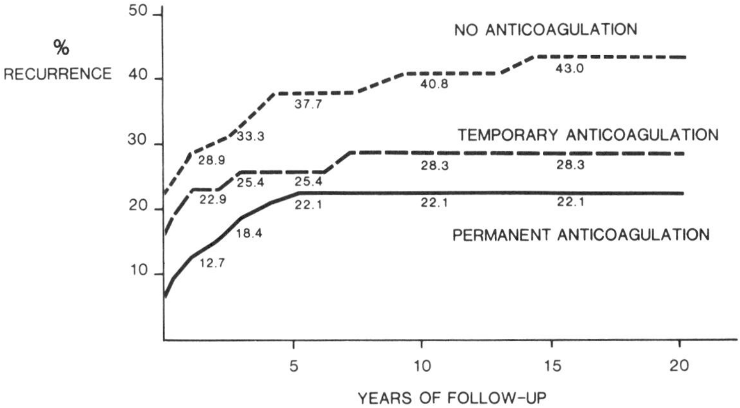

Fig 18–3.—Cumulative rate of recurrence of embolization in 215 survivors of initial embolic episodes with permanent anticoagulation (N = 97), temporary anticoagulation (N = 19), and no anticoagulation (N = 69). (Courtesy of Elliott, J. P., Jr., et al.: Surgery 88:833–845, December 1980.)

years, compared with 17 years for the general population. The most common cause of death was cardiac disease, usually atherosclerosis. One fourth of the patients receiving permanent anticoagulant therapy and only 3% of the others were alive at the end of the study.

Embolization from a cardiac source predominated in this series. A source for emboli was found in all but 11% of cases. Recurrent embolization was frequent, often multiple, and carried a poor prognosis. Permanent anticoagulant therapy, preferably with removal of the source of embolization, reduced the recurrence rate and, in general, decreased early and late morbidity and mortality rates. Indefinite anticoagulation, starting immediately postoperatively, is recommended. Early diagnosis and surgery will improve the outcome.

▶ [This well-studied, large series provides much meaningful data. The demonstration that within the range of 8 hours to 7 days the effect of delayed treatment had a linear relationship to the severity of the skin changes in the extent of favorable results runs counter to the data of Blaisdell et al. (*Surgery* 84:822–834, 1978). These authors have avoided embolectomy and thrombectomy where possible and have used heparin anticoagulation. Operation was deferred for the initial week and performed only when anticoagulation was contraindicated. The operation was best deferred for several weeks, but elective revascularization was done if indicated. Satiani et al. (*Ann. Surg.* 188:153–175, 1978) stressed another important point, limb salvage after embolectomy. These authors demonstrated that the absence of distal pulses postoperatively does not signify a poor result.—S.I.S.] ◀

18–12 **Hemodynamic Assessment of Transluminal Angioplasty for Lower Extremity Ischemia.** Treatment of arterial occlusive disease by percutaneous transluminal angioplasty (PTA) has been performed increasingly since introduction of the inflatable balloon-tipped catheter by Gruntzig and Hopff in 1974. Charles S. O'Mara, Harvey L. Neiman, William R. Flinn, Richard J. Herman, James S. T. Yao, and John J. Bergan (Northwestern Univ.) reviewed the results of PTA performed on 56 ischemic legs of 51 patients in a 9-month period. The 34 men and 17 women had an average age of 65 years. The indication

(18–12) Surgery 89:106–117, January 1981.

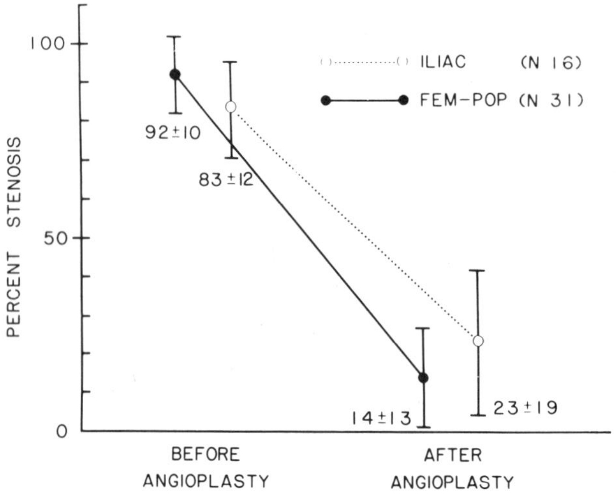

Fig 18–4.—Mean percent of stenosis before and after technically successful angioplasty. The 16 iliac dilatations are represented by open circles; 31 femoropopliteal dilatations are shown by closed circles. (Courtesy of O'Mara, C. S., et al.: Surgery 89:106–117, January 1981.)

was intermittent claudication in 46 instances and rest pain and ischemic ulceration in 5 cases each. Aspirin and dipyridamole were prescribed before balloon dilatation, which was performed under local anesthesia and with heparin and tolazoline injection.

Forty-two femoropopliteal and 17 iliac lesions were treated by PTA. The procedure was technically successful in all but 1 of the iliac segment lesions and in 31 of the 42 femoropopliteal lesions (Fig 18–4). All patients having technically successful angioplasty reported improvement in symptoms in the ischemic limb. More than half of the limbs having technically successful iliac angioplasty exhibited significant hemodynamic improvement, as did more than 80% of limbs with femoropopliteal lesions. On an average follow-up of 8 months, all iliac dilatations with initial hemodynamic improvement remained improved, but the pressure index returned to baseline in 44% of initially hemodynamically improved limbs with femoropopliteal lesions. Four complications occurred in the femoropopliteal group early in the series. No acute thrombosis or vessel perforation was observed.

Balloon dilatation is helpful in selected cases of leg ischemia. It appears ideal for short-segment lesions in a high-flow system such as the iliac artery. If claudication from femoropopliteal disease is disabling, bypass produces a better hemodynamic result than angioplasty and has a better early patency rate. The decision to perform angioplasty must be made jointly by the vascular surgeon and angiographer.

▶ [I would agree with all of the discussants in a strong endorsement of hemodynamic assessment of the results. Also essential is orientation to treat the patient rather than the angiogram. Colapinto et al. (*Radiology* 135:583–587, 1980) reported on the percutaneous transluminal dilatation in 109 iliac femoral and popliteal arteries; they achieved success in 96 of 109 attempted dilatations (88%). Iliac stenoses were the easiest to dilate, with a success rate of 96%. A 15-month follow-up showed that only 15 of 94 initial successes subsequently fail and, interestingly, no failure occurred in arteries that remained patent 7 months after dilatation.—S.I.S.] ◀

18–13 **Factors Contributing to Recurrent Lower Limb Ischemia Following Bypass Surgery for Aortoiliac Occlusive Disease, and Their Management.** Progressive or recurrent lower limb ischemia sometimes is observed after bypass surgery for aortoiliac atherosclerotic occlusive disease. John V. Robbs and Edwin J. Wylie (Univ. of California, San Francisco) reviewed the findings in 58 patients seen in 1977–1980 who required repeated surgery for recurrent ischemia after Dacron aortic bifurcation bypass surgery. The 30 male and 28 female patients had an average age of 58 years. The indication for initial surgery was claudication in all cases. The mean interval to repeated surgery was 3.8 years. Thirty-seven reoperations were done for relief of claudication, and 21 were performed because of threatened limb loss, 8 after acute occlusive episodes. Nine patients had a false aneurysm in the groin.

The chief etiologic factors are summarized in the table. More than half of the patients had progressive atherosclerosis impairing inflow to or outflow from the graft segment. Seven patients had severely compromised inflow caused by infrarenal aortic obstruction proximal to the aortic end of the graft. Twenty-five had progressive atherosclerotic outflow tract occlusion. Most of these patients had excision of the prosthesis with aortobifemoral grafting or a crossover graft between the patent graft limb and the opposite profunda artery. In patients with graft-related problems, there was a gross disparity in size between the graft and the outflow tract. Fibrous stenosis was managed by vein patch angioplasty or excision and graft replacement. In 15 cases, the original disease appeared not to have been adequately bypassed. In 30 cases, surgery was confined to the groins. All grafts in the 57 surviving patients were functioning at discharge. Six pa-

RECURRENT LOWER LIMB ISCHEMIA FOLLOWING AORTIC BIFURCATION GRAFTS (MAJOR ETIOLOGIC FACTORS IN 58 PATIENTS)

Etiologic Factor		Number of Patients
Progressive atherosclerosis		
inflow	7	32 (55.2%)
outflow	25	
Graft-related problems		
angulation	3	7 (12.0%)
mural thrombus fragmentation	4	
Fibroplasia		4 (6.9%)
Failure to bypass occlusion		
inflow and outflow	8	15 (25.9%)
outflow	7	
Total		58

(18–13) Ann. Surg. 193:346–352, March 1981.

tients had 8 complications after aortic reconstruction, and 5 had major complications after 30 local groin operations.

Aortic reconstruction might be reserved for patients with aortic inflow obstruction, infection of the graft body, or redundancy of the graft body causing enough angulation to produce obstruction.

▶ [This article brings to mind a report of Baird and associates (*Surgery* 82:785–793, 1978) pairing patients undergoing aortoiliac bypasses with those recieving aortofemoral bypasses. The superiority of aortofemoral reconstruction was shown, because subsequent downstream repair was necessary in 28% of the aortoiliac patients compared to 14% of the aortofemoral patients. The major difference was in the instances of subsequent repair to the arteries below the groin, i.e., 15% and 4%, respectively.—S.I.S.] ◀

18–14 **Popliteal Arterial Aneurysms: Their Natural History and Management.** Popliteal aneurysms are second only to abdominal aortic aneurysms with regard to potential serious complications. D. Emerick Szilagyi, Richard L. Schwartz, and Daniel J. Reddy (Henry Ford Hosp., Detroit) reviewed the management of 87 popliteal aneurysms in 62 patients in 1964–1979. All aneurysms but 1 were atherosclerotic in origin. More than 40% of aneurysms were asymptomatic; symptoms that did occur often imitated those of femoropopliteal occlusive disease. Physical findings of an aneurysm often were missed. About 45% of lesions were under 3 cm in diameter, and three-fourths were associated with other aneurysmal lesions or were bilateral.

Twenty-six patients were not operated on because of an aneurysm under 2 cm in size and 7 because of prohibitive risk factors; 4 patients

Fig 18–5.—Sketch of bypass procedure for popliteal aneurysm. (Courtesy of Szilagyi, D. E., et al.: Arch. Surg. 116:724–728, May 1981; copyright 1981, American Medical Association.)

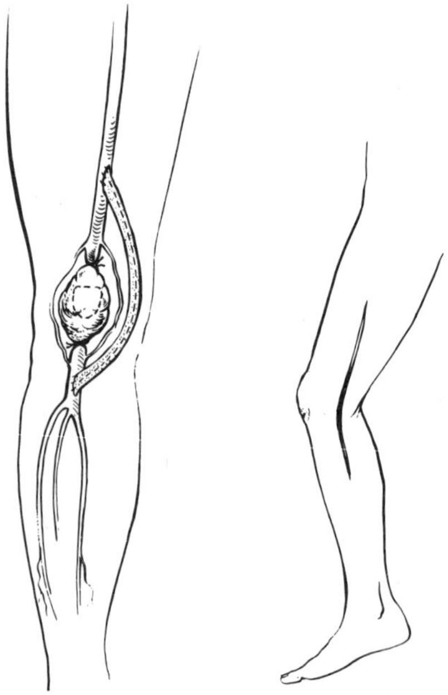

(18–14) Arch. Surg. 116:724–728, May 1981.

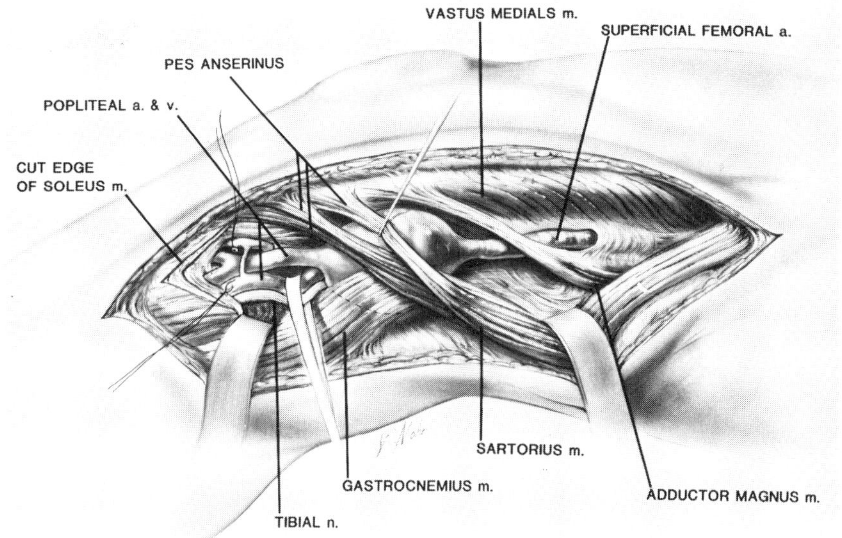

Fig 18–6.—Surgical anatomy of approach to bypass procedure for popliteal aneurysm; *a*, artery; *v*, vein; *n*, nerve; *m*, muscle. (Courtesy of Szilagyi, D. E., et al.: Arch. Surg. 116:724–728, May 1981; copyright 1981, American Medical Association.)

refused surgery. Twenty-nine aneurysms were managed by resection and grafting, 10 by bypass, and 11 by bypass and ligation. Autogenous vein grafts were used in 30 cases, and a Dacron prosthesis was used in 20 cases. The bypass procedure is illustrated in Figures 18–5 and 18–6. The immediate results of bypass and resection were com-

CUMULATIVE LATE RESULTS OF OPERATIVE CASES: PATENCY (N = 50)

Postoperative Period of Observation, yr	Cases at Risk	No. Patent	Cumulative Patency, %	Deaths
0-1	50	47	94	1
1-2	43	43	86	3
2-3	36	36	72	0
3-4	34	34	68	1
4-5	31	30	60	2
5-6	25	25	50	1
6-7	21	21	42	0
7-8	17	17	34	2
8-9	15	15	30	2
9-10	14	14	28	1
10-11	13	13	26	0
11-12	11	11	22	2
12-13	10	10	20	1
13-14	8	8	16	1
14-15	8	8	16	0
15-16	8	8	16	0
16 +	4	4	8	1
Total	...	...	...	**18**(36%)

parable, but operations with Dacron grafts appeared to be less successful. The late results are presented in the table. The greatest decrease in patency occurred in the second year of follow-up. There were no late amputations and no deaths attributable to surgery.

Unless there are specific contraindications, surgery is indicated for patients with popliteal artery aneurysms, even when symptoms are absent. The simplicity of the ligation and bypass procedure recommends it, but ligation must be carefully performed, and no potential collateral arterial branches should be left between the aneurysm and the ligature. Where the popliteal structures are compressed, the aneurysm must be at least unroofed and its contents removed. Autogenous material should be used in both the bypass and graft replacement procedures. Where the length of autogenous material is limited, reconstruction is easier if the sac is removed and an end-to-end anastomosis performed.

▶ [One can hardly argue with the data provided by this large and carefully followed series of patients. Popliteal artery aneurysms larger than 2 cm in diameter unequivocally represent lesions that demand surgical attention. Szilagyi points out in the discussion that the early results of the operation were such that the patency rate was 94% and there were no deaths during the first 30 postoperative days. There were no amputations necessary in patients whose grafts occluded. I would agree with Fry's discussion and the statement of the authors that the bypass procedure performed through the medial approach significantly reduces postoperative morbidity and is associated with equivalent results.—S.I.S.] ◀

18–15 **Morphological Structure of the Pedal Arch and Its Relationship to Patency of Crural Vascular Reconstruction.** The most critical factor in the success of crural vascular reconstruction is the integrity of the pedal arch; its roentgen image corresponds to the anatomic plantar arch. An intact arch consists of the arcade bridging the anterior and posterior tibial arteries and the pedal components of these vessels.

Aside from roentgen visualization with contrast medium, arch integrity can be additionally assessed during operation by sounding with a catheter and evaluation of the manual force required for injection of fluid. Although electromagnetic flow recording data correlate with the integrity of the pedal arch, this method is often imprecise; augmented flows with papaverine hydrochloride suggest intact arches, but contrast studies provide the optimal information. Pulse volume and Doppler recordings were not used in this study by Herbert Dardik, Ibrahim M. Ibrahim, Barry Sussman, Jutta Greweldinger, John Adler, Mark Kahn, and Irving Dardik (Englewood, N.J., Hosp.), as it was doubted the information would be more useful than that already obtained. A deficient arch could function as an intact arch if extensive arborization of the distal vessels in the foot was present.

Sixty-four arch studies obtained by adequate intraoperative angiography were categorized as intact, deficient, inadequate, or absent. Patency of crural reconstructions was obtained in 18 of 24 patients with intact arches as compared with 15 of 32 ($P < .06$) when the arch was deficient. Graft patency was a direct function of arch integrity, tibial

(18–15) Surg. Gynecol. Obstet. 152:645–648, May 1981.

or peroneal arborization, and artery size. Crural reconstruction when the arch was inadequate or absent resulted in predictable graft closure. Qualitative factors (size, calcium level, stenotic lesions) were related integrally to overall graft performance even with intact arches.

In patients with an absent or deficient arch with calcification, stenosis, or both, alternatives to bypass should be considered, including sympathectomy, continued nonoperative therapy, or primary amputation. In deficient arches with qualitative satisfactory vessels, predicting subsequent long-term graft patency has not been precise. A therapeutic alternative for a deficient arch currently under investigation with early promising results is the creation of an adjunctive arteriovenous fistula at the distal portion of the anastomotic site.

▶ [Roedersheimer et al. (*Am. J. Surg.* 140:591–595, 1980) studied the integrity of the pedal arch by hyperemic angiography preoperatively and then by intraoperative evaluation. Twenty of 21 patients with patent pedal arches who underwent vascular reconstructive procedures maintained patent grafts for 30 days; early patency was maintained in only 1 of 8 patients in whom the pedal arches were occluded. A significant percentage of patients with early patency related to patent pedal arches later obstructed their grafts within 18 months. This was related to extension disease and to poor selection of graft material; a higher percentage of occlusion occurred in patients in whom synthetic grafts were used for distal anastomoses.—S.I.S.] ◀

18–16 **Gangrene of the Toes With Palpable Peripheral Pulses: Response to Platelet Suppressive Therapy.** Most patients with peripheral gangrene have absent peripheral pulses. Of the exceptions, most patients have disorders associated with abnormal platelets and platelet function. Wyn Morris-Jones, F. Eric Preston, Martin Greaney, and Duleep K. Chatterjee (Sheffield, England) reviewed the findings in 35 patients seen in 1974–1979 who had gangrene or pregangrene of the feet associated with palpable peripheral pulses. The 21 men and 14 women were aged 47–72 years. Only 3 were cigarette smokers. All had very painful gangrene or pregangrene of one or more toes on one or both feet. All had had features of gangrene or pregangrene for at least 4 weeks, confined to the distal areas of the toes, and all had failed to respond to medical treatment. Two patients had had lumbar sympathectomy. Three patients were found to have essential thrombocythemia. None had diabetes, hypercholesterolemia, cryoglobulinemia, or aortic aneurysm.

Treatment was with 325 mg of aspirin and 100 mg of dipyridamole 3 times daily. Two patients who did not tolerate aspirin received 200 mg of sulfinpyrazone 3 times daily. Nineteen patients had relief of pain and disappearance of gangrene within 4–6 weeks of the start of therapy (table). Two other patients required amputations. Eleven patients improved after lumbar sympathectomy, whereas the other 5 have responded to naftidrofuryl therapy. Pain and some gangrene recurred within 6 weeks of discontinuance of aspirin-dipyridamole therapy in 5 cases, and the patients again responded to the drug therapy. The other patients have received continuous platelet suppressive therapy for up to 3 years. Spontaneous platelet aggregation was observed in 8 patients, 6 of whom responded well to platelet suppressive

(18–16) Ann. Surg. 193:462–466, April 1981.

RELATIONSHIP BETWEEN CLINICAL RESPONSE AND SPONTANEOUS PLATELET AGGREGATION AND ADP THRESHOLD PARAMETERS OF PLATELET SENSITIVITY

Patients		Spontaneous Platelet Aggregation	ADP Threshold (μM) <1	(Normal Range) 1–3.5	3.5+	Primary Aggregation Response Only
Responders	19	6*	9*	3	1	0
Nonresponders	16	2*	4*	6	2	2
Total	35	8*	13*	9	3	2

*Patients with sensitive platelets.

therapy. Nine of the 13 patients with increased sensitivity to ADP-induced platelet aggregation had a good response to therapy. Plasma β-thromboglobulin levels were higher than in normal subjects, but were comparable in the responders and nonresponders.

Abnormal platelet aggregation responses may be observed in patients with gangrene of the toes and palpable pulses, and may be associated with evidence of increased platelet activation. Antiplatelet drug therapy led to complete resolution of symptoms in more than half of the present patients. Many nonresponders had a good response to sympathectomy after medical treatment.

▶ [This subset of patients rarely received attention. A study of the pedal arches in these patients would have been of interest, particularly with the technique of hyperemic angiography. Antiplatelet drugs represent a logical approach, especially in view of the platelet hypersensitivity noted. Acute management could include Dextran, which coats the platelets and limits platelet aggregation.—S.I.S.] ◀

19. Veins and Lymphatics

19–1 **Heparin Therapy in Venous Thromboembolism.** In a study by James E. Wilson III, Lincoln J. Bynum, and Robert W. Parkey (Univ. of Texas, Dallas), 69 patients with pulmonary embolism and 45 with deep venous thrombosis were randomly assigned to receive either intermittent or continuous intravenous heparin therapy for 10–15 days. Lung scanning was used to document recurrent embolism.

The overall incidence of bleeding complications was 27% (major bleeding, 10%) and that of recurrent thromboembolism was 16%. For patients with a greater risk of bleeding, major bleeding was significantly more common during intermittent use of heparin; for patients without such risk factors, hemorrhage occurred with equal frequency during intermittent and continuous heparin therapy. For high-risk patients, the incidence of total bleeding episodes was 40%, compared to 17% for low-risk patients.

Adjustment of the heparin dose according to coagulation test results led to the administration of significantly larger daily doses of heparin with intermittent injections than with continuous infusion. When the intermittent route is used, significantly more heparin is required to keep the Lee-White clotting time or activated partial thromboplastin time 1½–2½ times the normal value immediately before the next dose is due. These test values were not statistically different for the group given heparin continuously and the group given heparin intermittently. Major bleeding complications with intermittent heparin therapy were significantly related to higher doses and a more prolonged Lee-White clotting time or activated partial thromboplastin time; 6 patients with major bleeding received a mean daily heparin dose of 45,450 ± 15,820 units/kg of ideal body weight, compared to the 36,660 ± 10,410 units/kg received by the 42 patients without major bleeding.

The patients who received continuous heparin therapy had recurrent thromboembolism significantly more often; there were no significant differences in average values for daily heparin dose, Lee-White clotting time, or activated partial thromboplastin time between patients with recurrences and those without. Of the 12 patients whose continuous heparin dose was adjusted according to coagulation test results, 8 who had 2 consecutive activated partial thromboplastin times of less than 45 seconds had a recurrence; the statistical significance was lost when patients receiving the standard dose of continuous heparin were included. The recurrence rate was no worse for patients receiving a standard dose of continuous heparin than when the continuous heparin dose was adjusted according to coagulation test re-

---

(19–1) Am. J. Med. 70:808–816, April 1981.

sults. However, the frequency with which coagulation test results were in the desired range was never more than 57% when control was attempted. Recurrence was not significantly associated either with absence of a precipitating cause or with previous venous thromboembolism.

The bleeding complications of intermittent heparin therapy could have been due to the higher dose, and the recurrences associated with continuous heparin therapy may have resulted from lower doses rather than from differences in the method of administration. In a small trial, lower heparin doses given intermittently (360 units/kg/24 hours), similar to the heparin doses given continuously, resulted in fewer bleeding complications and more recurrences.

For patients without risk factors for bleeding, the intermittent administration of heparin in higher dose is preferable, because there are fewer recurrences without increased hemorrhagic complications. For patients with a high bleeding risk, conventional heparin doses given continuously can reduce hemorrhagic complications but will result in more recurrences. It is suggested that major bleeding complications associated with intermittent intravenous heparin therapy are related as much to increased total dose as to peak blood levels. It is concluded that intermittent heparin therapy should be adjusted according to coagulation test results. It is recommended that the test used should be prolonged slightly, but not more than 1½ times normal, immediately before the next dose is due; a dosage of 480 units/kg/24 hours is usually sufficient.

The recurrence rate in this study was considered unacceptably high. Results of the small trial using 360 units/kg/24 hours of intermittent heparin therapy suggested that lower total dose was an important factor leading to recurrences. It is therefore recommended that the dose of intravenous heparin given continuously be pushed higher by attempting to keep the results of the coagulation test at least twice normal; a dosage of 480 units/kg/24 hours is frequently required.

▶ [There is now general agreement that the intravenous route of administration is preferred. The data in the present article that show some advantage to intermittent therapy certainly have a cost implication; many fusion pumps will become available. It would be interesting to compare the continuous and intermittent routes by monitoring thromboelastography and activated partial thromboplastin, as described by Lee et al. (*World J. Surg.* 4:323–330, 1980). These authors suggest that a more sensitive assessment is achieved and the dosage of heparin may be reduced.—S.I.S.] ◀

19–2 **Streptokinase Treatment of Deep Venous Thrombosis and the Postthrombotic Syndrome: Follow-up Evaluation of Venous Function.** The outcome of deep venous thrombosis (DVT) depends on the degree of thrombolysis and on the extent of restoration of valvular function. The results of streptokinase therapy, used to enhance lysis in DVT, have differed widely. Ulf Albrechtsson, Jan Anderson, Eibert Einarsson, Bo Eklöf, and Lars Norgren (Univ. of Lund) evaluated the results of streptokinase therapy by phlebography, foot volumetry, venous plethysmography, and intravenous femoral pressure measurements. Thirty-five patients with confirmed DVT were evalu-

---

(19–2) Arch. Surg. 116:33–37, January 1981.

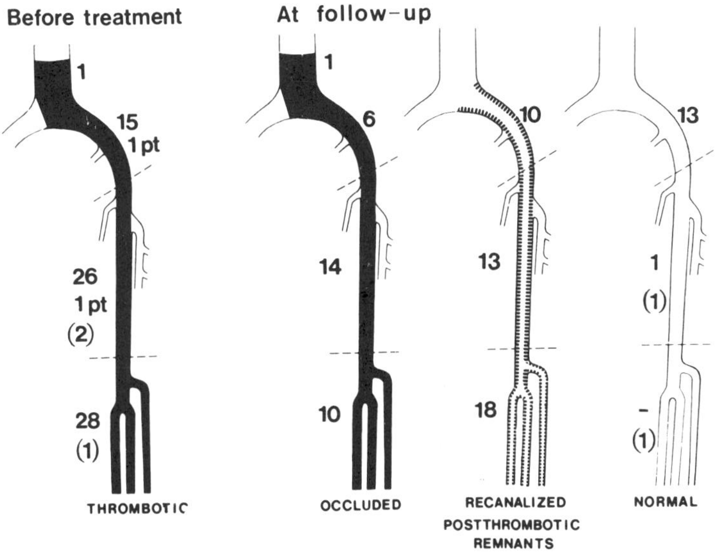

Fig 19–1.—Phlebographic findings in 28 patients (29 legs) before treatment and at follow-up. Number of legs with pathologic findings is shown for four parts of deep venous system: calf, femoral, and iliac veins, and inferior vena cava: Pt indicates postthrombotic changes. Numbers in parentheses indicate incomplete phlebogram. (Courtesy of Albrechtsson, U., et al.: Arch. Surg. 116:33–37, January 1981; copyright 1981, American Medical Association.)

ated 29 months after streptokinase therapy. An initial dose of 600,000 IU, given a mean of 3.7 days after the onset of symptoms, was followed by 100,000 IU/hour for up to 96 hours and then by heparin therapy. The 19 men and 16 women studied had a mean age of 54 years. Both legs were affected in 1 patient.

The phlebographic findings are shown in Figure 19–1. More than two thirds of the patients had leg symptoms at follow-up, and signs of venous insufficiency were found in 22 patients. Ten of 36 legs in 35 patients had good venous function by foot volumetry. Venous plethysmography indicated normal venous emptying in 6 of 36 legs examined. Femoral venous pressure was increased where iliac vein disease was present, especially during and after exercise. None of the patients had leg ulceration or severe postthrombotic syndrome.

None of these patients had a normal deep venous system at phlebography. Only 2 patients had normal plethysmographic and foot volumetric findings and were free of symptoms and abnormal physical findings. The phlebographic resolution of thrombi does not necessarily indicate that function has been restored. Relatively normal venous function and a good clinical outcome may be found where phlebography shows residual occlusion, if a good collateral circulation is present. Serious postthrombotic syndrome may be less likely to develop in patients with good venous function. Streptokinase therapy may save some venous valves and prevent severe postthrombotic syndrome, but treatment must be monitored more carefully with respect to dosage and time to obtain good results.

▶ [Each year there is a continuum in reports of streptokinase treatment of deep venous thrombosis, and each year the reports are characterized by extreme variability of results. The present article shows an absence of a normal deep venous system in any patient after therapy; a high rate of persistent occlusion is in keeping with most series. The authors' addition of plethysmography and foot volumetry provides added evidence for the lack of efficacy of this treatment. The authors make a most critical point that phlebographic resolution of thrombi does not mean that function is restored. Certainly, nobody is standing in line to get his supply of the medication to treat these disorders, and equivalent results have been achieved with simple early heparin therapy.—S.I.S.] ◀

19–3 **Greenfield Vena Caval Filter Experience: Late Results in 156 Patients.** Lazar J. Greenfield, Rodney Peyton, Stephen Crute, and Robert Barnes (Med. College of Virginia, Richmond) reviewed experience with use of the Greenfield caval filter in 156 patients followed up for an average of 23 months. There were 99 male and 57 female patients, with an average age of 53 years. Patients anticoagulated with heparin preoperatively had treatment resumed 12 hours postoperatively and generally received oral anticoagulation for at least 4 months. The filter insertion method was modified by attachment of an infusion line to the catheter carrier for continuous administration of heparinized saline, to avoid thrombus formation within the cylinder. The filter generally was discharged at the L3 level.

The most common indication for filter insertion was the inability to use anticoagulant therapy because of a significant contraindication. Forty-seven patients had had recurrent embolism during anticoagulant therapy. Twenty-seven were treated purely prophylactically. Access for filter placement was usually via the internal jugular vein. In 7% of cases, the filter was misplaced. No deaths were directly attributed to the procedure. In 19 instances, the filter was discharged in a tilted position. Recurrent embolism was suspected in 6 instances. The documented patency rate in 59 patients observed for up to 63 months by venacavography was 95%. Anticoagulant administration following the procedure was not correlated with subsequent caval patency.

Transvenous placement of a filter device now is the preferred means of preventing thromboembolism in all patients who require mechanical protection. The procedure is safe in patients who can hold their breath for a few seconds when the jugular vein is open. Sepsis has not contraindicated filter insertion. The incidence of recurrent embolism has remained low, probably in part because of continued filtration of caval flow. There is no evidence that the filter will jeopardize vena caval patency.

▶ [This represents a summation of experience at the center where it all began. The results are certainly encouraging and are in keeping with the study of Cimochowski et al. (*J. Thorac. Cardiovasc. Surg.* 79:358–365, 1980). Those authors reported that although the recurrence rate for nonfatal pulmonary emboli was the same with the Mobin-Uddin umbrella and the Greenfield filter, the occlusion rate was only 5% with the Greenfield filter as contrasted with 37% with the Mobin-Uddin umbrella. In discussion of Greenfield's paper, Mobin-Uddin points out that the new heparin-bonded filter may reduce the occlusion rate, and in his own experience this has been only 40%. Another point made in the discussion, and one that I strongly espouse, is that the need for use of any caval obstructive device should be quite minimal. Heparin remains the keystone of therapy, and at our own institution we do not occlude the cava in more than 4 patients per year.—S.I.S.] ◀

(19–3) Arch. Surg. 116:1451–1456, November 1981.

19-4 **Late Objective Assessment of Venous Valve Surgery.** Kistner recommended direct valve repair for femoral venous valve incompetence. Norris D. Johnson, Luis A. Queral, William R. Flinn, James S. T. Yao, and John J. Bergan (Northwestern Univ., Chicago) followed up 10 patients who underwent femoral valve transposition without saphenous vein stripping or ligation of perforators on 12 extremities, for 12–18 months. Successful surgery was confirmed by ascending and descending venography in these cases. Venous pressures were measured, and photoplethysmography was carried out. The operation was designed to transpose a valve-containing vein segment into the main deep venous flow stream at the groin level. A greater saphenous venous segment was used in 10 limbs, and a profunda femoris segment was used in 2.

At follow-up, persistent venous skin changes were seen in 9 limbs of 7 patients. All of these patients required elastic support to control venous stasis. Recurrent venous ulcers were present in 4 limbs. The venous refilling time was normal immediately after surgery in 11 limbs, but reversed to an abnormal level in 9 limbs at follow-up. Resting venous pressure and the pressure fall on exercise were unchanged after surgery and at follow-up. In 2 instances, repeated venography showed a patent reconstruction and a competent valve, but both limbs had severe postphlebitic changes of the femoral, popliteal, and calf veins.

In contrast to Kistner's cases, a direct surgical attack on the calf perforators was not made in the present patients. Far-advanced postthrombotic changes in the popliteal, calf, and superficial veins are not likely to benefit from femoral valve repair alone. In addition, the assessment of valvular incompetence by descending venography may not be totally accurate. Kistner's procedure is sound if venous insufficiency is primarily the result of femoral valve incompetence without femoral or popliteal occlusion, and with no or only minimal incompetence of communicating veins. However, isolated femoral valve incompetence is rare.

▶ [This represents a follow-up of the previous article reported by Queral et al. (*Surgery* 87:688–695, 1980) at the same institution. That article represented an affirmation of the procedure proposed by Kistner and Sparkle and was related to improvement in postexercise pressure recovery time and skin refilling time. The present article more appropriately addresses the central issue and is more negative. However, Kistner, the inventor of the procedure, emphasizes in the discussion that repair alone rarely reverses all the dynamics in the patient with chronic insufficiency. This suggests that the report merely emphasizes selectivity. Using criteria of selectivity, Kempczinski, in the discussion, has reported favorable results.—S.I.S.] ◀

19-5 **The Prognosis of Primary Lymphedema of the Lower Limbs.** Most patients with primary lymphedema can be controlled symptomatically by conservative measures, but it is not clear whether severe lymphedema will eventually develop in some. John H. N. Wolfe and J. B. Kinmonth (Univ. of London) examined the course of clinical lymphedema in a series of 372 patients seen with primary lymphedema of the legs in 1970–1978. Lymphography showed distal hypo-

---

(19–4) Arch. Surg. 116:1461–1466, November 1981.
(19–5) Ibid., pp. 1157–1160, September 1981.

plasia or aplasia in 91 cases; proximal hypoplasia in 60; both distal and proximal hypoplasia in 93; bilateral hyperplasia in 29; and the megalymphatic form of disease in 12. Forty-nine other patients did not have lymphography, and 38 did not have inguinal lymphography.

Congenital lymphedema was present in 10% of patients, whereas 19% had an onset after age 35 years. The course is shown in Figure 19–2; the median duration of disease at follow-up was similar in the various groups. Women constituted 72% of patients. Extension of lymphedema was unusual after the first year of symptoms and occurred after 5 years in only 3 patients. Lymphedema of the thigh did not develop after the first year of symptoms in any patient with distal hypoplasia. More than one third of patients showed a progressive increase in leg girth. This was most frequent in the groups with proximal obstructive hypoplasia and bilateral hyperplasia. Proximal obstructive hypoplasia was the likeliest form to cause severe edema; about one third of patients eventually required surgery (table). Distal hypoplasia appeared to be the least severe form of lymphedema. Recurrent cellulitis was most common in patients with evidence of proximal obstruction. Lymphedema of the entire extremity was present in more than 80% of patients with proximal obstructive hypoplasia but in only 2% of patients with distal hypoplasia.

Mild bilateral lymphedema associated with distal hypoplasia is well controlled by conservative measures. Some patients have a rapidly

Fig 19–2.—The progress of primary lymphedema of legs. (Courtesy of Wolfe, J. H. N., and Kinmonth, J. B.: Arch. Surg. 116:1157–1160, September 1981; copyright 1981, American Medical Association.)

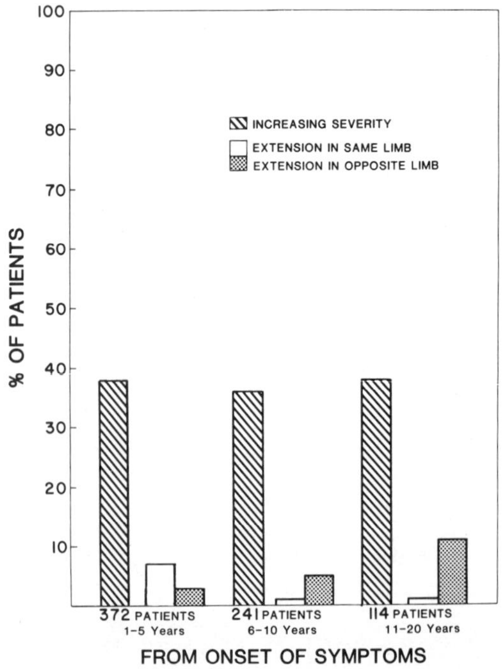

CLINICAL FEATURES RELATED TO LYMPHANGIOGRAPHIC CLASSIFICATION

	M/F Ratio	Unilateral Clinical Lymphedema, %	Whole-Limb Lymphedema, %	Leg-Reducing Surgery Required, %
Overall*	1:3	41	36	16
Hypoplasia				
Distal	1:9	30	2	1
Distal and proximal	1:3	54	49	22
Proximal obstructive	1:1	63	82	32
Hyperplasia				
Bilateral	3:2	10	24	3
Megalymphatics	3:2	83	75	25

*This group includes 49 patients who did not have lymphangiography and 38 patients with unclassified hypoplasia.

progressive disease starting in the pelvis, which may be controlled by lymphonodal venous shunt surgery or by a small bowel mesenteric bridge procedure.

▶ [The name "Kinmonth" is almost synonymous with lymphedema, because his contributions have been so extensive. The present work, therefore, truly represents a lifetime of clinical experience by one man. This categorization of patients is particularly important as far as prognosis is concerned and as a guide to which patients will require surgical intervention. For those patients in whom operation is required, the work of O'Brien and Shafiroff (*World J. Surg.* 3:3–15, 1979), which reports the results of microlymphaticovenous and resectional surgery in obstructive lymphedema, chronicles a modern approach. In keeping with the point made by Wolf and Kinmonth, the use of surgical intervention generally focuses on patients with obstruction of the proximal lymphatics and on those lymphatics located in the pelvis.—S.I.S.] ◀

19–6 **Microsurgical Treatment of Lymphedemas of the Limbs.** Many surgical methods have been proposed to treat lymphedema of the limb, but only rarely have the functional results been satisfactory. U. Fox, M. Montorsi, and G. Romagnoli (Univ. of Milan) performed 20 lymphaticovenous anastomoses for lymphedema of the limb in 1976–1980. The 18 women and 2 men were aged 15–71 years. Eight secondary and 12 primary lymphedemas were treated. Four secondary cases and 1 primary case affected the arm. Patients were followed up for 2 months to 4 years. Surgery was performed after a long period of antimicrobial and anti-inflammatory treatment and lymphography. A microsurgical technique was utilized. After dissecting tracts of lymphatic vessels and veins from the subcutaneous tissue, Degni's needle was used to introduce lymphatics in the vein and secure them to its wall with 8–0 monofilament stitches (Fig 19–3). The humeral vein is used in the arm, and the great saphenous vein is used in the leg. Positive pressure is applied to the operated limb starting on the second postoperative day.

Good results were obtained in 2 of 4 postmastectomy lymphedemas;

(19–6) Int. Surg. 66:53–56, Jan.–Mar. 1981.

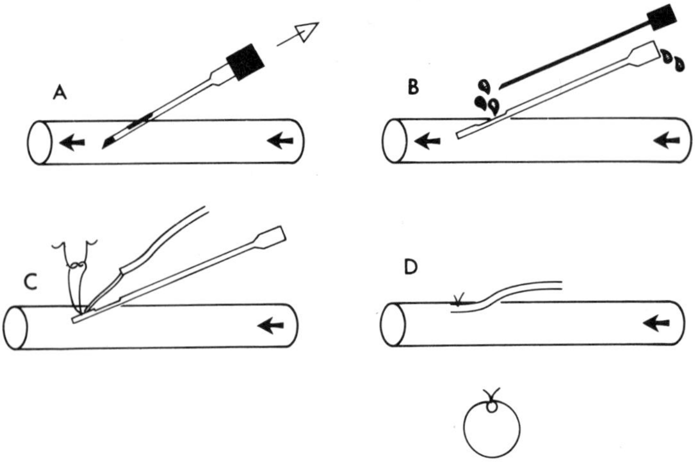

Fig 19–3.—**A,** needle is inserted into vein. **B,** mandril is removed. **C,** lymphatic is inserted into vein. **D,** lymphatic is secured to vein wall. (Courtesy of Fox, U., et al.: Int. Surg. 66:53–56, Jan.–Mar. 1981.)

the other 2 patients did not receive preoperative anti-inflammatory therapy and had attacks of lymphangitis in the early postoperative period. In secondary lymphedemas of the legs, a mean volumetric reduction of 50% was obtained, and the results have been stable. The best results were obtained in patients with primary lymphedemas, especially of a minor grade. Nine of 11 such patients had good subjective improvement (table). The decrease in limb tension and discomfort permitted the patients to resume their normal activities and return to work.

Lymphaticovenous anastomosis with Degni's needle is a relatively safe and brief procedure, with no morbidity. An attempt at surgery always is worthwhile in primary lymphedemas. The results at up to 4 years have been as good as the early results, with a persistent reduction in limb volume. In secondary lymphedemas of the arm, long-term preoperative anti-inflammatory and antimicrobial therapy is

RESULTS OF LYMPHATICOVENOUS ANASTOMOSES FOR SURGICAL TREATMENT OF LYMPHEDEMA OF THE LIMBS

		Good *	Fair **	Unchanged ***
Upper limbs	Secondary	2	1	1
	Primary		1	
Lower limbs	Secondary	3	1	
	Primary	9	1	1
Total		14	4	2

*Subjective and objective improvement.
**Subjective improvement.
***No improvement.

necessary to prevent lymphangitis that can compromise the results of surgery.

▶ [Most of the literature related to the therapy of lymphedema focuses on decreasing tissue bulk, using excision techniques employed in the Charles or Thompson procedures. Miller et al. (*Surg. Gynecol. Obstet.* 136:586, 1973) have reported favorable results after staged subcutaneous excision. The present report was an exciting experience. It parallels that published by O'Brien and Shafiroff (*World J. Surg.* 3:3–15, 1979) who combined a microsurgical and resectional segmental technique to treat lymphedema. A lipocutaneous resection with minimal underlining is performed, and at the same time a lymphaticovenous anastomosis is created by a direct vascular suture technique; an average of 3.9 anastomoses were performed in 35 evaluable patients. The widespread use of the dissecting microscope should allow expansion of this field. The present report represents an interesting simplification of the anastomotic procedure.—S.I.S.] ◀

20. Esophagus

20–1 **Lower Esophageal Sphincter Pressure as an Index of Gastroesophageal Acid Reflux.** Previous studies have not measured lower esophageal sphincter (LES) pressure and pH reflux simultaneously, and they involved placement of a fixed acid load in the stomach. George Ahtaridis, William J. Snape, Jr., and Sidney Cohen (Philadelphia) have recently measured LES pressure and esophageal pH simultaneously in 20 consecutive patients with heartburn and regurgitation, 4 of whom had peptic strictures, and in 35 asymptomatic volunteers with no history of gastrointestinal disease. After an overnight fast, measurements were recorded by using a multilumen polyvinyl manometry catheter during the gradual instillation of N/10 HC1 into the stomach.

The LES pressures obtained are shown in Figure 20–1. Symptomatic patients had a mean LES pressure of 7.5 mm Hg and refluxed at a mean acid volume of 140 ml. Asymptomatic refluxers had a mean pressure of 13.8 mm Hg and refluxed at a mean acid volume of 380 ml. The asymptomatic nonrefluxers had a mean LES pressure of 18.9 mm Hg and showed no reflux at an acid volume of 500 ml. Individual pressures overlapped, but the mean group pressures differed significantly, as did the mean acid volumes required to produce reflux. The overall correlation between these parameters was excellent and is shown in Figure 20–2. The continuous linear relation between pressure and volume suggested that competence of the antireflux mechanism was directly correlated with intrinsic LES pressure and the amount of acid in the stomach.

Results of a separate study of 7 subjects in which acid was infused at the same volume at which reflux first occurred correlated very well with those of the main study. At 100 ml, 60% of symptomatic patients and none who were asymptomatic exhibited reflux. At 300 ml, all symptomatic and 23% of asymptomatic subjects had reflux. Reflux was followed by a sustained elevation of LES pressure in asymptomatic subjects, and the increase was significant when compared with the prereflux pressure.

The LES pressure provides an accurate index of the strength of the gastroesophageal antireflux mechanism if the acid volume placed in the stomach is taken into account. In intermediate cases, factors other than LES pressure may be important in determining symptoms of gastroesophageal reflux.

▶ [Since Cohen and Harris originally pointed out the importance of the lower esophageal sphincter in the prevention of gastroesophageal reflux (*N. Engl. J. Med.* 284:1053, 1971), numerous investigators have been very critical of the use of lower

---

(20–1) Dig. Dis. Sci. 26:993–998, November 1981.

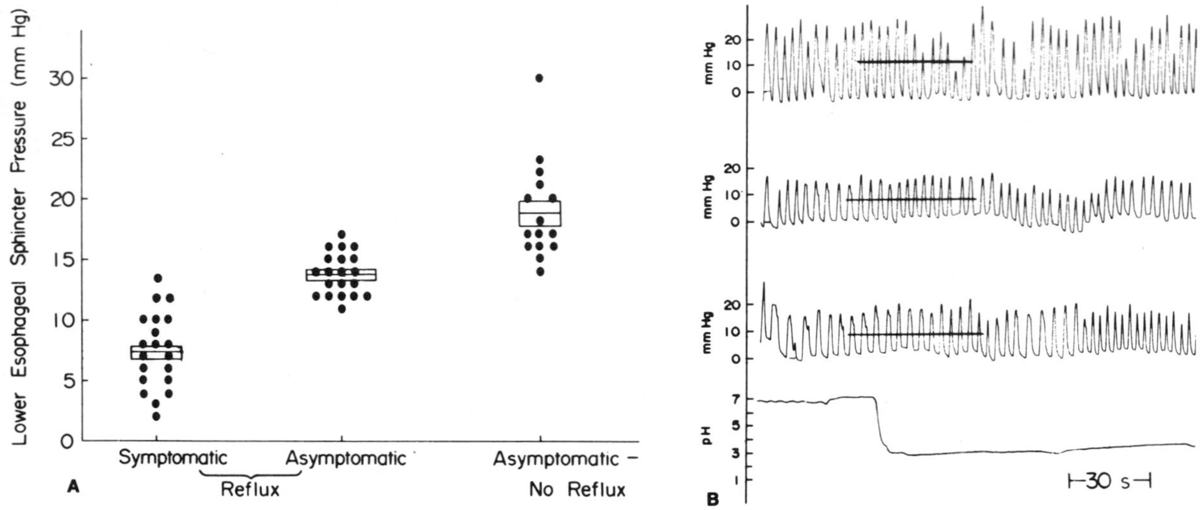

Fig 20–1.—A, LES pressure in all subjects and patients, who were divided into three major groups based on symptoms of reflux and presence of reflux during acid instillation into stomach. Although individual LES pressures showed overlap, mean LES pressure values for the three groups were significantly different. **B,** simultaneous recording of LES pressure and esophageal pH following instillation of 200 ml of acid into stomach. (Courtesy of Ahtaridis, G., et al.: Dig. Dis. Sci. 26:993–998, November 1981.)

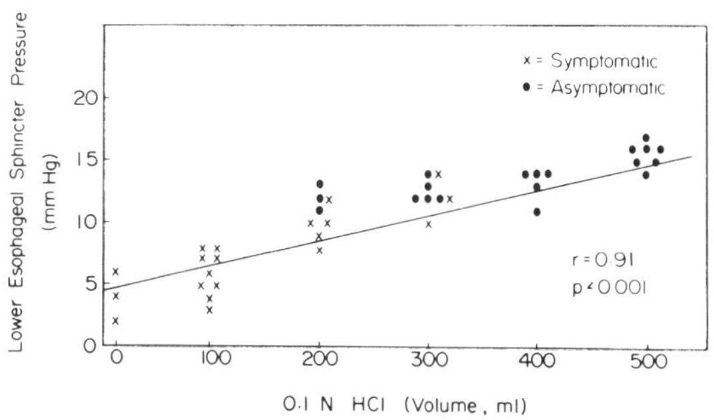

Fig 20–2.—Overall correlation between LES pressure and N/10 HCl acid volume at which esophageal reflux was first noted. Pressure and acid volume required to produce reflux showed excellent linear correlation for both symptomatic *(crosses)* and asymptomatic *(solid circles)* subjects showing reflux to a volume of 500 ml of acid. Symptomatic subjects had lower sphincter pressure and refluxed at lower acid volumes than asymptomatic individuals. (Courtesy of Ahtaridis, G., et al.: Dig. Dis. Sci. 26:993–998, November 1981.)

esophageal sphincter pressure as an accurate index of the gastroesophageal antireflux mechanism. For that reason, the 24-hour measurement of gastroesophageal reflux by an indwelling pH electrode has become very popular. In my opnion, the measurement of pH during a 24-hour period is probably too sensitive an index of gastroesophageal reflux and, basically, clinical decisions are really made on whether or not the patient has significant and serious symptomatic heartburn. The present study is an excellent one that puts into perspective the importance of the lower esophageal sphincter in protecting against gastroesophageal reflux, especially because the authors have demonstrated that patients with serious and symptomatic reflux generally do not respond to acid reflux with a reflex contraction of the lower esophageal sphincter, as do persons who do not have symptoms. For practical purposes, even though there may be methodologic problems associated with the measurement of lower esophageal sphincter pressure, pressures of lower than 10 mm Hg are almost invariably found in patients with symptomatic reflux, whereas pressures greater than that are not usually associated with symptoms. After all, the presence or absence of symptoms is really the major and important factor in our assessment of patients.—W.S.] ◀

20–2 **Gastric Acid Secretion (GAS) and Hiatal Hernia.**—*I. Relationship between GAS and esophageal reflux complications.*—Some studies show a relationship between GAS and esophageal reflux complications in patients with hiatal hernia and incompetent antireflux mechanism, and others do not. In most of these studies, however, factors other than GAS were not studied. Pantalei Gatzinsky, Göran Granerus, and Nils Sandberg (Univ. of Göteborg) took age and esophageal motility into account in a study of the relationship between GAS and esophageal reflux complications in 70 consecutive patients (45 men and 25 women aged 21 to 78 years) operated on for hiatal hernia and symptomatic gastroesophageal reflux.

There was no correlation between basal acid output (BAO) and peak acid output (PAO) in individual patients. High BAO was found in 16 patients and high PAO in 32. Patients with low BAO and PAO were generally older than those with normal and high BAO and PAO. Mean age of the 37 patients with severe reflux complications (ulcerative esophagitis, stricture, shortened esophagus) was higher than that of

(20–2) Acta Chir. Scand. 146:583–589, 1980.

patients without such complications. Mean age of the 31 patients with esophageal hypomotility was higher than that of those with normal motility. There was no significant difference in mean BAO or mean PAO between patients with and without severe reflux complications. High BAO occurred in 21% of patients with and in 25% of those without reflux complications, but high PAO occurred in 62% of patients with and in 27% of those without reflux complications.

There was no correlation between BAO and PAO, respectively, and esophageal motility. Esophageal hypomotility was found in 70% of patients with and in 15% of those without severe reflux complications, for a close correlation between esophageal hypomotility and severe reflux complications. There was no correlation between BAO or PAO and severe reflux complications in patients with esophageal hypomotility. In those with normal esophageal motility, however, there was a relationship between severe reflux complications and BAO and PAO, as reflux complications occurred in 50% of those with high PAO and normal esophageal motility compared with 16% of those with low and normal PAO. Severe reflux complications were clearly related to age.

The observed interplay between several factors means that the dominating factor in the development of severe reflux complications may be different in different patients, but esophageal hypomotility probably has a major role in the development of such complications. It appears that normal esophageal motility and younger age protect against the noxious action of refluxed gastric acid, but when this protective barrier is weakened or disappears, the risk of development of severe reflux complications is increased. Thus, increased GAS, as determined by measurement of PAO, is a significant risk factor for development of severe reflux complications in patients with hiatal hernia and incompetent antireflux mechanism, particularly after the age of 60 years.

20–3 *II. Relationship between GAS and clinical results after hernia repair.*—Gatzinsky, Granerus, and Sandberg studied the influence of gastric acid secretion (GAS) on the results of surgery in patients with hiatal hernia and symptomatic gastroesophageal reflux in order to assess the indications for gastric acid-reducing procedures in these patients.

Of 70 patients with hiatal hernia and symptomatic gastroesophageal reflux, 27 underwent surgical procedures that included division of vagal nerves (these patients were excluded from the study) and 43 underwent a modified Husfeldt hernia repair performed through a left-sided thoracotomy between the seventh and eighth ribs (Fig 20–3). The procedure included restoration of the abdominal esophagus, narrowing of the widened esophageal hiatus, restoration of the acute gastroesophageal angle, partial (180-degree) fundoplication, and partial fundodiaphragmopexy. None of these 43 patients underwent vagotomy or any other procedure aimed at reducing GAS or facilitating gastric emptying. Of the 43 study patients, 1 died postoperatively, 2

(20–3) Acta Chir. Scand. 146:591–595, 1980.

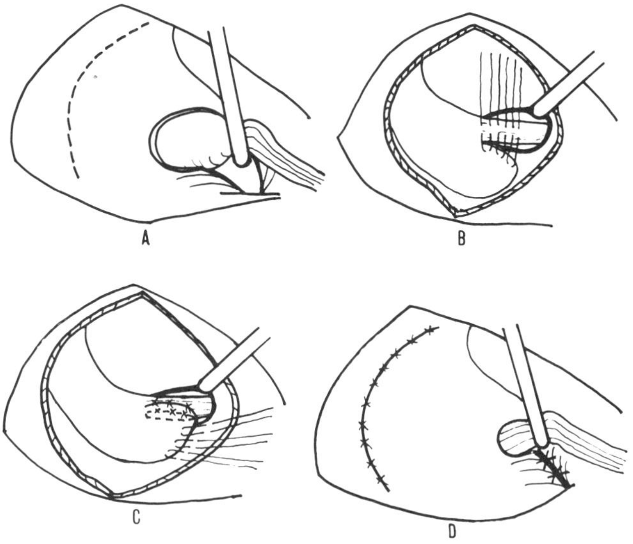

Fig 20–3.—Modified Husfeldt repair. **A,** herniated part of stomach and lower esophagus are mobilized. *Broken line,* diaphragmatic incision. **B,** abdomen is entered, cardia repositioned, and sutures for fundoplication are placed. **C,** fundoplication is completed and fundus sutured to inferior surface of adjoining diaphragm. **D,** incision is sutured and hiatus opening narrowed by posterior cruraplasty. (Courtesy of Gatzinsky, P., et al.: Acta Chir. Scand. 146:591–595, 1980.)

were lost to follow-up, and 40 (26 men and 14 women aged 21 to 68 years) were followed for 1 to 4 years.

Postoperatively, 27 patients were asymptomatic, 8 had occasional mild symptoms that did not require treatment, 2 were improved but needed some treatment, and 3 were unchanged or worsened. The clinical results depended on success or failure of correction of the pathologic gastroesophageal reflux. In 29 patients gastroesophageal reflux was not detected and in all the clinical results were satisfactory regardless of basal or peak acid output. The other 11 patients had gastroesophageal reflux of varying degree, and 5 of these had unsatisfactory clinical results.

Esophageal hypomotility was associated with poor clinical results. Of 5 patients with poor results, 4 had esophageal hypomotility. All 6 patients with gastroesophageal reflux and satisfactory results had normal esophageal motility. Gastric acid secretion did not influence the clinical results.

The main reason for unsuccessful clinical results after surgical repair of hiatal hernia was failure of the procedure to correct pathologic gastroesophageal reflux, indicating that high basal and peak acid output do not influence the results if the procedure has fulfilled its main objective of correcting pathologic gastroesophageal reflux. Thus, in patients in whom correction of gastroesophageal reflux is anticipated, a supplementary procedure aimed at reducing GAS is not indicated unless other indications (e.g., duodenal ulcer) are present.

▶ [The salient features of this article and the preceding one are worth reiteration. It seems quite clear that severe complications of esophageal reflux are related more closely to esophageal hypomotility and abnormalities in esophageal muscular function and also to increasing age than they are to acid secretion. In addition, the basal acid output seems to have very little relationship to preoperative symptomatology, whereas there seems to be a correlation between the peak acid output (PAO) and symptomatology only in patients who have normal esophageal motility. In other words, in those patients who had poor esophageal motility, there was no relationship between symptoms and PAO, whereas in those who had normal esophageal motility, there was such a relationship. Finally, it seems that there was no correlation between the clinical results of an antireflux operation and either the basal acid output or the PAO. It would appear that the success of the operation is solely dependent on whether reflux is prevented or not.

It should be emphasized that these authors did not carry out a complete fundic wrap, and therefore one could suggest that the outcome of the surgical procedure might be improved somewhat by increasing the degree of fundic wrapping. It is very clear, however, that the outcome of the surgical procedure is not at all influenced by the preoperative gastric acid secretion, whereas the esophageal hypomotility was associated with unsatisfactory clinical results in what appears to be a significant number of cases. I would agree completely with the suggestions of the authors that complementary acid reducing operations not be done in patients with symptomatic gastroesophageal reflux.

One of the most important questions that remains is whether the hypomotility of the esophagus is a primary disorder that results from increasing age or whether it is a disorder secondary to intense and prolonged gastroesophageal reflux. It is possible that the latter is operative because the worst results were encountered in those patients who had the poor esophageal motility. It seems evident that other studies are now showing that a very high incidence of esophageal motor abnormalities are present in these patients and that such motor abnormalities persist even after successful antireflux operations. This area certainly is deserving of further study.—W.S.] ◀

20–4 **Supradiaphragmatic Correction of Esophageal Reflux Strictures.** Severe fibrotic strictures of the esophagus secondary to reflux esophagitis develop in 5% to 20% of patients having operative correction of reflux. Their management is controversial. Timothy C. Pennell (Bowman Gray School of Medicine) evaluated intraoperative dilatation and an antireflux procedure in a monkey model of esophageal reflux and in patients. Reflux was produced in monkeys by making double pursestring gastrostomies, introducing barium sulfate solution, and increasing the intragastric pressure. A series of antireflux procedures was performed, including Hill median arcuate ligament posterior gastropexies, Belsey Mark IV procedures, and Nissen fundoplications. Reflux esophagitis was prevented most effectively by the Nissen fundoplication. The floppy Nissen fundoplication was as effective as the conventional procedure, whether done above or below the diaphragm.

Nineteen severely dysphagic adults with esophageal reflux and strictures were operated on. One patient underwent esophageal resection for adenocarcinoma. The others underwent transthoracic Nissen fundoplication after intraoperative dilatation. In 2 patients the fundoplications were placed subdiaphragmatically, whereas in 16 the antireflux valves were supradiaphragmatic. Seromuscular sutures were placed so as to prevent paraesophageal and other herniation. All 16 patients with a supradiaphragmatic Nissen fundoplication had good postoperative results, with no dysphagia or obstructive symptoms on taking a normal diet. The 2 patients having conventional fundopli-

(20–4) Ann. Surg. 193:655–665, May 1981.

cation procedures had esophageal bleeding from superficial ulcers at the fundic wrap, but did well after dilatation. No deaths or postoperative complications occurred. All but 2 patients were followed for over a year.

Transthoracic intraoperative dilatation followed by a supradiaphragmatic Nissen fundoplication is the preferred procedure for treating both annular and longitudinal esophageal strictures resulting from esophageal reflux.

▶ [It has been established beyond any doubt that Nissen fundoplication is an effective antireflux operation whether the repair is left within the thorax or whether it is placed below the diaphragm. The experimental findings of Pennell would also substantiate those of Butterfield in suggesting that this antireflux operation, as is true of all other effective antireflux procedures, produces an inanimate flap valve mechanism rather than altering anything inherent in the lower esophageal sphincter muscle.

On the one hand, Pennell and Woodward indicate that there is little adverse effect of leaving the Nissen fundoplication within the thoracic cavity. Pennell suggests that the lack of tension achieved by leaving such a repair within the thorax may be beneficial. On the other hand, other surgeons, such as Polk and Hatcher, have reported a high incidence of complications when the Nissen fundoplication is left within the thoracic cavity. It is entirely possible, if not likely, that small technical details may play a role in explaining the differences in outcome. It is important to point out that Pennell neither opens the diaphragmatic hiatus nor makes an incision in the diaphragm. Other authors are not quite so specific about the details of their operative procedure, and it is possible that the serious complications described by Polk and others, such as gastric ulceration and gastric stasis, might have been the result of large portions of the fundus of the stomach herniating into the chest through an enlarged hiatus or through an incision in the diaphragm. These are mere speculations, but some attempt must be made to explain the differences in these findings. I have encountered one instance of severe gastric stasis that resulted from poor emptying of a gastric pouch above the diaphragm after an intrathoracic Nissen procedure. We need more studies on this problem, and we need more interchange to find the explanation for these discrepancies in observations.—W.S.] ◀

0–5 **Principles of Surgical Treatment For Carcinoma of the Esophagus: Analysis of Lymph Node Involvement.** Hiroshi Akiyama, Masahiko Tsurumaru, Takeshi Kawamura, and Yoshimasa Ono (Tokyo) reviewed the findings from 354 cases of esophageal carcinoma seen in 1972–1981. Tumors of the hypopharynx and cervical esophagus and tumors of the esophagogastric junction were excluded from the study. All 354 patients had squamous cell carcinomas. A total of 210 patients underwent resections and reconstructions. Men constituted a large majority of patients; the peak age distribution was 60–69 years. The middle part of the esophagus was involved in 62% of cases. Care was taken to avoid damaging the recurrent nerves during dissection of the paratracheal nodes. Nodes around the ligamentum arteriosum, the left pulmonary hilar nodes, and the para-aortic nodes also were dissected.

Cancer-positive lymph nodes were found in 59% of the 205 patients who had systematic node dissection. Of all the nodes evaluated, 6.4% were positive. The findings are related to the site of tumor in Table 1. Pulmonary complications were the most common postoperative problem, followed by hoarseness (Table 2). Anastomotic leakage occurred in 5.2% of cases, but all leaks were minor. The operative mor-

(20–5) Ann. Surg. 194:438–446, October 1981.

TABLE 1.—Rate of Positive Lymph Nodes Related to Site of Tumor*

Group of Lymph Nodes	Location of Tumor: Upper Esophagus	Middle Esophagus	Lower Esophagus	Total
Thoracic				
superior mediastinal	29.4 (8.3)	11.4 (4.6)	9.8 (2.7)	
middle mediastinal	27.3 (7.7)	20.7 (4.7)	14.3 (2.4)	18.7 (5.2)
lower mediastinal	28.6 (7.8)	18.0 (4.9)	27.4 (9.5)	
Abdominal				
superior gastric	31.8 (3.0)	32.8 (6.6)	61.5 (14.1)	
celiac axis nodes	0 (0)	4.4 (2.9)	21.2 (11.6)	
common hepatic artery lymph nodes	0 (0)	2.0 (1.1)	9.8 (6.0)	18.9 (7.5)
splenic artery lymph nodes	0 (0)	6.3 (5.6)	15.0 (7.1)	

*Percentage of positive lymph nodes per number of patients (per number of lymph nodes examined).

tality was 1.4%. Survival is related to the nodal findings in Figure 20–4. Patients followed for 5 years or more had a much greater survival when the nodes were negative (53.8% vs. 15.3%). The overall 5-year survival rate was 34.6%.

Complete node dissection in the mediastinum and abdomen is necessary, regardless of the anatomical site of esophageal carcinoma. Total thoracic and abdominal esophagectomy with removal of the cardia and the proximal part of the lesser gastric curvature is a reasonable procedure. A right thoracotomy will provide a better exposure of the

TABLE 2.—Postoperative Complications After 210 Resections*

Complications	Number	Per Cent
Pulmonary complications	28 (1)	13.3
Hoarseness	24 (0)	11.4
Anastomotic leakage	11 (0)	5.2
Cardiac complications	9 (0)	4.3
Hepatic failure	1 (1)	0.5
Superior mesenteric thrombosis	1 (1)	0.5

*Operative mortality: 1.4%. Numbers in parentheses indicate number of operative deaths.

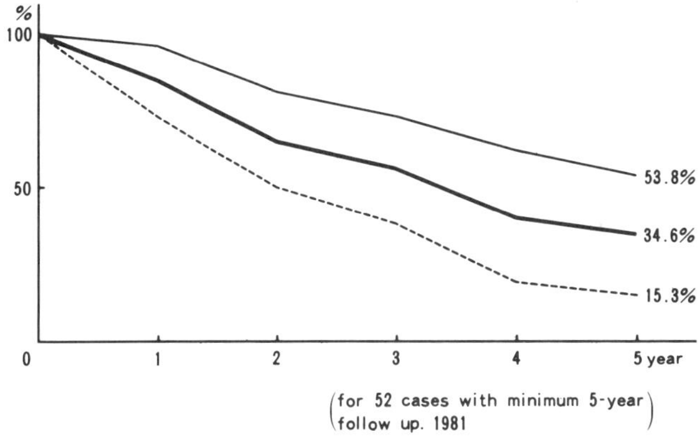

Fig 20–4.—Survival curve related to findings of lymph node involvement. *Thin solid line,* patients with negative lymph nodes. *Bold solid line,* overall survival. *Broken line,* patients with positive lymph nodes. (Courtesy of Akiyama, H., et al.: Ann. Surg. 194:438–446, October 1981.)

entire posterior mediastinum. Esophagotomy into the neck is useful to avoid a cancer-positive surgical margin. Staged surgery is recommended to reduce the risks, but satisfactory results have been obtained with one-stage surgery. Anastomosis routinely is performed in the neck. Esophageal replacement is performed in the retrosternal space. Radiotherapy, chemotherapy, and immunotherapy may be useful adjunctive measures.

▶ [The authors who have presented this extraordinary series of cases are to be congratulated not only for the extremely low mortality and morbidity but also for the superb 5-year survival. To my knowledge, there are no other series of cases of squamous cell carcinoma of the esophagus in which such outstanding results have been achieved. One of the important major findings of this study is that lymph node metastases may be very extensive in patients with squamous cell carcinoma of the esophagus. For example, even when the tumor was located in the upper esophagus, nodal metastases were present in the upper gastric area in almost one third of the cases. Conversely, when the tumor was located in the lower esophagus, involved lymph nodes were found in the superior mediastinum in roughly 10% of the patients. Perhaps these findings are the reasons that we have had such dismal failure in treating this disease both surgically and radiologically, because even radiologic treatment generally does not encompass all of the node-bearing areas that Akiyama and his coworkers have demonstrated to be involved. It is to be emphasized that approximately 40% of the patients encountered by the authors did not undergo the kind of resection described in this article, a point that is made by Akiyama in the discussion of the paper. The reasons for exclusion are not completely clear, although the presence of hepatic metastases and other blood-borne metastases are obvious indications for exclusion. It would have been nice, however, to know what other factors caused such exclusions, because it is vital that the criteria for selection be extremely clear. It is doubtful that every surgeon can achieve the low mortality and morbidity produced by Akiyama and his associates, but it is certainly a goal to be sought.—W.S.] ◀

-6 **Eradication and Palliation of Squamous Cell Carcinoma of the Esophagus With Chemotherapy, Radiotherapy, and Surgical Therapy.** Z. Steiger, R. Franklin, R. F. Wilson, L. Leichman, H. Seydel, J. J. K. Loh, G. Vaishamapayan, T. Knechtges, I. Asfaw, A. Dindogru, J. C. Rosenberg, T. Buroker, A. Torres, D. Hoschner, P.

(20–6) J. Thorac. Cardiovasc. Surg. 82:713–719, November 1981.

Miller, T. Pietruk, and V. Vaitkevicius evaluated combined chemotherapy and radiotherapy, followed by surgery where feasible, in 86 consecutive cases of proved squamous cell carcinoma of the esophagus. The 75 men and 11 women in the study had a mean age of 57 years. Two thirds of the patients had T2 N0 M0 (stage II) lesions. Chemotherapy consisted of administration of 5-fluorouracil and mitomycin C or, in more recent cases, cis-platinum. Administration of 3,000 rad was started at the same time as chemotherapy. Esophagectomy was done, when appropriate, 3–4 weeks after the completion of chemotherapy and radiotherapy. Further radiotherapy and chemotherapy were given if residual disease was found.

The mortality in 48 patients with esophagectomy was 10.4%. Four patients died later of sepsis. Two patients had late anastomotic strictures that required dilatation. Major complications were less frequent with cis-platinum than with mitomycin C therapy. Two of 29 patients with metastasis or a poor medical status survived more than 11 months, but died within 18 months. Three of 9 patients with good palliation who refused esophagectomy were still alive after 38 months. Eleven of the 33 patients who underwent esophagectomy and survived with residual disease are presently alive without disease after 36 months. Twelve patients without residual disease are alive after an average of 21 months.

Combined radiotherapy and chemotherapy relieves dysphagia in these patients, and often the mucosal lesion disappears. The 1-year survival rate in this series was 68%, which represented a distinct improvement. Hyperalimentation is necessary before surgery and during the immediate postoperative period.

▶ [The results achieved by these authors are very impressive, although not as good as those reported by Akiyama et al. It is obvious that case selection plays a major factor. It is my opinion that combination therapy will ultimately be the manner in which these patients are best treated. As yet, of course, this combination therapy is in its infancy, but series such as this one are promising.—W.S.] ◀

20–7 **Spontaneous Intramural Rupture and Intramural Hematoma of the Esophagus.** Spontaneous intramural rupture or intramural hematoma of the esophagus is a rare cause of acute chest and upper abdominal pain. It is much less ominous than spontaneous complete rupture, and seldom necessitates surgery. Mucosal rupture causing intramural hematoma and abscess formation may be produced by an ingested foreign body or by instrumentation, or may occur spontaneously. W. F. Kerr (Norwich, England) reports 5 new cases and reviews 15 previously described cases.

Woman, 77, being treated for pernicious anemia and myxedema, had pain in the anterior part of the chest shortly after eating and later awakened with a rasping cough and severe pain, which became worse despite antacids and analgesics. A barium swallow (Fig 20–5) showed an extensive intramural rupture of the esophagus. Severe pain persisted three days later, esophagoscopy showed a large amount of fluid regurgitated from the stomach into the pharynx and upper esophagus. A transverse laceration of the posterior and right wall was present at 32 cm. Thoracotomy showed the mediastinal pleura

---

(20–7) Thorax 35:890–897, December 1980.

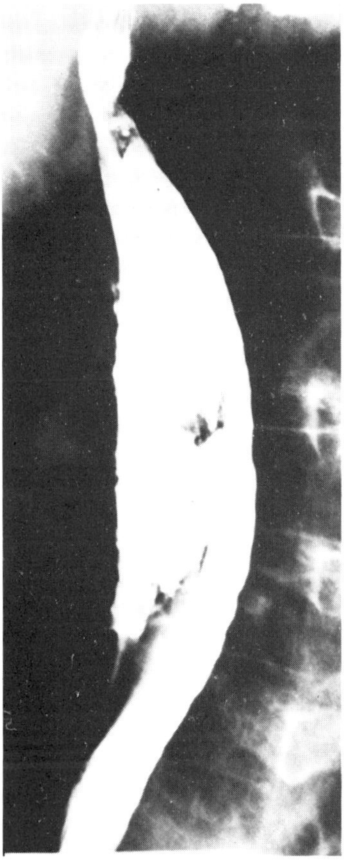

Fig 20–5.—Barium swallow on the fourth day. (Courtesy of Kerr, W.F.: Thorax 35:890–897, 1980.)

to be stained by old blood, most intensely at the level of the azygos vein. The thickened esophagus was mobilized, but the plane of dissection could not be located without incising the mucosa. The mediastinum was drained, and a feeding jejunostomy was established. The patient recovered slowly but completely.

All patients presented with severe, constant retrosternal or epigastric pain, and many had concomitant dysphagia. In 7 cases the pain was preceded or accompanied by vomiting. Ten cases appeared to be truly spontaneous. No patient had surgical emphysema, but all had abnormal Gastrografin or barium swallow studies, and esophagoscopy showed intramural hematoma formation with or without mucosal tearing. Fifteen patients recovered well on conservative management. One patient each had esophageal repair and abdominal exploration only, and 2 had drainage of the mediastinum when the false lumen was not found at thoracotomy. One patient died after emergency exploration and subsequent total esophagectomy.

This condition appears to be distinct from the Mallory-Weiss and Boerhaave syndromes. Conservative management usually results in rapid improvement and complete recovery. The condition probably is more common than generally is appreciated, and it should be considered when the cause of acute pain in the chest or upper abdomen is not obvious. If intramural rupture is suspected, the first study should be a Gastrografin swallow; esophagoscopy is not necessary.

▶ [This is an excellent clinical description of an entity that may be more common than generally has been recognized and that should be familiar to all surgeons. The discussion is an extremely thoughtful conceptualization of the possible pathogenetic mechanisms for this condition. I should like to add that exactly the same phenomenon can be seen as a result of injury by a foreign body that does not penetrate the full thickness of the esophageal lumen. One of the questions that arises in the so-called spontaneous group in the absence of foreign bodies is whether or not a mucosal tear is present. The presence of such a lesion would suggest that antibiotics be added to the nonoperative treatment regimen. Surely, patients who have the spontaneous variety of this entity and who vomit blood must indeed have such a mucosal injury, and perhaps the presence of hematemesis itself would indicate a requirement for antibiotic therapy without the need for endoscopy. Whether endoscopy should be done in persons who do not have hematemesis and in whom the radiologic diagnosis is clear is not readily apparent to me.—W.S.] ◀

21. Stomach and Duodenum

21-1 **Routine Early Endoscopy in Upper Gastrointestinal Tract Bleeding: Randomized, Controlled Trial.** Routine early endoscopy has been advocated for all patients with upper gastrointestinal bleeding on the assumption that early diagnosis will beneficially influence management. However, in most patients bleeding ceases during treatment regardless of the cause, limiting the need for therapeutic decisions and an accurate diagnosis. Walter L. Peterson, Cora C. Barnett, Herbert J. Smith, Michael H. Allen, and Desmond B. Corbett (Dallas) evaluated the practice of routine early endoscopy in patients with upper gastrointestinal bleeding that ceased during hospital treatment.

The subjects were 206 consecutive, unselected patients (mean age, 55 years) with untreated upper gastrointestinal bleeding in whom bleeding stabilized within 6 hours of beginning treatment. There was no contraindication to endoscopy, and all patients agreed to undergo endoscopy. One hundred underwent routine endoscopy within 4 hours of stabilization, and 106 underwent endoscopy only if bleeding recurred or if a gastric ulcer was found or a malignancy was suspected. All patients were treated with the same liquid antacid regimen, consisting of 80 mmoles of magnesium aluminum hydroxide or aluminum hydroxide hourly for the first 24 hours after stabilization, and then 1 and 3 hours after meals and at bedtime for 6 weeks.

There were no significant differences between the two groups in overall hospital deaths, recurrence of bleeding, number of transfusions needed to treat recurrent bleeding, deaths after recurrent bleeding, or duration of hospital stay (Table 1). During the 12 months after discharge, there were also no significant differences in frequency of

TABLE 1.—OUTCOME IN HOSPITAL IN THE TWO GROUPS*

VARIABLE	ROUTINE ENDOSCOPY	NO ROUTINE ENDOSCOPY
Recurrent bleeding (no. of patients)	33	32
Time after admission (days)	3.7±0.5	3.3±0.4
Transfusions (units)	7.4±1.2	6.3±0.7
Mortality during hospitalization (no.)†	8 (24)	5 (16)
Hospital stay (days)	13.0±1.0	14.7±1.2
Overall mortality (no.)	11	8

*None of the differences between groups was statistically significant at the 0.05 level. Mean data are reported ± SEM.

†Figures in parentheses denote percentages.

(21-1) N. Engl. J. Med. 304:925–929, Apr. 16, 1981.

TABLE 2.—RESULTS OF 12-MONTH FOLLOW-UP IN THE TWO GROUPS*

VARIABLE	ROUTINE ENDOSCOPY	NO ROUTINE ENDOSCOPY
	NO. OF PATIENTS	
Patients eligible	89	98
Follow-up available	82	91
Readmission to hospital	18	16
Upper-gastrointestinal-tract bleeding after discharge	7	6
Hemorrhage-related deaths	3	4
Gastrointestinal surgery	8	6
Gastric neoplasm	0	1

*None of the differences between groups was statistically significant at the 0.05 level.

hospital readmission, incidence of further gastrointestinal bleeding, number of hemorrhage-related deaths, or frequency of gastrointestinal surgery (Table 2). The incidences of pneumonia and myocardial infarction in the two groups were also similar.

Endoscopy should not be a routine procedure in patients with upper gastrointestinal bleeding that ceases during treatment. Although the observation that making a diagnosis did not influence outcome is contrary to classic medical teaching, it is not surprising, because therapy was not affected. If better, more specific therapeutic measures were available, making a diagnosis might be of greater value. Because the group of patients studied (i.e., those whose bleeding ceases) accounts for up to 90% of patients with upper gastrointestinal bleeding, the omission of routine endoscopy in such patients would save considerable physician time and patient expense.

▶ [This is a truly excellent randomized trial. It is essential to emphasize that the authors studied only those patients who came into the hospital with an upper gastrointestinal hemorrhage but then stabilized and stopped bleeding. This is obviously an important group, roughly 90% of all patients entering the hospital with gastrointestinal hemorrhage. Although it may seem anti-intellectual to suggest that making a diagnosis did not, in actuality, influence the outcome, this is true. The reasons for this dilemma may revolve around the fact that we do not have sufficiently outstanding therapeutic measures for many of the conditions that cause such bleeding. If we did, and especially if endoscopy was used for therapeutic purposes, perhaps the outcome might be more in favor of endoscopy. It is obvious that much money and time can be saved by comfortably excluding such patients from immediate or early endoscopy. On the other hand, this study was not designed to look at those patients who had continuing bleeding, in whom a therapeutic procedure such as surgical intervention needs to be considered. It seems self-evident that in the small group of patients with upper gastrointestinal hemorrhage who have continued or torrential hemorrhage, about 10% of all cases, endoscopy is probably of value in decision-making. Whether selection of patients for early operation by endoscopic demonstration of the "visible vessel" is valuable remains under consideration (see the following article).—W.S.] ◀

21–2 **Endoscopic Prediction of Recurrent Bleeding in Peptic Ulcers.** Bleeding that continues or recurs after hospitalization for an

(21–2) N. Engl. J. Med. 305:915–916, Oct. 15, 1981.

CLINICAL COURSES IN PATIENTS WITH PEPTIC ULCER ACCORDING TO FEATURES OF ULCER AT ENDOSCOPY*

ULCER FEATURE	TOTAL	FURTHER BLEEDING	EMERGENCY SURGERY	DEATH
		no. of patients (per cent)		
Visible vessel	34	19 (56)	17 (50)	5 (15)
Stigmata of bleeding other than a visible vessel	13	1 (8)	1 (8)	0
No stigmata of bleeding	40	0	0	0

*Ulcers inadequately visualized at endoscopy or given argon-laser treatment are not considered in this table.

acutely bleeding peptic ulcer is the single most important factor in an adverse prognosis. David W. Storey, Stephen G. Bown, C. Paul Swain, Paul R. Salmon, J. Squire Kirkham, and Timothy C. Northfield (London) conducted a prospective 1-year study of the prognostic importance of visible vessels in ulcer craters and other signs of recent bleeding in 292 consecutive patients with acute gastrointestinal bleeding. All endoscopies were done within 24 hours of admission. Ulcer craters were washed with standard washing catheters without precipitating arterial bleeding in any case. Careful washing usually showed whether or not a vessel was present.

Peptic ulcers were identified in 45% of patients. Full examination of the crater was possible in 117 patients, and a vessel was seen in 48% of this group. Other signs of recent bleeding were seen in 18% of cases. Arterial hemorrhage often was seen to start or stop spontaneously. The clinical course is related to the endoscopic findings in the table. In the patient in whom no vessel was seen at endoscopy but who had continued bleeding, a vessel was seen at operation.

A visible vessel in an ulcer crater has great prognostic significance, but other stigmas of recent bleeding do not. More than half of the patients with visible vessels in this study had further bleeding, compared to only 8% of those with other stigmas. Careful washing of ulcer craters after hemorrhage can demonstrate vessels much more often than previously thought. Further bleeding and mortality are almost entirely restricted to patients with ulcers having visible vessels, although only about half of these patients have further bleeding.

▶ [Because rebleeding after hospital admission is the one factor that both gastroenterologists and surgeons agree is a clear indication for operation in a patient with gastrointestinal hemorrhage, it becomes very important to identify, if possible, such patients before the second hemorrhage occurs. Griffiths et al. (*N. Engl. J. Med.* 300:1411, 1979) suggested that a visible vessel in the base of an ulcer was such an indicator. The present study, which is a very nice randomized trial, strongly supports the suggestion of Griffiths and his co-workers. Whereas Peterson and his group have found that endoscopy at a time when the hemorrhage has ceased does not alter the outcome, the findings of the present investigators and those of Griffiths et al. would suggest that early endoscopy may indeed alter the outcome if the visible vessel is used as an indicator for early operation. What needs to be done now is to look at the mortality rate in patients whose treatment is guided by the endoscopic finding. If mortality rates can be improved by early operation on patients with a "visible vessel," then the recommendations of Peterson et al. will need to be reconsidered.—W.S.] ◀

21-3 **National ASGE Survey on Upper Gastrointestinal Bleeding: Complications of Endoscopy.** Little is known of the risks of fiberoptic endoscopy in patients with upper gastrointestinal bleeding. David A. Gilbert, Fred E. Silverstein, and Francis J. Tedesco (Univ. of Washington, Seattle) report the findings in a national prospective survey conducted by the American Society for Gastrointestinal Endoscopy (ASGE) in 1978 in which 1,618 members were asked for information on at least 5 consecutive cases referred for evaluation of upper gastrointestinal bleeding. A total of 277 physicians reported data on 2,427 patients. A total of 2,097 patients underwent 2,320 upper endoscopic examinations.

The procedures were designated as emergencies in 65.5%. A complete examination was performed in about 85% of patients. At least one abnormality was found in 91.9% of examinations. Multiple lesions were found in one third of the patients. An actively bleeding lesion was seen in 32.6% of patients. Complications occurred in 0.9% of all endoscopies (table). Nine of the 12 major complications occurred during emergency endoscopies. The patients with aspiration pneumonia had a mean age of 78.3 years, which was more than 20 years older than the mean for the study population. All these patients had heart disease. One case of pneumonia proved fatal. All patients in whom endoscopy provoked bleeding had underlying liver disease with coagulation abnormalities. One patient exsanguinated during the procedure.

The complication rate in this survey was 0.9%. A major complication occurred in 1 of every 193 procedures. Previous studies included patients having endoscopy for a variety of less acute indications. These findings may prove useful in delineating cost risk-benefit factors for fiberoptic endoscopy in patients with upper gastrointestinal bleeding.

▶ [Upper gastrointestinal endoscopy has become so commonplace that it is ordered almost as freely as a blood test. Many of the young physicians who order endoscopy are unaware of its complications. This study certainly has to represent the best possible figures that are obtainable because it was conducted by persons who are expert at the technique. Therefore, it is very likely that, if anything, the incidence of complications in the hands of persons who are less competent will be somewhat greater. This must be kept in mind when such a test is ordered, although I would hasten to call to the attention of the reader that 65% of the procedures that were evaluated in this study were done as emergencies, therefore increasing the hazards of complica-

ENDOSCOPIC COMPLICATIONS IN 2,320 ENDOSCOPIES

*Major**		*Minor*	
Perforation	5	Mucosal tear	3
Aspiration	4	Medication reaction	3
Hemorrhage	3	Hypotension	1
		Atrial fibrillation	1
		Anoxic episode	1

*One death occurred in each of the major groups of complications.

(21–3) Dig. Dis. Sci. [Suppl.] 26:55s–59s, July 1981.

tions such as aspiration. This must be kept in mind in view of the recent data that indicate that patients with upper gastrointestinal hemorrhage who have had endoscopy after they have stopped bleeding have no lower mortality than do those who have not undergone endoscopy at all (See Peterson et al.: *N. Engl. J. Med.* 304:925, 1981).—W.S.] ◀

21–4 **Reflux Gastritis Syndrome: Mechanism of Symptoms.** Reflux gastritis occurs in up to one third of patients having gastric surgery. There has been speculation about the role of bile acids in the pathogenesis of gastric mucosal changes in this syndrome. Hooshang Meshkinpour, Jay W. Marks, Leslie J. Schoenfield, George G. Bonnoris, and Sylvia Carter attempted to determine whether administration into the stomach of autologous upper intestinal contents or artificial bile acid solutions can produce symptoms of reflux gastritis. The study group included 11 patients, mean age 49.5, with reflux gastritis and 10 asymptomatic patients, mean age 53, undergoing gastric surgery. The respective mean intervals since surgery were 6.2 and 7.3 years. Autologous intestinal contents, obtained after cholecystokinin injection, and normal saline were infused in a double-blind manner into the stomach. Two artificial bile acid solutions were evaluated in 8 patients in each group.

Ten of the 11 symptomatic patients had positive symptom responses to gastric infusion of autologous intestinal contents, as did 2 of the 10 asymptomatic patients, both of whom responded to saline infusion as well as to infusion of intestinal contents. No symptomatic patient had a positive response to saline. Abdominal pain and nausea best distinguished the two groups. The amount of bile acids in the intestinal contents was greater in the symptomatic patients (table). Only 1 symptomatic patient, but no asymptomatic patient, responded to infusion of artificial bile acid solution.

Proximal intestinal contents can produce symptoms of reflux gastritis in symptomatic patients, but not in asymptomatic patients following gastric surgery. The lack of response to infusion of artificial bile acids may be explained by a need for other compounds in the intestinal contents for symptoms to occur, or by the lack of a role for bile acids in symptom production in reflux gastritis syndrome. The latter possibility also may explain the ineffectiveness of cholestyra-

BILE ACID PROFILE OF INTESTINAL CONTENTS

	Symptomatic[a] (n = 11)	Asymptomatic[a] (n = 10)
Total bile acids[b]	2.74 ± 0.37	1.01 ± 0.24
Conjugated bile acids	2.72 ± 0.37	0.98 ± 0.25
Cholic acid	1.02 ± 0.17	0.33 ± 0.09
Chenodeoxycholic acid	0.96 ± 0.14	0.33 ± 0.10
Deoxycholic acid	0.66 ± 0.07	0.32 ± 0.07

[a]Values represent mean ± SE.
[b]μmoles/ml.

(21–4) Gastroenterology 79:1283–1287, December 1981.

mine in the symptomatic treatment of reflux gastritis. Bile acids still might contribute to production of histologic changes even though they have no role in producing symptoms.

▶ [Clear definition and diagnosis of reflux gastritis are extremely difficult. It is my impression that many patients with a variety of gastrointestinal symptoms after large number of different kinds of operative procedures have been subjected to diversionary procedures with a jejunal Roux-en-Y rather indiscriminately. There seems to be no single test or criterion on which the diagnosis can be based. However, the authors of this article have chosen very stringent criteria for inclusion of patients in the group identified as having reflux gastritis. I believe that if all physicians used such criteria, the diagnosis probably would be made much less often than it is now. In addition to the criteria of postprandial abdominal pain, bilious vomiting, and nausea, normal upper gastrointestinal series and oral cholecystogram, basal acid output less than 2 mEq/hour, endoscopic findings compatible with reflux gastritis, and endoscopic biopsy showing gastritis, the authors now have shown us that infusion of intestinal contents into patients with reflux gastritis will reproduce their symptoms in a fairly reliable manner. Thus, their suggestion may serve not only as the useful discriminant for the diagnosis but also as an implication that the pathogenesis of this condition is not related to the presence of bile salts in the refluxed material. We have had a small experience using 5 mM deoxycholate, which is roughly twice the concentration administered by these authors. In our experience, this has served as a useful test for the presence of reflux gastritis, but our series is small. This is an interesting study that deserves further investigation.—W.S.] ◀

21–5 **Delayed Gastric Emptying of Liquids and Solids Following Roux-en-Y Biliary Diversion.** A high rate of delayed gastric emptying has been noted after Roux-en-Y gastrojejunostomy. It is not clear whether this is unique to the procedure or the result of operating on patients with numerous postgastrectomy symptoms or an unrecognized gastric motility disorder. Michael P. Hocking, Stephen B. Vogel, Carlos A. Falasca, and Edward R. Woodward (Univ. of Florida, Gainesville) evaluated gastric emptying after Roux-en-Y diversion in vagotomized dogs undergoing antrectomy or subtotal gastrectomy. Four dogs having vagotomy and antrectomy with Roux-en-Y gastrojejunostomy were compared with 4 dogs who underwent vagotomy and antrectomy with a Billroth II gastrojejunostomy. Four other dogs had truncal vagotomy and 75% Roux-en-Y subtotal gastrectomy, while 4 had a Billroth II 75% subtotal gastrectomy with truncal vagotomy. The emptying of both solid food and normal saline solution containing phenol red dye was assessed.

The Roux-en-Y gastrojejunostomy after antrectomy was associated with a significant delay in gastric emptying of solid and liquid meals. The Billroth II antrectomy group also had delayed emptying compared with control animals but of a lesser degree than the Roux-en-Y procedure animals. Although gastric emptying after subtotal gastrectomy, vagotomy, and Billroth II reconstruction was somewhat delayed as compared with that of controls, it was more rapid than in dogs with Roux-en-Y reconstruction following subtotal gastrectomy and vagotomy.

Roux-en-Y diversion combined with truncal vagotomy delays the gastric emptying of solids and, to a lesser extent, liquids in comparison with Billroth II gastrojejunostomy. The cause of the delayed emp-

---

(21–5) Ann. Surg. 194:494–501, October 1981.

tying is unclear but transection of the proximal jejunum may be a contributing factor. The presence of both an afferent and efferent limb in a Billroth II gastroenterostomy may facilitate gastric emptying. In addition, reflux of duodenal secretions into the stomach may contribute to the gastric emptying of a solid meal. The delay in emptying appears to be dependent on complete vagal denervation, but it is more marked than that observed in traditional postvagotomy atony.

▶ [There is little doubt that delay in gastric emptying seems to occur with an alarmingly high frequency after Roux-en-Y reconstruction in patients who have reflux gastritis or in patients who are having Roux-en-Y reconstruction for other reasons such as malabsorption due to bacterial overgrowth in the afferent loop. Every single patient whom I have reconstructed has had an initial anastomosis done so that the afferent loop was placed to the greater curvature of the stomach and the efferent loop was toward the lesser curvature. In the discussion of this paper, the authors were asked how the anastomosis was found in the more than 100 patients who had undergone Roux-en-Y gastrojejunostomy in their institution, but, unfortunately, they could not give us those data. Part of the difficulty is that the use of the terms "isoperistaltic" and "anteperistaltic" is so confusing and thoroughly mixed up in the minds of most surgeons that a statement as to which is which is meaningless. Such terminology should be discarded. If we all would simply state that the afferent loop is put to the lesser or greater curvature, then we would understand each other. I am making a plea for doing so, because recently I have encountered a number of operative notes that even fail to make mention of anything about the relative position of the afferent and efferent loops. If we are going to make any headway in delineating more clearly the clinical syndromes that occur after gastrectomy—and, therefore, treat them more appropriately—we had better begin to clarify our terminology.

This experimental study suffers from many problems. The first is that gravity is an extremely important factor in emptying of the gastric remnant after gastrectomy. The authors of this paper freely admit this, and yet the use for such a study of the horizontal dog, which undoubtedly will be compared with upright man, is somewhat doubtful. Secondly, these animals were not used as their own controls and, in my view, this is a very important defect. Variations from animal to animal are sufficiently great that one wonders whether one can really draw the conclusions that the authors have made. I am fearful that some will extrapolate these results to man and begin to advocate higher gastric resection to solve the problem of the poor emptying. This may or may not do so.

I have little doubt that gastric emptying is delayed after many of these Roux-en-Y reconstructions, but I do not think that the authors of this paper have shown conclusively the mechanism by which that occurs, nor do I believe they have shown that it is, indeed, the Roux-en-Y reconstruction itself that has anything to do with such delay. We recently encountered a patient who 30 years previously had undergone a Billroth II gastrectomy with the afferent loop placed to the greater curvature. He required resection of the transverse colon for carcinoma, and even though the gastrojejunostomy was disturbed no more than that required to carry out the resection of the colon, he developed prolonged delay in gastric emptying for about 5 weeks after the colon resection. Had he had a Roux-en-Y reconstruction, one might have attributed that phenomenon to the Roux-en-Y. I believe that even minor changes in positioning of the gastrojejunostomy may play a role.—W.W.] ◀

21-6 **Serum Gastrin Response to Secretin After Vagotomy.** It may be difficult to diagnose Zollinger-Ellison syndrome (ZES) in vagotomized patients because the serum gastrin level often is elevated in vagotomized patients without ZES, and marked basal acid hypersecretion may be absent in ZES patients who have undergone vagotomy. Mark Feldman, John H. Walsh, and Charles T. Richardon measured gastrin responses to intravenously administered secretin in 13

(21–6) Dig. Dis. Sci. 25:921–923, December 1980.

vagotomized duodenal ulcer patients who had normal basal serum gastrin levels and acid secretion before vagotomy. Five patients with ZES who underwent vagotomy also were evaluated. Selective proximal vagotomy was done in all but 1 patient in each group. The duodenal ulcer patients were studied 6 weeks to 2 years after vagotomy.

Basal serum gastrin increased significantly after vagotomy in the duodenal ulcer patients without ZES, and was over 100 pg/ml in 5 cases. The serum gastrin increased in 12 of 13 patients after intravenous secretin in a dose of 0.44 μg/kg. The rise in gastrin after secretin was higher after vagotomy in all 5 subjects tested before and after operation. No rise of over 100 pg/ml was, however, observed. All 3 ZES patients who had secretin tests before vagotomy had positive results, and in each case the test remained positive after vagotomy. The secretin test was positive in both ZES patients who were not diagnosed until after vagotomy.

The means by which secretin increases the serum gastrin level is unknown, but the rise in gastrin may depend on the amount of gastrin-containing tissue present. Basal serum gastrin levels may not differentiate between vagotomized ZES patients and vagotomized ulcer patients without ZES, but the secretin test should help distinguish basal hypergastrinemia due to vagotomy from that due to ZES. A rise in gastrin of over 100 pg/ml after secretin is suggestive of ZES and should not be attributed to vagotomy itself.

▶ [The results of this paper are extremely important. I am aware of at least 1 and possibly 2 patients who underwent total gastrectomy under the erroneous impression that a gastrinoma was present, because a small rise in the serum gastrin level followed the administration of secretin in these patients with vagotomy and recurrent ulceration. We are indebted to Feldman and his colleagues for identifying so clearly for us the limits of the increase in serum gastrin induced by secretin in vagotomized individuals who do *not* have gastrinomas. The secretin test clearly remains the most critical discriminant for the presence or absence of gastrinomas in patients in whom the serum gastrin levels are borderline.—W.S.] ◀

21–7 **Elevated Serum Prolactin Level in Zollinger-Ellison Syndrome.** About one third of gastrinoma patients with the multiple endocrine neoplasia type 1 (MEN-1) syndrome have pituitary adenomas, usually chromophobe lesions, which traditionally have been considered nonfunctional in terms of hormonal secretion. The symptoms of pituitary prolactinoma may be nonspecific and the tumors may go undetected until the optic chiasm is compressed. Bruce E. Stabile, Edward Passaro, Jr., and Harold E. Carlson (UCLA School of Medicine, Los Angeles) estimated the prevalence of prolactinoma in a series of 36 adults with Zollinger-Ellison syndrome (ZES), all but 1 of whom had had a total gastrectomy and thorough exploration of the abdomen. A tissue diagnosis of tumor was made in 28 cases. Ten patients were known to have the MEN-1 syndrome; all 10 had parathyroid involvement, and 2 had adrenal involvement as well. Serum prolactin was measured by radioimmunoassay.

Eight of the 36 patients with gastrinoma had elevated serum prolactin levels. Four of them had well-documented MEN-1 syndrome,

---

(21–7) Arch. Surg. 116:449–453, April 1981.

and 1 had profound primary hypothyroidism as the cause of elevated prolactin. In 3 cases, hyperprolactinemia was the first suggestion of pluriglandular disease. All 5 patients given protirelin showed the blunted prolactin response characteristic of pituitary adenoma. Pituitary tumor was confirmed radiologically in 4 patients. Three of 4 men with elevated serum prolactin were impotent, and the fourth had loss of libido. Serum testosterone was low or borderline in the 3 men tested. One of 3 women had had secondary amenorrhea, but none had galactorrhea. Serum prolactin levels tended to rise over time in the 6 patients studied serially.

Seven of 13 patients in this study thought to have MEN-1 syndrome had elevated prolactin levels. Hyperprolactinemia appears to be second only to hyperparathyroidism as the most common endocrinopathy associated with ZES. Sexual dysfunction was prevalent in patients with prolactinoma. Polytomography of the sella will aid the early diagnosis of prolactinoma in this setting. The use of bromocriptine to restore ovulation is controversial because pregnancy may stimulate the growth of prolactinomas, but bromocriptine may be indicated for men with small lesions and sexual dysfunction, as well as for women with amenorrhea or galactorrhea who do not desire pregnancy.

▶ [This very nice contribution points out a method of assessing the presence of a pituitary tumor in patients with the multiple endocrine neoplasia syndrome before such tumors have become large enough to cause compression of the optic chiasm or erosion of the sella turcica. It seems clear now that prolactin levels should be ascertained in all patients in whom gastrinomas are detected. The incidence of pituitary involvement is second only to that of parathyroid involvement in the multiple endocrine neoplasia syndrome type I; therefore, it behooves us to identify the presence or absence of this problem.—W.S.] ◀

1–8 **Studies With Bombesin in Zollinger-Ellison Syndrome.** Bombesin is a potent stimulant of antral gastrin secretion and appears to stimulate gastrin in patients with Zollinger-Ellison syndrome (ZES). Nicola Basso, Emanuele Lezoche, Alberto Materia, Edward Passaro Jun, and Vincenzo Speranza measured total radioimmunoactive gastrin and determined the different molecular forms of gastrin after bombesin infusion in 16 patients with probable gastrinoma, 11 of whom had proved pancreatic gastrinoma and 2 of whom had proved duodenal gastrinoma. Gastric surgery had been done in 14 cases. Bombesin was infused at a rate of 8.9 pmole/minute/kg for 90 minutes. Gastric secretions were aspirated in 6 cases. After 2 to 4 days, 13 patients had calcium infused at a rate of 4 mg/kg/hour for 4 hours. In 5 patients the tests were repeated 2 to 4 weeks after total gastrectomy.

In patients with pancreatic gastrinoma, gastrin was elevated much more after calcium than after bombesin infusion (Fig 21–1). The reverse was true in patients with proved duodenal gastrinoma. Four of 5 patients who were restudied after total gastrectomy had comparable gastrin levels. Bombesin augmented the concentration of all gastrin components in all the patients studied.

(21–8) Br. J. Surg. 68:97–100, February 1981.

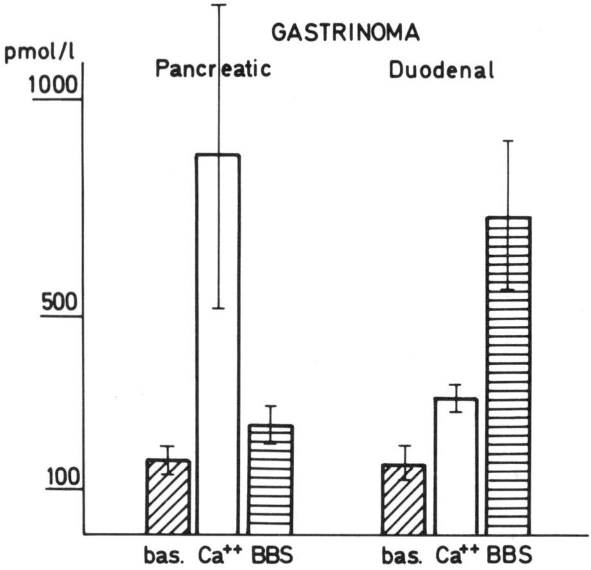

Fig 21–1.—Basal, calcium-, and bombesin-stimulated gastrin levels in 7 patients with pancreatic gastrinoma and 2 with duodenal gastrinoma. (Courtesy of Basso, N., et al.: Br. J. Surg. 68:97–100, 1981.)

Bombesin is more potent than calcium infusion in stimulating gastrin secretion in patients with retained antral mucosa and basal gastrin levels suggestive of ZES. Comparison between basal calcium-stimulated and basal bombesin-stimulated gastrin levels may help distinguish patients with pancreatic gastrinoma from those with retained antral mucosa or duodenal gastrinoma preoperatively. Gastrin-producing cells of duodenal gastrinomas may be more closely related to antral G cells, both morphologically and functionally, than to the gastrin-producing cells of pancreatic gastrinomas. Bombesin infusion enhances the absolute concentrations of all gastrin components, supporting the view that G34, G17, and the N-terminal G17 fragment are all present in gastrinomas.

▶ [These studies may prove to be of very great value in the practical clinical situation. If, indeed, the use of the ratio between bombesin-stimulated gastrin release and calcium-stimulated gastrin release can be used to distinguish between a duodenal and a pancreatic gastrinoma preoperatively, we will have made a great step forward. The number of duodenal gastrinomas in this series is small; nevertheless, the differences observed by these authors are great. In addition, the use of this same ratio to help us decide whether retained antrum is present in patients who have hypergastrinemia is also of great value, as pointed out by these authors. In other words, bombesin stimulates the release of antral gastrin in the presence of retained antrum as effectively as it does in patients with duodenal gastrinoma. The results of this study would suggest that the differences in the type of circulating gastrin do not seem to be of value in deciding whether a pancreatic or a duodenal gastrinoma is present.—W.S.] ◀

22. Small Intestine

22-1 **Intraoperative Determination of Small Intestinal Viability Following Ischemic Injury: Prospective, Controlled Trial of Two Adjuvant Methods (Doppler and Fluorescein) Compared With Standard Clinical Judgment.** The difficulty of accurately predicting intestinal recovery from ischemic injury has limited the successful management of patients with acute intestinal ischemic conditions. Gregory B. Bulkley, George D. Zuidema, Stanley R. Hamilton, Charles S. O'Mara, Peter G. Klacsmann, and Susan D. Horn (Johns Hopkins Med. Inst., Baltimore) compared the Doppler and fluorescein techniques with clinical judgments of viability in a prospective trial in 28 consecutive patients operated on for acute small bowel ischemic disease. Most had some form of strangulated intestinal obstruction due to an internal hernia or volvulus or to an incarcerated abdominal wall hernia. Four patients had acute mesenteric ischemia due to thromboembolism. Evaluation was made of 71 intestinal segments at least 15 minutes after reversal of the cause of ischemic injury. Judgments of the senior surgeon were compared with Doppler ultrasonic flowmeter measurements and with the results of fluorescein injection.

Viability was ascertained in 54 instances. The patterns of fluorescein reaction are shown in Table 1. In all categories, the fluorescein method proved superior in predicting viability and was without error in determinant segments. The accuracy of conventional clinical judgments was 89% but their predictive value was only 64% (Table 2).

TABLE 1.—PATTERNS OF FLUORESCEIN FLUORESCENCE

Pattern	Intensity	Texture	Predicted Outcome
Hyperemic	Increased	Uniform, "smooth"	Viable
Normal	Normal	Uniform, "smooth"	Viable
Fine granular	Normal to slightly decreased	Fine granular	Viable
Patchy	Decreased	Patches of nonfluorescence ≥5 mm diameter	Nonviable
Perivascular	Decreased	Only perivascular areas stained	Nonviable
Nonfluorescent	None	None	Nonviable

(22–1) Ann. Surg. 193:628–637, May 1981.

TABLE 2.—VIABILITY ASSESSMENT OF DETERMINANT SEGMENTS

Method	Sensitivity	Specificity	Predictive Value	Overall Accuracy
Standard clinical judgment	78 ± 27% (7/9)	91 ± 8% (41/45)	64 ± 28% (7/11)	89 ± 9% (48/54)
Doppler	63 ± 33% (5/8)	88 ± 10% (36/41)	50 ± 31% (5/10)	84 ± 10% (41/49)
Fluorescein fluorescence pattern	100% (9/9)	100% (45/45)†	100% (9/9)†	100% (54/54)*†

*Significantly better than clinical judgment by X_c^2 ($P < .04$).
†Significantly better than Doppler method by X_c^2 ($P \leq .05$).

Determination of viability with the Doppler probe was inferior to standard clinical judgment in all categories. No adverse reactions to fluorescein injection were observed.

Conventional clinical judgments are fairly accurate in assessing intestinal viability after surgery for ischemic injury, but a significant number of unnecessary resections may be performed to avoid leaving nonviable bowel in place. The Doppler ultrasound flow probe is not useful in this setting, but the fluorescein fluorescence pattern is a valuable adjuvant to clinical assessment. The fluorescein method provides a reliable means of evaluating borderline bowel segments in patients with acute small bowel ischemic disease.

▶ [This is the most carefully designed study I have seen to evaluate methods of assessment of intestinal viability. To my knowledge, there has never been an investigation of this problem that has so meticulously excluded bias in so far as it is possible to do so. Obviously, it is impossible to know whether resected segments ultimately would have survived or not, but the authors have done the best possible job of excluding error in this important group. Certainly, previous studies done with the Doppler flowmeter have not taken such pains, and it seems clear here that the fluorescein method is far better than the Doppler methods. One cannot help but wonder what the influence of antibiotics might be on the outcome of these findings. The authors do not mention whether all of these patients had antibiotics or not. Experimentally, intestine that clearly would not ordinarily be viable becomes so with the use of either intraluminal or systemic antibiotics. It would be nice to see a further study on this very point. It would also be of value to know what the operative mortality and morbidity were in this particular series.—W.S.] ◀

22–2 **Use of Intraperitoneal Xenon-133 for Imaging of Intestinal Strangulation in Small Bowel Obstruction.** Previous attempts at radionuclide imaging of ischemic small intestine have had only limited success because of limited access of isotope to devascularized tissue and because of the need for significant tissue necrosis for selective isotope uptake within ischemic tissue. Gregory B. Bulkley, Farid Gharagozloo, Philip O. Alderson, Susan D. Horn, and George D. Zuidema (Johns Hopkins Med. Inst., Baltimore) observed retention of sodium fluorescein dye in the injured bowel segment in a laboratory study of intestinal recovery after ischemic injury. It was suggested that the dye was absorbed passively across the peritoneal surface of the ischemic segment and retained because of lack of perfusion. Studies then were done in rats with obstruction of the terminal ileum. Anterior abdominal gamma camera imaging was performed following radioactive xenon injection into the peritoneum, 30 minutes after surgery.

Isotope washout was slowed significantly in the animals with strangulation. Camera images showed a complete absence of activity in control animals at 1 hour, with marked retention of localized activity in study animals for 90 minutes. The increased activity was most marked at 1 hour. The mean isotope concentration in strangulated tissue at 90 minutes was 266 times that in adjacent normal tissue, and 1,196 times that in tissue from rats with simple obstruction. Similar findings were obtained in dogs, in which gamma camera images also showed a marked difference between the strangulated and the control or simple obstructed state from 30 minutes on.

This method is based on differences in isotope clearance between perfused and nonperfused tissues and does not require the appearance of cell damage for production of a positive image. The model is highly reproducible; a 4-hour period of ischemia invariably results in recov-

---

(22–2) Am. J. Surg. 141:128–135, January 1981.

ery of the ischemic bowel segment. The test can be used to rule out ischemic bowel when one is planning to treat a patient conservatively with a long intestinal tube rather than undertaking laparotomy. It remains to be determined whether the adhesions associated with mechanical small bowel obstruction hinder the intraperitoneal distribution of isotope and alter washout. Use of the method to detect early mesenteric ischemia and portal vein thrombosis is under study.

▶ [This is an excellent, well-controlled study that could have important clinical implications. One of the problems that could limit the usefulness of this technique in patients with intestinal obstruction is the need to inject the ^{133}Xe into the peritoneal cavity. In patients who have obstruction of the small intestine, distension is often great and entry of a needle or angiocath into the intestinal lumen is as likely, if not more likely, to occur than entry into the peritoneal cavity when administration of the ^{133}Xe is to be done. Furthermore, one wonders whether the presence of adhesions would limit the access of the injected material to the ischemic segment of intestine. One could certainly envision the sequestration of an ischemic loop by adhesions that would not allow the xenon to enter that loop. Finally, the presence or absence of ischemia may not be at all important in patients in whom the diagnosis of intestinal obstruction is clear. All such patients probably should be operated on if a brief period of nonoperative treatment of a few hours is unsuccessful. On the other hand, a technique such as this, if it could overcome the objections raised above, might very well be of great use in patients in whom the diagnosis of obstruction itself is not evident. We look forward to further contributions by this group.—W.S.] ◀

22–3 **Complications and Results of 160 Baker Tube Plications.** Plication of the small bowel often is performed when there is an increased risk of adhesive obstruction after celiotomy. Baker tube plication decompresses distended bowel and is more rapid and simpler to perform than external plication. However, plication may be inadequate to prevent obstruction, and complications of the jejunostomy or indwelling tube are possible. John A. Weigelt, William H. Snyder III, and James L. Norman (Southwestern Med. School, Dallas) reviewed 160 plications done with the Baker tube in 154 patients in 1969 to 1974. Average patient age was 43 years. Six patients had a second procedure for recurrent obstruction within the 5-year review period. All but 4 patients had follow-up, for an average of 3.9 years. Tube plication was done for multiple, widespread areas of denuded enteric serosa. Adhesions were present in 87% of cases, purulence in 13%, and carcinomatosis in 10%. The tubes were introduced through jejunostomies, using the tunnel method described by Witzel. The tube was left as an indwelling stent for an average of 15 days.

Postoperative ileus persisted for an average of 4 days. Prolonged ileus occurred in 9 cases and enterocutaneous fistula in 10. Three patients with fistulas died of sepsis. There were 43 infectious complications, including 8 intra-abdominal abscesses. The hospital mortality was 13%. Of 96 patients in whom the jejunostomy was the only source of contamination, 21% had infection and 4 had intra-abdominal abscess formation. There were 10 minor tube complications and 1 major complication involving multiple intussusceptions over the tube in a patient who died 3 months later of sepsis and respiratory failure. Twenty patients had symptoms of recurrent small bowel obstruction; 13 required operative treatment.

(22–3) Am. J. Surg. 140:810–815, December 1980.

Morbidity from Baker tube plication includes intraoperative enteric contamination from the jejunostomy; obstruction or fistulization at the jejunostomy site; prolonged ileus, obstruction, or fistulization distal to the insertion site; and difficulty in removing the tube. It cannot be definitely concluded that Baker tube plication has reduced the rate of recurrent adhesive obstruction, but data from the literature suggest that this is the case.

▶ [This is one of the largest series of Baker tube plications for prevention of recurrent obstruction of the small intestine that has been reported to date. The basic defect of this study is that there is not an adequate control group, namely, a group who did not receive Baker tube plications but who had serosal injuries of the same extent. In order to ascertain whether the Baker tube is of any value at all, a prospective randomized trial must be done in which no stenting of any type is compared to the use of the Baker tube. The study by Brightwell et al. (Arch. Surg. 112:505, 1977) carries out such a comparison and concludes that the incidence of complications, was increased with the use of the tube and that postoperative hospitalization and recuperation were lengthier in patients who had the stent than in those who just simply had enterolysis. The incidence of intussusception was greater in those with the tube and that of infection, clearly so. In addition, the findings made the impression that recurrent obstructions were not prevented by the use of the stenting device.

The intestinal tract above an obstruction is a cesspool of bacteria as a result of overgrowth produced by the stasis of the obstruction. I have seen very serious septic complications as a result of only minimal contamination caused by an enterotomy in obstructed intestine. The seriousness and severity of such septic complications have not been sufficiently acknowledged. In view of the very real doubt that stenting can prevent recurrent obstruction, I do not recommend any type of plication. On the other hand, it is important that after any laparotomy, the intestinal loops be arranged within the abdominal cavity in a relatively normal position, making certain that loops of intestine that normally lie in the lower abdomen are not pulled into the upper abdomen by laparotomy pads removed during closure of the abdominal wound, and also making certain that the omentum covers the small intestine when it is present. In addition, unless a single point of obstruction can be defined clearly, it may be necessary to free up major portions, if not all, of the mesenteric small intestine. My hope is that we will develop pharmacologic means for preventing obstruction, but I doubt that tube plication has much of a place until then. Perhaps the use of a Leonard tube, which can be placed orally without contamination of the gastrointestinal tract, offers some advantage, although even this is a moot point.—W.S.] ◀

22–4 **Intraluminal Stenting in Management of Recurrent Intestinal Obstruction.** The Leonard tube, first described in 1961, is 10 ft long, has a coiled spring in its wall to give it body, and is designed for peroral placement. Rodney D. McMillin, Brack A. Bivins, and Ward O. Griffen, Jr. (Univ. of Kentucky) retrospectively reviewed the results in 23 male and 6 female patients aged 2–61 years (average, 35 years) in whom the Leonard tube was placed during operation for bowel obstruction during 1967–1972. Adhesions were the cause of bowel obstruction in 23 of the 25 patients who had had 1–5 previous abdominal operations.

In all cases the Leonard tube was passed perorally in the operating room with the abdomen open, according to the technique described by Leonard. In 3 patients the tube was used only for intraoperative suction decompression of the bowel and was removed before closure of the abdomen. In the other 26 patients the tube was left in place as an indwelling intestinal stent for 2–17 days (average, 9 days).

(22–4) Am. Surg. 47:74–77, February 1981.

Of the 22 postoperative complications, 16 were related to the indwelling tube; these included fever of unknown etiology that resolved when the tube was withdrawn, infiltrative pneumonia, aspiration, and pharyngitis. Five patients (17%) died postoperatively, and in 3 the indwelling tube contributed to death. The 21 surviving patients who had the tube in place for 48 hours or longer have been followed for 1–9 years (more than 100 cumulative patient-years). There have been no known recurrences of bowel obstruction (however, 1 patient required hospitalization and nasogastric suction for incomplete small bowel obstruction).

The Leonard tube is effective in preventing recurrent bowel obstruction, but the incidence of complications is high. Therefore, use of the tube as an indwelling stent should be reserved for patients who have had at least one previous episode of bowel obstruction requiring operative intervention or for patients with such extensive peritoneal injury (soilage or denuded surfaces) that severe adhesion formation is anticipated. When used as a stent, the tube is left in place 7–10 days to allow adhesion formation to fix the bowel in place. The tube is used most often for bowel decompression at the time of operation. Its use for decompression and removal before abdominal closure is very effective; none of the 3 patients in this series in whom this was done had recurrent bowel obstruction during follow-up.

▶ [It is very difficult to prove whether a splinting procedure such as that provided by the Leonard tube is or is not effective in the long-term prevention of recurrent intestinal obstruction. Obviously, one finds it difficult to carry out a controlled trial, and because this is a retrospective study, one can only raise the issue of why only 29 of 169 patients with intestinal obstruction between 1967 and 1972 at this particular medical center had placement of a Leonard tube. It would have been very interesting to have matched the 29 study patients with 29 patients who did not have a Leonard tube to see if, indeed, the incidence of recurrent small intestinal obstruction was lower in the splinted group. One cannot help but wonder whether the price paid for the presence of this very large tube in terms of postoperative complications is worth the benefit gained, and I have some doubt about that.

One of the most difficult aspects of the use of the Leonard tube is the passage of the tube itself. The authors do not allude to this problem, although 1 patient sustained a serosal tear during passage of the tube. Obviously, in the entire series of patients with intestinal obstruction, there must have been those in whom attempts to pass a Leonard tube failed. It would have been instructive to know what the actual incidence of successful intubation of the small intestine is in the hands of people who use this tube a great deal. I have been successful in only slightly over half of the instances in which intubation was attempted. The upper abdomen may be blocked off by adhesions, or the tube simply cannot be passed into the small intestine for other reasons. Clearly, if such can be done, the aseptic decompression of the small intestine may be of great benefit when closure of the abdominal wall is difficult because of severe distension. It remains to be proved whether prolonged intraluminal stenting will be important in the long-term prevention of recurrent intestinal obstruction.—W.S.] ◀

22-5 **Recurrence Rate After Primary Excisional Surgery for Crohn's Disease.** R. Hellberg, L. Hultén, C. Rosengren, and Ch. Åhrén (Univ. of Göteborg) prospectively studied recurrence rates in 132 consecutive patients undergoing primary excisional surgery for Crohn's disease

(22–5) Acta Chir. Scand. 146:435–443, 1980.

during 1968–1977 in whom all macroscopically involved gut had been resected, the lines of resection showed no histologic evidence of Crohn's disease, and postoperative survival was at least 1 year. All patients were operated on by the same team of surgeons. The policy was to remove the macroscopically diseased ileum along with 10–15 cm of healthy intestine on the proximal side and the smallest possible length on the colonic side.

The crude recurrence rates were generally lower than cumulative probability figures. The general pattern of recurrence for patients with exclusive ileal disease and those with combined disease was almost identical: most recurrences occurred during the first 2–3 years after operation, and the cumulative recurrence rate amounted to 40%–50% at the end of follow-up. The tendency toward recurrence in patients with exclusive colonic disease differed markedly, with a slow and even accumulation of recurrences over the years amounting to 25% at the end of follow-up. Although the total recurrence rate differed greatly, the likelihood of a second operation appeared not to be greater in classic Crohn's disease than in mainly or solely colonic disease. However, when the prognostic evaluation was based only on firmly established cases of Crohn's colitis, the cumulative proportion of recurrence at the end of follow-up was similar to that in classic Crohn's disease. Recurrence rates appeared to be higher in patients subjected to ileocecal resection than in proctocolectomy patients, but the difference disappeared when the calculation was based on the histopathologically "clear cases" only. Patients with extensive ileal involvement at primary operation had a worse prognosis. Age, sex, duration of disease prior to surgery, and whether the procedure was performed on an elective or urgent basis did not influence prognosis.

Previous conflicting results on the prognosis after surgery for Crohn's disease might be due, partly or entirely, to difficulties associated with the histopathologic diagnosis.

▶ [It is important to emphasize that this series was selected for those cases that showed no macroscopic or microscopic evidence of Crohn's disease at the lines of surgical resection. The series is also slightly unusual in that recurrences included not only cases proved at a second operation, but also those instances of radiologically demonstrable recurrent disease. The latter group has been excluded in most recent studies of this problem.

Of great interest to me was the finding that roughly 50% of the cases in this series classified as Crohn's disease of the colon were instances in which the pathologist could not clearly differentiate with certainty between Crohn's colitis and ulcerative colitis, a fact openly and clearly stated by the authors. One important message emanating from my hospital (Glotzer et al.: *N. Engl. J. Med.* 282:582, 1970) is that the pathologic criteria for differentiating between the two diseases overlap markedly. Many other investigators have suggested the same difficulties, and yet the belief is widely held that all one needs to do is ask the pathologist whether one is dealing with Crohn's colitis or ulcerative colitis in order to come up with a specific answer. In fact, these authors were sufficiently perceptive to evaluate the outcome with and without those cases that could not be identified clearly as Crohn's colitis. Such considerations make significant differences in the outcome, and it is very possible that these differences explain many of the discrepancies heretofore published in the literature. In terms of recurrence, these authors have confirmed findings in our own institution that patients with Crohn's colitis fare better than those with Crohn's ileitis.—W.S.] ◀

22–6 **Celiac Compression Syndrome: Myth or Reality?** Any causal connection between compression of the celiac artery by the median arcuate ligament, as seen on angiography, and upper abdominal pain remains obscure. Conflicting results of surgical division of the ligament have been reported. The celiac compression syndrome (CCS) is only vaguely defined, and its pathophysiology has not been elucidated. Gunnar Plate, Bo Eklöf, and Johannes Vang reviewed the results of division of the compressing ligament in 9 men and 6 women operated on between 1969 and 1976. Mean age was 36.5 years. All patients had a history of chronic, otherwise unexplained upper abdominal symptoms and angiographic demonstration of celiac artery stenosis. The mean duration of abdominal pains was 4.3 years. Eight patients had a history of mental illness, and 7 reported abdominal disease.

Moderate to severe eccentric stenosis of the proximal celiac axis was seen at lateral aortography in 14 patients. One patient had total celiac occlusion and stenosis of the superior mesenteric artery. Poststenotic dilatation was observed in 9 patients and increased flow in the pancreaticoduodenal arcade in 12. Initially, most patients were relieved of abdominal pain, however, at follow-up after a mean of over 6 years, only 2 patients were asymptomatic (table). The patients who were completely well at follow-up were the only ones who reported previous specific episodes of cramplike pains localized to the upper abdomen without mental or other abdominal illness. Both patients described the occurrence of symptoms during activities with the trunk bent forward. They had no postprandial pain.

Stenosis of the celiac axis itself, or stenosis with nonspecific abdominal symptoms, probably does not call for surgery, even when extensive studies fail to demonstrate another cause of symptoms. Some patients may experience cramplike upper abdominal pains, triggered by exercise or body position, which are causally related to angiographic celiac stenosis. In these patients, surgical division of the median arcuate ligament might be helpful.

▶ [It was my impression that Szilagyi et al. (*Surgery* 72:849, 1972) had very effectively dispelled the notion of the celiac compression syndrome or symptoms that could arise from celiac compression. The findings in the present study suggest great caution in attributing any symptoms whatever to compression of the celiac artery. The mechanism for such symptoms is hardly evident. Furthermore, as pointed out by the present authors, as many as 24% of individuals undergoing angiography will be found

Follow-up (1½–9½ Years, Mean 6.3)

	No. of patients
No complaints	2
Improved, but instead other abdominal symptoms	6
Unchanged	5
Worse	2

(22–6) Acta Chir. Scand. 147:201–203, 1981.

to have at least 50% stenosis of the celiac artery even in the absence of abdominal symptoms. The findings in this study are consonant with those of Szilagyi et al. Despite that, the authors do leave themselves an out in saying that compression of the celiac axis might be symptomatic in some cases, even though they have produced very little proof to support that statement. For now, it is probably best to avoid operation on the celiac axis with the hope of relieving abdominal symptomatology of a vague and poorly described nature.—W.S.] ◀

22–7 **Does "Intestinal Angina" Exist? A Critical Study of Obstructed Visceral Arteries.** Rodney J. Croft, G. P. Menon, and Adrian Marston (Univ. of London), after examining the incidence of atheromatous obstruction of the celiac axis and the superior and inferior mesenteric arteries, attempted to relate the pathology to symptoms and to patient survival. The mesenteric vessels were examined in 203 unselected autopsied adults aged 19–97; about 80% were aged 40–80 years. The male to female ratio was 1.2:1.

Severe atherosclerosis was present in 17% of aortas, and mild to moderate involvement in 60%. The mean stenosis of celiac axes was 21.9%, that of the superior mesenteric arteries was 27.3%, and that of the inferior mesenteric arteries was 30.5%. The respective rates of stenosis exceeding 50% were 3.4%, 4.9%, and 10.8%. All patients with such stenosis who had had gastrointestinal symptoms had other causes to explain the symptoms. The relation of stenoses to age is shown in the table. Of 41 patients with gastrointestinal symptoms, 6 had had undiagnosed abdominal pain for which no cause was found at autopsy. None of these patients had mesenteric stenoses exceeding 50%. One patient who had had superior mesenteric embolus removed, with no subsequent symptoms, had occlusion of all three vessels with a visible collateral circulation. Another patient had died after large bowel resection for acute obstruction, with less than 50% stenoses present at autopsy. Four patients with greater than 50% stenosis of two vessels had had no gastrointestinal symptoms. No collateral circulation was evident in these individuals.

"Critical" stenosis of the mesenteric arteries appears to be rare. No correlation between the degree of stenosis and previous gastrointes-

Distribution of Stenotic Lesions Either Greater Than or Less Than 50% Within Four Age Categories

Artery	Age group (yr) <40 (*n*=7)	40–60 (*n*=60)	61–80 (*n*=101)	>80 (*n*=35)
CA stenosis (%)				
<50	100	98·3	95·9	92·9
>50	0	1·7	4·1	7·1
SMA stenosis (%)				
<50	100	96·8	95·2	96·6
>50	0	3·2	4·8	3·4
IMA stenosis (%)				
<50	85·7	93·2	87·4	84·4
>50	14·3	6·8	12·6	15·6

(22–7) Br. J. Surg. 68:316–318, May 1981.

tinal symptoms was found in this autopsy study. Radiologic demonstration of stenosed or blocked visceral arteries remains of doubtful clinical significance. The relationship between surgically identified vascular disease and fatal intestinal infarction is uncertain. Intestinal angina almost certainly results from inability of the mesenteric vascular bed to increase its flow in response to food intake, but the critical degree and extent of stenosis are unknown.

▶ [The title of this paper is somewhat misleading because the text does not really address itself to the question of whether or not intestinal angina exists. In fact, the authors make allusion to a case or cases of intestinal angina with single-vessel occlusion that have been cured by revascularization—so, obviously, they believe that it truly does exist. The new and important observations in this study are that the authors very carefully measured the degree of stenosis of the splanchnic vessels, something that has not been done in previous studies. They found that although mild degrees of stenosis were common, the true incidence of critical stenosis is rather small. The fact that they found no correlation between the degree of stenosis and the presence of premortem gastrointestinal symptoms does not mean necessarily that angiographic examination of the patient with classic intestinal angina is not warranted. It is important to recognize that a wide variety of physiological and possibly pharmacologic perturbations might produce alterations in intestinal blood flow. When these physiological alterations are superimposed on the presence or absence of varying degrees of collateral circulation, it becames obvious that the risk of intestinal infarction for the patient under consideration cannot be assessed on the basis of an angiographic examination alone. Indeed, true intestinal angina is quite rare, and it is perfectly possible that not a single case of intestinal angina really was present in the 203 patients examined by these authors.

In the end, the indication for operation comes down to a classic history of cramping abdominal pain after ingestion of food, together with weight loss, in a patient who has angiographic evidence of critical stenosis of usually the superior mesenteric artery. As emphasized above, this constellation really does occur, although it is very rare.—W.S.] ◀

22–8 **Protein-Losing Enteropathy in Human and Experimental Rat Blind Loop Syndrome.** An increase in the bacterial population of the small intestine, termed the "stasis" or "blind loop" syndrome, can disturb the assimilation of various nutrients. Although depressed serum protein levels have been noted in this syndrome, the etiology of the protein metabolic abnormality is unknown. Charles E. King and Phillip P. Toskes (Univ. of Florida, Gainesville) suggest that protein loss may result from mucosal injury in the setting of small intestine bacterial overgrowth.

Studies were performed in 2 patients with protein-losing enteropathy and small intestine bacterial overgrowth. One had undergone Billroth II partial gastrectomy 3 months earlier. After both malabsorption and protein-losing enteropathy had been identified, 2 courses of antibiotic therapy over 2 months decreased the excessive ^{51}Cr fecal output to 4.2%; this was further decreased to normal (1.2%) with 3 more courses of antibiotics over the next 6 months. The other patient had bacterial overgrowth secondary to radiation-induced ileal stasis. Several courses of antibiotic therapy led to improvement in the bacterial overgrowth and partial reversal of a protein-losing enteropathy. These studies demonstrate for the first time antibiotic reversibility of protein-losing enteropathy in the human blind loop syndrome.

(22–8) Gastroenterology 80:504–509, March 1981.

Studies in rats with artificially created jejunal blind loops revealed depressed serum protein levels and excessive fecal excretion of intravenously administered ^{51}Cr as compared to nonoperated and surgical controls. Comparison of protein loss of rats who had had blind loops for varying lengths of time and paired comparison of rats tested for protein loss at 2 different times showed a relatively stable degree of protein loss once it was manifest. Reversal of protein loss with antibiotic therapy was accomplished in only a few rats, and in those only after prolonged therapy. Surgical extirpation of the blind loop from rats with protein-losing enteropathy consistently corrected the protein loss, although this correction was delayed up to 9 weeks from the time of extirpative surgery.

These studies demonstrate significant protein loss as one etiologic factor for protein metabolic disturbances in the human and experimental rat blind loop syndrome. Intestinal protein loss is a manifestation of functionally significant mucosal injury in the contaminated nonstagnant small bowel as well as the stagnant part of the small intestine affected by bacterial overgrowth. Functionally significant mucosal injury in the blind loop syndrome is difficult to reverse once it has been manifested. Excessive passage of endogenous protein to the bowel lumen may not be manifest with diminished serum protein levels unless the protein loss is massive or there are concomitant problems of digestion and absorption leading to incomplete reassimilation of protein lost to the lumen or inadequate compensation of serum protein synthesis after delivery of reabsorbed protein precursors to the liver.

▶ [Although it has been known for many years that protein metabolic disturbances occur in the human blind loop syndrome, the mechanism for those disturbances has been unclear. This study provides us with important new information emphasizing that bacterial overgrowth can indeed induce a protein-losing enteropathy that is reversible with long-term antibiotic treatment or by surgical resection. The mechanism by which the bacterial overgrowth causes such protein losing is not completely clear; nevertheless, we can now include the blind loop syndrome as one of the established causes of protein-losing enteropathy that should be sought in patients with hypoalbuminemia.—W.S.] ◀

23. Colon and Rectum

23–1 **Delayed Primary Wound Closure in Gangrenous and Perforated Appendicitis.** Wound sepsis is the most common cause of morbidity after surgery for perforated or gangrenous appendicitis. Delayed primary wound closure has been reported by some researchers to reduce wound sepsis in various clinical settings. Ross A. Pettigrew (Univ. of Auckland) compared the morbidity after delayed primary wound closure with that after primary closure in a prospective study of 122 patients with perforated or frankly gangrenous appendicitis. The patients were placed in three groups. In group A, 41 patients with a mean age of 26.5 years had primary closure alone. In group B, 39 patients with a mean age of 24.5 years had primary closure with topical ampicillin administration, and in group C, 42 patients with a mean age of 24.9 years had delayed primary wound closure on the fifth postoperative day. All closures were done with monofilament nylon sutures, and all groups were clinically comparable.

A significant reduction in wound sepsis was observed in group B patients compared with group C. Primary closure with topical ampicillin administration was superior to delayed primary closure, and marginally superior to primary closure alone (table). Infection occurred in 45% of all wounds with positive cultures at surgery. Anaerobic bacteria colonization of wounds decreased in the interval between surgery and delayed closure; however, 7 wounds became colonized with *Staphylococcus aureus,* and 4 of these patients had wound infection. Intra-abdominal abscesses developed in patients in all groups. Group B patients had the shortest hospital stay and group C had the longest. Several patients found delayed primary closure intolerable. Patients with more serious perforations had a reduction in wound sepsis when antibiotics effective against *Bacteroides fragilis* were administered systemically.

Delayed primary wound closure was not well accepted by patients in this study and failed to reduce wound sepsis. In some cases, exog-

INFECTED WOUNDS IN GROUPS OF PATIENTS

	Group A	Group B	Group C	Total
No. of patients	41	39	42	122
No. of infected wounds	15	7	23	45
Percentage of infected wounds	37	18	54	37

(23–1) Br. J. Surg. 68:635–638, September 1981.

enous organisms such as staphylococci contaminated wounds in the interval between surgery and closure. Systemic antibiotics effective against *B. fragilis* reduce the wound sepsis rate. The need for topical ampicillin therapy when such systemic treatment is used is questionable.

▶ [There is an increasing tendency in the United States to leaving highly contaminated wounds open. Recently, delayed primary closure has become popular, presumably as a means of decreasing the morbidity associated with allowing wounds to heal by secondary intention. This nice study confirms my prejudices, which are based on clinical experiences that have been purely anecdotal, but are forceful in their impact nevertheless. Pettigrew has shown what I have preached for many years, namely, that open wounds indeed do become secondarily contaminated and occasionally infected by organisms not originally present. I believe that such secondary infections often are not recognized as such. Open granulating wounds obviously cannot develop a collection of purulent material, but I have encountered many patients who become febrile, feel poorly, and have increased wound pain and a change in the type of discharge that clearly represents infection in open wounds. Such patients often need systemic antibiotics, although often, because the wound is open, the surgeon looks for other, more ethereal, causes for the febrile course and lack of well-being of the patient. If one looks very carefully, one will find that leaving a wound open does not confer immunity against secondary infection by any stretch of the imagination. While I am not opposed to leaving highly contaminated wounds open, I think we must recognize that secondary infections do occur in such wounds and we must treat them appropriately when they do.—W.S.] ◀

23–2 **Neutropenic Typhlitis in Adults.** The term "typhlitis," or inflammation of the cecum, has been used recently to describe a lesion developing in leukemic patients, especially children. Robert W. Ikard (Vanderbilt Univ.) describes findings in an adult with typhlitis whose disease was successfully managed by a two-stage surgical procedure.

Woman, 64, with recent onset of refractory anemia and excess blast cell formation, was treated with fluoxymestrone, folic acid, and furosemide. After 3 days of vague abdominal pain, nausea and vomiting, and fever, the patient was hospitalized. A rigid abdomen and fever of 38.3 C were noted. Rebound tenderness was most marked in the right lower quadrant; bowel sounds were absent. The white blood cell count was 200 cu mm. Tobramycin and ticarcillin were given in preparation for surgery. The cecum and proximal ascending colon were diffusely inflamed. An ileocecectomy was carried out, with ascending colostomy and ileostomy. White blood cell infusions were given for 4 days postoperatively. Several wound complications occurred, as well as erysipelas. The operative specimen exhibited vascular thrombosis, edema and infarction of the cecum, and extensive infiltration of the cecal wall by gram-positive rods and cocci. Only the serosal surface of the appendix was inflamed. The patient's nutritional and hematologic status improved markedly postoperatively. The colostomy and ileostomy subsequently were taken down uneventfully.

The cecum can be involved in any inflammatory bowel condition. Leukemic patients have a high incidence of gastrointestinal tract complications. Patients with cecal necrosis associated with granulocytopenia usually have localized peritonitis. The white blood cell count is an unreliable index of disease progress. Usually, a barium enema study is not necessary before abdominal exploration. The frequently identified invading organism is *Pseudomonas*. Immunosuppressive therapy has been implicated as a cause of typhlitis in some instances.

(23–2) Arch. Surg. 116:943–945, July 1981.

It is not clear why the cecum is the usual target organ in neutropenic enterocolitis. Six of 9 adults have had successful results from surgery. Indications for surgery are essentially the same as in patients with a normal immune system, because affected patients probably will not live without removal of the necrotic process.

▶ [It is my opinion that we are going to see an increasing incidence of this disorder as more and more potent chemotherapeutic measures are used. The one recurrent background theme in these cases is leukopenia, and this, of course, makes these patients much graver operative risks. Nevertheless, the lesion must be treated by resection. Clearly, those patients in whom resections were not done did not survive. The reasons for selection of the cecum for this process are unknown.—W.S.] ◀

23–3 **Solitary Ulcer of the Rectum—Or Is It? Report of 6 Cases.** Solitary rectal ulcer is an uncommon condition that may mimic more serious rectal pathology such as Crohn's disease, ulcerative colitis, or carcinoma. G. Thomson, A. Clark, J. Handyside, and G. Gillespie (Glasgow) report 6 cases of so-called solitary ulcer of the rectum seen in 1969 to 1979. The clinical features are summarized in the table. These lesions need not be either solitary or ulcerous. The classic appearance is that of a discrete, "punched-out" shallow ulcer with a gray base, hyperemic edge, and surrounding induration, usually on the anterior rectal wall. A preulcerative phase also is described, with polypoid, hypertrophic, or hyperemic mucosa. Overt ulceration has not appeared for over 2 years in 1 of the present cases. The lesions were variable in both site and number, in different patients and at different times in the same patient.

The cause of this disorder remains obscure. Rutter found a defect in normal reflex relaxation of the puborectalis muscle during defecation in some patients and related it to the flap valve theory of fecal continence proposed by Parks et al., which holds that the puborectalis maintains continence through preserving the anorectal junction at a 90-degree angle. The lesions might be due to trauma from the anterior rectal mucosa being forced against the tightly contracting bar of muscle during defecation, possibly through ischemia. Alexander-Williams suggested that the solitary ulcer syndrome is due to preexisting rectal prolapse. No satisfactory treatment for the condition is known, but all patients in the present series have been managed without de-

SUMMARY OF PRESENTATION AND PROGRESS

Case no.	Age/sex	Presentation	Sigmoidoscopic appearance	Initial diagnosis	Progress
1	26 M	Rectal bleed	Ulcer	Carcinoma	Chronicity
2	22 M	Rectal bleed	Multiple polyps	Benign polyp	Chronicity
3	43 F	Rectal bleed	Inflammation + multiple ulcers	?	Healed
4	27 M	Rectal bleed	Nodular mass	Carcinoma	Chronicity
5	46 F	Rectal bleed, pain, tenesmus, mucus	Anterior mucosal prolapse + ulcer	Carcinoma	Chronicity
6	20 F	Rectal bleed, pain, frequency, mucus	Ulcer	Irritable colon	Chronicity

(23–3) Br. J. Surg. 68:21–24, January 1981.

finitive surgery. Longer follow-up of affected patients is needed to obtain a clearer picture of the natural history of the condition.

▶ [The condition of solitary ulcer of the rectum is rare and its pathogenesis is enigmatic. I doubt, however, that this report will enhance our understanding of the causation of this condition, or even serve to do anything but confuse us. The authors have accepted the pathologist's diagnosis of solitary ulcer of the rectum in at least 2 cases in which no ulceration could be seen either grossly or microscopically. In 1 of the cases, which has been followed for 2 years, ulceration has never developed. This blind acceptance of a pathologist's diagnosis has plagued surgery in many spheres. One has only to look to the problems encountered by the pathologic interpretation of parathyroid lesions, breast lesions, and many other conditions in which precise definition of the pathology is lacking. Although Madigan and Morson (*Gut* 10:871–881, 1969) have suggested that this disease has a preulcerative stage, and, indeed, described its picture, they make no claim that the findings were completely specific. In addition, solid evidence is lacking that such changes are always followed by the development of an ulcer, and one wonders how one can call this "solitary ulcer of the rectum" in the absence of ulceration. It would be far better to simply acknowledge our ignorance over this matter, rather than to confuse the issue in this way. These are interesting cases, but we need much more information about the causation of this condition, and we need less confusion about its microscopic aspects. If, indeed, Thomson and his co-workers can show us that the nonulcerative lesions went on to ulceration, then we would be happy to acknowledge that these *are* cases of solitary ulcer of the rectum.—W.S.] ◀

23–4 **Randomized Prospective Evaluation of EEA Stapler for Colorectal Anastomoses.** The EEA stapler was designed to perform inverted end-to-end anastomoses and offers many improvements over its predecessor, the Russian stapler. Robert W. Beart, Jr., and Keith A. Kelly (Mayo Clinic) conducted a randomized prospective study of the EEA stapler in patients undergoing anterior anastomosis of peritonealized sigmoid or descending colon to nonperitonealized rectum for such conditions as rectosigmoid tumor, rectal prolapse, and diverticulosis. Either a stapled anastomosis or a two-layered, hand-sewn anastomosis was carried out. Thirty-five patients were randomly assigned to each of these procedures. The average age was 64 years. The study and control groups were similar in diagnoses, biochemical profiles, and estimated intraoperative blood loss.

Sixty percent of hand-sewn anastomoses and 36% of stapled anastomoses were considered technically difficult. Postoperative biochemical findings and stool consistency were comparable in the two groups. One patient in the stapled group had wound infection. One patient in each group had pelvic infection, and 1 had anastomotic dehiscence. The 1 death was of a patient in the stapled group who had anastomotic dehiscence. The time for anastomosis averaged 11 minutes in the stapled group and 19 minutes in the hand-sewn group. The postoperative course was generally similar in the two groups. There were 3 significant intraoperative complications with use of the staple technique and none with the hand-sewn technique.

Postoperative roentgenography now is done on all patients having stapled anastomoses; if there is evidence of discontinuity of the staple ring, a protective loop colostomy is done. A single-layered anastomosis was not considered in the present series, but this type of anastomosis is technically easier. The EEA stapler can save several rectums

(23–4) Am. J. Surg. 141:143–147, January 1981.

that otherwise might have to be removed because of technical inability to perform a hand-sewn anastomosis. This may have been the case for all 10 patients excluded from the present study as being unsuitable for randomization.

▶ [This is a fine randomized study. We would be very interested in a subsequent trial that compared single-layer anastomoses with the stapler, particularly in regard to the level at which the anastomosis could be accomplished. Obviously, if the distal pursestring suture is placed transanally, as has been suggested by Goligher, one certainly can carry out a lower anastomosis with the stapler. However, if the pursestring suture is placed from the abdominal approach, it would be interesting to know whether, in fact, a lower anastomosis could be achieved with the stapler. I feel that the differences might not be as large as one might have predicted.

It is surprising to me that the surgical literature continues to be overly preoccupied with the length of a given operation. In this modern era, it is hardly conceivable that the 8 additional minutes required for the hand-sewn anastomosis could make any difference whatever in terms of outcome, even though the difference in time was statistically significant.

I have always been slightly uncomfortable with the fact that once the stapler is activated and the procedure carried out, there is very little that the surgeon can do to correct a poor anastomosis if the anastomosis is in the very depths of the pelvis. It is one thing to be able to correct a faulty esophagogastric anastomosis by using a layer of sutures on the outside, where this can be readily accomplished, but it is clearly another when the one-shot affair is over and a faulty anastomosis cannot be corrected. Therefore, excessive emphasis cannot be placed on the proper placement of the pursestring suture. If the rectal wall is extremely thick, I have found that occasionally the cuff that is to be cut by the stapler may be somewhat excessive and may interfere with the proper placement of the staples. For that reason, we need to develop methods to assure ourselves that very distally placed anastomoses are intact. In addition to the suggestion proposed by these authors that an x-ray film be taken to ascertain the completeness of the stapled ring while the patient is on the operating table, I would propose that the rectum be irrigated with a tinted saline solution through a preoperatively placed rectal catheter to make certain that the anastomosis is watertight. This maneuver has been exceedingly helpful. Also, I would suggest that a covering colostomy be performed if any question arises as to the watertight nature of the anastomosis. We have found that the staples may be difficult to see on an x-ray film taken in the operating room.—W.S.] ◀

23–5 **Reversible Ischemic Colitis in Young Adults.** Ischemic colitis is well recognized in older patients, but its occurrence in patients younger than age 30 is rare. Terence J. Duffy (Cambridge, England) reports 4 cases of transient ischemic colitis in patients under age 30.

Man, 20, presented after 2 days of lower abdominal pain, vomiting, diarrhea, and passage of fresh blood rectally. The lower abdomen was diffusely tender, and the sigmoid was very tender. Bright red blood was found in the rectum. The hemoglobin level was 15.4 gm/dl; the sedimentation rate was 43 mm/hour. Proctoscopy showed a normal rectal mucosa but reddened mucosa above, with shallow ulcers up to 5 cm across, some with purulent exudate. A barium enema study showed persistent spasm of a long segment of colon with "thumbprinting." Intravenous Pro-Banthine failed to relax the spastic segment. Stool cultures revealed normal flora. The patient was virtually asymptomatic 3 days after admission, and was discharged after 6 days without symptoms. Sigmoidoscopy done 2 weeks after discharge showed no abnormalities to 20 cm.

Transient ischemic colitis is characterized by lower abdominal pain, diarrhea, and sudden rectal bleeding. The features clear rapidly on nonspecific management. There was no direct evidence proving the

(23–5) Br. J. Surg. 68:34–37, January 1981.

ischemic basis of transient colitis in these cases. The present patients were younger than previously described patients, had a short course, and recovered rapidly and completely. Roentgenographic findings included thumbprinting of the colon and mucosal irregularity. No patient had abnormal fecal flora, and this, along with the site of the lesion, helps distinguish the condition from infective colitis, inflammatory bowel disease, and ischemic colitis.

The outcome was satisfactory in all the present cases. One patient had laparotomy because of signs of peritonitis. The other 3 patients became asymptomatic within 4 days without specific treatment. Reported cases indicate a benign course when there is no predisposing cause, but laparotomy may be necessary when the clinical signs progress.

▶ [It is difficult to accept these 4 cases as unequivocal examples of ischemic colitis. The diagnosis rested mainly on "thumbprinting" shown on barium enema study, the clear reversibility of the lesions, and the fact that the lesions were found in individuals in whom no ordinary pathogens could be detected in the stool. Absolute positive evidence for ischemia by biopsy is not at hand. I have seen a *Salmonella* infection of the colon that produced a radiologic picture identical to that seen in ischemic colitis or in any of the cases shown by this author. I am not suggesting that these cases were examples of salmonellosis or disease caused by other known pathogens, because none was found. However, the author does not mention that *Yersinia* infection was excluded, and such things as *Campylobacter* and other more unusual types of bacterial infection certainly are much more likely than ischemia as a cause for the observations in these patients. The medical profession unfortunately responds in a reflex fashion to certain catch terms, so that the minute the term "thumbprinting" is used, one needs necessarily to assume that ischemia is present. I am fascinated by the fact that films that show classic thumbprinting can be displayed to physicians, but if the word "thumbprinting" is not used, then ischemia often does not come to mind. The usual causes of ischemic colitis in young individuals, previously clearly described in the literature, have been severe hypotension, drug abuse with sepsis, and oral contraceptive. Just as "all that glitters is not gold," all that thumbprints is not ischemic.—W.S.] ◀

23–6 **Proctitis and Colitis Following Diversion of Fecal Stream.** Donald J. Glotzer, Michael E. Glick, and Harvey Goldman (Harvard Med. School) observed inflammation limited to excluded segments of the colon in 6 men and 4 women aged 26–83 years (mean 65 years), with no prior inflammatory bowel disease, who had undergone fecal diversion because of complications of diverticular disease (6 patients), fecal incontinence secondary to neurologic disorders (2), drug-induced colonic ileus (1), or protection of low anterior rectal anastomosis (1). Four patients had loop or end sigmoid colostomy, 5 had loop transverse colostomy, and 1 had an end ileostomy. Several other patients with prior fecal diversion did not show proctitis on sigmoidoscopy.

Nine patients were asymptomatic when the lesion was discovered by endoscopy 10 weeks to 3 years after fecal diversion; the 10th complained of mucoid rectal discharge 7 years after colostomy. The proctoscopic findings appeared similar to those of mild ulcerative colitis. In 8 of the 10 patients the inflammatory changes were confined to the distal few centimeters of the rectum, while 2 had inflammation in the entire excluded segment. Microscopic alterations were focal and in-

(23–6) Gastroenterology 80:438–441, March 1981.

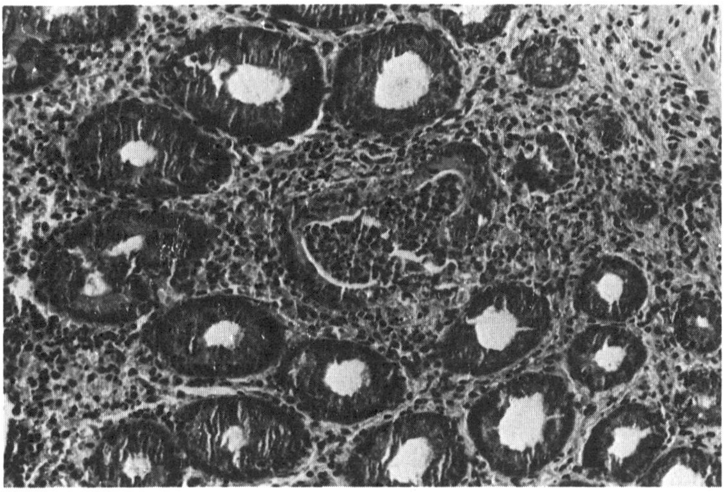

Fig 23–1.—Rectal mucosal biopsy in man, aged 49, with loop sigmoid colostomy for free perforation of a sigmoid diverticulum, shows a discrete crypt abscess *(center)* with marked inflammation in the crypt wall and adjacent lamina propria. Normal crypts are seen at the periphery. Hematoxylin-eosin; ×250. (Courtesy of Glotzer, D.J., et al.: Gastroenterology 80:438–441, March 1981.)

cluded crypt abscesses, epithelial cell degeneration, acute and chronic inflammation in the lamina propria, and regenerative changes in the crypts (Fig 23–1).

Of 5 patients who have not had restoration of intestinal continuity 2–8 years (mean, 5 years) after diversion, 2 became symptomatic with abdominal cramps and purulent rectal discharge. All of the 4 patients in whom follow-up endoscopy of the excluded segment was performed showed ongoing inflammation. Five patients had restoration of intestinal continuity 2½–6 months after discovery of proctitis, despite the presence of inflammation in the excluded segment. These patients had no anastomotic complications, and each remains asymptomatic. Each of the 4 in whom sigmoidoscopy was performed 2–36 months after colostomy closure showed resolution of the colitis.

The inflammation in these patients probably resulted from diversion of the fecal stream and was not a recognized form of specific or idiopathic colitis. Diversion-related colitis must not be confused with other forms of inflammation, since this may result in improper therapy or delay in treatment of the condition for which fecal diversion was performed.

▶ [This is a very important contribution. I personally have seen at least 2 instances of this entity. In 1 case, an unfortunate patient was subjected to subtotal colectomy with ileostomy for this condition, which was thought to be inflammatory bowel disease. This is one of the most important points that can be made about the discovery of this previously undescribed disorder. Its pathogenesis is completely unclear at present. Its true incidence is unknown, because the total number of cases undergoing diversion from which the 2 reported cases were drawn is unknown. Obviously, it is important to investigate the true incidence of this phenomenon. At the same time, all surgeons who undertake diversionary procedures must be aware that the presence of a mild proctitis and colitis in the defunctionated segment should not be misconstrued to indicate necessarily the presence of inflammatory bowel disease.—W.S.] ◀

23–7 **Colectomy with Rectal Mucosectomy and Ileoanal Anastomosis in Young Patients: Its Use for Ulcerative Colitis and Familial Polyposis.** Martin et al., in 1977, described the use of total colectomy with mucosal prostectomy and preservation of rectal continence. The rectal mucosa is completely removed with the muscular rectal wall and sphincters being retained; the terminal ileum is then pulled through the muscular cuff and sutured to the pectinate line. Robert L. Telander and Jean Perrault (Mayo Clinic and Found.) performed colectomy with rectal mucosectomy and ileoanal anastomosis in 25 patients, 22 with chronic ulcerative colitis and 3 with familial polyposis, from 1977 to 1980. The mean age was 16.5 years, and the mean follow-up was 14½ months. Total parenteral nutrition was used rather extensively in initial patients. The rectal dissection now is limited and similar to that in the Swenson procedure (Fig 23–2). The mucosectomy is done via a perineal approach, leaving a short rectal muscular cuff (Fig 23–3). A temporary loop ileostomy is made in the right lower quadrant (Fig 23–4). Balloon catheter dilations of the

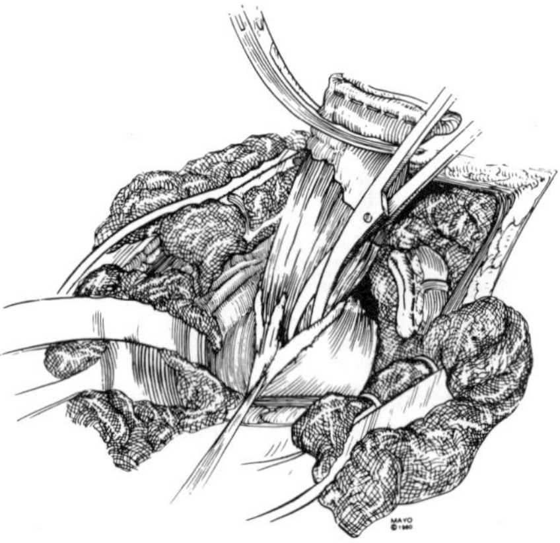

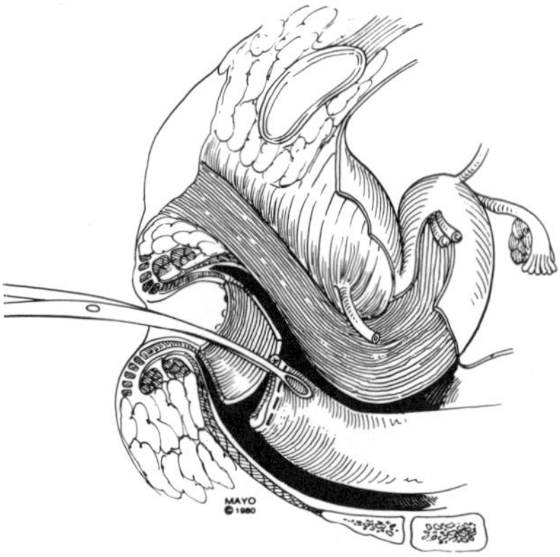

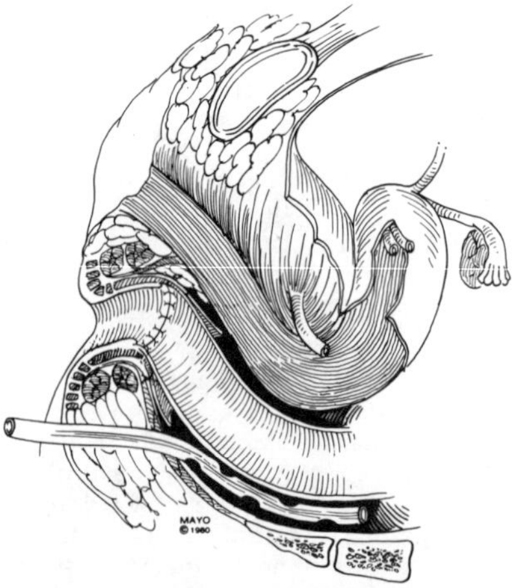

Fig 23–2 (above left).—Removal of rectum, with dissection directly on rectal wall.

Fig 23–3 (above).—Removal of anorectal mucosa. Mucosa is excised at dentate line with dissection of it away from underlying distal 8 cm of rectal muscularis.

Fig 23–4 (left).—Ileoanalanastomosis completed. Silastic catheters are used to drain rectal cuff and pelvis. (Courtesy of Telander, R.L., and Perrault, J.: Arch. Surg. 116:623–629, May 1981; copyright 1981, American Medical Association.)

(23–7) Arch. Surg. 116:623–629, May 1981.

neorectum now are done; the ileostomy is closed 8–12 weeks after the pull-through procedure.

No deaths and no abscess formation have occurred, but 1 patient had a vesicoenteric fistula several months postoperatively. There were no abdominal wound infections. Two patients required lysis of adhesions causing small bowel obstruction. The ileostomy has been closed in all patients but 1. Eleven patients had an excellent result, with a satisfactory stooling pattern and no perineal discomfort. Seven had good results, 3 had fair results, and 3 had a poor outcome. All patients presently are at school or work. Perineal discomfort and excoriation generally resolved over time. The patients have learned to distinguish gas from liquid stool. Three patients have undergone further surgery. All but 1 of 8 patients followed for at least a year were above the 25th percentile in height and weight. Also, all 7 patients in whom the determination was made had normal vitamin B_{12} levels.

All of the patients in this series had good anal sphincter tone and voluntary rectal continence after colectomy with rectal mucosectomy and ileoanal anastomosis. The prodedure is recommended for selected young patients with chronic ulcerative colitis and familial polyposis.

▶ [The results achieved by these authors are extremely promising. However, from a functional standpoint, they are not yet perfect. Whether the use of a J-shaped ileal reservoir pouch, advocated by some surgeons, will improve the outcome in patients such as this remains to be seen. It is rather surprising that these authors were able to excise all the diseased mucosa without problems in patients with ulcerative colitis, because this portion of the operative procedure has offered much difficulty to other surgeons. The outcome of this study suggests cautious optimism and further study of this problem, with the use of variations of the procedure that might improve the functional results.—W.S.] ◀

23–8 **Prognosis of Ileorectal Anastomosis in Crohn's Disease.** Colectomy with ileorectal anastomosis has been advocated for selected patients with Crohn's colitis. Peter Buchmann, Irene T. Weterman, Michael R. B. Keighley, Salvador A. Peña, Robert N. Allan, and John Alexander-Williams reviewed the results of this procedure in 105 patients operated on electively for Crohn's colitis in 1958 to 1978. Patients with very severe rectal disease, severe perianal lesions, or incontinence were excluded. Ten patients had a defunctioning ileostomy and 9, an end-ileostomy with either closure of the rectal stump or a mucous fistula with the intention of early reoperation and ileorectal anastomosis.

In 1978, 70% of patients still had a functioning ileorectal anastomosis. Twenty patients had had an ileostomy, 8 had died, and 3 were lost to follow-up. Mean follow-up was 7.6 years. The outcome was not influenced by the presence of active terminal ileal disease at the time of surgery or by the presence of perianal disease. Fewer ileorectal anastomoses remained functioning when proctitis was present at the time of colectomy. The risk of reoperation increased linearly after primary operation (Fig 23–5). There was 1 postoperative death due to intra-abdominal abscess formation and septicemia. Only 3 patients with a functioning ileorectal anastomosis reported significant prob-

---

(23–8) Br. J. Surg. 68:7–10, January 1981.

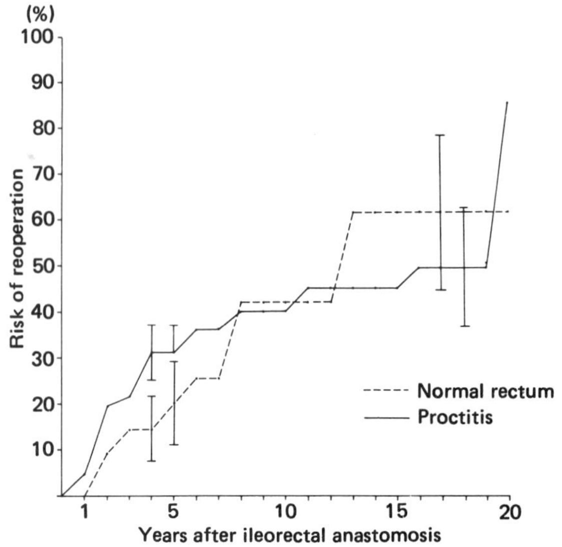

Fig 23–5.—Cumulative risk of needing reoperation for recurrent Crohn's disease in patients with or without preoperative proctitis. Excluded are 17 patients with unknown preoperative findings. (Courtesy of Buchmann, P., et al.: Br. J. Surg. 68:7–10, January 1981.)

lems. Many patients passed stools frequently but coped quite well with this. The renal mucosa appeared abnormal in fewer than half of the patients having sigmoidoscopy. All 8 perianal fistulas and 4 rectovaginal fistulas were quiescent. Ten perianal abscesses were drained either spontaneously or surgically, and 3 fistulas were opened during follow-up. In both patients in whom incontinence led to failure of the operation, severe perianal disease was present.

Ileorectal anastomosis after colectomy has an important role in the management of patients with Crohn's disease, even if proctectomy and ileostomy are required later. Performing a defunctioning ileostomy is not necessary. Only patients with severe proctitis, severe perianal disease, or incontinence need be excluded from ileorectal anastomosis. Most patients having ileorectal anastomosis will tolerate an increased frequency of defecation in preference to an ileostomy.

▶ [This is a very interesting and optimistic report of the outcome of treatment of colonic Crohn's disease by ileorectal anastomosis. Our own results, in a much smaller series of patients followed from 9 to 25 years, indicate that about 25% of patients with anastomotic procedures will stay in good health for a prolonged period, whereas 75% will ultimately have proctectomy and ileostomy. The reasons for the differences in outcome between our own series and those depicted in this report are not clear. Nevertheless, the conclusions that can be drawn from this study, and the position that we have taken in regard to ileorectal anastomosis, are virtually identical. We feel, as do the authors, that ileorectal anastomosis should be used with confidence, particularly in younger patients with an intense aversion to ileostomy and especially where the rectum is normal or near normal. We would exclude those patients with severe proctitis or rectal strictures, and especially those with serious perianal disease or incontinence. Our practice has been not to perform ileorectal anastomosis where significant rectal disease is present, but the results of this study suggest that this is successful in some patients, albeit less so than when the rectum is normal.—W.S.] ◀

23–9 **Elective Postoperative Radiotherapy After Incomplete Resection of Colorectal Cancer.** Incompletely resected colorectal cancer has a high local recurrence rate. N. A. Ghossein, E. C. Samala, S. Alpert, F. R. DeLuca, H. Ragins, S. S. Turner, P. Stacey, and H. Flax (Albert Einstein College of Medicine, New York) conducted a prospective study of the value of elective postoperative irradiation in patients undergoing either complete or incomplete resection of colorectal cancer. Between 1972 and 1978, radiotherapy was given to 78 patients with rectal or rectosigmoid cancer and to 47 with colonic cancer above the midsigmoid. The former patients received 4,600 rad through an inverted T-shaped field over about 5 weeks; the para-aortic extension was cut after 4,000 rad. An additional 1,000–1,500 rad was delivered to patients with residual disease. Those with tumors above the midsigmoid received treatment to the entire abdomen by the moving strip technique, a tumor dose of about 2,100 rad being given in 8 days. Patients with residual disease received an additional 1,000–1,500 rad through a coned-down field. Megavoltage therapy was given in all cases.

Nodal involvement was present in 60% of patients, and 85% had at least a stage T_3 lesion. Residual disease was present in 25% (Table 1). Two thirds of the patients with rectosigmoid cancer and 60% of those with colonic cancer are alive without disease after an average of 38 months. Local control is related to the degree of postoperative residual disease in Table 2 and to adjacent organ involvement in Table 3. Four patients had complications from pelvic irradiation, and 3 had complications from whole abdominal radiotherapy; 1 died of radiation enteritis.

Moderate doses of postoperative irradiation will eradicate most subclinical colorectal cancers still present after attempted resection. Patients with gross residual cancer in the present series had a worse prognosis, but half of them were free of local recurrence and over a third were alive without disease at follow-up. Radiation complications do not appear to be a deterrent to this type of treatment. Longer fol-

TABLE 1.—DISTRIBUTION OF PATIENTS ACCORDING TO DEGREE OF RESIDUAL DISEASE AFTER RESECTION

Surgical Procedure	R0	R1	R2
Abdominoperineal resection	16	2	9
Anterior resection	40	6	5
Hemi or partial colectomy	38	5	4
TOTAL	94 (75 Per Cent)	13 (10 Per Cent)	18 (14 Per Cent)

(23–9) Dis. Colon Rectum 24:252–256, May–June 1981.

TABLE 2.—LOCAL CONTROL* ACCORDING TO POSTOPERATIVE RESIDUAL DISEASE

R0	R1	R2	Total
81†/94 (86 Per Cent)	11/13 (84 Per Cent)	9/18 (50 Per Cent)	101/125 (81Per Cent)

*Patients in whom treatment failed either locally or locally and distantly were considered to have local failure.
†One patient lost to follow-up was considered to have local and distant failure.
Follow-up: minimum, 12 months; maximum, 84 months; average, 38 months.

TABLE 3.—LOCAL CONTROL* AFTER ELECTIVE POSTOPERATIVE RADIOTHERAPY IN 39 PATIENTS WITH ADJACENT ORGAN INVOLVEMENT

	Residual Disease		
	Gross	Microscopic	Completely Resected
Line of resection	1/1	5/6	—
Bladder and/or prostate	2/5	1/1	1/1
Rectovaginal septum	—	1/1	1/1
Abdominal and/or pelvic wall	4/6	3/3	—
Pararectal tissues (including presacral and ischiorectal spaces)	2/6	—	—
Fallopian tube and/or small bowel	—	—	4/6
Liver	—	1/2	—
TOTAL	9/18 (50 Per Cent)	11/13 (84 Per Cent)	6/8 —
	20/31 (65 Per Cent)		

*Patients in whom treatment failed locally or locally and distantly were considered to have failure.
Follow-up: minimum, 12 months; maximum, 84 months; average, 47 months.

low-up is necessary to determine whether postoperative irradiation increases the survival of patients undergoing incomplete resection of colorectal cancer.

▶ [This is an impressive study. The results are quite startling in view of the far-advanced nature of the lesions treated. Although, unfortunately, there are no prospective randomized trials available that evaluate postoperative radiotherapy in patients with colorectal cancer, the preliminary results achieved in this series strongly suggest that such a trial is highly warranted. In the meantime, if postoperative radiation therapy can be delivered with as low mortality and morbidity as that achieved by these authors, serious consideration should be given to advising such treatment in patients with far-advanced lesions.—W.S.] ◀

23–10 **Repair of Postirradiation Damage to Colorectum: Progress Report.** Eugene M. Bricker, William D. Johnston, and Ramesh V. Patwardhan (Columbia, Mo.) report the results of 21 operations for

(23–10) Ann. Surg. 193:555–564, May 1981.

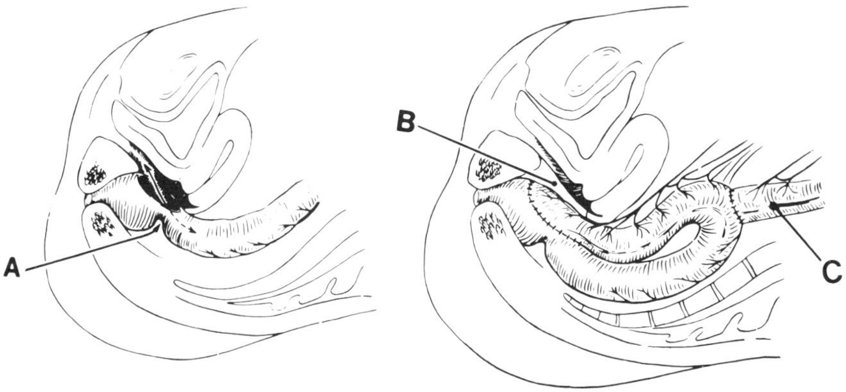

Fig 23–6.—Type I repair. **A,** web stricture at level of the fistula is typical. **B,** pedicle graft of labium majus with fat pad used to substitute for the vagina to cover suture line of reconstruction. **C,** segment of proximal colon, always attached to the reconstruction, ensures that all anastomoses and suture lines are completely healed before colostomy closure. (Courtesy of Bricker, E.M., et al.: Ann. Surg. 193:555–564, May 1981.)

the repair of rectovaginal fistula or stricture secondary to irradiation for pelvic cancer. The procedures are based on the use of proximal unirradiated colon for the repair. Both the type I, or "patch" repair (Fig 23–6), and the type II, or "fillet and foldover" repair (Fig 23–7), are based on the use of bypassed sigmoid colon distal to a previous colostomy. In type III repairs (Fig 23–8) there either is no previous colostomy or the bypassed colon is not usable; therefore, normal colon is mobilized and brought into the pelvis for use as a patch or as a

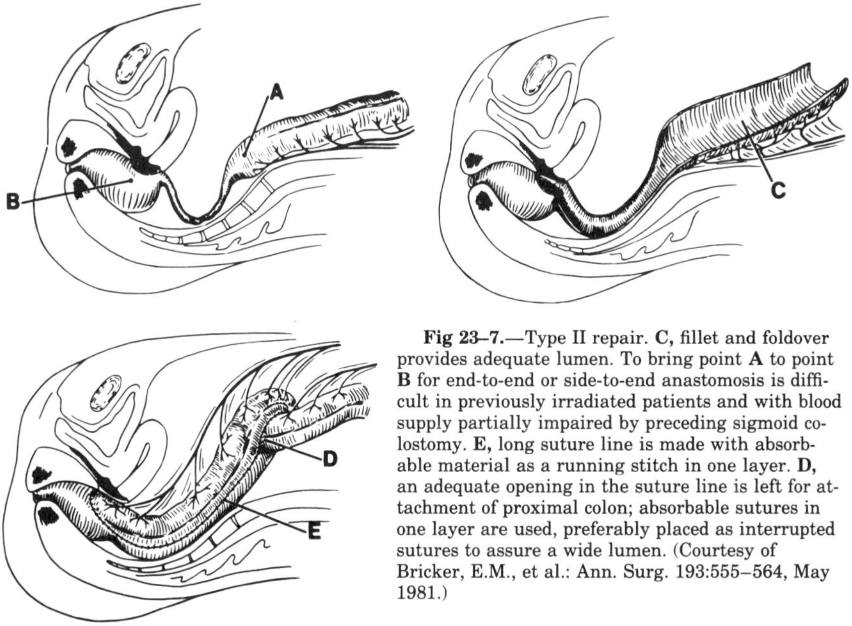

Fig 23–7.—Type II repair. **C,** fillet and foldover provides adequate lumen. To bring point **A** to point **B** for end-to-end or side-to-end anastomosis is difficult in previously irradiated patients and with blood supply partially impaired by preceding sigmoid colostomy. **E,** long suture line is made with absorbable material as a running stitch in one layer. **D,** an adequate opening in the suture line is left for attachment of proximal colon; absorbable sutures in one layer are used, preferably placed as interrupted sutures to assure a wide lumen. (Courtesy of Bricker, E.M., et al.: Ann. Surg. 193:555–564, May 1981.)

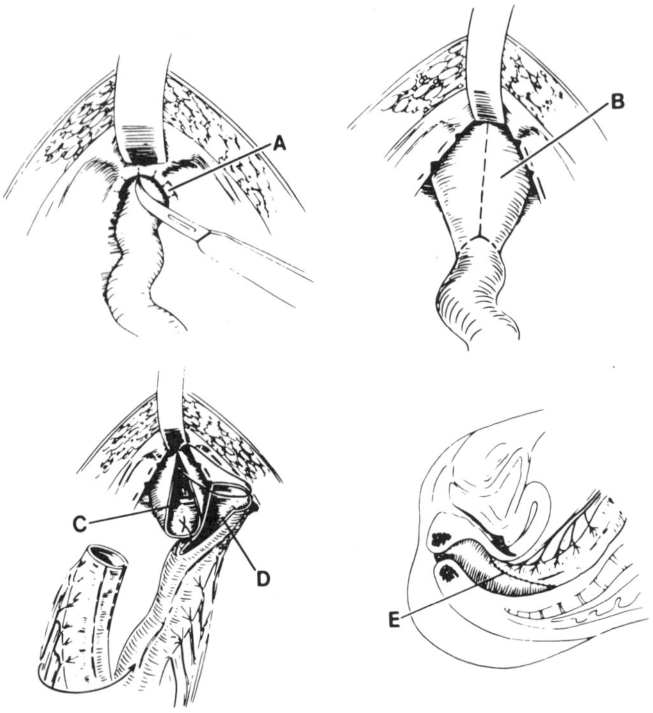

Fig 23–8.—Type III repair. **A,** shortened and constricted uterosacral arch is characteristic. **B,** ampulla of rectum is exposed and incised longitudinally, with amputation of the scarred rectosigmoid, leaving a widely open lumen for anastomosis **(C).** **D,** proximal colon is brought down and slit to fit the open ampulla, with completion of anastomosis using a single row of absorbable interrupted sutures. **E,** wide open anastomosis results, with less chance for suture line stricture. (Courtesy of Bricker, E.M., et al.: Ann. Surg. 193:555–564, May 1981.)

wide anastomosis to the anterior wall of the rectal ampulla. Most patients with fistulas have required a combined abdominovaginal procedure (Fig 23–9). A proximal defunctionalizing colostomy is always created. Size 24 sump suction catheters are used in the depth of the pelvis for 48–72 hours to prevent hematoma formation. Meticulous preparation of the colon and rectum is essential.

All 21 patients who underwent colostomy closure have normal or essentially normal rectal function, except for 2 total failures, 1 death from small bowel complications, only partial continence in 1, intermittent diarrhea in 1, and moderate intermittent abdominal discomfort in several patients. Complications are listed in the table. Two residual rectovaginal fistulas required vaginal reoperation. A patient with a recurrent rectovaginal fistula required repeat colostomy and vaginal repair of the fistula. One patient required a second operation for repair of a stricture at the anastomotic site. Both total failures occurred in patients having type III repairs. No symptoms were positively related to the use of antiperistaltic colonic segments.

These results show promise. Whatever type of operation is used, the segment of colon used in the repair must have a good blood supply.

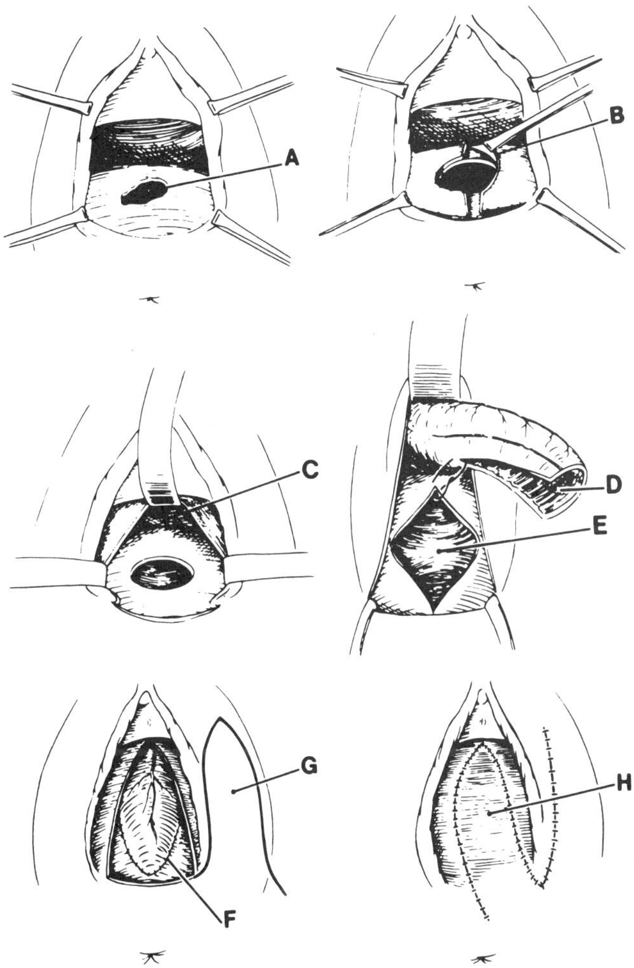

Fig 23–9.—Combined abdominovaginal procedure. **A,** vaginally, fistula is freshened by conservative excision of scarred edges, after which posterior vaginal wall is incised longitudinally and separated from rectum **(B).** Dissection is extended laterally and superiorly to meet plane of dissection from above **(C).** Colon patch **(D)** is sutured in place with interrupted absorbable sutures. If web structure **(E)** is present, it may be relieved by a longitudinal incision and transverse closure. **F,** approximation is done with two rows of sutures if possible. **G** and **H,** if posterior vaginal wall cannot be expected to heal due to irradiation and scar tissue, it is trimmed away and defect filled with pedicle graft of labium majus and fat pad. (Courtesy of Bricker, E.M., et al.: Ann. Surg. 193:555–564, May 1981.)

When a colostomy is necessary, it should be done high enough in the sigmoid so that 15–20 cm of normal colon are bypassed, on the chance that a reconstruction may become possible. It is helpful to bring out the bypassed proximal colon as a small mucous fistula in order to evaluate the disease by retrograde contrast study.

▶ [This is an extraordinary series of cases with absolutely superb results. The problems encountered in this group of patients are extremely difficult, and many investigators have considered them insoluble. Bricker and his colleagues are to be congratulated for offering us a new and improved method of dealing with this situation.

TOTAL EXPERIENCE

	Number
Total patients	21 (one male)
stricture plus fistula	7
fistula alone	2
stricture alone	12
Approach to operation	
abdominal alone	10
abdominovaginal	10
abdominoperineal	1 (male)
Types of operation	
Type I	7
Type II	5
Type III	9
Complications	
residual fistula, corrected vaginally	2
recurrent fistula requiring repeat colostomy and vaginal repair	1
stricture of anastomosis at site of colostomy requiring abdominal operation for correction	1
total failures	2
death due to small intestinal complications (one of total failures)	1
Functional results (19 patients)	
satisfactory to excellent	18
poor (incontinence)	1

The basic principles are important and are well described in the manuscript. It is clear that uninvolved normal intestine must be used for the reconstruction. A proximal colostomy as a complementary procedure is also mandatory. We are much indebted to Bricker and his colleagues.—W.S.] ◀

23–11 **Occurrence and Outcome After Primary Treatment of Anal Fistulas in Crohn's Disease.** Fistulas occur commonly in association with Crohn's disease, and anal fistulas are a major treatment problem. G. Hellers, O. Bergstrand, S. Ewerth, and B. Holmström (Stockholm) examined the incidence of anal fistulas in a series of 826 patients seen in 1955 to 1974 with Crohn's disease. There were 379 male and 447 female patients in the series. The mean observation time was 9.4 years. Anal fistulas were recorded in 184 patients (23%). They occurred in 33% of male and 22% of female patients, a significant difference. Most fistulas appeared within 6 months before diagnosis or after the time of definite diagnosis of Crohn's disease.

The risk of an anal fistula developing increased with the distal extent of the intestinal lesion (Table 1). Of 40 patients with small bowel lesions only, 22 had local surgery for anal fistula before curative intestinal surgery. Eight of these fistulas (38%) failed to heal before curative intestinal surgery. The recurrence rate was 43% in patients with ileocolic disease and 83% in those with large bowel involvement only. The outcome of primary curative intestinal resection is shown in Table 2. All but 4 of 40 patients with fistulas and small bowel disease had healed at follow-up. One had had a proctocolectomy, and 3 had an open fistula. Many of the healed patients had had repeated

(23–11) Gut 21:525–527, June 1980.

TABLE 1.—FREQUENCY OF FISTULAS IN RELATION TO SITE OF INTESTINAL LESION

Site of intestinal lesion	Patients (no.)		
	Total	With fistulae	
		(No.)	(%)
Small intestine	339	40	12
Combined ileocolic	341	51	15
Large intestine			
No rectal involvement	68	28	41
With rectal involvement	71	65	92

TABLE 2.—SPONTANEOUS HEALING OF ANAL FISTULAS IN RELATION TO SITE OF INTESTINAL LESION AFTER PRIMARY CURATIVE RESECTION OF INTESTINAL LESION

Site of intestinal lesion	Patients (no.)		
	Total	Healed	Recurrence*
Small intestine	14	9	4
Combined ileocolic	25	10	3
Large intestine			
No rectal involvement	4	1	0

*Recurrence: reopening of the fistula after primary spontaneous healing.

local operations. Four of 51 patients with combined ileocolic disease had an open fistula, and 1 had had proctocolectomy. Eight of 28 patients with large bowel disease but not rectal involvement had healed. Seven had an open fistula, and 13 had had proctocolectomy. Of 65 patients with rectal involvement, 4 had healed, 3 had an open fistula, and 58 had undergone proctocolectomy.

Local surgery is well worth trying in patients with Crohn's disease and an anal fistula when intestinal resection is not planned and when small bowel or ileocolic involvement is present. In patients with colonic disease, however, local surgery is not followed by healing. If curative resection is planned, local surgery can be postponed, if feasible, to await possible spontaneous healing. The poor prognosis for patients with rectal involvement and anal fistulas might be altered by the more frequent use of a diverting colostomy.

▶ [This important article gives us some perspective on the development of anorectal fistulas in a very large series of patients with Crohn's disease. The results also suggest which patients should undergo operative treatment, namely, those in whom the intestinal disease is more proximally located, especially after adequate treatment of such disease. The dismal outcome in those persons with fistulas who have colonic Crohn's disease makes one wonder whether, in fact, the fistulas are really a manifestation of the presence of Crohn's disease in the anorectal area itself. This important question has not yet been resolved. Microscopic assessment of tissue from this area is not always as definitive as one might hope in regard to this important point. If one were able to delineate those patients who had Crohn's disease of the anorectal region, it seems clear that they would not be the ones amenable to surgical treatment of the fistula itself, short of excision of the rectum. Perhaps more sophisticated electron microscopic studies may help us to define that group.—W.S.] ◀

23–12 **Randomized Trial To Compare Rubber Band Ligation With Phenol Injection for Treatment of Hemorrhoids.** F. Greca, M. M. Hares, E. Nevah, J. Alexander-Williams, and M. R. B. Keighley (Genl. Hosp., Birmingham, England) conducted a prospective randomized trial of rubber band ligation and phenol injection in 82 consecutive patients (50 men and 32 women; mean age, 45 years) referred for the first time with symptomatic hemorrhoids. The patients had no additional pathology and a maximal resting anal pressure less than 120 cm of water.

Rubber band ligation was performed using the Barron applicator to the mucosa above the 2 largest hemorrhoids; no more than two sites were ligated at the first visit, and patients were told that a second application of bands to any residual hemorrhoids might be necessary. Phenol injection was with 2–3 ml of a 5% solution in almond oil injected into the mucosa just above the 3 primary hemorrhoids.

The 39 patients receiving rubber band ligation and the 43 receiving phenol injection were similar with respect to age, sex, degree of prolapse, and initial symptoms. The symptomatic results in all patients 12 months after treatment were similar, 64% being improved after rubber band ligation compared to 70% after phenol injection (Table 1). Complications of treatment were recorded in 5 patients after rubber band ligation, 3 of whom required hospitalization; there was only 1 minor complication after phenol injection. However, repeated treatment was necessary in 13 patients after phenol injection and in only 4 after rubber band ligation. Additional treatment was necessary in 6 patients from each group, including 75% of all patients with third-degree prolapse (Table 2).

Rubber band ligation and phenol injection provide similar results in patients with hemorrhoids, but rubber band ligation is more liable to complications when performed by inexperienced operators. Phenol

TABLE 1.—Patients' Assessment of Symptomatic Relief

	Rubber band ligation						Injection therapy					
	1 mth (n = 33)		4 mth (n = 33)		1 yr (n = 28)		1 mth (n = 37)		4 mth (n = 33)		1 yr (n = 33)	
Excellent	14	} 79%	18	} 72%	13	} 64%	13	} 84%	14	} 76%	15	} 70%
Better	12		6		5		18		11		8	
No better	4		3		4		2		3		4	
Withdrawn	3		6		6		4		5		6	

TABLE 2.—Patients Requiring Additional Therapy

	Rubber band ligation		Injection therapy	
	Number	Additional therapy	Number	Additional therapy
First degree	3	—	4	—
Second degree	33	4	34	2
Third degree	3	2	5	4

(23–12) Br. J. Surg. 68:250–252, April 1981.

injection is the treatment of choice for patients with first and second-degree hemorrhoids. Neither method is recommended for those with third-degree lesions.

▶ [This is a welcome trial because a comparison between rubber band ligation and phenol injection in a carefully controlled study had not been done previously. It is somewhat surprising to me that the phenol injections fared as well as they did, because my own personal experience has been that rubber band ligation is preferable for comparable hemorrhoids because repeated injections are not necessary. The findings in this study would support this position, although if you are willing to be persistent about injections, you obviously can achieve the same sorts of results as with rubber band ligation. It is to be emphasized that these studies were carried out in patients who had relatively low anal sphincter pressures. Therefore, patients with high sphincter pressures might differ in their response to these two treatments, and this must be kept in mind. Because sphincter pressures tend to be lower in older individuals, this study is applicable mainly to the more aged population.—W.S.] ◀

23–13 **Treatment of Anal Fissure by Lateral Subcutaneous Sphincterotomy Should Be Under General Anesthesia.** Lateral subcutaneous sphincterotomy would seem to be a logical treatment for anal fissure, because the condition is associated with an overactive internal sphincter; however, recurrent or persistent fissure is more frequent after surgery with the use of local anesthesia than after anal dilatation. Division of the sphincter may be inadequate in a tense patient undergoing surgery on the anal canal. M. R. B. Keighley, F. Greca, E. Nevah, M. Hares, and J. Alexander-Williams (Birmingham, England) attempted to determine whether the results of sphincterotomy can be improved by using general anesthesia. New patients with anal fissure were allocated to receive lateral subcutaneous sphincterotomy under local lidocaine anesthesia or general anesthesia. The 34 patients having local anesthesia and the 37 having general anesthesia were clinically comparable. All patients but 4 had a posterior fissure.

Nine patients had early complications, 6 after local and 3 after general anesthesia. Three of the 4 patients with an unhealed fissure 1 month postoperatively had local anesthesia (table). At 4 months, 14 other patients treated with the use of local anesthesia had evidence of recurrent fissure. No further recurrences were noted at 1 year in

SYMPTOMATIC RESULTS

	Local anaesthetic (n = 34)			General anaesthetic (n = 37)		
	1 mth	4 mth	1 yr	1 mth	4 mth	1 yr
Improved						
No symptoms	18	10	7	20	22	18
Minor symptoms	13	17	6	16	11	9
No better	3	17	19	1	4	4
Incomplete follow-up	—	—	2	—	—	6
Recurrent fissure (cumulative)	3	17	17	1	1	1

(23–13) Br. J. Surg. 68:400–401, June 1981.

either group. Comparable reductions in anal pressure were observed after surgery with local or general anesthesia in the 11 patients studied before and 4 months after surgery.

A general anesthetic of short duration for lateral subcutaneous sphincterotomy to treat anal fissure is associated with better results than surgery done with local anesthesia. Probably a more extensive division of the sphincter is possible with general anesthesia. Only 1 patient having general anesthesia in this series had a recurrent fissure. A prospective study is needed comparing lateral subcutaneous sphincterotomy with the use of general anesthesia with anal dilatation in patients with acute uncomplicated anal fissure.

▶ [It is likely, as the authors suggest, that internal sphincterotomy done with the use of local anesthesia is not nearly as complete as that done with the use of general anesthesia. This would offer a very reasonable explanation for the differences in outcome between the two techniques. This study offers compelling evidence for carrying out subcutaneous sphincterotomy with the use of general anesthesia. One rather unusual point is that the authors indicate that they treated 71 consecutive patients with *acute* anal fissure. In the United States, at least, acute anal fissure usually is treated by nonoperative means, and surgery is reserved for chronic anal fissure. Therefore, it is a bit surprising that the authors undertook to treat patients with acute anal fissures operatively.—W.S.] ◀

23–14 **Creation of Anal Sphincter Mechanism by Bilateral Proximally Based Gluteal Muscle Transposition.** Fecal incontinence due to the absence of normally functioning anal musculature is a major medical and social problem. Sphincteroplasty is not possible if no intact innervation or functioning sphincter muscle remains. Both reinforcement of the puborectal sling and creation of a sphincter by transposing the gracilis muscles have been described. Hajo A. Bruining, Kurt E. Bos, Eduard G. Colthoff, and David E. Tolhurst (Rotterdam, The Netherlands) describe an improved technique of gluteus maximus transposition to produce active anal continence in the absence of a functioning puborectal sling and of both the internal and external anal sphincters.

Girl, 17, incurred multiple limb fractures, compound pelvic fractures, and a deep posterior perineal wound in a bicycle accident. The rectum was not recognizable, and there was no sign of the anus. A diverting sigmoidostomy was performed, the perineal wound was packed, and the fractures were stabilized. The patient was ventilated for severe respiratory distress syndrome. A rectocutaneous fistula 5 mm in diameter remained 13 months after injury. The perineal skin defect healed secondarily. A new rectal stump had formed, with no active sphincteric movements and no electromyographic activity. Passive rectal filling was felt by the patient, but partial perineal anesthesia prevented early sensing of fecal loss.

Scarred skin in the perineum was excised along with granulation tissue in the anal remnant. The neorectum was mobilized and the stricture incised posteriorly. A transposition flap from the buttock was dissected free (Fig 23–10). Transposition of the distal gluteus maximus muscles is illustrated in Figure 23–11. A firm, sphincter-like ring that could be contracted at will was present 6 weeks postoperatively. Sphincter competence was considered adequate after 4 months of training, when sigmoidorectostomy was carried out. The patient gradually became continent during the ensuing 6 weeks, even

---

(23–14) Plast. Reconstr. Surg. 67:70–73, January 1981.

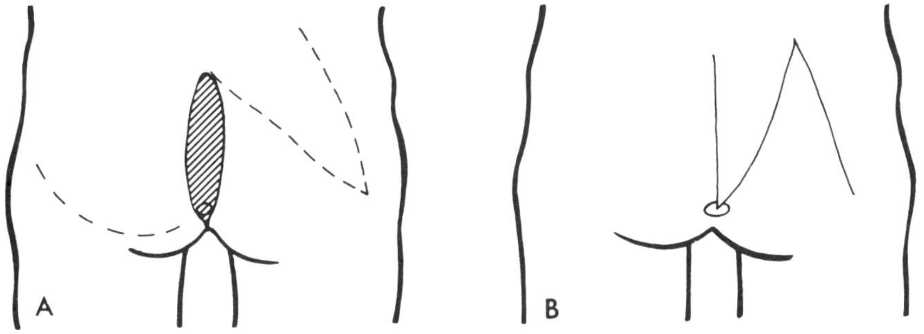

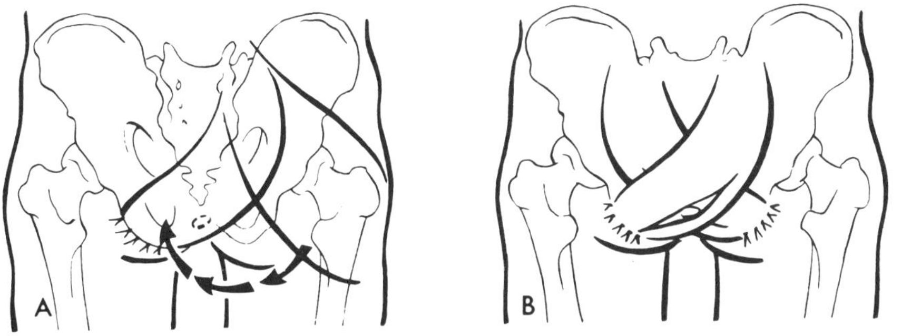

Fig 23–10 (top).—A, skin incisions. Routine approach to gluteus maximus on left. Transposition flap for closure of defect *(shaded)* and correction of stricture on right. **B,** flap transposed and anal stricture corrected with tip of flap.

Fig 23–11 (bottom).—A, mobilization and transposition of distal half of gluteus maximus muscles. **B,** muscles are split longitudinally to create a double scissor-like diaphragm and fixed to the ischial tuberosities.

(Courtesy of Bruining, H.A., et al.: Plast. Reconstr. Surg. 67:70–73, 1981.)

during an episode of diarrhea. Frequency of defecation decreased to twice daily.

Creation of a double scissor-like diaphragm of gluteus maximus muscle fixed to the ischial tuberosities produces a firm muscle ring that can be contracted voluntarily more forcefully than a normal sphincter. This procedure may be preferable to the gracilis-plasty in smaller children and in patients who have difficulty with muscular coordination. This method, with a pull-through procedure, may be useful after abdominoperineal rectal amputation.

▶ [This report contains an ingenious method for reconstruction of a totally destroyed anal sphincter mechanism. There is much to commend the use of this method, but one question not addressed by the authors is that of impairment of function as a result of loss of the normal gluteal muscle function. Although the authors do not specifically mention the extent to which each gluteal muscle is used in this procedure, it would appear from their illustrations that at least half of the gluteal musculature is left intact. In addition, I presume that the authors would have suggested some dysfunction had it been present, although this is by no means certain.

An additional possible use for this technique is that of filling the space of a persistent perineal sinus after it has been unroofed. The gracilis muscle has been used for this purpose, but the ready availability of the gluteus maximus in close proximity to the perineal wound makes it much more convenient as a filling material. Certainly, the potential use of the gluteus for this purpose should be considered.—W.S.] ◀

24. Liver and Spleen

24–1 **Intra-Abdominal Packing for Control of Hepatic Hemorrhage: Reappraisal.** David V. Feliciano, Kenneth L. Mattox, and George L. Jordan, Jr. (Baylor College of Medicine, Houston) describe currently available techniques for control of hepatic hemorrhage, including the approach they used from July 1978 to September 1980 in the treatment of 10 patients with extensive injuries who had continued hepatic parenchymal oozing following all attempts at surgical control. Insertion of intra-abdominal packing around the liver was used as a last desperate measure. Multiple laparotomy pads were used in 6 cases and appeared to be the most effective tamponading agent; reoperation was necessary for their removal. Vaginal packs were used in 2 cases and Kerlix rolls in another 2. Suction drains usually were placed beneath the packs to allow for continued autotransfusion.

Packing was removed from 8 hours to 10 days (average 5.2 days) after the last operation to control hepatic hemorrhage. The timing for removal of intra-abdominal packing did not appear to be critical. Packing was removed at relaparotomy in 4 cases and through abdominal drain sites in 5.

Nine patients survived. There were no instances of renewed bleeding after removal of the packing. Intra-abdominal complications following removal of packing required reoperation in 2 cases: 1 patient had a late subphrenic abscess after incomplete drainage through an old drain tract, and 1 had a small infected subhepatic hematoma. In 2 other cases, late purulent perihepatic collections were drained through old drain tracts while the patients were under general anesthesia.

A "second-look" operation is valuable in the care of certain patients with hepatic trauma, because it allows further debridement of nonviable tissue, irrigation of subphrenic and subhepatic spaces, and insertion of clean perihepatic drains. Intra-abdominal packing for control of exsanguinating hepatic hemorrhage can be lifesaving in cases of extensive subcapsular hematoma or extensive bilobar injuries and in cases in which coagulopathy, hypothermia, and acidosis would make further surgical efforts likely to increase hemorrhage.

▶ [For years, a dictum was proposed stating that a pack should not be left in place for control of hepatic hemorrhage. This was historically related to the findings of Madding and Kennedy in World War II when they showed that the simple insistence on drainage of all liver wounds and prohibition of long-term packing of such wounds reduced the mortality significantly. The reintroduction of packing of liver wounds as a lifesaving device is totally appropriate and has been addressed by Calne et al. (*Br. J. Surg* 66:338–339, 1979), who reported 4 consecutive cases of potentially lethal liver trauma in which packing with gauze rolls was lifesaving. The concept is particularly

(24–1) J. Trauma 21:285–290, April 1981.

meaningful for surgeons practicing away from a major center. The important follow-up to this approach is that the definitive procedure, i.e., a laparotomy and reexploration and removal of the pack and control of bleeding, should be carried out within a short time so that significant bacterial overgrowth does not occur.—S.I.S.] ◀

24–2 **Nonoperative Management of Subcapsular Hematomas of the Liver.** Hepatic injury from blunt abdominal trauma continues to carry significant mortality and morbidity. Patients with a parenchymal tear and subcapsular hematoma formation can be identified by hepatic scintiscanning and may be managed nonoperatively. James E. Cheatham, Jr., E. Ide Smith, William P. Tunell, and Ronald C. Elkins (Univ. of Oklahoma) describe 5 patients seen in 1978–1979 with subcapsular hematomas of the liver after blunt abdominal trauma.

Woman, 30, incurred several left rib fractures with pulmonary contusion and cerebral contusion, as well as a fractured pelvis, in an automobile accident. The abdominal findings were negative on admission, but right upper quadrant pain was noted 24 hours later, and a liver-spleen scan showed an irregular 10-cm defect in the posterolateral surface of the right lobe of the liver. The patient's condition remained stable during treatment with bed rest, broad-spectrum antibiotics, and nasogastric suction. The hematocrit reading fell to 32%, with a total bilirubin level of 2 mg/dl. The patient was discharged after 11 days with normal liver function, and was well a year later. A repeated liver scan showed nearly complete resolution of the defect.

These patients are a small proportion of those with blunt abdominal trauma. However, subcapsular hematomas will be recognized more often with technetium imaging of the liver. The results of lavage are usually negative in these cases. Scanning will show lesions as small as 1–2 cm and is a relatively rapid procedure. All of the present patients reported abdominal pain and had an increased serum glutamic oxalacetic transaminase level. The wounds may be diffuse, and attempted evacuation may lead to massive bleeding, possibly necessitating extensive resection. An alternative is bed rest in an intensive care unit with the use of gastrointestinal tract decompression and antibiotic coverage. The patients have had no postoperative complications. Possible complications include delayed rupture of a subcapsular hematoma, hepatic abscess formation, and hemobilia.

In selected cases, nonoperative management is preferable for patients with subcapsular hematoma of the liver.

▶ [The subcapsular hematoma is a very uncommon lesion, but it is appropriate to stress that many of these cases can be managed nonoperatively. Several of the technetium scans are unequivocal, but some in this article are open to question, and it is known that a high incidence of false positive and false negative results is associated with the scanning technique. We have felt more secure using angiography, even though it is more evasive, in defining the lesions in these patients and in other patients with hepatic trauma. Using the angiographic technique and assessing the amount of intraperitoneal rupture, we have also managed nonoperatively patients with parenchymal tears that have traversed Glisson's capsule and caused intraperitoneal bleeding.—S.I.S.] ◀

24–3 **Ultrasonography and Amebic Liver Abscesses.** Intestinal amebiasis, which is endemic in Egypt, is complicated in about 8% of cases by amebic liver abscess. Mahmound Helmy Abul-Khair, Mohamed M.

(24–2) Am. J. Surg. 140:852–857, December 1980.
(24–3) Ann. Surg. 193:221–226, February 1981.

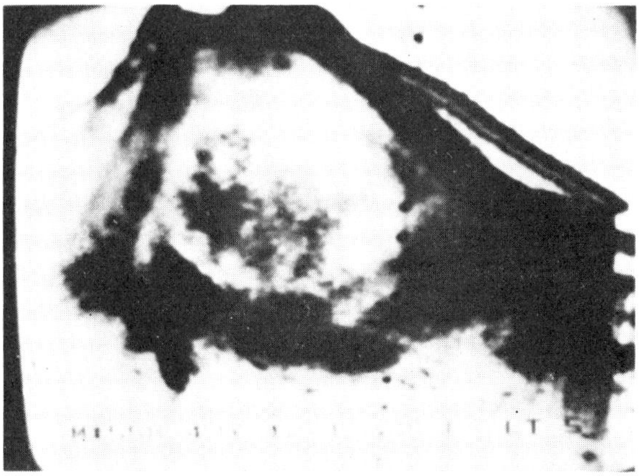

Fig 24–1.—Left lobe abscess with coarse internal echoes. Note the good through transmission of sound waves and posterior acoustic enhancement. (Courtesy of Abul-Khair, M.H., et al.: Ann. Surg. 193:221–226, February 1981.)

Kenawi, Ezz El-Din A. Korashy, and Nabil M. Arafa (Cairo Univ.) evaluated the usefulness of ultrasonography in the diagnosis of amebic liver abscess in 21 men and 3 women aged 20–70 years (mean, 33 years), with suspected liver abscesses. The patients underwent clinical examinations, stool specimen analyses for cysts and trophozoites of *Entamoeba histolytica,* radiologic examinations, routine liver function tests, and ultrasonographic examination using the gray-scale imaging technique.

Ultrasonography demonstrated amebic liver abscesses in 20 patients. The presence of abscesses was verified by aspiration biopsy in 19 patients (95%); the 1 patient with a false positive ultrasonogram had a degenerated hepatoma. Of the 19 abscesses, 63% were located in the right lobe and 37% in the left. The two most common sonographic patterns were the lack of a definite abscess wall and the presence of both fine and coarse (Fig 24–1) internal echoes amid an echo-free pattern, indicating the presence of fibrinous masses or thick pus.

The site, size, and nature of the pus in the abscess could be determined by ultrasonography, helping in the management and technique of aspiration biopsy. Follow-up data were more detailed using ultrasonography. Ultrasonographic examination is a noninvasive, safe, accurate, and rapid method of diagnosis. It is recommended highly as a routine procedure in all cases of suspected amebic liver abscesses in the pretreatment and posttreatment stages of the disease and as an indicator of complete cure at follow-up examination.

▶ [Ultrasound diagnosis of amebic liver abscess has been so successful that even if aspiration does not confirm the diagnosis, open surgical treatment is justified. Ultrasonographic examination is also a valuable guide to follow the progress of treatment.—E.E.P.] ◀

4–4 **Resection of Primary Solid Hepatic Tumors.** Martin A. Adson and Louis H. Weiland (Mayo Clinic and Found.) reviewed experience

(24–4) Am. J. Surg. 141:18–21, January 1981.

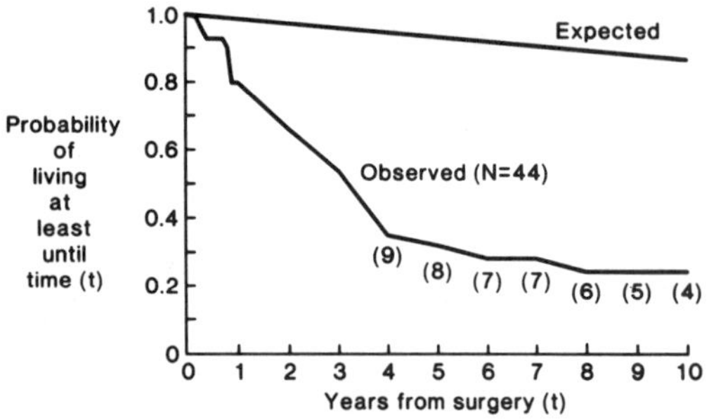

Fig 24–2.—Survival after resection for malignant primary hepatic tumor. (Courtesy of Adson, M.A. and Weiland, L.H.: Am. J. Surg. 141:18–21, January 1981.)

with the surgical management of 60 solid hepatic tumors. The presenting clinical features were related chiefly to the size of the lesions. Forty-one patients presented with pain, and 24 had a palpable mass. There were 33 women and 27 men in the series. Forty-six lesions were malignant; 43 were hepatocytic cancers and 3, cholangiocarcinomas. Two patients had huge hamartomas, and 12 had hepatocytic adenomas. Twelve benign tumors were in women, 8 of whom used oral contraceptives. Malignant tumors in women occurred most often in the middle or later years.

Half of the patients underwent hemihepatectomy, 20% had trisegmentectomy or extended right hepatic lobectomy, and 15 patients had segmentectomy or very large wedge resections. The average lesion size was 13 cm. Nine of the 57 hospital survivors required hospitalization for more than 3 weeks. Complications were related to bleeding from the operative site in early convalescence, bile leakage, and sepsis associated with either of these complications. Survival rates are shown in Figure 24–2. Patients with malignancies had 5- and 10-year survival rates of 36% and 33%, respectively. All patients having benign tumors resected are well and have no evidence of residual or recurrent disease.

Aggressive treatment of primary hepatic malignancy appears to be warranted by the acceptable operative risk and the significant palliation or improved survival that results. The safety of major hepatic resections depends in part on adequate exposure. Thoracic extension of an upper abdominal oblique incision is favored with large lesions of the right lobe of the liver. Most primary solid tumors of the liver encroach on the hepatic hilus, making preligation or division and suture of branches supplying the lobe to be resected advisable. Some patients with focal nodular hyperplasia have been observed, but patients with hepatocytic adenoma are at risk of both malignant transformation and bleeding.

▶ [This represents the report of a large personal experience. The statement that the risk of routine or standardized hepatic resection is less than 3% relates to that operation performed by an experienced surgeon. Hepatic resection should not be a once-yearly endeavor conducted in any hospital in the community. The authors' report that 80% of the patients evaluated surgically were found to have resectable lesions relates to their use of preoperative angiography. We have recently reported that optimal preoperative information be achieved by a combination of angiogram and computed tomography scan; these studies should be carried out before any exploration is undertaken (Gutierrez and Schwartz, at the International Radiologic Association, Brussels, 1981).—S.I.S.] ◀

24–5 **Screening for Liver Metastases From Colorectal Cancer With Carcinoembryonic Antigen and Alkaline Phosphatase.** The presence of liver metastasis influences the management of patients with colorectal cancer, but liver scanning is an expensive and inconvenient screening measure and involves radionuclide exposure. Paul I. Tartter, Gary Slater, Irwin Gelernt, and Arthur H. Aufses, Jr. (Mount Sinai School of Medicine, New York) devised a sensitive, economical screening regimen based on serum alkaline phosphatase and carcinoembryonic antigen (CEA) determinations. Information was reviewed on 327 patients operated on for colorectal cancer between 1977 and 1979. Liver scanning was done preoperatively in 179, and 190 patients had CEA immunoassays.

Liver metastases were detected by scanning preoperatively in only 69% of 35 cases, and there was a false negative rate of 6%. The false positive rate was 2%. Alkaline phosphatase determination was 77% sensitive in detecting liver metastasis. The false positive rate was 34% and the false negative rate, 4%. The CEA concentration exceeded 5 ng/dl in 81% of 26 patients with and in 24% of patients without liver metastasis. The false negative rate was 2%. When a CEA concentration of over 10 ng/dl and an alkaline phosphatase value above 135 were used, 23 of 26 patients with liver metastases fulfilled these criteria, for a sensitivity of 88%. The false negative rate was 2% and the false positive rate, 12%.

A 12% false positive rate, as found by using a CEA concentration of over 10 ng/dl and an alkaline phosphatase value above 135 IU, is acceptable for a screening measure. Patients meeting such criteria may undergo liver scanning to verify suspected liver metastasis from colorectal carcinoma. This approach reduces the expense, inconvenience, and radionuclide exposure associated with detection of liver metastasis in patients with colon cancer.

▶ [The need to develop sensitive and economic methods for screening becomes more meaningful in light of expanding interests in resectional surgery for liver metastases from colorectal cancer. Present protocol uses both the CEA and alkaline phosphatase determinations as screens, and, in the face of significant elevations, we will subject the patient to angiographic evaluation and to computed tomography scan. To date, the screening technique has uncovered 5 patients who subsequently have undergone partial hepatic resection for metastatic disease. One of these patients is alive and well 5 years after a 75% hepatic resection. The CEA assay has been particularly helpful in following patients after resection, in that significant elevation of the antigen level almost invariably has meant recurrence of the hepatic metastasis.—S.I.S.] ◀

24–6 **Congenital Hepatic Fibrosis in Children.** Congenital hepatic fibrosis is an autosomal recessive disease that carries risks of both gastrointestinal bleeding from portal hypertension and cholangitis related to bacterial infection of dilated intrahepatic bile ducts. Renal abnormalities are present in virtually all cases. F. Alvarez, O. Bernard, F. Brunelle, M. Hadchouel, A. Leblanc, M. Odièvre, and D. Al-

(24–5) Ann. Surg. 193:357–360, March 1981.
(24–6) J. Pediatr. 99:370–375, September 1981.

agille (Bicetre, France) reviewed experience with 27 children having this disease who were seen in 1960–1980. The histologic findings included bands of fibrous tissue, dysmorphic bile ducts of varying size, and the presence of mucinous material or inspissated bile in the bile duct lumens. Data supporting autosomal recessive transmission were obtained in 8 cases.

The most common presenting features were hepatomegaly and hematemesis. Four patients had hepatosplenomegaly, 1 had splenomegaly, and 4 had polycystic kidneys associated with hepatomegaly at presentation. Liver function was normal in all children. Eighteen patients had thrombocytopenia consistent with hypersplenism, and 11 had hematemesis. Varices were confirmed by esophageal endoscopy in all but 1 of 22 patients with splenomegaly. Splenoportography showed duplication of the intrahepatic branches of the portal vein in 16 of 21 cases. Portal thrombosis was present in 1 case. Seventeen patients underwent portal-systemic shunt surgery, 6 of them prophylactically. At present, all of these patients are well, except those presenting with renal failure. Cholangitis was diagnosed in 3 children. Ten patients had obvious polycystic kidney disease.

Congenital hepatic fibrosis now can be diagnosed noninvasively in early childhood. Patients with major dilatation of extrahepatic bile ducts may benefit from resection of the dilated ducts. Portal-systemic shunting was generally successful in the present cases. The risk of renal failure is unknown; patients with minimal renal lesions should have regular pyelography or sonography as well as renal function tests.

► [This represents a large series of cases of an unusual pathologic entity. Results of surgery are excellent, as has long been emphasized. Also to be noted is that there is no overt sign of encephalopathy in any of these patients. This represents another example in which encephalopathy does not develop in patients without hepatic dysfunction who undergo major shunting procedures.—S.I.S.] ◄

24–7 **Noncirrhotic Portal Hypertension in Adults.** Most adults with portal hypertension prove to have cirrhosis that ultimately results in intrahepatic portal bed block. William V. McDermott, Albert Bothe, Jr., Melvin E. Clouse, and Murray M. Bern (Boston) reviewed data on 366 patients, aged 16 and older, seen in a 15-year period, with portal hypertension and found 41 in whom the cause was unrelated to cirrhosis or hemochromatosis. In 37 cases a cause for portal hypertension was identified. An extrahepatic portal bed block was found in 21 patients and an intrahepatic block in 7, whereas 7 patients had typical Budd-Chiari syndrome. Two patients had portal hypertension resulting from an arteriovenous fistula. Shunting, portal-azygous disconnection, or direct operation was necessary to control portal hypertension in 23 patients. Thirteen of 15 shunts succeeded in controlling portal hypertension. In all, 20 of 23 operations were completely effective in controlling the presenting clinical problem, whether gastrointestinal hemorrhage or intractable ascites.

Of 21 patients with portal hypertension secondary to occlusion of the prehepatic venous inflow to the liver, 4 had had portal hypertension since infancy. Only 1 patient in this group died of causes related

(24–7) Am. J. Surg. 141:514–518, April 1981.

to portal hypertension or operation. Most patients with a presinusoid intrahepatic block had idiopathic hepatic fibrosis. Splenorenal shunts were made in these patients, with no mortality, subsequent bleeding, or postshunt encephalopathy. Nine patients had a postsinusoid block, usually with severe, intractable ascites. Two patients had an intrahepatic block; 1 had a primary hepatoma and 1 had veno-occlusive disease. Two patients had Budd-Chiari syndrome due to suprahepatic obstruction of hepatic venous outflow by retroperitoneal and retrohepatic extension of metastatic malignancy. Four others had occlusion of the major hepatic veins by thrombus secondary to a hypercoagulable state.

In the absence of rapidly fatal primary disease, portal hypertension in the adult is not a threatening problem and may be controlled by appropriate surgery with minimal mortality. Angiography and venography are important in diagnosis of noncirrhotic portal hypertension. A hypercoagulable state should be considered.

▶ [This represents an interesting group of patients. In our experience with extrahepatic portal hypertension (Grauer and Schwartz: *Ann. Surg.* 189:566–574, 1979), the patients rarely required an emergency procedure and some patients have been followed for long periods into adulthood without operative intervention. Although multiple bleeding episodes occur, they are rarely fatal. This article points out that no postshunt encephalopathy occurred, not did it develop in patients with idiopathic hepatic fibrosis in whom there was no hepatocellular dysfunction. This absolutely parallels our experience. The control of massive ascites associated with the Budd-Chiari syndrome by peritoneal venous shunt parallels LeVeen's experience. The intrahepatic venous shunts, causing portal hypertension, have represented our most difficult problems. We have attempted to embolize these with little success. On two occasions we performed resections; one was successful and the other patient died of intraoperative hemorrhage during an attempt to remove a large lesion from the middle of the liver.—S.I.S.] ◀

24–8 **Gastrointestinal Hemorrhage From Left-Sided Portal Hypertension: An Unappreciated Complication of Pancreatitis.** In the past 10 years, Alex G. Little and A. Rahim Moossa (Univ. of Chicago) have encountered 16 patients having splenic vein thrombosis caused by pancreatitis. Of 92 patients seen in 1969–1979 with suspected or proved pancreatitis, 36 were evaluated for suspected pancreatic carcinoma, pseudocyst, chronic pancreatitis, or gastrointestinal blood loss. Twenty patients had no evidence of blood loss and no angiographic evidence of venous abnormality. The study patients were 9 men and 7 women with a mean age of 45.2 years. Seven were being studied for possible pancreatic carcinoma and 9, for gastrointestinal blood loss.

Most of the 16 study patients had a history suggestive of pancreatitis, and 10 had known chronic pancreatitis. Three patients had massive gastrointestinal blood loss, and arteriography showed splenic vein thrombosis with bleeding gastroesophageal varices and a normal portal vein. They were treated by splenectomy and gastrotomy with oversewing of the bleeding varices. Similar angiographic findings were obtained in the 3 patients with moderate bleeding. All of these patients had gross evidence of previous pancreatitis. All underwent splenectomy, and 1 also has cystogastrostomy for a pancreatic pseu-

---

(24–8) Am. J. Surg. 141:153–158, January 1981.

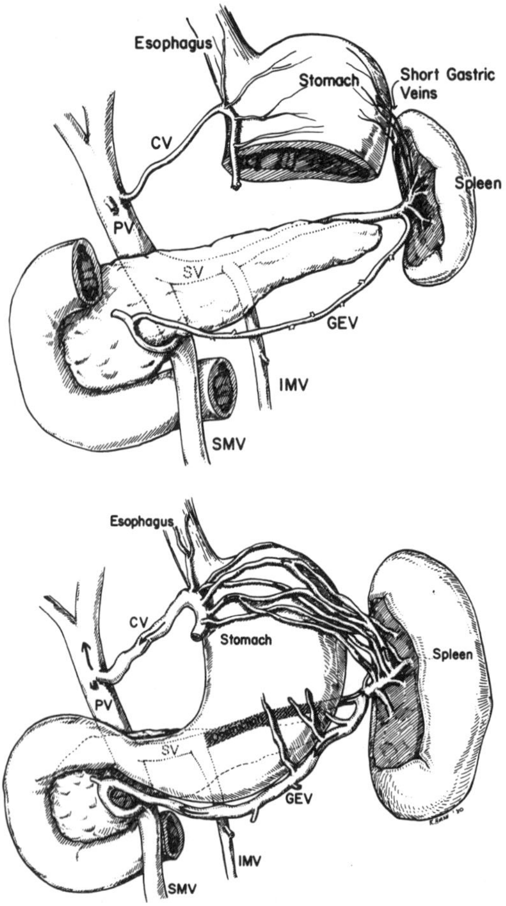

Fig 24–3.—Top, normal venous anatomy. The splenic vein *(SV)* is posterior to the pancreas and in direct contact. **Bottom,** splenic vein thrombosis. Reversed flow direction is indicated. Left-sided portal hypertension leads to gastric varices and dilatation of the short gastric, gastroepiploic *(GEV),* and coronary veins *(CV).* The portal vein *(PV)* is patent. IMV and SMV indicate interior and superior mesenteric veins, respectively. (Courtesy of Little, A.G., and Moossa, A.R.: Am. J. Surg. 141:153–158, January 1981.)

docyst. All 5 patients with occult bleeding had clinical pancreatitis at some time. Angiography showed splenic vein thrombosis with normal portal veins. Operative treatment varied in this group. All specimens showed changes of pancreatitis. Five patients had no evidence of blood loss. All of the operative specimens exhibited chronic or acute pancreatitis. There was no operative evidence of cirrhosis or generalized portal hypertension. All patients are alive after a mean follow-up of 35 months. None have had evidence of gastrointestinal blood loss.

Any significant pancreatic inflammation will involve the splenic vein (Fig 24–3). Inflammatory changes in the vein wall induce spasm, venous stasis, and intimal damage, predisposing to thrombosis. Thrombosis, in turn, leads to increased flow and pressure in the stomach wall veins and gastric varix formation. Esophageal varices may develop if the coronary vein drains into the splenic vein. Angiography is necessary to establish the diagnosis. The definitive treatment is splenectomy. Transgastric ligation of varices is also necessary if active bleeding is present. None of the present patients have had recurrent bleeding.

▶ [This article reports results of a large series of patients with pathologic features of the most readily correctible portal hypertension. As the authors point out, angiography is mandatory to establish the operation preoperatively; in this circumstance, percutaneous splenoportography most readily defines the lesion. In the discussion, Denis Bourbeau reports an experience with 38 patients with left-sided portal hypertension, 20% of whom had massive upper gastrointestinal bleeding. The causes included pancreatitis, basal carcinoma of the stomach and pancreas, retroperitoneal fibrosis, and aneurysm of the splenic artery.—S.I.S.] ◀

24–9 **Success of Medical and Surgical Management of Acute Variceal Hemorrhage.** Surgical portal decompression is clearly the most definitive treatment of variceal bleeding over the long term, but the timing of shunt surgery is controversial. John M. Holman, Jr., and Layton F. Rikkers (Univ. of Utah) have performed emergency operation only when Pitressin infusion and Sengstaken-Blakemore tube tamponade failed to control bleeding. Data were reviewed on 36 patients seen between 1978 and 1980 with active bleeding from varices and an average blood requirement of over 10 units. Laennec's cirrhosis was present in 83%. The 30 men and 6 women had a mean age of 51 years. Pitressin was infused at a rate of 0.4 unit per minute, followed after 24 hours by 0.2 unit per minute for 24 hours and then 0.1 unit per minute for 12 to 24 hours. Balloon tamponade was used when Pitressin infusion failed to control bleeding.

Hemorrhage stopped after gastric lavage alone in 4 patients. Pitressin infusion controlled bleeding in 19 of 31 patients, but 10 rebled before elective operation. Pitressin infusion controlled bleeding again in 5 of these patients. Ten patients had emergency shunt operations, and 10 had intubation because of initial failure to control bleeding with Pitressin. Balloon tamponade controlled hemorrhage in 11 of 14 instances. Conservative management led to complete control of bleeding in 69% of cases. No major morbidity resulted from either conservative procedure. Nutritional support was maximized during conservative management, and ascites was treated intensively. The Child score improved significantly by the time operation was performed. Overall operative mortality was 15%; mortality after elective operation was 8%. Patients with better hepatic reserve had fewer postoperative complications.

Management of variceal bleeding with intravenous Pitressin infusion, Sengstaken-Blakemore tube tamponade, or both is effective in most cases. Improvement in liver function in poor-risk patients leads to decreased postoperative morbidity. Emergency portasystemic shunt operations should be performed only on a selective basis, and variceal hemorrhage should initially be controlled nonoperatively.

▶ [This article substantiates my own personal prejudice because it shows that most

(24–9) Am. J. Surg. 140:816–820, December 1980.

acute variceal hemorrhages can be controlled medically and improved hepatic function may be achieved. In our own experience (Resnicoff and Schwartz: *Arch. Surg.* 97:317, 1968), the operative mortality associated with the shunt in a nonbleeding patient was 5%, contrasted with approximately 50% in an acutely bleeding patient. Recently, I had the opportunity of visiting Professor Myburgh's unit at the Witwatersrand Hospital in Johannesburg, South Africa. The group there has achieved a near 0% 30-day operative mortality after portacaval shunts by adopting a policy of medical control of bleeding and continued hospitalization for as long as 2 months to achieve improvement in hepatic function and a period of imposed abstinence from alcohol.—S.I.S.] ◀

24–10 **Prospective Study of Portasystemic Encephalopathy After Emergency Portacaval Shunt for Bleeding Varices.** Fear of post-shunt encephalopathy has deterred physicians from recommending definitive therapy for bleeding esophageal varices. Richard H. Bell, Jr., Paul V. B. Hyde, William P. Skivolocki, John E. Brimm, and Marshall J. Orloff (Univ. of California Med. Center, San Diego) reviewed data on 180 patients who underwent emergency portacaval shunt surgery for bleeding varices in 1963–1978. No patients were treated medically during this period. Direct portacaval anastomosis was performed in all but 3 cases. Ninety-five patients were discharged. If an 80-gm protein diet was tolerated postoperatively, the patient was discharged on a 60-gm diet. Five patients have been lost to follow-up. Encephalopathy was managed with neomycin and magnesium sulfate.

Encephalopathy developed in 31.5% of the patients discharged from the hospital after shunt surgery. The 30 affected patients required a total of 108 hospitalizations in 130 patient-years of follow up. The most common predisposing factor was dietary indiscretion with respect to protein. Continued alcohol abuse was implicated in 29% of hospitalizations. Encephalopathy was considered severe in 7% of patients. Preoperative encephalopathy is related to the development of encephalopathy during follow-up in Figure 24–4. Good liver function was predictive of a low rate of follow-up encephalopathy. A higher serum glutamic oxaloacetic transaminase level at the time of shunt

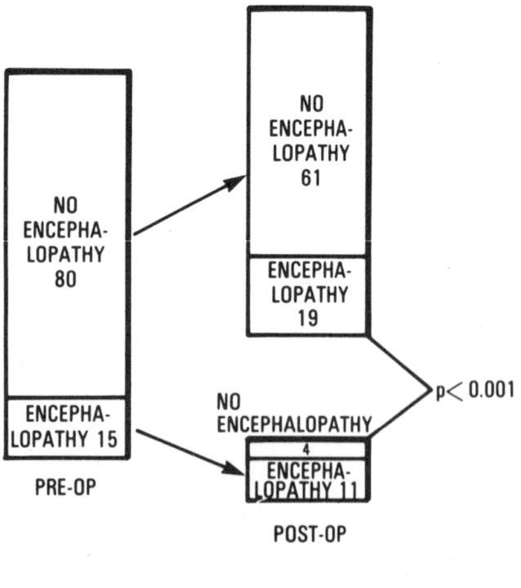

Fig 24–4.—Relationship of preoperative encephalopathy to development of encephalopathy in follow-up period. (Courtesy of Bell, R.H., Jr., et al.: Am. J. Surg. 142:144–150, July 1981.)

(24–10) Am. J. Surg. 142:144–150, July 1981.

surgery was associated with more frequent encephalopathy during follow-up. Encephalopathy also was related to a return to alcoholism. Survival of patients who experienced encephalopathy was lower than that of the other patients; the difference was significant after 5 years.

Portacaval shunting remains the best protective measure in patients with variceal bleeding. Encephalopathy usually follows a departure from the postoperative dietary regimen, often in conjunction with resumption of alcohol intake, and these problems are potentially reversible. Frequent follow-up aimed at alcoholic rehabilitation and frequent counseling in dietary matters is essential.

▶ [This article brings into focus the incidence of encephalopathy after portacaval shunt; the figures are similar to those in other reports. Langer and associates (*Surg. Gynecol. Obstet.* 150:45–48, 1980) reported that 5 of 28 patients had severe encephalopathy. Our own incidence is in the range of 15%. If one further discounts patients who have had encephalopathy preoperatively, the incidence of severe encephalopathy requiring protein restriction is really quite small. It is this group that is at issue in reference to the appropriateness of the selective splenorenal shunt. There is little question in my mind that there is a subset of patients, certainly those with schistosomiasis, in whom a selective splenorenal shunt is mandated. In cases of portal hypertension associated with alcoholism, the selective shunt really is directed at 15% of the shunted population, at most.—S.I.S.] ◀

24–11 **Results of 12-Year Randomized Trial of Portacaval Shunt in Patients With Alcoholic Liver Disease and Bleeding Varices.** The role of portacaval shunting in the management of patients with bleeding esophageal varices remains uncertain. T. B. Reynolds, A. J. Donovan, W. P. Mikkelsen, A. G. Redeker, F. L. Turrill, and J. M. Weiner (Univ. of Southern California, Los Angeles) entered 89 patients with alcoholic liver disease and at least one severe upper gastrointestinal hemorrhage from esophageal varices in a randomized trial of medical therapy versus end-to-side portacaval shunt surgery between 1967 and 1974. These patients were followed for at least 5 years. Shunting was performed in 41 patients. Four others randomized to surgery were not operated on. The two groups were clinically comparable. Seven patients assigned to medical management eventually underwent portacaval shunt surgery.

Gastrointestinal bleeding in the 2 treatment groups is compared in Table 1. Bleeding was attributed to varices in most instances. Ten deaths were attributed to bleeding and 13 to liver failure precipitated by bleeding, all in the medical group. No shunt thrombosis occurred.

TABLE 1.—GASTROINTESTINAL BLEEDING AFTER THERAPY ASSIGNMENT

	Surgical	Medical
Number of episodes	11	190
Pints of blood transfused	18	589
Deaths ascribed		
to bleeding	0	10
to bleeding + hepatic failure	0	13

(24–11) Gastroenterology 80:1005–1011, May 1981.

TABLE 2.—CAUSES OF DEATH

	Surgical	Medical
Operative	3	0
GI bleeding	0	10
GI bleeding + hepatic failure	0	13
Hepatic failure	18	3
Other	4	2
Unknown	1	1
	26	29

Shunt patency was confirmed at autopsy in all 13 patients evaluated. Hepatic encephalopathy developed without an obvious precipitating cause in 18 surgical patients, being severe in 8. About two thirds of patients in each group returned to some degree of active alcoholism. Causes of death are listed in Table 2, and survival curves are shown in Figure 24–5. Analysis of patients as initially assigned to treatment did not alter the difference in survival curves between the medical and surgical groups.

Portacaval shunting may reduce the frequency of bleeding from alcoholic gastritis. Routine shunting is not recommended in patients having a single episode of upper gastrointestinal tract bleeding from esophageal varices. It is hoped that better selection will be possible through hemodynamic studies such as measurements of functional portal flow, hepatic artery flow, or the response to portal vein occlusion.

▶ [This is a very serious attempt to study the difficult problem of the proper treatment of gastrointestinal hemorrhage resulting from esophageal varices due to alcoholic liver disease. As in the case of the preceding three well-controlled and randomized studies, it appears that the differences in outcome between operative and nonoperative treatment are extremely small when one is considering survival alone. Clearly,

Fig 24–5.—Survival in patients randomized and receiving prescribed regimen. Diminishing sample size allowed curves to be drawn for only 10 years. (Courtesy of Reynolds, T.B., et al.: Gastroenterology 80:1005–1011, May 1981.)

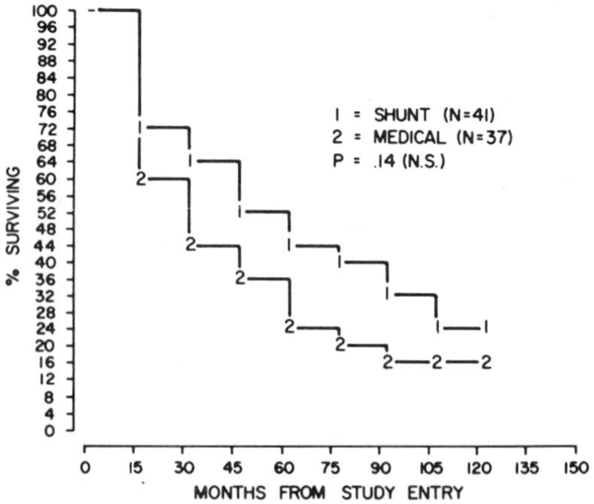

in this study, as in the others, the incidence of gastrointestinal hemorrhage in the surgical group was reduced markedly, as was the need for transfusions. Perhaps one can regard this as the most positive and clear-cut effect of the shunting procedures. It is surprising at the same time, however, that the need for hospitalization did not seem to be reduced by the surgical procedure, given the fact that these data were not quite as precise as the authors would like them to have been. Postshunt patients frequently were hospitalized for encephalopathy or episodes of hepatic decompensation related to alcoholic intake. We are still left, then, with a very real problem in knowing whether to recommend a shunt for a patient who has bled once from esophageal varices. Furthermore, and unfortunately, there did not seem to be any factors that would be helpful in selecting patients for either operative or nonoperative treatment.—W.S.] ◀

24–12 **Selective Transsplenic Decompression Procedure: Changes in Technique After 300 Cases.** W. Dean Warren and William J. Millikan, Jr. (Emory Univ.) reviewed experience with more than 300 patients undergoing selective transsplenic decompression (distal splenorenal shunt) since 1971. This approach has proved to be superior to nonselective shunt (portacaval-mesocaval shunt) in maintaining portal perfusion, preventing postshunt encephalopathy, and preventing recurrent variceal hemorrhage. The ideal patient is a stable cirrhotic without ascites who is not actively bleeding and has good liver function. Introduction of the LeVeen valve and careful preoperative and postoperative care have eliminated mild and moderate ascites as a contraindication to selective shunt surgery.

Antibiotic prophylaxis is used empirically, and parenteral high-dose corticosteroid treatment is begun preoperatively and continued for 24 hours. Cimetidine also is administered. A hockey stick incision 1 to 2 cm below the costal margin is used. The gastrocolic ligament is divided inside the gastroepiploic arcade to reduce collateralization by this route. The pancreas must be mobilized along its entire lower border to expose the splenic vein adequately. Care must be taken to avoid injuring the tail of the pancreas. The posterior surface of the splenic vein is dissected first, after removal of the adventitia. The splenic vein-portal vein junction is controlled. The splenic vein usually is ligated flush with the superior mesenteric vein. It should approach the renal vein from left to right, usually from a cephalad and anterior position. An end splenic-side renal anastomosis is usually done in the region of the divided adrenal vein. The coronary vein is ligated at its origin along the superior margin of the splenic vein or as it originates from the portal vein. Postoperative fluids are restricted to free water and salt-poor albumin. Aldactone is begun when the patient is taking fluids. Fat is restricted to 20 gm daily for 30 days.

Portal perfusion decreases over time as retroperitoneal collaterals develop between the portal system and the splenorenal shunt. The goal of operation is to decompress varices and preserve portal perfusion by aggressively performing portal vein-coronary vein disconnection.

▶ [This article is a classic and one that surgeons at all levels pray for: the description of technique based on long experience and modifications that have evolved during

---

(24–12) Contemp. Surg. 18:11–32, March 1981.

that experience. This is the best description I have seen for this operation. For me, the most important part of the article relates to the coronary azygos disconnection at the junction between the coronary vein and the splenic or portal vein; the authors' method of interruption certainly facilitates the procedure.—S.I.S.] ◀

24–13 **Long-term Loss of Warren's Shunt Selectivity: Angiographic Demonstration.** Distal splenorenal shunting with gastrosplenic-mesenteric disconnection has been accepted widely as the operation of choice for portal hypertension caused by cirrhosis. It is assumed that esophageal varices are decompressed while the portal supply to the liver is maintained. Jacques Belghiti, Philippe Grenier, Olivier Nouel, Henri Nahum, and François Fekete (Clichy, France) found that the selectivity of Warren's operation is lost a few months after surgery. Twenty patients had the operation for cirrhosis and ruptured esophageal varices in 1976–1979, and 18 survived the postoperative period. One had recurrent bleeding a week after surgery due to ruptured varices associated with thrombosis of the splenorenal shunt. Ten of the other 17 patients experienced transient ascites. Four had small gastrointestinal bleeds unrelated to ruptured varices 3–5 months postoperatively. Angiography showed a patent shunt in 15 patients and an occluded shunt in 2 others. Collateral circulation from the portomesenteric to the gastrosplenic system through enlarged venous channels was observed in all patients when evaluated 3–36 months postoperatively. A decrease in portal flow was evident in all cases

Fig 24–6.—Diameter of portal vein before and after shunt at venous phase of superior mensenteric arteriography. (Courtesy of Belghiti, J., et al.: Arch. Surg. 116:1121–1124, September 1981; copyright 1981, American Medical Association.)

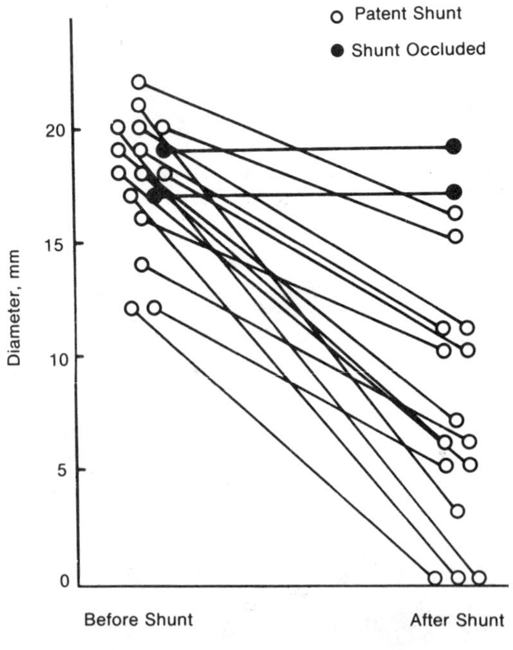

(24–13) Arch. Surg. 116:1121–1124, September 1981.

PORTAL PERFUSION JUDGED BY VENOUS PHASE OF SUPERIOR MESENTERIC ARTERIOGRAPHY

	Portal Perfusion Grade*			
	1	2	3	4
Before shunt (n = 15)	7	6	2	0
After shunt (n = 15)	2	3	7	3

*Values of grades 1 and 2 and of grades 3 and 4 were significantly different ($P < .05$) when compared with each other.

from degradation of portal perfusion of the liver and/or a decrease in diameter of the portal vein (Fig 24–6). In 2 cases, the portal vein was thrombosed. Changes in portal perfusion, as assessed from superior mesenteric angiography, are given in the table.

This study showed that, in all patients with a patent distal splenorenal shunt, a collateral circulation from the portomesenteric to the gastrosplenic system developed a few months postoperatively. This produces decreased portal perfusion of the liver. Distal splenorenal shunting appears not to differ hemodynamically from side-to-side portacaval shunting. The intestinal bleeding noted in some patients in the late postoperative phase could be a result of the large venous collateral circulation reconnecting.

▶ [The present study represents an affirmation of the previously reported work by Mallard et al. (*Surgery* 86:663–671, 1979) and Widrich (*Radiology* 134:341–345, 1980). In work recently presented at the Southern Surgical Association, and to be included in the 1983 edition of the YEAR BOOK OF SURGERY, Warren and his associates have demonstrated continued adhepatic flow in the portal veins of a significant number of patients over a long period of time after selective splenorenal shunt. Warren and his associates also emphasize that there are other factors related to the splanchnic venous circulation that might reduce the incidence of encephalopathy in patients subjected to the selective shunt. The various series are difficult to reconcile. Most series concerned with randomization of the selective distal splenorenal shunt have showed improved encephalopathy, e.g., Langer et al. (*Surg. Gynecol. Obstet.* 150:45–48, 1980), whereas Conn and associates, in a prospective double-blind study, showed no statistically significant difference in the rate of encephalopathy between patients subjected to the selective splenorenal shunt and those patients subjected to the more classic procedures.—S.I.S.] ◀

24–14 **Effect of Portacaval Anastomosis on Hypersplenism.** Cirrhosis often is associated with manifestations of hypersplenism, but the effects of portacaval anastomosis (PCA) on the hematologic abnormalities are unclear. Milton G. Mutchnick, Emanuel Lerner, and Harold O. Conn (Yale Univ.) determined the occurrence of hypersplenism in 52 control patients who were not operated on and 38 patients with a patent prophylactic PCA. Each patient had a histologic diagnosis of cirrhosis and an endoscopic diagnosis of esophageal varices with no previous bleeding. Another 39 patients undergoing therapeutic PCA were also studied. Follow-ups were 54.7 months for controls, 54.5 months for the prophylactic shunt group, and 59.9 months for the therapeutic shunt group. The control and prophylactic shunt groups

(24–14) Dig. Dis. Sci. 25:929–938, December 1980.

were hematologically similar at the outset and had similar cumulative survival rates.

There was no significant difference in the prevalence of hypersplenism between the control and the prophylactic shunt groups during follow-up. Hemolytic anemia resolved in all 4 affected controls but appeared during follow-up in 2 others and in 3 patients who had a PCA. One therapeutic shunt patient had hemolytic anemia that persisted after operation; 7 others developed hemolytic anemia after PCA. Leukopenia and thrombocytopenia developed in comparable proportions of the groups. Splenomegaly appeared more often in the control group than in the prophylactic shunt group during follow-up. Hypersplenism resolved in all 5 affected controls, but it appeared in 11 other patients during follow-up. It resolved in 4 of 5 prophylactic shunt patients but appeared in 9 others (24%). In the therapeutic shunt group, hypersplenism resolved in 1 of 2 patients after PCA and developed in 8 other patients (22%).

Hypersplenism appears not to be affected by prophylactic creation of a PCA. None of these patients had hemolysis severe enough to require transfusions. It seems clear that PCA reduces portal hypertension and spleen size, and it therefore would be expected to improve hypersplenism, but no significant change was seen in this study.

▶ [Over the years, we have come to anticipate a basic iconoclasm in Doctor Conn's reports. The question that the surgeon asks is what is the effect of a shunt on hypersplenism. Hutson and associates (*Ann. Surg.* 185:605–612, 1977) responded that the selective splenorenal shunt improved the leukopenia and thrombocytopenia in a series of patients in whom the portal venous system was decompressed successfully. Most series have indicated that 60% of patients with hypersplenism associated with portal hypertension have improvement in their hypersplenism subsequent to a shunting procedure. The point to be stressed, however, is that hypersplenism does not constitute an indication for a decompressive procedure, and the patients who maintain the hypersplenism subsequent to the decompressive procedure rarely have difficulties related to this disorder.—S.I.S.] ◀

24–15 **Portacaval Shunt for Familial Heterozygous Hypercholesterolemia.** Portacaval shunting reduces the serum cholesterol concentration, but its use for the treatment of heterozygous type 2 hypercholesterolemia is controversial. Peter N. Madras (Univ. of Toronto) describes 2 patients with extensive premature cardiovascular disease who underwent portacaval shunting and have had no major complications after 30 months.

CASE 1.—Woman, 29, with crescendo angina and xanthelasmas, remained disabled after coronary bypass. The cholesterol concentration fell from a mean of 375 to a mean of 213 mg/dl after portacaval shunting.

CASE 2.—Woman, 30, with crushing retrosternal pain and cholesterol concentrations above 600 mg/dl, underwent portacaval shunting after bypass surgery. The average serum cholesterol concentration fell 59% from the preoperative values present during cholestyramine treatment and a low-cholesterol diet. A further decline was found at 30 months. The patient lost 30 lb postoperatively. Slight fatty infiltration of the liver was seen 8 months after operation.

These patients had unstable cholesterol concentrations preopera-

---

(24–15) Surg. Gynecol. Obstet. 152:187–190, February 1981.

tively, and neither was rigorous about adhering to treatment or diet. Neither had clinical evidence of encephalopathy. Patient 1 reported insomnia and depression a year after portacaval shunting and had a serum ammonia concentration of 86 μg/dl. In neither case was protein restricted, and the postoperative symptoms in Patient 1 did not improve with a low-protein diet. In both patients portacaval shunting reduced the cholesterol concentrations by about 40%. No adverse effects were observed. Xanthelasmas regressed partially in Patient 1.

Portacaval shunting is an effective means of reducing serum cholesterol concentrations in young patients with heterozygous type 2 hypercholesterolemia in whom cardiovascular complications pose a major threat to life. The benefits of the procedure outweigh the risk in this setting.

▶ [This report substantiates Starzl's findings (*Arch. Surg.* 113:71, 1978). The fact that these patients did not have any evidence of encephalopathy with the end-to-side portacaval shunt supports the contention that encephalopathy is related to hepatic dysfunction and not to the shunting of blood per se. The important difference in the present report is that the maximal reduction of serum cholesterol level occurred immediately postoperatively, unlike the experience of other authors. Additional studies are required to resolve this difference.—S.I.S.] ◀

24–16 **Renal and Hemodynamic Effects of the Peritoneovenous Shunt: II. Long-Term Effects.** The peritoneovenous shunt is effective in the management of intractable hepatic ascites, but the mechanism of its persistent beneficial effect is unclear. P. D. Greig, L. M. Blendis, B. Langer, B. R. Taylor, and R. F. Colapinto (Univ. of Toronto) investigated 11 patients up to 29 months postoperatively. They were among 24 patients given a peritoneovenous shunt for intractable hepatic ascites in 1975–1979. Nine patients had micronodular cirrhosis, 1 had polycystic liver with portal hypertension, and 1 had Budd Chiari syndrome with persistent ascites after portacaval shunting. Sodium balance studies were done in 7 patients who were not receiving diuretics. Hemodynamic studies were done in 8 patients before and late after operation.

The results of sodium balance studies are shown in Figure 24–7. Responses to sodium challenge with 100 mEq daily were variable, but 6 of 7 patients showed sodium retention. Plasma renin activity and serum aldosterone levels were reduced on the higher sodium intake. The mean creatinine clearance was 104 ml/minute. Portal pressure fell by a mean of 12 mm Hg on shunting, but portal hypertension persisted. Free hepatic vein pressure did not change significantly; the corrected sinusoidal pressure decreased significantly. No significant changes in liver biochemistry findings were observed. Two patients had major variceal bleeds, despite the relief of ascites and a fall in portal pressure. Both of these patients died.

Continued patency of the peritoneovenous shunt is observed in patients without clinical ascites. Improved sodium excretion permits a greater dietary salt intake and the reduction or elimination of diuretics. The improvement may be related to a persistent increase in cre-

---

(24–16) Gastroenterology 80:119–125, January 1981.

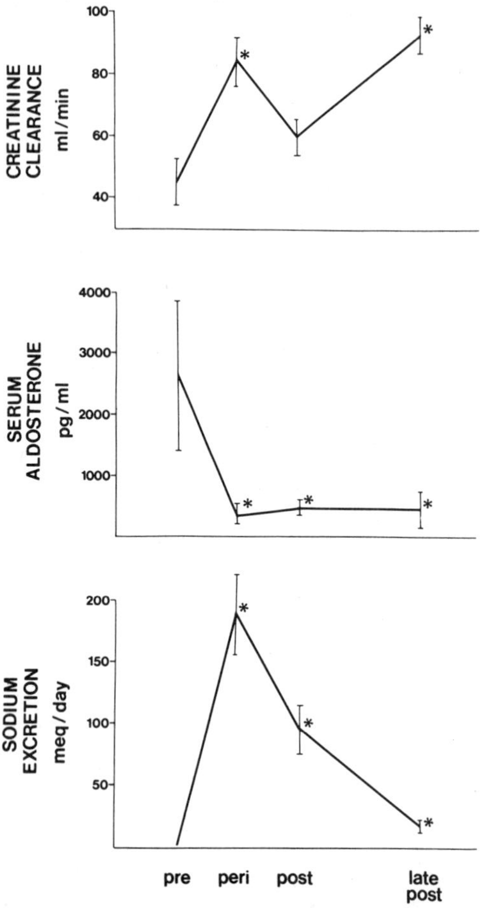

Fig 24–7.—Changes in creatinine clearance, serum aldosterone level, and sodium excretion on the 20-mEq sodium diet in 7 patients receiving the peritoneovenous shunt. The preoperative status *(pre)* is compared with the postoperative status at 72 hours *(peri)*, at 2 weeks *(post)*, and from 3 to 30 months *(late post)*. (Courtesy of Greig, P.D., et al.: Gastroenterology 80:119–125, January 1981.)

atinine clearance and normalization of the renin activity and aldosterone level, as well as a fall in portal pressure. However, sodium retention is not completely reversed, and most patients will not tolerate an unrestricted sodium diet without ascites reaccumulating. Persistent portal hypertension leaves these patients still at risk of esophageal variceal bleeding.

▶ [This is an extension of previous studies by this group emphasizing that sodium retention in cirrhosis is multifactorial and that the shunt can reverse the sodium retention. It must be stressed, however, that the overwhelming majority of patients with ascites secondary to sodium retention cirrhosis do not require surgical intervention and a shunting procedure and can be managed medically. Also, there is an increasing literature concerning the dangers associated with a peritoneovenous shunt. Major variceal hemorrhage has been noted by other investigators, as have significant coagulopathy, infection, and shunt obstruction. At present, there is an ongoing study to determine whether the benefits outweigh the complications and to find out specifically when a shunt is indicated in the cirrhotic patient.—S.I.S.] ◀

24–17 **Injuries Associated With Splenic Trauma.** The spleen is the most frequently injured organ in blunt abdominal trauma, and also is often injured in cases of penetrating trauma to the upper part of the abdomen or lower left part of the chest. Audrey C. Traub and John F. Perry, Jr. (St. Paul-Ramsey Med. Center) reviewed experience with 258 patients treated for splenic injury in a 5½-year period. Blunt trauma was present in 241 cases and penetrating injuries were noted in 17 patients. More than two thirds of patients with blunt trauma were in the second and third decades of life. Only 27 patients presented with isolated splenic trauma, and 135 patients had both intra- and extra-abdominal injuries as well as splenic trauma. Male patients predominated in a ratio of 3:1. Peritoneal lavage was 96.5% accurate in showing the presence of splenic injury in patients with blunt abdominal trauma.

Hypotension was present at admission in more than one third of patients. A capsular tear was present in 32.5% of patients, and hilar injury was seen in 45.7% of cases. Ten of 13 splenic transection injuries occurred in children younger than age 16 years. Splenic avulsion was present in 11 patients, fragmentation in 12, a subcapsular hematoma in 3, and a ruptured solenic cyst in 1. Associated injuries are summarized in the table. Complications occurred in 42% of patients with blunt trauma and in 53% of those with penetrating injuries. Pulmonary complications were most frequent; thromboembolism was rare. Isolated splenic injury did not cause death (Fig 24–8), but mortality was increased in pedestrians, patients older than age 65 years, and patients with associated injuries, especially combined intra-abdominal and extra-abdominal injuries. Hypotension at admission also was associated with increased mortality.

Peritoneal lavage enhances the diagnosis and management of splenic

Fig 24–8.—Mortality in splenic trauma with associated injuries: *S*, splenic injury only; *S-I*, splenic injury with concomitant intra-abdominal injury; *S-E*, splenic injury with concomitant extra-abdominal injury; *S-I-E*, splenic injury with concomitant intra- and extra-abdominal injuries. (Courtesy of Traub, A.C., and Perry, J.F., Jr.: J. Trauma 21:840–847, October 1981.)

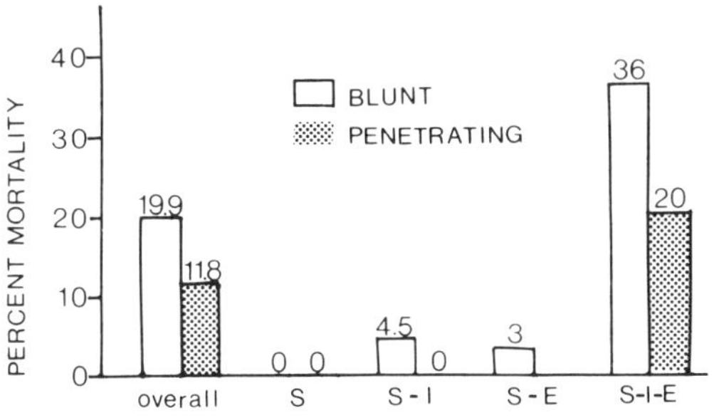

(24–17) J. Trauma 21:840–847, October 1981.

ASSOCIATED INJURIES IN PATIENTS WITH SPLENIC TRAUMA

Extra-abdominal	Blunt (193 patients)	Penetrating (10 patients)
Head injury	117	
Chest	109	10
Spine	27	
Extremity	70	2
Pelvic	42	

Intra-abdominal	Blunt (147 patients)	Penetrating (16 patients)
Gastrointestinal	52 (22)*	15 (15)
Liver	58 (34)	6 (5)
Pancreas	11 (4)	8 (7)
Mesentery	37 (14)	3 (1)
Diaphragm	18 (18)	8 (8)
Genitourinary	72 (29)	5 (4)
Retroperitoneal hematoma	79 (2)	4 (0)
Other	33 (31)	5 (5)

*The first number denotes total number of injuries in each category; second number (in parentheses) denotes number of injuries in each category that required surgical repair.

injuries. More than one third of patients with splenic trauma will require surgery for serious concomitant intra-abdominal injury, making splenic repair feasible. Suturing has been effective in adults as well as in children. Preservation of splenic function will reduce the problems of postsplenectomy sepsis.

▶ [This article addresses one of the important issues to be considered in patients undergoing conservative, nonoperative management. In reference to diagnostic peritoneal lavage, unquestionably it is extremely accurate in assessing the presence of splenic injury. The question would be raised regarding the importance of peritoneal lavage in defining the need for operative intervention. Most of the clinicians who have been subscribing to a nonoperative approach in most patients base operative intervention on a continuing decrease in hematocrit and hypotension. If such is the case, peritoneal lavage would add little. This one criticism does not detract from the importance of the message of the article that monofocal determination to avoid an operation and avoid splenectomy might prove more deleterious than laparotomy in a group of patients who have associated intra-abdominal injuries.—S.I.S.] ◀

24–18 **Selective Management of Injured Spleen.** Denis R. King, Thom E. Lobe, Gerald M. Haase, and E. Thomas Boles, Jr. (Ohio State Univ.) reviewed experience over 6 years with splenic trauma in 68 consecutive children aged 1–16 years. Blunt trauma was implicated in 97% of cases. About 40% of children were in shock at admission, and 20% were unresponsive because of closed head injury. In the first 2 years of the study period, paracentesis was done promptly in most children, and all 15 lavages were positive. Nuclide scanning now is the basic diagnostic study. No false positive scans have been obtained. Two thirds of the patients received transfusions. More than half of the children had associated injuries.

(24–18) Surgery 90:677–682, October 1981.

Twenty-two children had splenectomy, 16 had splenic repair, and 30 were managed nonoperatively. Good results were obtained in all of these groups. Two children (3%) died of their injuries; both had massive closed head injuries. Seven early postoperative complications occurred in 5 splenectomized children, and 2 patients had complications after splenic repair. No patients having repair or managed nonoperatively have had late complications. One splenectomy patient required enterolysis for small bowel obstruction on 2 occasions. Another survived an episode of overwhelming pneumococcal sepsis 6 months postoperatively.

Nonoperative management is preferred to splenic repair in children with spleen injuries, and the latter is preferable to splenectomy. Following this plan, 86% of 49 patients treated since 1977 have had splenic salvage. Splenic laceration now can be diagnosed with considerable accuracy, and patients can be managed with minimal risk and with salvage of splenic function in a large majority of cases. Splenectomy may be reserved for severe penetrating injuries and devascularization or fragmentation of the spleen.

▶ [This article presents a spectrum of treatment permeating the pediatric surgical experience. Nobody questions the fact that asplenic sepsis exists in a given number of pediatric patients; most patients, however, have hematologic disorder, and the incidence of splenectomy associated with trauma is really quite small. The incidence is even smaller in an adult population. A growing concern is arising as to whether insistence on a nonoperative approach or the necessity for splenic preservation may, in itself, result in death. Pressure may result in more patients dying than would be salvaged by splenic preservation. Nielsen and associates (*Scand. J. Haematol.* 27:51–56, 1981) have pointed out that splenosis was detected in 22 of 45 patients splenectomized after abdominal trauma or accidental lesions of the spleen during operation. In their experience, the only patient with overwhelming infection was a girl in whom splenectomy was performed for hereditary spherocytosis, and she recovered from sepsis. They feel that it is this splenosis that may account for a lessened tendency to overwhelming sepsis after posttraumatic splenectomy.—S.I.S.] ◀

24–19 **Is Splenic Salvage Safe in the Traumatized Patient?** Armando E. Giuliano and Robert C. Lim, Jr. (Univ. of California, San Francisco) have managed selected patients with severe, often multiple injuries by splenic salvage methods. Review was made of data on 92 patients operated on for splenic injury in 1978–1979. Fifty-nine patients underwent splenectomy, whereas 33 had splenic salvage procedures. The mean age was 32.9 years. Twenty-five male and 8 female patients had splenic salvage surgery. Blunt injury was the most common cause of splenic damage in these cases, and was most often caused by motor vehicle accidents. Eleven patients had stab wounds, and 1 had a gunshot wound. Eighteen of the 33 study patients had associated injuries.

Hemostatic agents were used in 26 cases. Six patients had suture repair, and 1 underwent hemisplenectomy. Most often, hemostasis was achieved with a combination of electrocautery, microfibrillar collagen, or absorbable gelatin sponge plus thrombin, and gentle pressure. Occasionally, devitalized splenic tissue was debrided. Hemostasis was satisfactorily achieved in all cases. Drains were not used unless the

---

(24–19) Arch. Surg. 116:651–656, May 1981.

tail of the pancreas was injured. No patient required reoperation for control of bleeding on subsequent splenectomy. Eleven patients had major complications, the most common being pneumonia and respiratory failure. No complications were related to the splenic repair, and there were no subphrenic abscesses.

Splenic salvage may be attempted in children and young adults, who probably have a higher rate of long-term complications from splenectomy. Isolated splenic injuries may be repaired in older patients. In general, undue risk should not be taken in order to attempt to save a spleen, but in appropriate circumstances splenic salvage can be carried out safely and should prevent the adverse effects of splenectomy. The simplest approach is to control bleeding with gelatin sponge and thrombin or, preferably, microfibrillar collagen, and by applying gentle pressure with packs.

▶ [By now, I think everybody has the message that it is possible to save part of the spleen in a traumatized patient. A reasonable sequence for managing these patients would begin with: (1) observation, because we now appreciate that many patients do not require laparotomy, (2) laparotomy with suture, (3) laparotomy with partial splenectomy, (4) removal of the spleen with implantation of portions into the omentum. There is little question that an occasional asplenic patient in whom splenectomy has been performed for trauma will develop massive sepsis and die. A case can be made for avoiding this circumstance. The message of the article, however, relates to the "selectivity." As G. Hugh Lawrence points out in the discussion of this article, there are patients who have to be returned to the operating room for complete splenectomy after attempted salvage. Also, the salvage rate in this report is 36%. Some traumatized spleens will require splenectomy, and more deaths will arise from the concept that splenic salvage must be effected in all cases. Splenectomy may still represent the most conservative approach in trauma patients for surgeons who have not had experience with splenic preservation.—S.I.S.] ◀

24–20 **Splenectomy for Immune Thrombocytopenic Purpura.** Although steroids are considered the initial treatment of choice for patients with immune thrombocytopenic purpura (ITP), splenectomy continues to be useful in the management of this state. Steven J. Mintz, Scott R. Petersen, Bruce Cheson, Linda J. Cordell, and Ralph C. Richards (Univ. of Utah) reviewed the results of splenectomy in 71 patients with ITP, operated on in 1965–1979. Only 4 patients were lost to follow-up. The mean length of follow-up was 4.8 years. The 35 male and 36 female patients had a mean age of 27.2 years; 22 were younger than age 16 years. The mean duration of disease before splenectomy was 15 months. Nearly all patients received prednisone before splenectomy, in an initial dose of 40–60 mg. The indication for splenectomy usually was failure to respond to steroids or inability to taper the dosage after a 3- to 6-month trial.

Nearly 60% of evaluable patients had an elevation of platelet counts on preoperative steroid therapy. Accessory spleens were found in 20 cases. Eighteen patients received platelet transfusions. All patients but 1 survived splenectomy. The complication rate was 14%; 4 patients had thromboembolic complications. Complete remission occurred in 77% of the 66 patients who were followed up, and 5 others had a good response. Two patients had "late" remissions 5 and 10

(24–20) Arch. Surg. 116:645–650, May 1981.

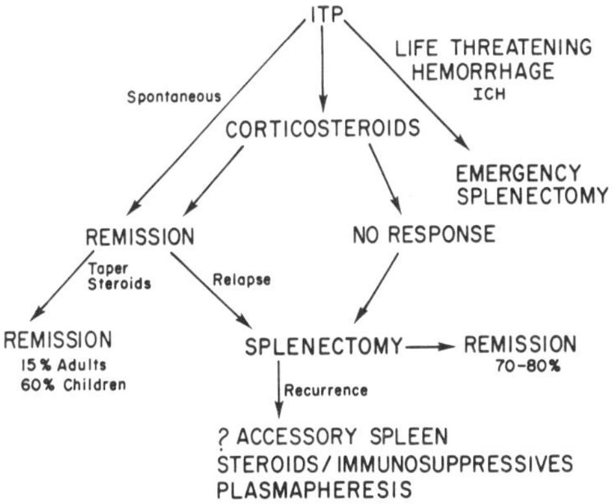

Fig 24–9.—Protocol for treating patients with ITP includes initial trial of corticosteroids. If patient does not respond with elevation of platelet count, splenectomy is performed. If patient does respond, steroid dosage is tapered. If thrombocytopenia recurs after remission with corticosteroids, operative management is indicated. Life-threatening hemorrhage demands emergency splenectomy. Patients unresponsive to splenectomy should be assessed for presence of accessory spleen. Immunosuppressive agents or plasmapheresis may be useful in patients whose disease is refractory to splenectomy and corticosteroids: ICH indicates intracranial hemorrhage. (Courtesy of Mintz, S.J., et al.: Arch. Surg. 116:645–650, May 1981; copyright 1981, American Medical Association.)

years after splenectomy. Four patients had no response, and 6 others relapsed after an initially favorable response to splenectomy. Complete remission was more frequent in children than in adult patients. Ten patients have required continued steroid and/or immunosuppressive therapy after splenectomy. A preoperative response to steroids was predictive of remission after splenectomy.

These findings confirm the value of splenectomy in patients with ITP. The response to splenectomy is correlated with a platelet response to preoperative steroid therapy. The authors' protocol for managing patients with ITP is shown in Figure 24–9. Immunosuppression may be useful in patients in whom other reticuloendothelial organs continue to sequester platelets. Emergency splenectomy is indicated in patients with life-threatening hemorrhage or those who continue to have profound thrombocytopenia despite high doses of steroids.

▶ [The figures are in keeping with our own experience, with the exception that we failed to note any significant difference in patients who did not respond to the steroids prior to splenectomy (Schwartz et al.: *Surgery* 88:497–506, 1980). One of the interesting features that is not stressed in the literature relates to those patients who fail to respond with a significant increase in platelet counts; this is about 15% of the splenectomized population. In those patients, improvement is frequently achieved, because it is rare for splenectomized patients to develop recurrence of petechiae, ecchymosis, or significant bleeding. The other statistic emphasized by the present article that is in concert with our findings is that there was no correlation between postoperative thromboembolic disease and the postoperative platelet count.—S.I.S.] ◀

24–21 **Thrombosis of the Portal Vein Following Splenectomy for Myeloid Metaplasia.** Patrick J. Broe, C. Lockard Conley, and John L. Cameron (Johns Hopkins Med. Inst.) reviewed the records of 28

(24–21) Surg. Gynecol. Obstet. 152:488–492, April 1981.

patients (18 women) who underwent splenectomy for myeloid metaplasia between 1952 and 1979. Mean age was 56 years. Most patients had some degree of hypersplenism, and this was the chief indication for splenectomy in 19. In 8 the main indication was symptomatic splenomegaly. One patient had protracted fever of unknown origin. Mean interval from diagnosis of myeloid metaplasia to splenectomy was 5.8 years.

One patient died of portal vein thrombosis 9 days after splenectomy. Thromboembolic complications were documented or suspected in 9 patients, remotely from splenectomy in 5. One patient had two episodes of pulmonary embolism associated with high platelet counts. Two patients developed thrombophlebitis shortly after operation, and another did so 18 months postoperatively. Two patients died of pulmonary embolism about 2 years postoperatively; in 1, multiple pulmonary emboli were documented in the immediate postoperative period. Portal vein thrombosis was documented in 3 patients and strongly suspected in 2 others. Four of these 5 patients died. The 5 patients had a mean preoperative platelet count of 121,000/cu mm and a mean count of 254,000/cu mm a week after operation. The 3 patients living at 3 months had a mean count of 417,000/cu mm. Postsplenectomy thrombocytosis occurred in 7 patients, in 2 of whom thrombotic episodes developed.

Thrombocytosis may be a cause of portal vein thrombosis in some patients undergoing splenectomy, but this complication may occur in others operated on for myeloid metaplasia who have normal or low platelet counts postoperatively. Platelet function abnormalities may be more important in predisposing patients to portal vein thrombosis. Stasis in the splenic vein may also be a factor. The prophylactic use of anticoagulants and antiplatelet drugs should be strongly considered in this setting, and long-term maintenance therapy may be indicated. An attempt should be made to ligate the splenic vein as close as possible to its junction with the inferior mesenteric vein to eliminate a diverticulum and decrease the low-flow state in the splenic vein. Systemic and portal hypotension should be avoided postoperatively.

▶ [The authors make some extremely important points regarding a potentially devastating complication of splenectomy for hematologic disease. The first point is that thrombosis of the splenic vein extending to the portal and mesenteric veins is an extremely uncommon complication after splenectomy for diseases other than myeloproliferative disorder. However, it does occur with sufficient frequency following splenectomy for myeloproliferative disorder, as reported by Gordon et al. (*Arch. Surg.* 113:713, 1978), that specific attention is required. Since that article, we have managed 9 patients with myeloproliferative disorders undergoing splenectomy by using prophylaxis with antithrombotic drugs. Under this circumstance, the complication has not occurred. The authors make an important point that thrombocytosis is not present in most of these patients. An interesting study by Boxer et al. (ibid., pp. 808–809) showed no association between postsplenectomy thrombocytosis and thromboembolism.—S.I.S.] ◀

24–22 **Splenectomy for Hypersplenism in Malignant Lymphomas.** It has been suggested that splenic overactivity often complicates the

---

(24–22) Br. J. Surg. 68:29–33, January 1981.

course of malignant lymphomas. P. G. Gill, R. G. Souter, and P. J. Morris (Univ. of Oxford) report that, since 1975, splenectomy was performed in advanced malignant lymphomas in an effort to correct hematologic cytopenias in 41 patients—30 with non-Hodgkin's lymphoma and 11 with Hodgkin's disease.

In all but 1 patient with Hodgkin's disease, the disease was stage III or IV; in 15 non-Hodgkin's lymphoma patients, there was liver, widespread nodal, and bone marrow disease. In 4 patients, prior splenic irradiation failed to reverse cytopenia. Excess splenic sequestration of red blood cells or platelets was not regarded as a necessary indication for splenectomy. Operation was considered only in those who had exhausted normal avenues of therapy or in whom therapeutic options were curtailed by a serious hematologic defect. The spleen was palpable in all cases of non-Hodgkin's lymphoma and in 8 of Hodgkin's disease.

The spleen was not involved by disease in 2 patients with Hodgkin's disease and 1 with non-Hodgkin's lymphoma. Splenectomy was associated with a 90% overall hematologic correction. When chemotherapy was resumed after splenectomy, worthwhile remission was achieved in 87.5% of the patients. All patients with Hodgkin's disease had their cytopenia completely corrected and resumed treatment in full doses. Of non-Hodgkin's lymphomas, the hematologic abnormality was corrected in 26 patients (87%). Bone marrow infiltration did not preclude correction; 2 Hodgkin's disease patients had infiltration as did 19 non-Hodgkin's lymphoma patients, in whom it was frequently extensive. Of these, the cytopenia was reversed in 16 cases. Of patients with non-Hodgkin's lymphoma, 19 resumed full chemotherapy doses and 17 achieved remission (7 had no further treatment after splenectomy corrected the cytopenia).

There were no postoperative deaths. Morbidity was considered acceptably low; complications occurred in less than 25% of the cases. Changes in some patients after splenectomy—decreased size of lymph nodes, decrease in peripheral lymphocyte numbers, and resolution of fever—suggest that splenectomy may alter the course of malignant lymphomas other than by solely correcting hypersplenism.

It is concluded that splenectomy is a valuable adjunct to treatment in advanced malignant lymphomas and should be considered at the first suggestion of splenic overactivity and reduced marrow reserves. The nature of the underlying condition influenced whether a good result was obtained, the majority of such cases having nodular or diffuse well-differentiated lymphocytic histologic features of chronic lymphatic leukemia; however, splenectomy is worthy of consideration even in the more malignant variants of non-Hodgkin's lymphoma.

▶ [Splenectomy is being performed with increasing frequency in patients with lymphomas and chronic lymphocytic leukemia in situations in which the organ is enlarged and in severe cytopenias where residual bone marrow function is present. In patients with very large spleens, as in chronic lymphocytic leukemia, improvement may be substantial even with reduced numbers of normal hematopoietic cells in the bone marrow. However, if the spleen is only slightly enlarged, reduced bone marrow cellularity may indicate a reduced probability of benefit from the operation. Between

1969 and 1975, we operated on 18 patients with lymphoma; the indication for the procedure was splenomegaly in 8 cases and hypersplenism in 10. Eight of these patients have died, but 10 are alive and well 6 months to 5 years later and most have expressed sentiment that the procedure has been helpful. During the same period 12 patients with chronic lymphatic leukemia were operated on for similar reasons; 10 improved temporarily.—S.I.S.] ◀

25. Biliary Tract

25–1 **The Place of Hepatobiliary Isotope Scanning in the Diagnosis of Gallbladder Disease.** The trend toward more aggressive surgical management of acute cholecystitis has prompted a search for more accurate diagnostic methods. Andrew W. Hall, M. L. Wisbey, F. Hutchinson, Robert A. B. Wood, and Alfred Cuschieri examined the reliability of hepatobiliary imaging with ^{99m}Tc-pyridoxylideneglutamate (^{99m}Tc-PG) in 99 patients presenting in an 18-month period with acute right-sided upper abdominal pain. Four other patients were studied before surgery for morbid obesity. The mean age was 55 years. Patients were imaged with a gamma camera interfaced with a computer after a fast of at least 2 hours and the injection of 2 mCi of ^{99m}Tc-PG, or 5 mCi if clinical jaundice was present. A 1-hour dynamic study was recorded. Contrast studies were performed in 87 patients.

Acute cholecystitis was diagnosed in 23 patients, while 31 had no evidence of gallbladder disease. All patients with acute cholecystitis had positive scans, and all those without gallbladder disease had negative scans. No consistent pattern was obtained in patients with other gallbladder disease. The relative efficacy of hepatobiliary scanning and radiology is compared in the table. The predictive value of a negative hepatobiliary scan was 100%. A positive scan appeared to be a good indicator of the presence of gallbladder disease. However, the

COMPARATIVE VALUE OF VARIOUS TESTS IN THE DIAGNOSIS OF GALLBLADDER DISEASE

	Sensitivity (%)	Specificity (%)	Predictive value: Test positive (%)	Predictive value: Test negative (%)
Diagnosis of acute cholecystitis				
Hepatobiliary scan	100	70	50	100
Radiology (all)	75	63	44	80
Intravenous cholangiography	69	59	44	73
Oral cholecystogram	100	67	50	100
Diagnosis of gallbladder disease				
Hepatobiliary scan	68	100	100	58
Radiology (all)	79	87·5	94	62
Intravenous cholangiography	72	89	94	52
Oral cholecystogram	100	75	90	100

(25–1) Br. J. Surg. 68:85–90, February 1981.

scan was inferior to contrast radiology, particularly oral cholecystography, in excluding gallbladder disease in general.

Hepatobiliary scanning is useful for excluding acute cholecystitis and cystic duct obstruction in the emergency setting. A positive scan confirms gallbladder disease but does not distinguish between acute cholecystitis and a nonfunctioning gallbladder due to chronic disease. The scan will not replace contrast radiology in the elective management of gallbladder disease. Its greatest value probably will lie in the rapid diagnosis of acute right upper quadrant pain.

▶ [This represents a significant addition to the diagnostic armamentarium. Our present diagnostic protocol for biliary tract disease in patients with acute right-sided upper abdominal pain in whom the diagnosis is equivocal has included the use of the PIPDA or HIDA scan. Suarez et al. (*Ann. Surg.* 191:392–396, 1980) have reported equivalent results. In the face of enthusiastic acceptance of a new technique, it is important to stress the authors' point that cholecystography should continue to represent the standard technique for the routine diagnosis of chronic gallbladder disease. With the advent of radionuclide scans, endoscopic retrograde cholangiopancreatography, and percutaneous transhepatic cholangiography, it may well be that the use of intravenous cholangiography will become a test of the past. The technetium scan has a distinct advantage over ultrasound; one of the major problems associated with ultrasonography is the false negative result in a patient who has cystic duct obstructed by a small stone.—S.I.S.] ◀

25–2 **Choledochal Cyst: Survey by the Surgical Section of the American Academy of Pediatrics** is reported by Samuel H. Kim (Boston). A total of 188 cases of choledochal cyst have been reviewed. The most common type is dilatation of the common bile duct, and often the hepatic ducts as well, which was present in 175 cases. Biliary atresia was present in 23 of these cases, and in 1 of 10 cases of common duct diverticulum. Three patients had a choledochocele, or dilatation of the intraduodenal common bile duct. Of the 135 female and 53 male patients, 71 presented in the first year, and only 19 were seen after age 12. The most common clinical features were jaundice, abdominal pain, dark urine, hepatomegaly, and acholic stools. Intravenous cholangiography was diagnostically more useful than oral cholecystography. The most useful laboratory values were serum bilirubin, alkaline phosphatase, and the Rose Bengal scan.

A total of 240 operations were done in 185 patients, the most common being Roux-en-Y choledochocystjejunostomy and choledochocystduodenostomy. Hepatic cirrhosis was present in 61 patients, and cholelithiasis was seen in 14. Relatively few postoperative complications occurred. Recurrent cholangitis necessitated reoperation in 14 cases. Seventeen patients had portal hypertension. A total of 115 patients are alive without evident liver disease; 23 have liver disease. Six patients died of progressive liver failure caused by inoperable biliary atresia. A total of 24 patients had biliary atresia. Eleven of 22 patients are alive without liver disease.

▶ [It is helpful to have a survey by the American Academy of Pediatrics on this subject. An interesting change in therapy has occurred over the past several years. This has focused on the appropriateness for removing the cyst because of a true incidence of carcinoma in that region. Powell et al. (*Ann. Surg.* 139:666–674, 1981) re-

---

(25–2) J. Pediatr. Surg. 16:402–407, June 1981.

ported on the management of adult choledochal cyst and conducted an extensive review of the literature, encompassing a total of 1,337 patients. Todani et al. (*Cancer* 44:1134, 1979) reported an increase in frequency of carcinoma arising in choledochal cyst with a report on a total of 63 patients. This represents an incidence of 4.7%.—S.I.S.] ◀

25–3 **Chenodiol (Chenodeoxycholic Acid) for Dissolution of Gallstones: The National Cooperative Gallstone Study: A Controlled Trial of Efficacy and Safety** is reported by Leslie J. Schoenfield, John M. Lachin, and the Steering Committee of the National Cooperative Gallstone Study Group. Gallstones are a major medical and economic problem in the United States. Dissolution of gallstones by oral administration of bile acid mixtures was first reported in 1937. A double-masked study now has been done to determine the efficacy and safety of chenodiol, in daily doses of 750 and 350 mg, compared with placebo in 916 patients treated for 2 years for dissolution of radiolucent gallstones.

The results are shown in Figure 25–1. Complete dissolution was confirmed in 13.5% of patients given 750 mg of chenodiol daily, in 5.2% of those given the lower dose, and in 0.8% of placebo patients. Partial (more than 50%) or complete dissolution was confirmed in 40.8%, 23.6%, and 11.0% of these groups, respectively. Nearly 40% of high-dose patients showing partial dissolution at 9 months showed complete dissolution at 2 years. Dissolution was more frequent in women, thin patients, and patients with small or floating gallstones or a serum cholesterol level of 227 mg/dl or above. The presence of biliary pain did not influence the rate of dissolution significantly.

Fig 25–1.— Life-table analyses of confirmed complete dissolution. Tabular insert shows cumulative percentages of patients with dissolution and numbers of patients in whom dissolution could be (or previously had been) observed. (Courtesy of Schoenfield, L.J., et al.: Ann. Intern. Med. 95:257–282, September 1981.)

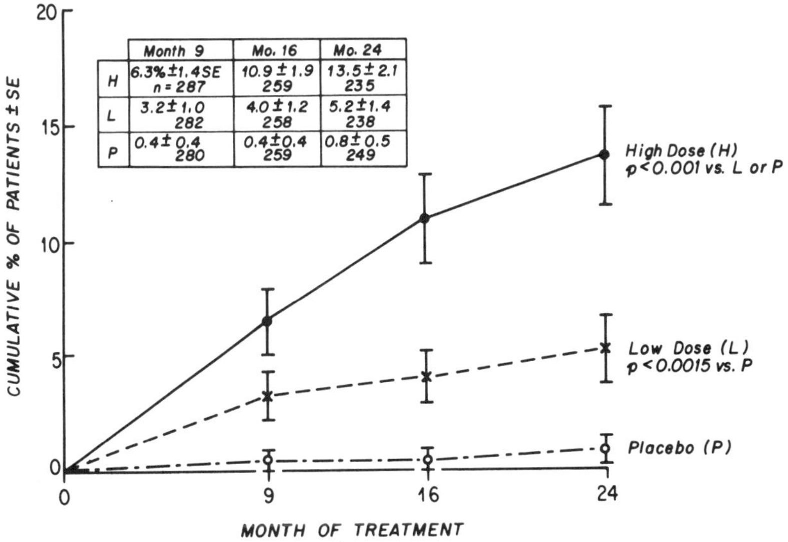

(25–3) Ann. Intern. Med. 95:257–282, September 1981.

Clinically significant hepatotoxicity occurred in 3% of the high-dose group, 0.4% of the low-dose group, and 0.4% of placebo patients. It always was biochemically reversible. Majorities of both groups had elevations of the serum cholesterol level, mainly low-density lipoproteins, of 10% or more. Dyspepsia was less frequent during the first year of treatment in all groups. Clinically important diarrhea was significantly more frequent in the high-dose chenodiol group.

It is concluded that chenodiol, in a daily dose of 750 mg for up to 2 years, is appropriate treatment for the dissolution of gallstones in selected patients. However, chenodiol has not reduced biliary symptoms or the need for cholecystectomy during the treatment period, and there is a risk of hepatotoxicity and also a chance of cholesterol level elevation. No deaths have been attributed to chenodiol administration.

▶ [The data made available in this excellently conducted national cooperative study will become part of the dialogue of surgeons interested in biliary tract disease. The study selects out those patients in whom a protocol would be more efficacious. It comes to an appropriate conclusion that chenodiol has a role in treatment of *selected* patients with gallstones. From the surgical point of view, it also points out that the medication did not reduce biliary symptoms or the need for cholecystectomy during the treatment.—S.I.S.] ◀

25–4 **Biliary Tract Surgery Concomitant With Other Intra-abdominal Operations.** The risks of biliary tract surgery done in conjunction with other intra-abdominal procedures have not been defined. Charles K. McSherry and Frank Glenn (New York Hosp.-Cornell Med. Center) reviewed information on 253 patients who had biliary tract surgery performed at the same time as other intra-abdominal operations between 1932 and 1979. They represented 2.1% of all patients having operations for nonmalignant biliary tract disease during this time at the authors' institution. Biliary tract operations were performed primarily in 51 patients and incidentally to other operations in 137, whereas 65 patients had both procedures planned preoperatively.

The patients having incidental biliary tract surgery had a mean age of 62.5 years. Ten patients had two nonbiliary diseases requiring operation. The large bowel, stomach, and duodenum were most frequently involved. A large majority of patients had chronic cholecystitis, and cholecystectomies were done in 93 patients. Morbidity was 15%. Three complications were directly related to biliary tract surgery. Operative mortality was 7%. The patients undergoing planned biliary tract and other procedures had a mean age of 51.6 years. Chronic cholecystitis was present in 62 of these 65 patients. Morbidity was 20% and mortality, 2%. The patients who had planned biliary tract surgery and other incidental and unplanned procedures had a mean age of 54.9 years. Fifteen operations were done for gastroesophageal lesions. There were no deaths in this group. Morbidity was 11.8%.

It is feasible to perform cholecystectomy or cholecystostomy for stone disease in patients operated on for nonbiliary tract diseases and to perform definitive operations for most gastrointestinal diseases found incidentally to a planned cholecystectomy. Concomitant procedures

(25–4) Ann. Surg. 193:169–175, February 1981.

requiring choledochotomy are not recommended in most circumstances. The patient's condition must permit the added operative stress, and exposure must be adequate to operate safely on the gallbladder.

▶ [This provides an interesting and meaningful data base that enforces the recommendation that the gallbladder should be palpated during all intra-abdominal procedures and removed if calculi are defined. I would take issue with the statement about concomitant operations requiring choledochotomy. Deliberate planned choledochotomy should not increase the morbidity too significantly. The point regarding an increased incidence of retained stones is not a meaningful argument because, with the T tube left in place and the use of radiographic solution, the problem can be resolved with operative intervention.—S.I.S.] ◀

25–5 **Biliary Enteric Fistula** is manifested by air in the biliary tract, intestinal obstruction, and a gallstone in the intestine, usually in the terminal ileum. The most common site of these fistulas is between the gallbladder and duodenum. Most patients have symptoms resembling those of chronic cholecystitis and cholelithiasis. Frank Glenn, Carolyn Reed, and William R. Grafe (New York Hosp.–Cornell Med. Center), reviewed 105 cases of biliary enteric fistula seen in 1932–1978. The rate of correct preoperative diagnosis was 43%. In over half the cases, a gallstone was impacted in the terminal 50 cm of the ileum. The duration of biliary symptoms varied greatly. The diagnosis was confirmed at surgery or autopsy in 99 of the 105 cases. There were 81 cholecystoduodenal and 16 cholecystocolic fistulas.

Ninety-eight patients had a total of 109 operations. Forty underwent cholecystectomy, choledochotomy, and repair of the fistula, and 37 had cholecystectomy with fistula repair and operative cholangiography. Thirteen patients had ileotomy only for removal of stones causing intestinal obstruction. Ileus due to gallstones was proved in 22 cases. Eleven patients died, 6 of them postoperatively. Subphrenic abscesses developed in 3 patients and subhepatic abscesses in 3. One had ascending cholangitis. The overall morbidity rate was 14.7%.

Primary repair of biliary enteric fistula usually can be performed in patients without obstruction. Cholecystectomy, excision of the fistula, common duct exploration, and operative cholangiography are recommended. Where the fistula involves the colon, choledochotomy followed by cholecystectomy and, lastly, division of the fistula, should reduce the extent of contamination. A similar sequence is indicated in patients in whom a fistula is not suspected preoperatively. Broad-spectrum antibiotic therapy is indicated in cases of unsuspected cholecystocolic fistula. Intestinal obstruction due to gallstones should be treated initially, and correction of the fistula should be deferred to a later time.

▶ [This represents a large experience from an institution with a long-time interest in problems of the biliary tract. I would feel negligent if I didn't point out that Frank Glenn continues to contribute in a lucid fashion at age 80. The authors add the recommendation of treatment of gallstone ileus presenting with intestinal obstruction by correction of the biliary enteric fistula at an elective second stage of operation. Day and Marks (*Am. J. Surg.* 129:552–558, 1975) reported that only 3 of 25 patients who were treated by enterotomy alone had recurrent symptoms of biliary disease. In selected patients, however, it was shown that one-stage cholecystectomy, fistula repair, and enterotomy did not result in a higher mortality than enterotomy alone.—S.I.S.] ◀

(25–5) Surg. Gynecol. Obstet. 153:527–531, October 1981.

25–6 **Radiation Hazard to Operating Room Personnel During Operative Cholangiography.** The potential danger of diagnostic irradiation and the need to minimize any exposure are well recognized. Dimitrios A. Linos, Joel E. Gray, and Donald C. McIlrath (Mayo Clinic) reviewed the radiation hazards associated with operative cholangiography, which is performed by some surgeons several times every week. Phantom measurements of scattered radiation indicated that a surgeon standing at the patient's side during cholangiographic filming would receive 3.2 mR per film, while exposure would be reduced to 0.5 mR if the surgeon stepped back 2.5 feet from the patient. This would reduce the monthly exposure of a surgeon performing 4 studies a week from about 205 to 32 mR (Fig 25–2). If a surgeon must inject the dye while taking films, he still could reduce exposure by stepping back about 1 m. Interposing a portable lead barrier also would appreciably reduce the amount of radiation exposure.

The radiation risk from fluoroscopy is much greater than with roentgenography. Typical exposures of about 5,000 mR/minute involve exposure to about 10 times more radiation during 1 minute of fluoroscopy than from 1 conventional roentgenographic procedure. The new electronic videodisc recording systems minimize the time the x-ray beam is on. A 1-second exposure results in a patient dose of about 80 mR, or 5 times less than a roentgenographic exposure. During fluoroscopy or with procedures requiring the surgeon to make more than 5 roentgenograms, all operating room staff should use portable lead barriers or protective lead aprons. Surgeons also are exposed to radiation from other diagnostic exposures and to background radia-

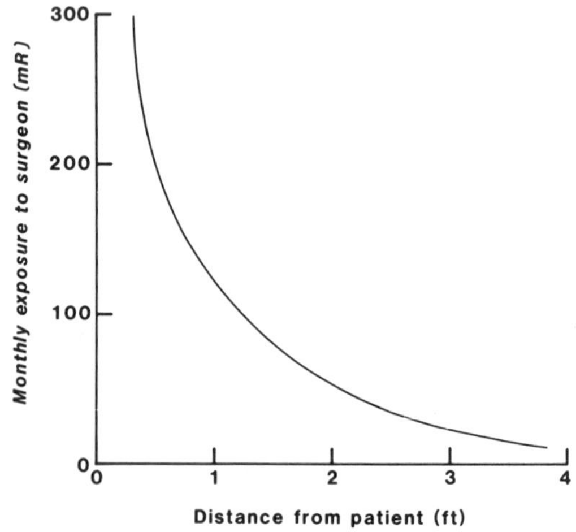

Fig 25–2.—Monthly radiation exposure to surgeon as function of distance from patient during operative cholangiography. (Courtesy of Linos, D.A., et al.: Arch. Surg. 115:1431–1433, December 1980; copyright 1980, American Medical Association.)

(25–6) Arch. Surg. 115:1431–1433, December 1980.

tion. Occupational exposure should be kept as low as possible. For most medical staff a monthly dose of 50 mR or less can be reasonably achieved.

▶ [I would concur completely in the recommendations made by the authors of this important paper. The problem of radiation to the surgeon during these procedures has received inadequate attention. I should like to emphasize, as do Linos et al., that the exposures may be made well after the operating surgeon has stepped away from the operating table, something I have done for many years, with excellent quality of films being achieved.—W.S.] ◀

25–7 **Impact of Choledochoscopy on Management of Choledocholithiasis: Experience With 499 Common Duct Explorations at the Massachusetts General Hospital** was reviewed by David W. Rattner and Andrew L. Warshaw (Harvard Med. School). Choledocholithiasis is present in nearly 15% of patients operated on for gallstones. Stones are missed in at least 5% of patients when standard methods of duct exploration and operative cholangiography are used. A total of 499 choledochotomies were done for stone disease by more than 45 surgeons in 1974–1978. Postexploration intraoperative cholangiography was done in more than 60% of cases. All patients but 2 had T-tube cholangiograms performed 1–2 weeks after surgery. The Storz choledochoscope, a rigid right-angle instrument, was used in all cases. In about 80% of cases, it was passed into the duodenum. Seventy-eight patients underwent sphincteroplasty or biliary-enteric bypass procedures.

Stones were found in 56% of cases by standard exploratory techniques. Three of 23 retained stones were knowingly left behind. Choledochoscopy was done in 144 patients, including 43 with negative exploration and cholangiography. Additional stones were found in 34 cases (24%), including 3 of 43 cases in which exploration had been negative. Retained stones occurred in 6 patients undergoing choledochoscopy; all of them had had a positive exploration. Intraoperative postexploration T-tube cholangiograms failed to identify missed stones. Additional operative procedures effectively prevented further difficulties with retained stones. Choledochoscopy added little to the operating time. No common duct injuries resulted from the procedure. Four patients required reoperation for retained stones, and 1 of them died shortly after the second operation.

Choledochoscopy can help reduce the number of retained stones if the biliary tree is systematically examined and the instrument is passed into the duodenum. Fiberoptic instruments have not been shown to be superior to the rigid choledochoscope. Endoscopy may aid the removal of difficult stones, and unsuspected bile duct tumors may be discovered and undergo biopsy. Bile duct strictures can be inspected and undergo biopsy.

▶ [Routine choledochoscopy during bile duct exploration is a reasonable consideration because it then prepares the operator or resident to use the modality under those circumstances when the yield is significant. The rigid choledochoscope continues to be the one most frequently used, but there is an increasing satisfaction re-

---

(25–7) Ann. Surg. 194:76–79, July 1981.

ported for the new generation of flexible choledochoscopes. Bauer and associates (*Ann. Surg.* 194:161–166, 1981) recently reported an experience with a flexible fiberoptic endoscope in 52 patients. The modern instruments are designed to accommodate a wide variety of accessory equipment, including balloon-tipped catheters, basketing forceps, and stone-grabbing and biopsy forceps. It is of interest to note that the earliest report of choledochoscopy was in 1923 by Bakes, who used a rigid instrument.—S.I.S.] ◀

25–8 **Retained Biliary Tract Stones: Nonsurgical Treatment With Capmul 8210, a New Cholesterol Gallstone Dissolution Agent.** Retained common duct stones are found in 2% to 6% of patients after cholecystectomy. Mechanical extraction is not possible in some cases. Capmul 8210, consisting mainly of glyceryl 1-mono-octanoate, is a good cholesterol solvent in vitro and is quite safe in primates. Eberhard Mack, Emmons P. Patzer, Andrew B. Crummy, Alan F. Hofmann, and Vigen K. Babayan evaluated Capmul 8210 in 20 patients

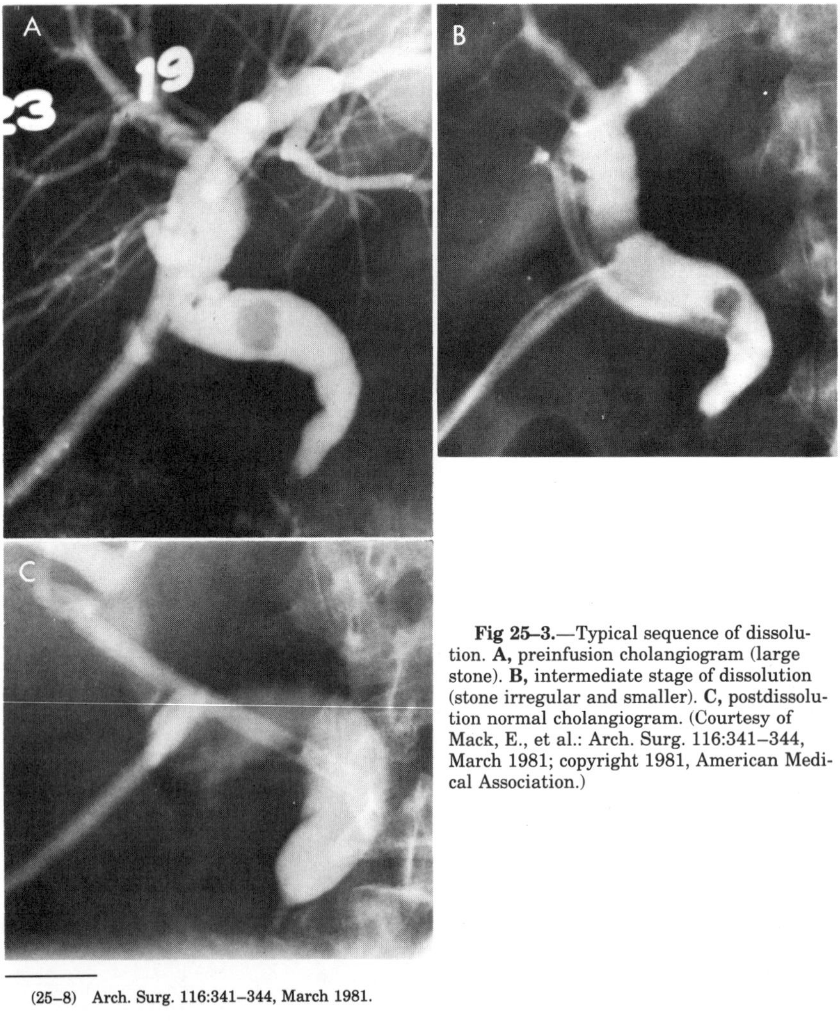

Fig 25–3.—Typical sequence of dissolution. **A,** preinfusion cholangiogram (large stone). **B,** intermediate stage of dissolution (stone irregular and smaller). **C,** postdissolution normal cholangiogram. (Courtesy of Mack, E., et al.: Arch. Surg. 116:341–344, March 1981; copyright 1981, American Medical Association.)

(25–8) Arch. Surg. 116:341–344, March 1981.

having a total of 43 retained common duct stones. Eight patients had more than 1 stone present. Therapy was begun a month or more after common duct exploration. An infusion catheter was passed through the T-tube tract to the common duct, and Capmul 8210 was infused at an average rate of 4 ml/hour. In 5 patients, residual stones subsequently were extracted using a Dormia basket.

A single retained common duct stone dissolved completely in 10 of 12 cases (Fig 25–3). Complete dissolution also was obtained in 3 patients with 3 stones each and in 1 patient with 4 stones. A total of 79% of stones were dissolved with Capmul 8210 therapy. Seven of the 9 stones not completely dissolved were removed or crushed with a basket. The mean duration of therapy for complete single-stone dissolution was 4 days. The infusions were reasonably well tolerated. About half of the patients showed a transient rise in serum glutamic oxaloacetic transaminase and alkaline phosphatase levels. Amylase levels showed a tendency to decline.

Capmul 8210 infusion appears to be useful for the treatment of postoperative choledocholithiasis. Further trials under well-controlled conditions with this or similar solvents are needed. Studies of means of dissolving gallstones within the gallbladder itself are in progress and may lead to a purely endoscopic approach to the treatment of gallbladder stones with Capmul 8210 in selected patients.

▶ [Capmul 8210 has proved to be a significant addition to the surgeon's armamentarium. The particular advantage over sodium cholate relates to a more potent solvent effect coupled with fewer side effects. Gadacz (*J. Surg. Res.* 26:378–380, 1979) reported success with this technique. We have had experience in 3 patients in whom Capmul was passed into the hepatic duct proximal to a point of stenosis and dissolution of the stones with the small hepatic ducts was effective within 4 to 6 days.—S.I.S.] ◀

25–9 **Gallstone Pancreatitis: Biliary Tract Pathology in Relation to Time of Operation.** The precise mechanism of nonalcoholic acute pancreatitis remains unclear, since an impacted gallstone is seldom found within 1–2 days of the onset, and pancreatic inflammation may continue and even become worse after passage of a stone. H. Harlan Stone, Timothy C. Fabian, and William E. Dunlop (Univ. of Tennessee) performed biliary tract exploration in 36 patients within 73 hours of admission and in 29 others 3 months after remission was induced nonoperatively. Cholecystectomy, transduodenal sphincteroplasty, and pancreatic duct septotomy were performed, and major bile ducts were cleared of stones by passing a Fogarty catheter up the sphincteroplasty. All patients received cefamandole intravenously. The average age was 59 years. Most patients were obese. Forty-three patients had a history consistent with a previous attack of pancreatitis. The initial serum amylase level averaged 1,158 units.

Common duct stones were found in two thirds of operative cholangiograms at early surgery but in only 18% of those obtained during delayed surgery. Common duct stones were retrieved in 75% and 28% of the groups, respectively. In 31% of the early surgery group, gallstones were found free within the duodenum, usually in the third or

(25–9) Ann. Surg. 194:305–312, September 1981.

fourth portion. Acute cholecystitis was present in 31% of the early surgery group and in 3% of patients operated on later. Ampullary, terminal common duct, and/or duodenal inflammation was much more frequent in the early surgery group. A sudden gush of clear pancreatic juice nearly always issued from the dilated or cut ampulla at early surgery, but this was infrequent at later operation. No patient became worse after early surgery. No patient had recurrent pancreatitis on an average follow-up of 14.3 months. Mortality and morbidity were comparable in the 2 groups. The overall mortality was 5%. Total hospitalization times and costs were greater in the delayed surgery group.

Early surgery for gallstone pancreatitis appears to be as safe as delayed surgery, and results in savings of both time and money. The pancreatitis appears to be caused by ampullary edema, with or without gallstone impaction, and early transduodenal sphincteroplasty can obviate the need for a second hospital admission.

▶ [The argument as to whether one should perform early operative intervention in patients with this disorder continues to rage. Osborne and associates (*Br. J. Surg.* 68:758–761, 1981) reviewed the clinical course of 47 patients with gallstone-associated acute pancreatitis who had surgery during the same admission. In 37 patients, the signs and symptoms of pancreatitis settled down under conservative management, and then biliary tract surgery was performed safely without mortality. By contrast, when the operation was carried out as an urgent affair, the mortality was 50%. Ranson (*Ann. Surg.* 189:654, 1979) provided guidelines contributing to the selection of a therapeutic regimen. There was no relationship between prognosis and the initial serum amylase level, and in most instances a conservative approach is justified. I would also agree with the comment made by Moody in the discussion of the present paper that an operation on the papilla is not mandated in all these patients. Cholecystectomy and operative cholangiography can be carried out, and, if the cholangiogram is normal, one does not have to perform a papillotomy, which is certainly associated with increased morbidity.—S.I.S.] ◀

25–10 **The Role of Chiba-Needle Cholangiography in the Diagnosis of Possible Acute Pancreatitis With Cholelithiasis.** Many patients with acute abdominal pain associated with gallstones and elevated serum amylase levels have no gross evidence of pancreatitis at early surgery, and morbidity and mortality are increased if intra-abdominal surgery is done early in the acute stage of illness. Gene F. Coppa, Richard LeFleur, and John H. C. Ranson (New York Univ. Med. Center, New York) have attempted to follow a course of initial nonoperative management in patients suspected of having acute gallstone pancreatitis. Percutaneous transhepatic cholangiography was performed using the Chiba needle in 14 such patients. Nine had a final diagnosis of acute pancreatitis, and 5 had a diagnosis of acute biliary disease.

The biliary ducts were opacified in all cases. The cholangiographic findings are presented in the table. All patients showed free emptying of the common bile duct into the duodenum, and all who had not had cholecystectomy exhibited patency of the cystic duct. Five patients had findings suggestive of acute pancreatitis. Abdominal surgery was deferred in 8 of the 9 patients with acute pancreatitis and was avoided

(25–10) Ann. Surg. 193:393–398, April 1981.

RADIOGRAPHIC FINDINGS OF CHIBA-NEEDLE CHOLANGIOGRAPHY IN PATIENTS WITH ACUTE PANCREATITIS OR ACUTE BILIARY DISEASE

	Calculi		Obstruction		
	Gall-bladder	Common Bile Duct	Cystic Duct	Common Bile Duct	Pan-creatitis
Acute pancreatitis (Group A)					
Patient					
1	+	–	–	–	+
2	+	–	–	–	–
3	+	+	–	–	+
4	*	–	*	–	+
5	–	–	–	–	–
6	+	–	–	–	–
7	+	–	–	–	+
8	–	–	–	–	–
9	–	–	–	–	+
Acute biliary disease (Group B)					
Patient					
1	+	+	–	–	–
2	–	–	–	–	–
3	+	+	–	–	–
4	*	+	*	–	–
5	+	+	–	–	–

*Previous cholecystectomy.

in 1 patient who did not have stone disease. The patients with acute biliary disease had definitive surgery 3–13 days after cholangiography. Small stones were not detected in 1 patient with acute biliary disease. The one complication of transhepatic puncture was a subphrenic hematoma, which was evacuated at the time of cholecystectomy and common duct exploration.

Most patients with either acute gallstone pancreatitis or acute biliary disease and hyperamylasemia respond well to early nonoperative management. Where early laparotomy may be considered necessary to diagnose or treat possible life-threatening biliary disease but is considered undesirable because of possible acute pancreatitis, percutaneous transhepatic Chiba-needle cholangiography is useful for determining the anatomical status of the biliary tree. The usefulness of ^{99m}Tc-HIDA scanning in acute pancreatitis is unclear, but scanning does not provide absolutely reliable information on the status of the common bile duct.

▶ [It is my opinion that ultrasound and either HIDA or PIPDA scan should be carried out first because they are noninvasive and a successful definition of the common duct can be achieved. Certainly, Chiba needle cholangiography provides a definition of the biliary tree, and this may be required in some of these patients. In patients with significant jaundice and evidence of calculi within the common duct, we feel that despite the elevation of the amylase level, early intervention should be carried out. We have noted that many of these patients show no evidence of pancreatitis at operation (Adams et al.: *Surgery* 63:877–884, 1968).—S.I.S.] ◀

25–11 **Late Result of Sphincteroplasty in the Treatment of Primary Cholangitis.** Tat K. Choi, John Wong, Kam H. Lam, Thuan K. Lim, and Guan B. Ong (Univ. of Hong Kong) reviewed data on 342 patients with primary cholangitis who underwent sphincteroplasty in 1964–1977. The peak incidence was in the fifth and sixth decade of life. Surgery was done on an emergency basis in 31 cases. Eighty-four patients had previously had emergency drainage procedures for acute primary cholangitis. The indication for sphincteroplasty was an impacted lower common duct stone in 122 cases; a thickened, rigid common duct dilated up to the sphincter of Oddi in 97; periampullary stricture in 75; and pancreatitis in 48. After incising the sphincter of Oddi, the edges of the common bile duct and posterior duodenal wall were anastomosed, stones were removed, and the ductal system was irrigated.

The operative mortality was 4.7%; it was 12.9% in emergency cases. Of 271 patients followed up for an average of 7½ years, 83.4% were asymptomatic following discharge, and another 8.5% had a fair result. Seventeen patients were operated on for cholangitis; 2 others refused surgery. Recurrent stones or mud were found in 8 of these cases. Four patients had a sphincteroplasty stricture, and did well after being converted to a choledochojejunostomy. Two patients had a liver abscess, and 2 had empyema of the gallbladder. Most of the patients requiring reoperation had enteric bacteria cultured from the bile.

The most common indication for sphincteroplasty in this series was the presence of impacted stones at the lower end of the common duct that could not be removed from above. Periampullary stricture and a rigidly dilated common duct were other indications. Sphincteroplasty is an effective and safe means of treating primary cholangitis where specific indications exist. Many failures of sphincteroplasty can be managed successfully by appropriate corrective procedures.

▶ [The literature from the Orient provides much meaningful data on this disorder because that region experiences such a high incidence. In considering the treatment of refractory primary common bile duct stone disease, Braasch and associates (*Am. J. Surg.* 139:526, 1980) report that best results were achieved in those patients who underwent lithotomy plus end-to-side or side-to-side anastomosis between the duct and the duodenum or jejunum. Endoscopic papillotomy has added a new dimension to the therapy for this disease. Saharia et al. (*Am. Surg.* 177:185, 1978) reported that a properly performed papillotomy will permit the duct to evacuate itself of stones over a long period of time.—S.I.S.] ◀

25–12 **Choledochoduodenostomy, Choledochojejunostomy or Sphincteroplasty for Biliary and Pancreatic Disease.** David P. Vogt and Robert E. Hermann (Cleveland Clinic) reviewed the results of these procedures in 153 patients operated on in 1962–1979, 147 of whom were available for follow-up. Choledochoduodenostomy was performed in 91 patients with a mean age of 60 years. The indications included bile duct obstruction by unresectable cancer, bile duct stricture, biliary fistula, recurrent bile duct stones, stenosis of the sphincter of Oddi,

(25–11) Arch. Surg. 116:1173–1175, September 1981.
(25–12) Ann. Surg. 193:161–168, February 1981.

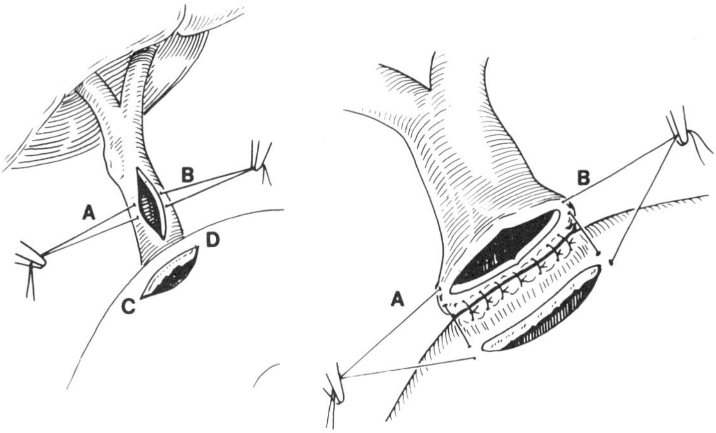

Fig 25–4.—Incisions are placed longitudinally in the bile duct and duodenum, and a two-layered anastomosis is constructed. (Courtesy of Vogt, D.P., and Hermann, R.E.: Ann. Surg. 193:161–168, February 1981.)

and choledochal cyst. The operative approach is illustrated in Figure 25–4. Choledochojejunostomy using a Roux-en-Y loop was performed in 25 patients with a mean age of 54 years, for biliary obstruction of benign or malignant nature. Sphincteroplasty was performed in 37 patients with a mean age of 50 years for pancreatitis, recurrent or impacted bile duct stones, or choledochal cyst.

Good results were obtained in 84% of the patients, fair results in 10%, and poor results in 3%. The mean follow-up time was 8 years. Four patients died postoperatively, all after choledochoduodenostomy for malignant bile duct obstruction. All patients with recurrent bile duct stones had good results from choledochoduodenostomy. Cholangitis followed this operation in 4 patients. Two patients required revision for recurrent stricture. All patients had significant palliation after choledochojejunostomy. None of 10 patients having sphincteroplasty for bile duct stones had further stones during follow-up. No postoperative pancreatitis was observed.

Choledochoduodenostomy appears to be a safe and effective procedure. Choledochojejunostomy and sphincteroplasty are also effective in the management of patients with difficult or recurrent biliary and pancreatic problems. These operations complement one another. Choledochoduodenostomy has been preferred for most patients with bile duct obstruction. Choledochojejunostomy is performed where the duodenum is scarred or obstructed, or cannot be mobilized for a safe anastomosis. It is preferred for difficult or recurrent bile duct structures. Sphincteroplasty is preferred for sphincter stenosis and impacted bile duct stones.

▶ [The two procedures should not represent competitive operations, but each should have specific indications. Choledochoduodenostomy should be performed only in the face of a dilated duct. The large series by Degensheim (*Surgery* 76:319, 1974) provides testimony to the efficacy of the procedure and to the low incidence of complications. I would agree that sphincteroplasty is preferred for sphincteric stenosis and for stones impacted in that region and also in patients who have a history that raises the question of pancreatitis, so that, if necessary, the pancreatic duct can be explored at the same time.—S.I.S.] ◀

25–13 **Biliary Tract Surgery and Cirrhosis: A Critical Combination.** Seymour I. Schwartz (Univ. of Rochester) reviewed the records of 33 cirrhotic patients who underwent cholecystectomy or surgery for bile duct obstruction in 1965–1980. Twenty-one had cholecystectomy, 7 underwent cholecystectomy during a shunt procedure, and 5 had surgery on the common bile duct. Review also was made of data on 100 noncirrhotic patients who had cholecystectomy during the same period; 50 cirrhotic patients who had shunt surgery for bleeding varices; and 25 noncirrhotic patients who had common duct surgery.

Nine of the 21 study patients having cholecystectomy for gallbladder disease had an uncomplicated course, but 12 others had excessive bleeding of more than 1,500 ml. Seven of these patients required 3–4 units of blood and 5 required more than 4 units. Only 2 of 100 noncirrhotic patients having cholecystectomy received transfusions. Cholecystectomy did not add significantly to transfusion requirements in 6 of the 7 study patients having portacaval decompression, even when the coagulation time was prolonged or platelet counts were reduced. All 5 cirrhotic patients having biliary tract surgery bled massively and died within 2 weeks of surgery. Four of these patients had biliary cirrhosis, and 1 had alcoholic cirrhosis. The 25 noncirrhotic control patients had a mean blood requirement of 500 ml.

Surgical preparations regarding bleeding for cirrhotic patients undergoing cholecystectomy are even more important in those having reconstructive surgery on the common bile duct, especially in the face of secondary biliary cirrhosis and hepatic dysfunction. Increased bleeding should be anticipated in these patients if surgery is necessary. Extensive intrahepatic dissection should be avoided. Intraoperative infusion of vasopressin and an antifibrinolytic agent may be considered. Both a beef pancreas extract that blocks fibrinolysis and ε-aminocaproic acid have been used in this setting.

▶ [As pointed out in the text of this article, the work had its genesis in several conversations reflecting experiences with surgeons throughout the United States that emphasized the problem. It is of interest that we were unable to uncover a single article specifically dealing with the subject. As pointed out by Folk in the discussion, parallel experience has been reviewed at the Veterans Administration Hospital, Hines, Illinois, and an 88% mortality was noted in the group of patients with prothrombin time values that were not correctable.—S.I.S.] ◀

25–14 **Biliary Carcinoma Associated With Methyldopa Therapy.** Biliary carcinoma has a poor prognosis, and it appears to be increasing in frequency in Sweden. Lowenfels suggested that the bile acids, under the influence of *Clostridia* organisms, are degraded to form carcinogenic substances, indicating that bacterial overgrowth might be related to this carcinoma. A possible association with oral contraception and with isoniazid has been described. G. Brodén and L. Bengtsson (Stockholm) reviewed data on 82 patients seen in 1968 to 1976 with

(25–13) Surgery 90:577–583, October 1981.
(25–14) Acta Chir. Scand. [Suppl.] 500:7–12, 1980.

biliary carcinoma other than gallbladder carcinoma. Sixty-one had extrahepatic carcinoma and 21, intrahepatic carcinoma. Medication also was assessed in 58 age- and sex-matched control subjects.

The incidence of gallstones was not higher than expected, but 18% of cases were associated with use of a drug having a known potential for causing liver toxicity, compared with 1.7% of the control group. All levels of methyldopa consumption were associated with an excess risk of biliary carcinoma. Methyldopa was associated with 8 cases of biliary carcinoma, chlorpropamide with 3, and oral contraceptives, indomethacin, hydrochlorothiazide, and chenodeoxycholic acid with 1 case each.

A causal connection between methyldopa and biliary carcinoma appears probable from these findings. Methyldopa is an extensively used antihypertensive drug that has a limited enterohepatic circulation. Adverse effects of the drug may have an immunologic basis, but the histologic findings suggest a toxic reaction. Only a minority of treated patients have adverse effects, indicating that an inborn metabolic error converting methyldopa to toxic substances may exist. Electrophilic reactive molecules may be related to both nonspecific toxic effects and, through an unknown factor, specific effects such as carcinogenicity. None of the present patients had a history of methyldopa hepatitis. Further studies of a possible association between methyldopa and biliary carcinoma are necessary.

▶ [The number of serious side effects produced by the panoply of drugs currently available for the treatment of medical conditions is staggering, and it is very likely that we do not yet appreciate their magnitude. Methyldopa is a very commonly used antihypertensive drug that is very well known to cause serious hepatotoxicity, including cholestatic jaundice, acute massive necrosis, chronic active hepatitis, and cirrhosis. All surgeons who see patients with biliary tract disease should be aware of these side effects, and, more importantly, we must document a careful drug history in our patients who have biliary ductal carcinoma.—W.S.] ◀

5–15 **Carcinoma of the Gallbladder.** Jarley Koo, John Wong, Frank C. Y. Cheng, and G. B. Ong (Univ. of Hong Kong) reviewed data on 100 patients seen in 1960–1979 with carcinoma of the gallbladder. The 59 female and 41 male patients had a median age of 68 years. Most patients were seen with advanced disease. Pain was the most common feature, followed by an abdominal mass and jaundice. Anorexia and weight loss were significant in half of the cases. The mean duration of symptoms was 4.6 months. Thirty-five patients presented with obstructive jaundice, and 33 had right hypochondrial inflammatory complications, usually empyema of the gallbladder. The results of various studies are presented in Table 1.

Cholecystectomy, with or without common duct exploration, was done in 36 cases, and in 20 cases was considered to be curative. Six patients had radical en bloc resection. Biliary-enteric bypass surgery was done in 26 cases; external drainage was used in 12 cases. In only 20 cases was gross tumor involvement outside the gallbladder not noted at operation, and microscopic extension was found in 6 of these cases. Biliary tract stones were present in 34 cases, usually in the

(25–15) Br. J. Surg. 68:161–165, March 1981.

TABLE 1.—INVESTIGATIVE PROCEDURES AND RESULTS

Procedures	No. of patients	Results
Oral cholecystography and intravenous cholangiography	18	10 non-functioning 3 gallstones 3 primary cholangitis 1 extrahepatic biliary stone 1 non-filling of body and fundus
Percutaneous transhepatic cholangiography and endoscopic retrograde cholangiopancreatography	15	All extrahepatic biliary obstruction
Radioisotope liver scan	20	7 space-occupying lesions 6 exaggerated gallbladder impression 7 normal
Peritoneoscopy	19	11 hepatic tumour 5 carcinoma of gallbladder 1 normal 2 carcinoma of pancreas
Hepatic and coeliac angiography	11	9 tumour neovascularity 5 hepatic tumour 2 retroperitoneal tumour 2 gallbladder tumour 2 normal
Ultrasonography	3	All non-diagnostic

TABLE 2.—SURGICAL PROCEDURES AND SURVIVAL

	No. of patients	Median survival (range)
No operation	16	4 wk (10 d–3 mth)
Biopsy only	14	4 wk (1 d–9 mth)
Radical resection	6	2 wk (1 d–1 mth)
Hepatic artery ligation	2	5 wk (4 wk–6 wk)
Internal drainage (+cholecystectomy in 6)	14	8 wk (2 d–8 mth)
External drainage	12	3 wk (2 d–2 mth)
Cholecystectomy		
Palliative	16	8 wk (3 wk–10 mth)
Curative	20 (7*)	1 yr (1 mth–2·5 yr)
Total	100	

*Still alive and excluded from calculation.

gallbladder. Seven of the 99 patients followed up were alive. All had had "curative" cholecystectomy. Survival is related to the various surgical procedures in Table 2. Internal biliary drainage gave better palliation than external drainage in patients with obstructive jaundice. Seven patients had substantial relief of jaundice and lived for 2 to 8 months.

Survival in this series is similar to that in other reported series of patients with gallbladder carcinoma. Radical surgery has given uniformly poor results. Cure by cholecystectomy can be expected only when carcinoma in situ or a small mucosal lesion is found incidentally at operation. Where gross tumor extension beyond the gallbladder is present, radical surgery is associated with very high hospital mortality. Biliary-enteric bypass, preferably by the internal route, is worthwhile in patients presenting with obstructive jaundice.

▶ [The results with this lesion continue to be miserable, and a 5-year cure represents a rarity. If a carcinoma is found incidentally at the time of cholecystectomy and it is located on the peritonealized surface away from the gallbladder, cholecystectomy alone should be sufficient. If the lesion is located in juxtaposition to the hepatic bed, a segment of the adjacent liver should be removed, but a radical hepatic resection is not called for because the cure rates are essentially negligible. Evander and Ihse (*Br. J. Surg.* 68:158–160, 1981) reviewed the records of 44 consecutive patients with carcinoma of the gallbladder. In 10, resection of the tumor was carried out; all microscopic tumor was excised in 6 patients and a liver resection was carried out in 4. Median survival was 4 months, and the authors concluded that radical surgery by itself did not confer any advantage. A case should be made for opening the gallbladder routinely at the operating table in order to define the presence or absence of a tumor and its location, in view of different management regimens for patients with tumor of the gallbladder. Cures will occur in patients who have a small tumor found incidentally at operation.—S.I.S.] ◀

25–16 **Prognostic Factors in Bile Duct Carcinoma: Analysis of 96 Cases.** Ronald K. Tompkins, David Thomas, Alan Wile, and William P. Longmire, Jr. (Univ. of California, Los Angeles) undertook a computerized analysis of prognostic variables in 96 proved cases of extrahepatic bile duct carcinoma treated in 1954–1978. All patients but 1 underwent surgery. The average age at the time of definitive surgery was 59.9 years. The male-female ratio was 1.6:1. Most lesions were in the upper third or confluence of the right and left hepatic ducts and common hepatic duct. Seven patients had diffuse lesions or multicentric extensive ductal involvement. The average postoperative follow-up was 23.3 months. Patients were operated on an average of about 5 months after the onset of symptoms, which were chiefly jaundice and pain. The mean total serum bilirubin level at presentation was 18 mg/dl. Transjugular and transhepatic cholangiography were more accurate in diagnosing these cases than either ultrasonography or endoscopic retrograde cholangiopancreatography.

A total of 171 operations were performed in 95 patients. The operative mortality was 12%; it was similar for resectional and palliative procedures. Cumulative survival was 50% at 9 months after definitive surgery and 8% at 5 years. Patients with lower-third lesions had the best 5-year survival (28%). Survival is related to the type of operation done in Figure 25–5. No significant effect on survival was seen in the 30 patients given treatment of some type after operation. Location of the lesions appeared to be the factor most responsible for differences in survival rates. Lower-third lesions were more often resectable than the others, and more of them were papillary tumors or well-differentiated lesions.

Patients with bile duct malignancy of the lower third of the ducts that can be resected by a Whipple procedure have the best outcome,

---

(25–16) Ann. Surg. 194:447–457, October 1981.

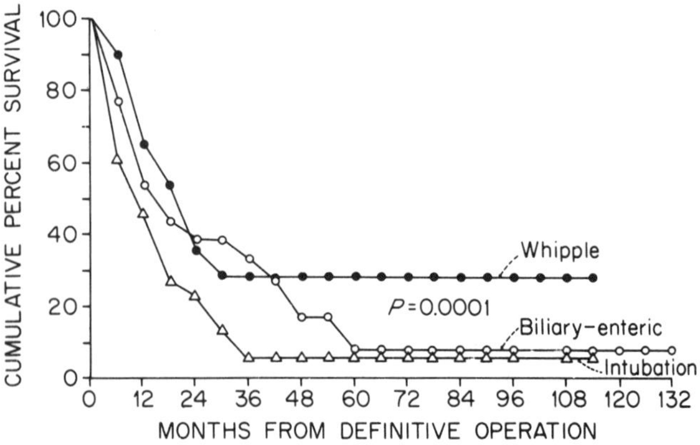

Fig 25–5.—Postoperative survival curves according to type of operation performed. When Whipple's procedure could be done for middle- or lower-third lesions, survival was significantly better. (Courtesy of Tompkins, R.K., et al.: Ann. Surg. 194:447–457, October 1981.)

especially when a papillary type of lesion is present and the patient is seen within 3 months of the onset of symptoms. Resection is indicated, if at all possible. Further studies of newer chemotherapeutic agents and radiotherapy are needed in patients who cannot undergo curative resection.

▶ [Our own experience, as reported by Rodgers et al. (*Surgery* 90:596, 1981), is quite similar. The best prognosis was achieved with pancreaticoduodenectomy for lesions of the lower third of the duct, including the ampulla. There was general dissatisfaction with lesions of the upper third, i.e., Klatskin lesions, and the authors' figure of 0% survival at 5 years is in keeping with the reported literature. Forty-six percent of our patients with this lesion had lymph node or liver metastasis at the time of the operation. Presently, we have embarked on a study of combining transhepatic drainage with adjunctive radiation for these lesions that are usually not resectable and rarely curable by surgical extirpation. A similar approach has been adopted by a group at the Cleveland Clinic (Lees et al.: *Surg. Gynecol. Obstet.* 151:913–198, 1980).—S.I.S.] ◀

25–17 **Carcinoma of the Hepatic Duct Junction** is an uncommon but well-recognized cause of jaundice. It often goes undetected. Phyllis A. George, Colin Brown, and Robert T. E. Foley (London) reviewed 54 cases of hepatic duct carcinoma seen in 15 years. The 28 women and 26 men were aged 33 to 78 years. Increasing jaundice was the usual presenting feature. Pain was a major symptom in 17 cases, and in 6 it preceded jaundice. Percutaneous cholangiography was done in 43 cases. Thirty-nine patients had been explored previously without the correct diagnosis being made. Three patients died before operation. Patients were explored an average of 4½ months after onset of jaundice. Three patients had radical and 42 had palliative operations. In most of the latter a tube was placed in the left hepatic duct.

The mean bilirubin concentration was 277 μmole/L, and the mean alkaline phosphatase value was 624 IU/L. Liver scans showed nonspecific changes of extrahepatic obstruction. Percutaneous cholangiography typically showed widely dilated intrahepatic ducts with a

(25–17) Br. J. Surg. 68:14–18, January 1981.

block in the region of the porta hepatis. Both scirrhous mucus-secreting tumors and papillary or simple mucus-secreting tumors were observed. One of 3 patients was well for 4 months after tumor resection before being lost to follow-up. Jaundice was relieved in most patients treated palliatively. There were 3 postoperative deaths. Eighteen patients died 1 month to 3 years after operation, whereas 7 are alive 3 months to 12 years postoperatively.

The diagnosis of cancer of the hepatic duct junction should be improved by ultrasound and computed tomography. All patients operated on for unexplained jaundice should have operative cholangiography. Palliative measures appear to be indicated, since only a few of these tumors are resectable, and radical resection has not resulted in longer survival times. The role of radiotherapy in the management of these tumors remains to be established.

▶ [This lesion, also known by the eponymic term "Klatskin," is one of the most difficult to treat. This tumor has received attention somewhat out of proportion to its frequency because of the general need for palliation, the poor prognosis despite small tumor size, and a recently more aggressive attitude toward resection. In a recent review by Rodgers et al. (*Surgery* 90:596–601, 1981) of 23 cases, all patients were jaundiced and the diagnosis was best achieved by percutaneous transhepatic cholangiogram. Resection rarely was carried out, and the patients with resection died within 2 years. There were no 5-year survivals. As early as 1965, Quattlebaum and Quattlebaum (*Ann. Surg.* 161:876–889, 1975) championed an aggressive approach. We would certainly agree that surgical management may become increasingly conservative, and with the advent of radiographic improvement, we are presently managing a group of patients in whom an internal stent was passed via the percutaneous transhepatic route with administration of supplementary radiotherapy and chemotherapy. Although the tube frequently requires changing, with the use of radiographic control this has not been a problem, and we have several patients who have survived longer than 6 months.—S.I.S.] ◀

25–18 **Cholangitis due to Malignant Obstruction of Biliary Outflow.** M. J. O'Connor, M. L. Schwartz, D. G. McQuarrie, and H. W. Sumner (Minneapolis) reviewed the findings in 21 patients with malignant obstruction of the biliary tree, among 65 seen in 1957–1980 with cholangitis. Fourteen patients had no history of previous biliary disease or operative manipulation of the biliary tree. Fourteen had carcinoma of the head of the pancreas, 4 had common bile duct carcinoma, and 3 had carcinoma of the hepatic ducts. Cholangitis was present in 12.7% of all patients seen in the 23-year period with carcinomatous obstruction of biliary outflow.

Eleven patients presented with clinical features of cholangitis. Seven of 10 patients with a previous diagnosis of carcinoma had had operative manipulation of the biliary ductal system. All patients were men. The mean age at the time of cholangitis was 64.8 years. The mean peak serum bilirubin level during episodes of cholangitis was 12.8 mg/dl, and the peak serum glutamic oxaloacetic transaminase level was 83.1 IU/dl. Bile cultures were positive in 8 of the 21 patients; the most common organism was *Escherichia coli*. Thirteen patients had surgery to relieve biliary obstruction during episodes of cholangitis. Six of them had postoperative liver abscess, and 5 had recurrent cholangitis. Two patients had bile leakage postoperatively.

(25–18) Ann. Surg. 193:341–345, March 1981.

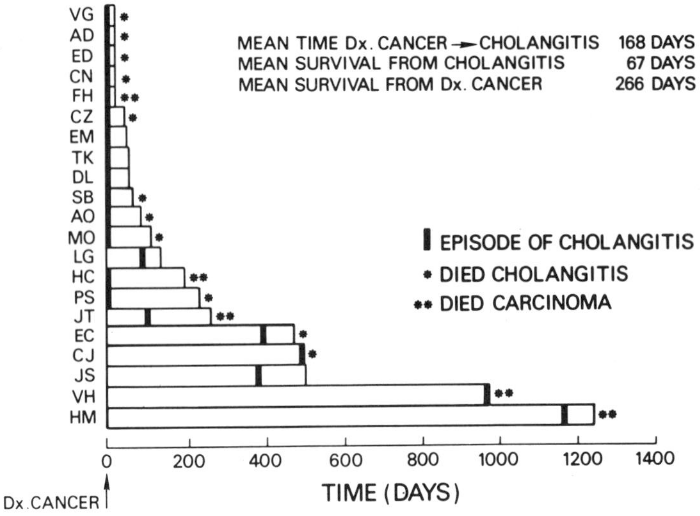

Fig 25–6.—Course from time of diagnosis of carcinoma to episode of cholangitis or death. (Courtesy of O'Connor, M.J., et al.: Ann. Surg. 193:341–345, March 1981.)

One had a wound infection. The course of the patients is shown in Figure 25–6. Fifteen of the 21 patients died during their first hospital admission. The chief cause of death was biliary sepsis, followed by carcinomatosis. The mean survival from the episode of cholangitis was 67 days.

Acute bacterial cholangitis occurs in association with pancreatic and extrahepatic biliary carcinoma and is highly lethal. More than half of the present patients who had some form of drainage recovered from cholangitis, and one-third were able to return home. Early operative treatment of cholangitis in patients with biliary malignancy may be worthwhile in terms of resolving cholangitis and prolonging life.

▶ [An early aggressive approach in these patients may well achieve some palliation, but will not necessarily alter the cure rate. An alternative approach in these poor-risk patients would be percutaneous transhepatic drainage coupled with antibiotics. This regimen satisfies the tenets of therapy; it deals with the stasis of obstruction and the treatment of the general sepsis. Because catheter drainage will be effected, roentgenographic demonstration of the diagnosis can be achieved via the percutaneous route, and cholangitis due to multiple calculi can be ruled out.—S.I.S.] ◀

25–19 **Preoperative Percutaneous Transhepatic Biliary Decompression Lowers Operative Morbidity in Patients With Obstructive Jaundice.** Excessive hyperbilirubinemia appears to be a risk factor for patients having surgery for benign and malignant causes of obstructive jaundice. Theoretically, percutaneous biliary decompression should reduce hyperbilirubinemia and decrease operative morbidity and mortality. David A. Denning, E. Christopher Ellison, and Larry C. Carey (Ohio State Univ.) examined the effects of preoperative biliary decompression in a series of 57 patients with obstructive

(25–19) Am. J. Surg. 141:61–65, January 1981.

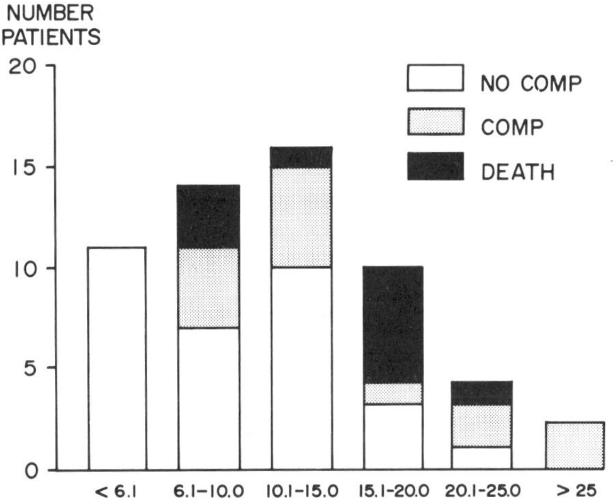

Fig 25–7.—Preoperative bilirubin level (milligrams per deciliter) in relation to complications and mortality. The number of complications increases as the preoperative bilirubin level increases. (Courtesy of Denning, D.A., et al.: Am. J. Surg. 141:61–65, January 1981.)

jaundice and a bilirubin level exceeding 5 mg/dl who were operated on in 1975–1979. Twenty-five patients had transhepatic drainage catheters placed preoperatively, whereas 32 underwent surgery without preoperative biliary decompression. All patients had obstructive jaundice. The average time of preoperative biliary drainage was 13 days.

Complications associated with the drainage catheter were minor. Operative morbidity and mortality in the two groups are compared in the table. All but 1 of the patients who died had malignancies. Sepsis was the chief postoperative complication. Significantly fewer patients having preoperative biliary decompression had complications, but there was no difference in operative mortality in the two groups. The preoperative bilirubin level was significantly lower in the patients having drainage, and alkaline phosphatase levels also were lower in this group. Operative morbidity and mortality increased with the preoperative serum bilirubin level (Fig 25–7).

Operative Morbidity and Mortality in Patients With and Without Preoperative Biliary Decompression (PBD)

	Drainage			No Drainage		
	No.	PBD	Death	No.	PBD	Death
Benign	3	0	0	6	4	1
Malignant	22	7	4	26	14	7
Curative resection	3	1	1	6	4	3
Palliation	14	6	3	15	7	3
Biopsy	5	0	0	5	3	1
Total	25	7	4	32	18	8

Percutaneous transhepatic biliary decompression appears to be the safest way of reducing hyperbilirubinemia preoperatively. Percutaneous transhepatic drainage catheters can be left in place for up to a year with minimal complications. At times, it is not possible to reduce the serum bilirubin level to below 6 mg/dl, but with adequate decompression, the bilirubin level will reach a plateau level. Warshaw questions the need for decompression unless the bilirubin level exceeds 20 mg/dl. Long-term catheterization of a duct that may be used for an anastomosis may be unwise.

▶ [The improvement in operative morbidity and mortality in patients with preoperative biliary decompression is quite convincing, but because there is essentially no change with bilirubin levels less than 6 mg/dl, it would seem that there is no point to decompress unless there is a profound elevation in the serum bilirubin level. Long-term catheter drainage also has the theoretic disadvantage of contaminating an area of subsequent anastomosis. The authors state that this will permit hepatic function to return to more normal states preoperatively. This however, is not defined, and the only statement that can be made is that it will decrease the levels of bilirubin and alkaline phosphatase. Their own data indicate that the transaminase level shows no significant difference in the drained and not-drained group.—S.I.S.] ◀

25–20 **Successful Long-Term Percutaneous Decompression of the Biliary Tract.** Percutaneous transhepatic biliary drainage is used most often for preoperative biliary decompression and relief from jaundice, but it also has been reported to be a satisfactory primary treatment for inoperable or poor-risk patients. Brian F. Smale, Ernest J. Ring, David B. Freiman, Juan A. Oleaga, Robert Reichman, James L. Mullen, and Ernest F. Rosato (Univ. of Pennsylvania) evaluated the efficacy of drainage for over 3 months in 35 patients seen between 1977 and 1979. Percutaneous transhepatic cholangiography was done before or at placement of the drainage catheter. External drainage was performed for at least 48 hours before being converted to internal drainage. Broad-spectrum antibiotic coverage was given all patients. Twenty-five patients had malignant and 10 had benign causes of obstruction.

Mean duration of percutaneous transhepatic biliary drainage was 9.3 months. In 2 patients the catheter could not be advanced through the obstruction, necessitating external drainage from the proximal intrahepatic duct system. The bilirubin and alkaline phosphatase concentrations fell markedly after successful institution of percutaneous drainage. All patients but 4 had a 50% or greater fall in serum bilirubin concentration. Few complications occurred, and no deaths were related directly to drainage or to the presence of the drainage catheter. Four patients had septic episodes that were managed successfully with antibiotics and catheter drainage, without untoward sequelae.

Percutaneous transhepatic biliary drainage appears to be a safe and effective means of decompressing the biliary tract for longer than 3 months, especially in poor operative risks and patients with metastatic or unresectable malignancy. The procedure provides access to the biliary tract for percutaneous dilation of common duct or anasto-

---

(25–20) Am. J. Surg. 141:73–76, January 1981.

motic strictures. The procedure may be used temporarily in debilitated patients being prepared for reconstructive biliary tract surgery.

▶ [Long-term decompression of the biliary tract, preferably by internal self-contained stents, is particularly applicable to patients with carcinoma of the hepatic duct confluence. This can be combined with radiation therapy as definitive treatment for patients with this lesion, because results of resection therapy leave much to be desired. These catheters have a tendency to plug, but can be changed readily under radiographic control. The radiographic techniques presently used are such that the old concepts of the U tube are no longer necessary. In managing benign strictures, surgical reconstruction is to be preferred if the patient can tolerate the procedure. In this circumstance, a mucosal-to-mucosal anastomosis that generally can be performed extrahepatically or a modified Hepp procedure with side-to-side anastomosis between the Roux-Y of jejunum and the left hepatic duct carried out extrahepatically may be done. As the authors point out, the tubes have a propensity to plug and to require frequent drainage. The other complication of hemobilia, although reported in approximately 15% of cases, rarely requires therapeutic intervention.—S.I.S.] ◀

5-21 **Ampullary Disconnection During the Course of Biliary and Duodenal Surgery.** The major pancreatic duct, distal common bile duct, or ampulla of Vater can be injured during any operation for ulcer or other disease of the proximal duodenum. Michael G. Florence, Michael J. Hart, and Thomas Taylor White reviewed 12 cases of injury or transplantation of the ampulla of Vater seen in the Seattle area in a 31-year period. Nine patients had a primary diagnosis of peptic ulcer disease, and 4 of them had had previous surgery that had failed to cure the ulcer. One of the ulcer patients and 1 of those without ulcer disease had duodenal diverticula. Other patients had a duodenal polyp and a duodenal hemangioma.

Most morbidity occurred within the first year after injury. Eight patients were doing well after 2–24 years. Four required a second operation. Two deaths were secondary to leakage and sepsis, 1 to acute pancreatitis, and 1 to chronic pancreatitis with depression and suicide. Only 2 of the 10 accidental injuries went unrecognized at the time of injury. All patients had some initial morbidity.

Analysis of 84 cases indicated that the usual cause of disconnection of the ampulla is dissection between the duodenum and pancreas at gastric resection for ulcer disease in the presence of severe scarring, shortening of the duodenum, or an abnormally located ampulla. Pa-

Fig 25–8.—We prefer this method of correction by duodenal advancement as advocated by Santy and Duroux. Heavy black lines in ducts represent polyvinyl drainage tubes. (Courtesy of Florence, M.G., et al.: Am. J. Surg. 142:100–105, July 1981.)

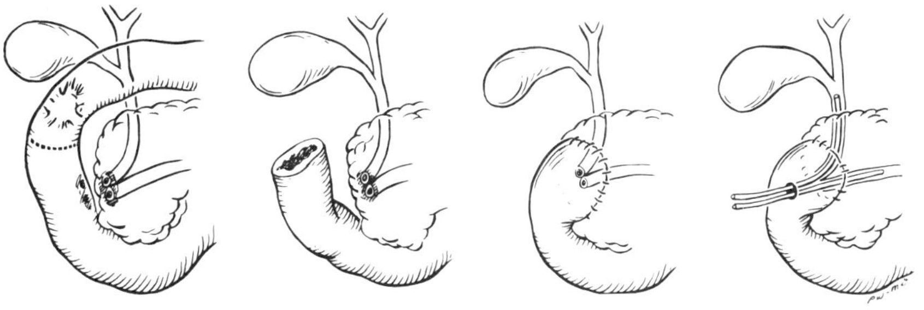

(25–21) Am. J. Surg. 142:100–105, July 1981.

surgeons talk about major portions of the pancreas having sloughed out, only for them to find that upon recovery of the patient, no pancreatic exocrine or endocrine insufficiency was evident. As Leger et al. pointed out, the process is often very extensive outside the pancreas at the same time that the necrotic process is very mild in the pancreas. The ability to assess this at operation is poor.—W.S.] ◀

26–2 **Chlorpromazine Treatment of Experimental Acute Fulminant Pancreatitis in Pigs.** Acute fulminant pancreatitis often is associated with fatal changes in remote organs, including the lungs. It has been suggested that phospholipase A_2, which is released mainly from the pancreas and is present in the serum in high levels in pancreatitis, is important in the development of respiratory distress, possibly through hydrolysis of the alveolar surfactant phospholipids with resultant alveolar collapse. T. Schröder, M. Lempinen, S. Nordling, and P. K. J. Kinnunen (Univ. of Helsinki) used a pig model to test the effect of chlorpromazine, a potent inhibitor of phospholipase A_2 in vitro, on the development of pulmonary dysfunction in association with pancreatitis. Pancreatitis was induced by injecting sodium taurocholate and trypsin into the pancreatic duct and giving secretin intravenously. Chlorpromazine was given intravenously 3 times daily for a week in a dose of 1.5 mg/kg of body weight. Hypovolemia was corrected with physiologic saline and a dextran solution.

Hemorrhagic pancreatitis developed within a few minutes of the induction procedure. Serum amylase levels increased after the first 5 hours and remained elevated in chlorpromazine-treated animals; serum lipase levels also remained high until the animals were killed. Serum phospholipase A_2 levels rose continuously in untreated pigs, but declined after 5 hours in treated animals. Untreated animals had a sharp fall in Po_2 after 3 hours. Blood glucose levels rose significantly in both groups, and serum calcium concentrations declined significantly. Mortality was significantly lower in the chlorpromazine-treated group. Pancreatic changes were less extensive and more chronic in treated animals that lived for more than 24 hours than in controls. Changes in the lungs also were less extensive in chlorpromazine-treated animals.

These findings support the view that phospholipase A_2 is an important pathophysiologic factor in acute pancreatitis. Chlorpromazine does not prevent the pancreatic process itself in this highly traumatic model of pancreatitis, but appears to have protective effects against certain severe systemic changes.

26–3 **Early Prediction of Severity of Acute Pancreatitis Using Peritoneal Lavage.** The severity of some attacks of acute pancreatitis, including eventually fatal ones, is unrecognized at the time of admission, and early intensive treatment probably would improve the outcome of such attacks. A simple, rapid means of diagnosing severe pancreatitis early in its course is needed. The Ranson approach may not yield a diagnosis until circulatory, renal, or respiratory failure has developed. Michael J. McMahon, Ian R. Pickford, and Michael J. Playforth (Leeds, England) evaluated diagnostic peritoneal lavage in

---

(26–2) Eur. Surg. Res. 13:143–151, 1981.
(26–3) Acta Chir. Scand. 146:171–175, 1980.

TABLE 1.—CHARACTERISTICS OF ASPIRATED FREE PERITONEAL FLUID AND LAVAGE RETURN FLUID IN 98 ATTACKS OF ACUTE PANCREATITIS*

Characteristics found during diagnostic lavage procedure		Severe attacks (n=21)	Mild attacks (n=68)
Free fluid volume	>10 ml	13	3
	<10 ml	8	65
Free fluid colour	Brown	8	1
Lavage fluid colour	mid-straw or darker	12	0
	clear to pale straw	9	68
Multiple criteria: (*a*) brown coloured free fluid	1 criterion only present	5	4
(*b*) >10 ml free fluid	At least 2 of the criteria present[a]	11	0
(*c*) mid-straw or darker lavage fluid	All 3 criteria present	7	0

*Figures refer to the number of attacks in the mild or severe categories displaying the features indicated.
[a]Three deaths and all patients who received therapeutic lavage were in this group.

168 consecutive attacks of acute pancreatitis seen in 1975 to 1979. Attacks considered severe resulted in over 2 weeks' hospitalization, complications such as renal or respiratory failure, or death. Diagnostic lavage was attempted in 96 attacks of acute pancreatitis and in 1 patient with suspected pancreatitis in whom the diagnosis was incorrect. The procedure utilized 1 L of warmed physiologic saline.

Lavage was successful in 93% of attempts. Most failures were due to the cannula not being correctly located in the peritoneal cavity. The 1 complication was penetration of the stomach where the stomach had not been emptied; no peritoneal contamination resulted. Lavage was done a mean of 7 hours after admission, but more recently

TABLE 2.—COMPARATIVE PERFORMANCE OF DIAGNOSTIC LAVAGE AND CLINICAL ASSESSMENT TO PREDICT SEVERITY IN ACUTE PANCREATITIS*

	Percentage predicted successfully by	
Attack	Lavage	Clinical assessment
Severe (n=21)	76	38
Mild (n=68)	94	100

*Lavage criteria of severity were more than 10 ml of free fluid, brown-colored free fluid, or straw-colored lavage fluid. Clinical assessment was carried out immediately before lavage by 1 of 3 investigators.

in the later cases. Characteristics of the aspirated peritoneal fluid and the lavage return are given in Table 1. Sixteen of 21 attacks considered severe by clinical criteria were recognized as such by lavage, on the basis of brown-colored free fluid, more than 10 ml of free fluid, or a straw-colored or darker lavage return fluid. None of the 5 other attacks involved shock or its sequelae. Only 4 attacks classed as mild exhibited any lavage criteria of severity; 3 were in patients with probable alcohol-associated pancreatitis. Lavage and clinical assessment are compared in Table 2.

Clinical assessment is unreliable in predicting severe acute pancreatitis. Diagnostic peritoneal lavage is the best means of selecting patients who may benefit from therapeutic lavage through the removal of noxious ascitic fluid.

▶ [The authors of this article seem to have delineated some characteristics of the peritoneal fluid in patients with pancreatitis that indicate the presence of a severe attack. Many investigators have attempted to define the severity of attacks in order to determine which patients should be subjected to vigorous management. To date, the most vigorous and acceptable management for these severe attacks has been the use of peritoneal lavage, but its efficacy has not yet been established unequivocally. Ranson and Spencer (*Ann. Surg.* 187:565, 1978) were unable to demonstrate an advantage in terms of mortality rate in the use of therapeutic peritoneal lavage, although Stone and co-workers, using a slightly different technique of peritoneal lavage, have indeed demonstrated an improvement in outcome (*Surg. Cynecol. Obstet.* 150:878, 1980). In view of the conflicting reports of the results of use of peritoneal lavage, we need further studies to establish or refute its efficacy. In any case, it would appear that the criteria identified by these investigators would suggest the use of lavage, because we have nothing better at present. It is not completely clear as to how the authors of this article selected the features of the peritoneal fluid that reflect a severe attack, except by retrospective analysis. There is no quarrel with that means of identification, if such criteria hold up as accurate predictive factors in other series. Certainly, the procedure of aspiration of peritoneal fluid advocated by these authors seems to be a safe one, and it would appear that further use of this technique is warranted.—W.S.] ◀

26–4 **Myocardial Function in Acute Pancreatitis.** A myocardial depressant factor found in circulatory shock has been demonstrated in experimental hemorrhagic pancreatitis and in patients with pancreatitis. Katsuki Ito, Gerhart Ramirez-Schon, Pravin M. Shah, Nanakram Agarwal, Louis R. M. Delguercio, and Benedict M. Reynolds (New York Med. College) assessed cardiopulmonary function in 15 patients with acute pancreatitis on 68 occasions. The patients, mean age 36.9 years, were resuscitated with intravenous fluids to maintain an adequate urine output. The mean serum amylase level was 1,529 IU. Ten patients had confirmed hemorrhagic pancreatitis, and in 2 of them abdominal abscesses subsequently developed. Sixty-one studies were done in nonseptic postoperative patients without cardiopulmonary disease and 113 in 41 cirrhotic patients without pancreatitis.

The cardiac index and arterial pressure were increased in the group with pancreatitis, but left ventricular stroke work was decreased. No significant differences in total peripheral resistance or arteriovenous

---

(26–4) Ann. Surg. 194:85–88, July 1981.

oxygen content were noted. Oxygen consumption was increased in the study group. Pulmonary vascular resistance was increased, but this could not be attributed to heart failure. Sarnoff curves showed myocardial depression in patients with pancreatitis in comparison with findings in controls and the hyperdynamic cirrhotic patients. The patients with pancreatitis increased their oxygen consumption along with the cardiac index, in contrast to findings in cirrhotic patients, whose hemodynamic impairment is at the capillary level rather than at the cardiac level.

Acute pancreatitis is accompanied by myocardial depression. The peripheral vasculature in these patients reacts as in healthy persons, in contrast to what occurs in cirrhotic patients, in whom the opening of arteriovenous shunts robs the tissues of a nutritive blood supply. The myocardial depression presumably is due to a myocardial depressant factor elaborated in the pancreas.

▶ [The results of this study done in human patients with acute pancreatitis confirms the experimental observations that a myocardial depressant factor is released in hemorrhagic pancreatitis. The cardiovascular dynamics found in these patients are quite different from the hyperdynamic state in cirrhotic individuals, and these authors make a strong case for the development of significant myocardial depression in pancreatitis as demonstrated by the ventricular function curves. This, of course, raises the question of cardiac support in patients with acute pancreatitis, an area to which we possibly have not paid sufficient attention and to which we will direct some efforts in the future.—W.S.] ◀

26–5 **A Study of Chronic Pancreatitis by Serial Endoscopic Pancreatography.** Atsuo Nagata, Tatsuji Homma, Kozo Tamai, Kazuya Ueno, Katsuhide Shimakura, Hisao Oguchi, Seiichi Furuta, and Masayuki Oda (Shinshu Univ., Matsumoto, Japan) obtained satisfactory serial endoscopic retrograde pancreatograms in 16 control patients with hepatobiliary disease who were not alcoholics and had no clinical signs of pancreatitis; 31 patients with chronic pancreatitis, which was related to alcoholism in 15 cases; and 32 patients with suspected chronic pancreatitis but not a definite diagnosis.

On a mean follow-up of 2.3 years, 2 of 16 control patients had simple dilatation of the main duct and 1 developed mild irregularity of the main duct wall at the tail of the pancreas. The serial findings in patients with chronic alcoholic pancreatitis, who were followed up for a mean of 2.4 years, are shown in Figure 26–1. Eleven of 12 patients with marked changes on initial study showed progressive changes in the main duct, usually dilatation, stenosis, or irregularity of the duct wall. Most patients who reduced their drinking or abstained showed progressive ductal changes. The serial findings in patients with chronic nonalcoholic pancreatitis, who were followed up for a mean of 3.6 years, are shown in Figure 26–2. Progressive changes in the main duct developed in only 3 patients in this group. Seven of the 32 patients with suspected chronic pancreatitis had progressive changes on serial endoscopic pancreatography. Definite chronic pancreatitis developed in 2 of 5 patients who were alcoholics. One had progressive

---

(26–5) Gastroenterology 81:884–891, November 1981.

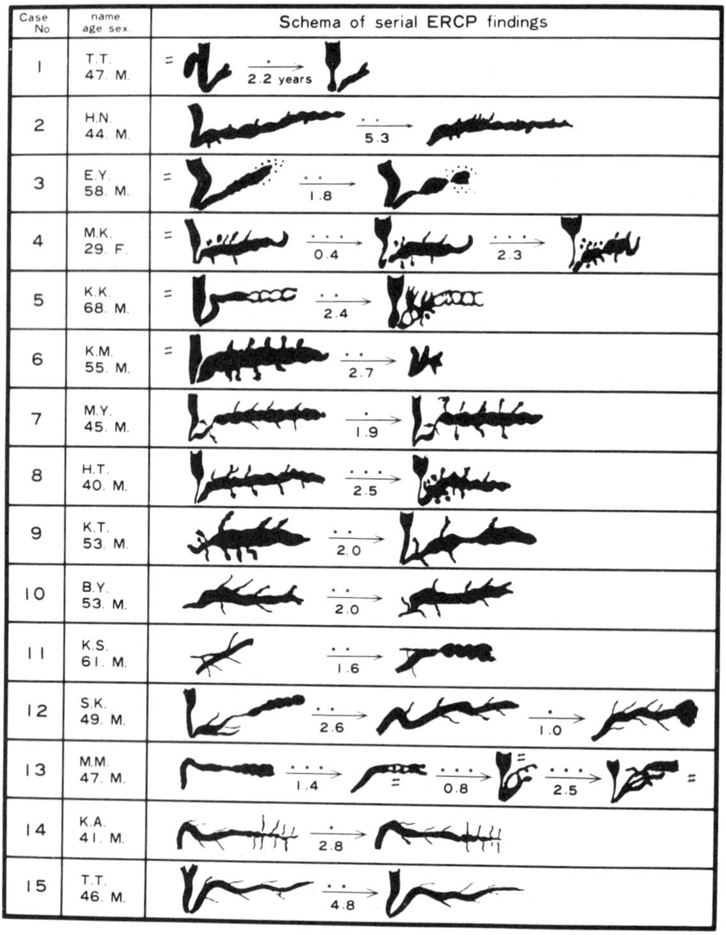

Fig 26–1.—Schema of findings in serial endoscopic pancreatography in patients with chronic alcoholic pancreatitis. Drinking habits: *asterisk,* abstinence, *double asterisk,* reduced, *triple asterisks,* continued. One patient had calcification of pancreas (#). (Courtesy of Nagata, A., et al.: Gastroenterology 81:884–891, November 1981.)

ductal alterations at 5 years 10 months, after initial examination, and 1 had stenosis, irregular wall, and large cystic formation in the main duct 4 years 4 months after initial examination.

Serial endoscopic pancreatography showed marked and progressive changes in patients in this study with chronic alcoholic pancreatitis, even after a reduction or cessation of drinking, but no remarkable changes developed in patients who were not alcoholics and had definite or suspected chronic pancreatitis. The findings suggest that pancreatic duct lesions are important in the development and progression of chronic alcoholic pancreatitis, in contrast to chronic nonalcoholic pancreatitis.

▶ [We are now beginning to see patients in whom several endoscopic retrograde cholangiopancreatographic examinations have been done previously. Occasionally,

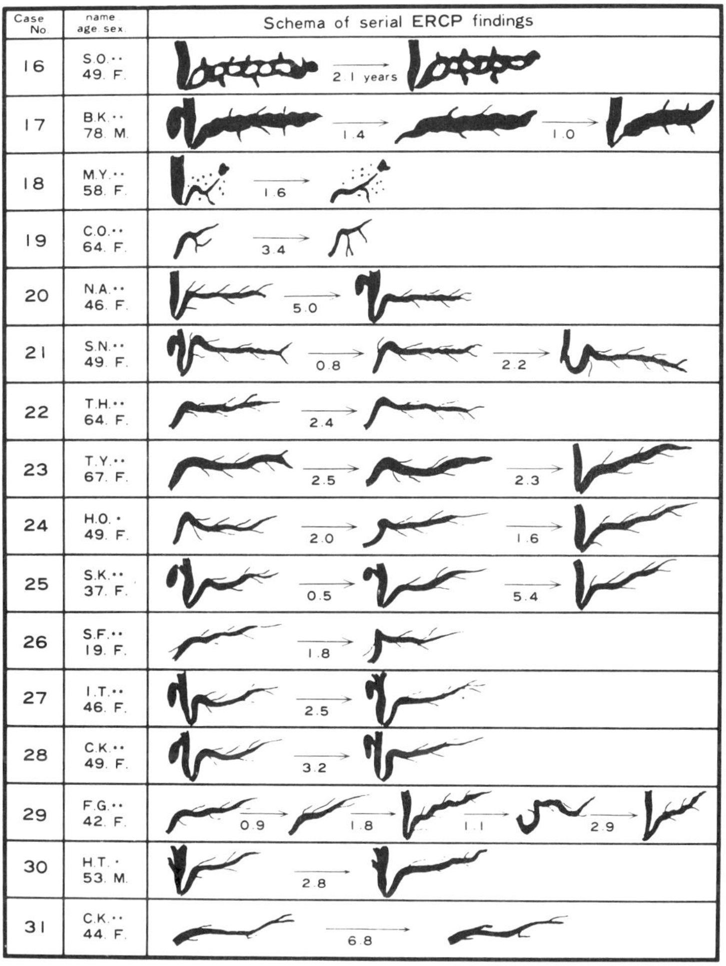

Fig 26–2.—Schema of findings in serial endoscopic pancreatography in patients with chronic nonalcoholic pancreatitis. Etiology: *asterisk,* biliary; *double asterisks,* idiopathic. (Courtesy of Nagata, A., et al.: Gastroenterology 81:884–891, November 1981.)

the etiology of the pancreatitis in such patients is unclear, and, therefore, studies such as this one are very helpful in giving us enough information to assess such patients. Findings correspond very nicely with the clinical observation that gallstone pancreatitis almost never produces serious and progressive pancreatitis.—W.S.] ◀

26–6 **Clinical Relevance of Isolated Ventral Pancreas.** Failure of union of the dorsal and ventral pancreatic duct systems during development results in an isolated ventral pancreas (Fig 26–3). The anomaly has been recognized in up to 8% of cadavers. M. H. Thompson, R. C. N. Williamson, and P. R. Salmon (Univ. of Bristol) found 11 cases (1.3%) of isolated ventral pancreas in a total of 850 endoscopic retrograde cholangiopancreatographic studies done over 7 years. Diagnosis was based on the demonstration of a short, branching duct

(26–6) Br. J. Surg. 68:101–104, February 1981.

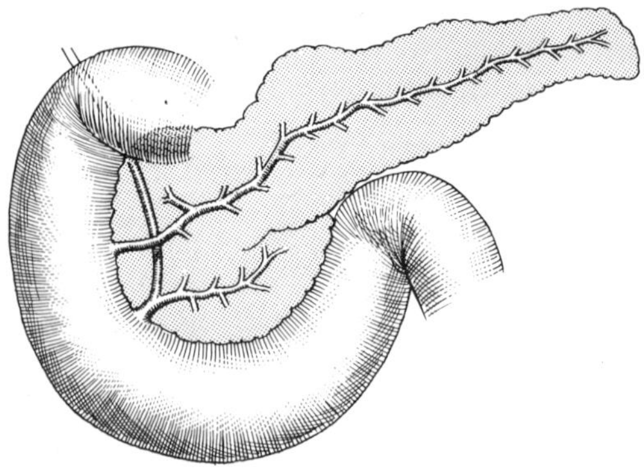

Fig 26–3.—Anatomy of the pancreatic ducts in isolated ventral pancreas. The duct of Santorini drains through the minor papilla proximally in the duodenum, and the isolated ventral pancreas drains through the major papilla with the bile duct. (Courtesy of Thompson, M.H., et al.: Br. J. Surg. 68:101–104, February 1981.)

system cannulated at the main ampulla in conjunction with the common bile duct. Only cases with complete separation of 2 duct systems were included.

The 8 women and 3 men had a mean age of 44 years. All presented with upper abdominal pain that was associated with transient jaundice in 2 cases and with possible mild acute pancreatitis in 3 cases. Average duration of symptoms was 4.1 years. Four patients had exploration before the diagnosis was made or its significance was appreciated. Five patients were operated on because of severe pain requiring frequent doses of opiates. Pancreatograms were normal in all these cases, but histologic study showed pancreatitis in 2 cases, with marked periductal fibrosis. The patients secreted low volumes of pancreatic juice in response to secretin. Duodenal bicarbonate concentration and tryptic activity were substantially lower in patients with established chronic pancreatitis; values were generally normal in patients with isolated ventral pancreas.

In cases of isolated ventral pancreas, the small accessory drainage system might result in partial functional obstruction and eventual obstructive pancreatitis in the distal part of the dorsal pancreas; however, operative pancreatography has shown a free flow of contrast into the duodenum without obvious signs of ductal dilation. Operative treatment may be necessary for abdominal pain. Laparotomy permits direct examination of the pancreas and the exclusion of concomitant gastrointestinal disease. Pancreatic resection probably should be reserved for patients with definite chronic pancreatitis. Further experience is needed to determine whether this anomaly is a clinically important finding.

▶ [This article was chosen for review primarily because other publications have suggested that the so-called isolated ventral pancreas or pancreas divisum is an important cause of upper abdominal pain and is significant pathogenetically in the development of pancreatitis. I believe that these contentions have yet to be proved, and this article would support that view. In the absence of any new and startling information, it is very difficult to understand why this simple rearrangement of the ductal system should produce symptoms. Until clear-cut evidence of the causation of the pain and pancreatitis in patients with isolated ventral pancreas has been ascertained, these patients should probably not be operated on simply because of the presence of this anomaly. One can hardly construct a rational therapeutic surgical procedure for a condition with such an ethereal pathogenesis.—W.S.] ◀

26–7 **Endoscopic Sphincterotomy Before Pancreaticoduodenectomy for Ampullary Carcinoma** is reported by D. Alderson, M. I. Lavelle, and C. W. Venables (Newcastle upon Tyne, England). Pancreaticoduodenectomy is the operation of choice for carcinoma of the ampulla of Vater, but the presence of severe jaundice in almost all patients with ampullary neoplasia is a major factor contributing to the high incidence of complications and hospital mortality after operation. Thus, it has been suggested that to reduce operative mortality, biliary decompression should be performed before definitive resection is undertaken. Until recently, the only way of achieving preliminary bile drainage was by surgical decompression, which meant a two-stage operation. With the advent of endoscopic retrograde cholangiopancreatography and its therapeutic offshoot, endoscopic sphincterotomy, an accurate preoperative diagnosis can be made and adequate biliary drainage can be provided without an intra-abdominal procedure.

In 5 consecutive patients with obstructive jaundice but without abdominal pain (Table 1), endoscopic sphincterotomy was performed at

TABLE 1.—CLINICAL DETAILS AND RESULTS OF INVESTIGATIONS*

Case No	Sex	Age (years)	Duration of history (weeks)	Weight loss (kg)	Results of investigations
1	M	75	3	6	Ultrasonography: dilated intrahepatic ducts; dilated common bile duct ERCP: ulcerated ampullary tumour
2	M	63	8	20	Ultrasonography: technically unsuccessful PTC: grossly dilated system; complete obstruction near termination of common bile duct ERCP: ulcerated ampullary tumour
3	M	58	12	10	Ultrasonography: dilated intrahepatic ducts; distended gall bladder; common bile duct not identified with certainty ERCP: irregular enlarged papilla, macroscopically neoplastic
4	F	50	3	0	Ultrasonography: distended gall bladder; biliary tree not identified otherwise with certainty PTC: unsuccessful (unable to cannulate) ERCP: ulcerated ampullary tumour
5	F	77	8	8	Ultrasonography: dilated intrahepatic duct; dilated common bile duct ERCP: deeply ulcerated ampullary tumour

*PTC, percutaneous transhepatic cholangiography; ERCP, endoscopic retrograde cholangiopancreatography.

(26–7) Br. Med. J. 282:1109–1111, Apr. 4, 1981.

TABLE 2.—ENDOSCOPIC SPHINCTEROTOMY IN 5 PATIENTS

Case No	Ducts entered	Ease of procedure	Haemorrhage at time of procedure	Complications after procedure	Time to operation (days)
1	Common bile duct	Easy	Slight	None	20
2	Pancreatic duct, common bile duct	Easy	Very slight	None	20
3	Pancreatic duct, common bile duct	Difficult ("precut")	None	Increased amylase activity	11
4	Common bile duct	Slight difficulty	Moderate	None	21
5	Common bile duct	Easy	Moderate	None	36

the time of endoscopic retrograde cholangiopancreatography. Biliary drainage was successfully achieved in all cases, and the procedure was without appreciable morbidity (Table 2). All 5 patients underwent pancreaticoduodenectomy 11–36 days later, the interval to operation being decided by the speed of resolution of the jaundice. Minor pancreatic leaks in 2 patients were the only complications. Patients were discharged 20–40 days postoperatively, and all 5 were well 6 weeks after hospital discharge.

Endoscopic sphincterotomy should be performed at the time of duodenoscopy if an obstructive ampullary tumor is found.

▶ [This is an interesting suggestion and merits further investigation. Sphincterotomy has been accomplished surgically in patients with ampullary carcinoma with reasonably good results, and it therefore seems reasonable to suggest that endoscopic sphincterotomy might be temporarily advantageous in patients with ampullary carcinoma. Because no external drainage is needed, secondary infection of the biliary tree may be somewhat less likely with this procedure than with transhepatic drainage. Clearly, the procedure deserves further study. On the other hand, it should be emphasized that patients with lesions arising in the head of the pancreas would likely be unsuitable for such a procedure, and, therefore, careful selection of patients for this technique is warranted.—W.S.] ◀

26–8 **Surgical Principles for Pancreatic Cancer: Regional Total and Subtotal Pancreatectomy** are discussed by Joseph G. Fortner (Meml. Sloan-Kettering Cancer Center, New York).

Regional total, or type I, pancreatectomy involves removal of the pancreatic segment of portal vein and end-to-end anastomosis without a graft. The base of the transverse mesocolon and a generous margin of soft tissue around the pancreas with regional lymph nodes are removed en bloc with the pancreas and portal vein segment. The vena cava and aorta are skeletonized, and all tissues are removed en bloc. The common hepatic bile duct is transected just below its bifurcation. Regional pancreatectomy type I is recommended for all cancers of the pancreas and periampullary region, for invasive ampullary cancers that have not spread beyond the immediate pancreatic region, and in patients who are good surgical risks.

Involvement of the celiac axis, superior mesenteric artery, or hepatic artery can be treated with arterial resection and reconstruction in addition to the type I operation; this is termed a type II operation (Fig 26–4). A type O regional pancreatectomy refers to the same op-

(26–8) Cancer 47[Suppl.]:1712–1718, Mar. 15, 1981.

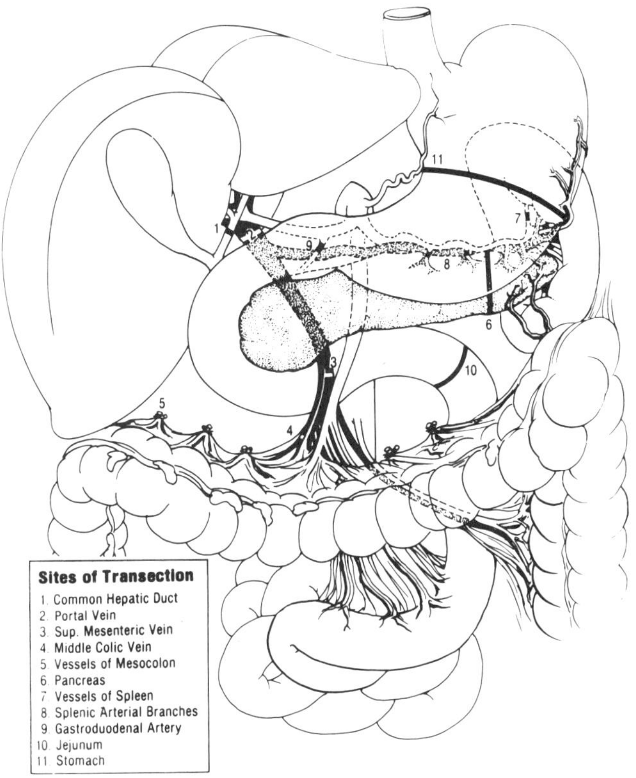

Fig 26–4.—Sites of transection for regional subtotal pancreatectomy. (Courtesy of Fortner, J.G.: Cancer 47 [Suppl.]:1712–1718, Mar. 15, 1981.)

eration as type I but without removal of the pancreatic segment of portal vein. This is reserved for cases in which the tumor is in the distal body or tail of the pancreas, and the region near the portal vein is completely normal. Regional subtotal pancreatectomy refers to the operation in which the distal (approximately 5 cm) part of the pancreas is left intact.

In 151 patients treated according to these approaches, the resectability rate was 32% (48 of 151). Regional pancreatectomy was performed in 40 patients, 36 with periampullary or pancreatic cancer and 4 with benign diseases. In these 40 patients the 30-day postoperative mortality rate was 7% (2 of 29) for regional total type I, 29% (2 of 7) for type II, and 50% (2 of 4) for regional subtotal type I, for an overall rate of 15% (6 of 40). The causes of death are shown in Table 1. Of the 30 patients with cancer who survived the operation, 10 are alive up to 58 months postoperatively (Table 2), 12 died of disease, and 8 died of other causes. Analysis of treatment failures from recurrent disease after regional pancreatectomy shows that the error was in patient selection, not with the operation.

There appears to be a small group of patients with cancer of the pancreas of periampullary region whose cancer is localized at the

TABLE 1.—CAUSES OF DEATH AFTER REGIONAL PANCREATECTOMY

Total pancreatectomy	Postop day
Type I	
Myocardial infarction	3
Necrosis of common bile duct and thrombosis of portal vein	14
Type II	
Pulmonary embolus	2
Thrombosis of hepatic artery and liver infarction	3
Subtotal pancreatectomy	
Type I	
Exsanguination via abdominal drains	10
Monilial esophagitis with hemorrhage	18

TABLE 2.—LENGTH OF SURVIVAL (MONTHS) OF 10 SURVIVING PATIENTS

	Pathologic stage of disease and survival		
	I	II	III
Adenocarcinoma of the pancreas	—	10,13 m	—
Other tumors	6,13,17 36,58 m	18,26 m	5 m

time of diagnosis and in whom surgical procedures that conform to basic surgical oncologic principles should result in cure. The frequency of late deaths from causes other than recurrent cancer can be decreased by dealing with the immune deficient state that many patients show, perhaps due to postpancreatectomy zinc deficiency.

▶ [The author describes a surprisingly low overall mortality of 15% (6 of a total of 40 cases). Closer perusal of the article indicates, however, that this was the mortality 30 days postoperatively. Another sentence in the article indicates that only 30 patients survived the operation. Therefore, another 4 persons must have died after the 30-day cut-off period. Inclusion of these 4 cases would increase the operative mortality to 25%, which, admittedly for this kind of procedure, is not altogether excessively formidable. However, one must take into account the causes of death that were unrelated to malignancy. Among 6 of the 8 patients who died of causes other than malignancy, death was due to hepatic failure (1), hepatitis (1), hypoglycemia (1), staphylococcal pneumonia (1), gastrointestinal hemorrhage (1), or inanition (1). Careful review of these clearly indicates that these complications must ultimately be attributable to the operative procedure itself. Although we are told that 33% of the patients who survived operation are still alive (i.e., 10 of the initial 40 patients), we are not given actuarial figures. The follow-up in some of these patients was as short as 5 months, and how many of these patients were alive less than 1 year after operation is not stated clearly. Therefore, it would appear that we must await better and more detailed information from the author of this article in order to evaluate the validity of the concept of regional pancreatectomy.—W.S.] ◀

26–9 **Pancreatic Fistula Complicating Pancreatectomy for Malignant Disease.** Pancreatic fistula, the most common complication of

(26–9) Br. J. Surg. 68:238–240, April 1981.

TABLE 1.—INCIDENCE OF PANCREATIC FISTULA

Procedure	No.	Fistula No.	Fistula %
Pancreatoduodenectomy	70	37	52·8
Pancreas ligated	37	26	70
With sutures	34	24	70
With staples	3	2	67
Pancreas anastomosed			
To jejunum	33	11	33
End-to-end	27	9	37
End-to-side	9	3	33
Distal pancreatectomy	108	8	7·4
Total	178	45	25

pancreatectomy, is caused by extravasation of pancreatic fluid secreted by the remaining part of the gland. The fistula predisposes to subphrenic abscess formation, dehiscence of visceral anastomoses, and erosion of blood vessels near the pancreas, thereby causing high operative mortality. Because active treatment rarely alters the course of a pancreatic fistula, prevention is important. Dimitrios N. Papachristou and Joseph G. Fortner (Meml. Sloan-Kettering Cancer Center, New York) review results with 178 patients with malignant tumors who underwent pancreatoduodenectomy or distal pancreatectomy.

Fistulas developed in 45 patients (25%). The incidence depended on the type of pancreatectomy and the technique used for management of the remaining pancreas (Table 1). Thus, the incidence was 52.8% after pancreatoduodenectomy and only 7.4% after distal pancreatectomy; in patients who underwent pancreatoduodenectomy it was 33.3% with pancreatojejunostomy and 70.2% with ligation and closure of the remaining pancreas. The use of intraductal stents did not prevent development of fistulas. Fistulas were rare in patients who had dilated pancreatic ducts. All but 19 fistulas were minor and required no active treatment other than local wound care. Ten patients with fistulas underwent surgery, usually because of life-threatening complications; only 3 survived.

The course of pancreatic fistulas was influenced by the type of pancreatectomy. Fistulas that developed after distal pancreatectomy ceased draining within 1 month in all patients except 1, whereas 38% of those that developed after pancreatoduodenectomy lasted more

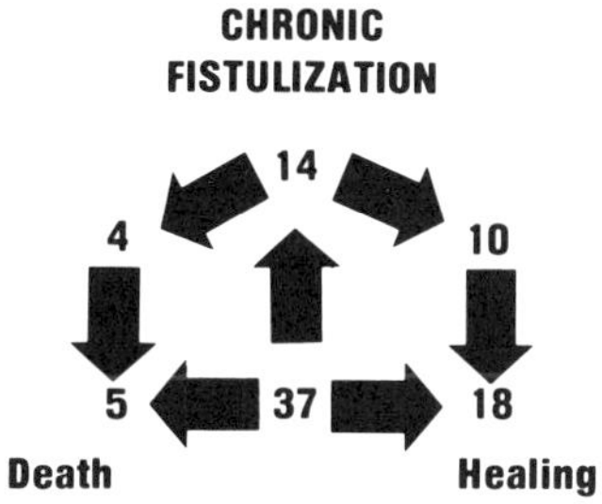

Fig 26–5.—Course of 37 pancreatic fistulas that complicated pancreatoduodenectomy. (Courtesy of Papachristou, D.N., and Fortner, J.G.: Br. J. Surg. 68:238–240, April 1981.)

TABLE 2.—MORTALITY FROM PANCREATIC FISTULA

Procedure	Operative mortality No.	%	Deaths caused by fistula No.	%	Lethal fistula No.	%
Pancreatoduodenectomy	13/70	18*	9/13	69	9/37	24
Pancreas ligated	7/37	19	5/7	71	5/26	19
Pancreas anastomosed to jejunum	6/33	18	4/6	66	4/11	36
Distal pancreatectomy	4/108	8*	1/4	25	1/8	12
Total	17/178	9	10/17	59	10/45	22

than 1 month (Fig 26–5). Chronicity was not always associated with a benign course because 9 of those patients required reexploration and 4 died. Pancreatic fistula was the most dangerous complication of pancreatectomy (Table 2). Of all secondary complications precipitated by pancreatic fistulas, hemorrhage in 5 patients, and subphrenic abscess in 16 were the most serious.

To prevent fistula development, ligation and closure of the pancreatic remnant should be avoided in pancreatoduodenectomy, which, as practiced today, leads to a prohibitively high incidence of fistulization. Pancreatojejunostomy is preferable particularly in the presence of pancreatic obstruction and ductal dilation. Pancreatojejunostomy does not protect from fistulization if the pancreatic duct is not dilated. Radiation to the pancreas may be an alternative to other treatment attempts if the fistula persists.

▶ [It is no great surprise that pancreatic fistulization after distal pancreatectomy is far less frequent than after pancreaticoduodenectomy. After all, the pancreatic juice has an alternate means of drainage into the duodenum after distal pancreatectomy, and, in addition, there is rarely an activation of the pancreatic juice by intestinal content, because the isolated pancreatic remnant does not communicate with the intestinal tract except at the papilla of Vater. The authors have clearly defined the major problem that follows pancreaticoduodenectomy. Unfortunately, they do not make any specific recommendations that would enable the surgeon to deal definitively with the problem of pancreatic fistula after this operation. The number of cases that responded to radiation therapy is small, and this therapy is unlikely to be an important advance in the management of this problem. Because mortality is so high, one cannot help but wonder whether a very aggressive approach should be taken once fistulization has occurred, especially if hemorrhage is a complicating feature. Removal of the distal pancreas after pancreaticoduodenectomy, together with adequate ligation of the bleeding vessel in normal tissues, should, indeed, adequately care for the problem of pancreatic fistula after pancreaticoduodenectomy. Consideration should be given to this means of treatment once this very serious complication occurs.—W.S.] ◀

26–10 **Gastrointestinal/Pancreatic Hormone Concentrations in the Portal Venous System of Nine Patients With Organic Hyperinsulism.** B. Glaser, G. Valtysson, S. S. Fajans, A. I. Vinik, K. Cho, and N. Thompson (Univ. of Michigan) used percutaneous transhepatic blood sampling of the portal venous system in an attempt to localize

(26–10) Metabolism 30:1001–1010, October 1981.

hormone-secreting tumor in 9 patients with fasting hypoglycemia and hyperinsulinism. All patients had a diagnosis of symptomatic hypoglycemia due to organic hyperinsulinism and underwent pancreatic angiography with pharmacoangiography.

In 6 cases, pancreatic angiography, abdominal computed tomography, and ultrasound studies failed to identify a single tumor later found at operation. All these tumors were localized by the peak hormone level in the portal venous system. Three were in the neck, and one each in the head, body, and tail of the pancreas. Nesideoblastosis was confirmed in a patient with findings suggestive of multiple areas of insulin hypersecretion. One patient with a tumor shown by angiography had findings suggesting a multicentric or diffuse process. Another with a large tumor in the head of the pancreas had confirmatory hormonal findings. No patient has had recurrent symptoms of organic hyperinsulinism. In the patients with single small adenomas, elevated levels of immunoreactive insulin were not always restricted to an area close to the tumor.

Percutaneous transhepatic sampling of portal venous blood has successfully localized small angiographically-negative insulinomas in several cases. The procedure appears to be relatively safe, and it can be recommended for use in patients with proved organic hyperinsulinism but negative pancreatic angiograms and those with recurrent hypoglycemia due to multiple tumors or multiple endocrine neoplasia type I. More recently, two more single insulinomas have been demonstrated by this technique in patients with negative angiographic findings.

▶ [There has been much recent interest in superselective angiographic sampling of the pancreatic venous drainage for the localization of insulinomas and other islet tumors that produce various hormones. As reported in the 1981 YEAR BOOK OF SURGERY (p. 464), the data in the literature are not all that convincing to those who would peruse them carefully and critically. I am afraid that the data in this article fall into the same category. In the tables, the authors report only the gradient between the level of insulin in portal venous blood and that in arterial blood. Such gradients really are not extremely useful. Perusal of the figures of each of the cases indicates, however, that there are many aberrant values for insulin levels. At best, it seems to me that the surgeon could only be directed to one rather gross area for special attention during the exploration. Taken as such, this technique may, indeed, be of some value. However, the crux of the issue is: What does the surgeon do if the tumor is not palpable? More careful palpation might have ensued as a result of levels of insulin that suggest a given area of the pancreas. But failing to find the lesion, I wonder whether the authors would be willing, for example, to perform pancreaticoduodenectomy in a patient in whom no lesion is palpable in the head of the pancreas if the insulin levels were high only in that region. I doubt that they would, and I certainly would not. The solution is very easy if the high values are on the left side of the pancreas, because then a distal pancreatectomy can be done relatively simply and safely, but the big payoff comes if, indeed, the surgeon is willing to resect the head of the pancreas with the use of pancreaticoduodenectomy based on these insulin levels alone.

The vagaries of the venous drainage of the pancreas are great. The absolute level of insulin in the venous blood will depend on the proximity of the sampling catheter to the tumor and the amount of dilution of the venous blood from the tumor by veins that do not drain a tumor-bearing area. The data produced by the Scandinavian workers in the 1981 YEAR BOOK OF SURGERY are completely unconvincing in terms of the insulinomas, and the data are far from completely convincing in this article from the University of Michigan. Furthermore, I think it would be very dangerous to assume that hyperplasia of the islets was present in a patient who had diffusely elevated levels. We obviously still need better methods for localization of insulinomas, and more particularly for definition of those patients who have either nesideoblastosis or hyperplasia of the islets.—W.S.] ◀

27. Endocrine Glands

27–1 **The Relationships Among Surgical Histometry, Outcome and Pretreatment in Graves' Disease.** Both the size of the thyroid remnant left after subtotal thyroidectomy and the extent of lymphocytic infiltration of the thyroid are thought to influence the outcome in patients with Graves' disease. T. J. Wilkin, A. Gunn, M. Al Moussa, T. E. Isles, J. Crooks, and J. Swanson Beck (Dundee, Scotland) attempted to determine by quantitative histometry whether the extent of lymphocytic infiltration influences the outcome and whether pretreatment affects the epithelial content of the thyroid. Studies were done in three groups of patients: 73 patients with Graves' disease who were given carbimazole and triiodothyronine for 6 months before surgery, 38 patients pretreated for up to 6 weeks with propranolol, and 32 patients given Lugol's iodine as well as propranolol for 10 days before surgery. The control group consisted of 107 patients without known thyroid disease who were examined at autopsy.

No significant relationship was found between the surgical outcome at 18 months and the proportion of either lymphocytes or epithelium in resected tissue. These two histologic measurements were not significantly correlated in the patients pretreated with carbimazole and triiodothyronine. The proportion of epithelium was less in propranolol-iodide-pretreated patients than in those given propranolol alone. The proportion of lymphocytes was significantly greater in the patients pretreated with carbimazole and triiodothyronine than in the control group.

The outcome of surgery for Graves' disease could not be related to the proportion of lymphocytes in the resected specimens from patients in this study who were pretreated with carbimazole and triiodothyronine. This finding is contrary to the view that lymphocytic infiltration is a major determinant of postoperative hypothyroidism. No relationship with the proportion of epithelium was observed. Several factors strongly favor the spontaneous restoration of euthyroidism after thyroidectomy, including the naturally cyclical nature of primary thyrotoxicosis and the presence of adequate epithelium in even a small remnant of thyroid tissue.

▶ [The major thrust of this article is that the variation in the epithelial content of the thyroid is so great that even if the surgeon were able to judge accurately the anatomical mass of the thyroid remnant, he or she would still have little or no idea of the functional mass of that thyroid remnant. Therefore, the outcome after subtotal thyroidectomy for Graves' disease may have very little bearing on how much actual anatomical mass the surgeon leaves behind in the neck. In other words, the surgeon, unfortunately, may have very little control in directing the ultimate outcome in the surgical treatment of Graves' disease. It seems clear from this study, for example,

(27–1) Acta Endocrinol. (Copenh.) 98:43–49, September 1981.

that there is no correlation between the size of the lymphoid infiltrate and the epithelial mass of the resected thyroid, so that simple lymphocytic infiltrations probably do not replace thyroid tissue, as was once thought. The claims of some surgeons that one technique or another may ensure a very low incidence of recurrence or hypothyroidism need to be scrutinized carefully. Natural factors, such as a strong tendency in the patient to spontaneous remission, may favor the restoration of euthyroidism after thyroidectomy, and the surgeon's role probably should be viewed in this light. I tend to err on the side of radicalism in determining the amount of gland to be resected, simply because I feel that the worst possible outcome is that of recurrent hyperthyroidism. Those factors that dictated the use of surgical treatment in preference to radioactive iodine usually are still present when the recurrence develops, and one is then faced with a serious dilemma in the patient who has received previous surgical treatment. It is far easier to give thyroid substance to a hypothyroid patient than it is to treat a recurrence. I generally leave a total of 4 or 5 gm of thyroid tissue equally divided between the two sides of the neck.—W.S.] ◀

27-2 **Influence of Surgery on Plasma Propranolol Levels and Protein Binding.** Many patients undergo surgery while receiving long-term medication. In addition to the influence of these drugs on the response to surgery and anesthesia, the influence of surgery and anesthesia on the handling of these drugs by the body must be considered. John Feely, Alexander Forrest, Andrew Gunn, William Hamilton, Ian Stevenson, and James Crooks (Univ. of Dundee) studied the influence of surgery and anesthesia on plasma propranolol levels in 25 hyperthyroid and 5 euthyroid patients undergoing thyroidectomy. The mean age of the 30 patients was about 44 years; 26 were women.

Hyperthyroid patients were prepared for surgery with propranolol alone (160–480 mg/day) for at least 1 week. Each patient was given propranolol approximately 3 hours before surgery and continued after

Fig 27–1.—Perioperative plasma propranolol levels in hyperthyroid patients, 20 of whom received propranolol orally and 5 through a nasogastric tube, and in 5 euthyroid patients. (Courtesy of Feely, J., et al.: Clin. Pharmacol. Ther. 28:759–763, December 1980.)

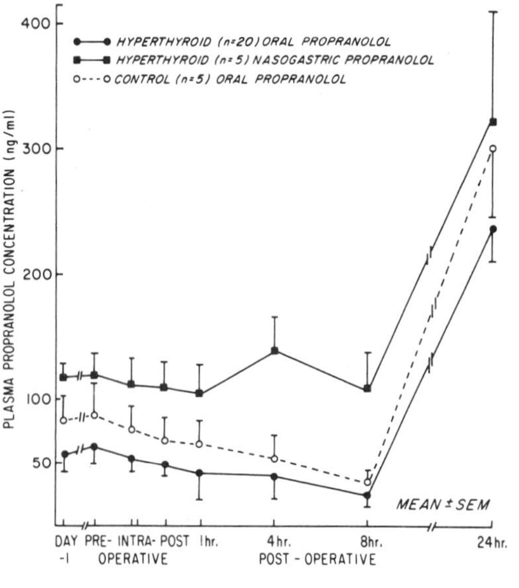

(27–2) Clin. Pharmacol. Ther. 28:759–763, December 1980.

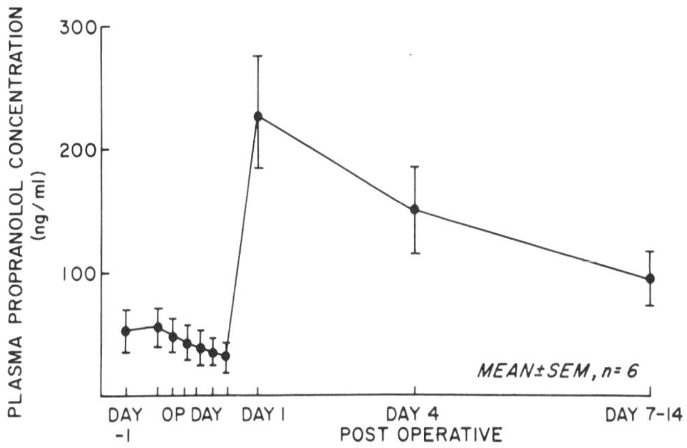

Fig 27–2.—Plasma propranolol levels in patients before surgery (when hyperthyroid), after surgery, and when euthyroid on days 7–14. (Courtesy of Feely, J., et al.: Clin. Pharmacol. Ther. 28:759–763, December 1980.)

surgery on the same dosage schedule for 7–14 days. The initial 5 patients received 40 mg 4 times a day, did not have the response to propranolol therapy objectively assessed, and received propranolol orally after surgery. The other 20 patients had the dosage of propranolol individually titrated to produce a high degree of β-adrenoceptor blockade at the end of a dosing interval, both as outpatients and as inpatients on the day before surgery. Of these 20 patients, 5 required 80 mg 4 times a day. After surgery they received the 80-mg dose through a nasogastric tube, beginning 30 minutes after surgery and continuing for 24 hours. The other 15 patients received their propranolol (mean, 229 mg/day) orally after surgery, with the preoperative dosage schedule. The euthyroid patients were treated hyperthyroid patients who were undergoing elective thyroidectomy for relapse after treatment with antithyroid drugs. They received 40 mg of propranolol orally 4 times a day and 5 mg of carbimazole with 20 μg of triiodothyronine 3 times a day for at least 1 month. The last two drugs were not given after surgery. The surgical technique was identical in all groups; a thyroid remnant was left, which was equal in size to a 10-gm section of the excised gland.

Propranolol levels fell markedly after surgery because of poor drug ingestion in the immediate postoperative period, due largely to patient nausea, somnolence, and inability to swallow. The drug was not detectable in the plasma of 3 hyperthyroid patients 8 hours after surgery. When propranolol was given through a nasogastric tube, values were satisfactory throughout (Fig 27–1). Compared with preoperative levels, all patients showed a twofold to threefold rise in total and free propranolol levels 24 hours after surgery (Fig 27–2), suggesting decreased hepatic clearance of the drug. The degree of plasma protein binding of propranolol also had increased on the day after surgery, leading to a 30% reduction in free propranolol.

Although thyroid storm did not occur in any patient, propranolol levels in the immediate postoperative period were often inadequate regardless of preoperative dosage titration. Propranolol should be administered nasogastrically when patients are somnolent or unable to swallow.

▶ [This article provides eloquent testimony and data to support a fear I have voiced in previous years (1980 YEAR BOOK OF SURGERY, p. 469). We have been concerned about the propriety of preparing hyperthyroid patients with propranolol alone. Whereas this indeed can be accomplished, these patients are not euthyroid, and the omission of a dose in error or changes in blood levels that result from operation may be fraught with the considerable hazard of thyrotoxic crisis and storm. The data produced by these authors clearly support this fear. It seems prudent to operate on a euthyroid patient, if that is at all possible, and to fall back on propranolol alone only if antithyroid drugs cannot be utilized. In cases in which propranolol alone must be used, the variations in blood levels or propranolol demonstrated in this article are important. Propranolol probably should be administered nasogastrically in the perioperative period.—W.S.] ◀

27–3 **Serum Thyroglobulin in Thyroid Cancer.** Thyroglobulin (Tg) is present in the serum of most healthy persons. Elevated levels have been found in patients with various thyroid disorders, including differentiated carcinoma. E. G. Black, A. Cassoni, T. M. D. Gimlette, C. L. Harmer, M. N. Maisey, G. D. Oates, and R. Hoffenberg assayed serum Tg at various stages of treatment in 274 patients with differentiated thyroid carcinoma. A double antibody radioimmunoassay and a serum anti-Tg assay were used. Cases of medullary cancer were not included in the study. Of the 266 patients who had a thyroidectomy, 183 had received ablative radioiodine therapy. Patients treated with thyroxine had received at least 100 μg daily for 8 weeks or longer.

The findings are shown in the table. In patients who did not receive thyroxine, the serum Tg levels correlated with the presence or absence of cancer; a criterion of 5 μg/L was used in 83% of cases. Six patients who were thought to have residual cancer had a serum Tg level below 5 μg/L, whereas 22 patients with higher levels had no clinical evidence of disease. Concordance was 97.5% in patients who received thyroxine. The findings in patients studied with and without thyroxine administration are shown in Figure 27–3. Only 1 false positive result was obtained in a thyroxine-treated patient. Anti-Tg was

THYROGLOBULIN VALUES IN PATIENTS WITH OR WITHOUT CANCER ON OR OFF THYROXINE TREATMENT*

	Off T4		On T4	
—	With cancer	Without cancer	With cancer	Without cancer
Tg <5 μg/l:				
Patients	6	85	3	128
Samples	11	169	6	336
Tg >5 μg/l:				
Patients	51	22	26	1
Samples	131	56	75	5

*Reproduced from Lancet 2:443–445, Aug. 29, 1981.

(27–3) Lancet 2:443–445, Aug. 29, 1981.

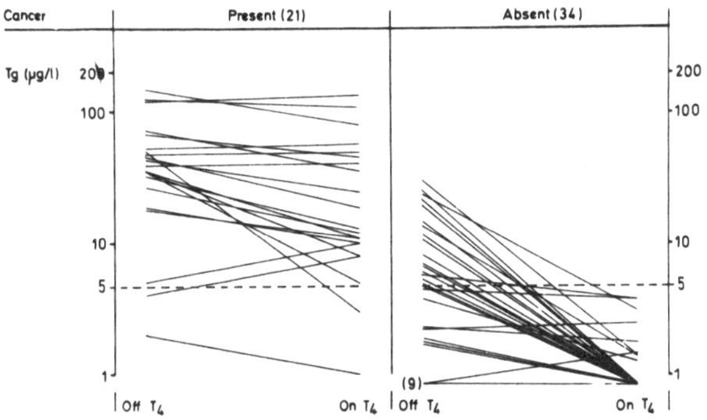

Fig. 27–3.—Thyroglobulin values in patients with or without cancer studied before or after administration of thyroxine. (Courtesy of Black, E.G., et al.: Lancet 2:443–445, Aug. 29, 1981.)

found in the serum of one fourth of the patients studied. Its presence did not affect the serum Tg assay in patients with or without residual cancer.

The serum Tg level provides an excellent marker of the presence or absence of differentiated thyroid cancer in patients treated with thyroxine, even if anti-Tg antibodies are present. It should now be possible to perform scans only when the serum Tg level remains above 5 µg/L despite thyroid hormone therapy or when there is clinical evidence that suggests recurrence. Some tumors may not produce Tg, or tumors may produce abnormal molecular forms not recognized by the antibody used. Monitoring by assay of serum Tg may, however, supplant routine radioiodine scanning of the neck or whole body in patients who were operated on for thyroid cancer.

▶ [The need to withdraw exogenous thyroid replacement for 4 weeks in order to carry out radioactive iodine uptake studies in patients with thyroid cancer is extremely devastating to a patient who must undergo such testing. I believe that physicians who order such tests have not recognized adequately the disruptive effect of such a plan on a patient with thyroid cancer, especially if such studies are to be repeated at intervals of 6 months or 1 year. Some of these patients cannot work effectively near the end of the period of withdrawal of exogenous thyroid therapy. Therefore, any kind of test that will avoid this is highly desirable. I wholeheartedly agree with the conclusion of these authors that monitoring of the serum thyroglobulin level should supplant routine assessment by radioactive iodine scans of the neck or whole body. Although this test is by no means perfect, it is undoubtedly as good as the radioactive iodine scan. It is especially pleasing to note that the test is even more effective when patients are placed on exogenous thyroid treatment. Obviously, if a rise in the level of serum thyroglobulin occurs, then radioactive iodine uptake studies are indicated for possible therapeutic purposes.—W.S.] ◀

27–4 **Familial Hypocalciuric Hypercalcemia: Recognition Among Patients Referred After Unsuccessful Parathyroid Exploration.** Hypercalcemia persists or recurs after 4% to 14% of initial parathyroidectomies. A high failure rate has been reported in 2 large kindreds with an autosomal dominant syndrome of hypercalcemia without hypercalciuria, familial hypocalciuric hypercalcemia, which has a generally mild course when untreated. Stephen J. Marx, John

(27–4) Ann. Intern. Med. 92:351–356, March 1980.

DIVALENT CATION METABOLISM IN HOMOGENEOUS GROUPS WITH HYPERCALCEMIA*

	Typical Primary Hyperparathyroidism	Familial Hypocalciuric Hypercalcemia	Hypercalcemia with Suppression of Parathyroid Glands
Patients, *no.*	24	6	4
Serum calcium, *meq/L*	6.10 ± 0.51	5.72 ± 0.33	5.83 ± 0.32
Serum magnesium, *meq/L*	1.64 ± 0.21	1.91 ± 0.12	1.70 ± 0.21
Creatinine clearance, *mL/min·1.73 m²*	72 ± 28†	84 ± 16†	21 ± 16
Logarithm (calcium:creatinine clearance ratio)‡	−1.63 ± 0.16†	−2.25 ± 0.28§	−0.88 ± 0.19

*Excludes patients receiving drugs known to have major effects on divalent cation metabolism. Data are expressed as means ± 1 SD.

†Differs from group with suppression of parathyroid glands.

‡Antilogarithmic back-transformation of these data provides the mean and 95% confidence ranges (in parentheses) for calcium-creatinine clearance ratios: typical primary hyperparathyroidism, 0.023 (0.011–0.049); familial hypocalciuric hypercalcemia, 0.0056 (0.0015–0.020); and hypercalcemia with suppression of parathyroid glands, 0.13 (0.055–0.32).

§Differs from group with primary hyperparathyroidism and group with suppression of parathyroid glands.

L. Stock, Maurice F. Attie, Robert W. Downs, Jr., David G. Gardner, Edward M. Brown, Allen M. Spiegel, John L. Doppman and Murray F. Brennan (Natl. Inst. of Health) have now reviewed the findings in 67 patients referred after unsuccessful surgery for presumed primary hyperparathyroidism in 1976 to 1978.

Fig 27–4.—Renal calcium-creatinine clearance ratio in hypercalcemic patients. Each datum point represents a different patient. Data are shown for the same patients as in the table; patients receiving drugs known to have major effects on divalent cation metabolism were excluded. (Courtesy of Marx, S.J., et al.: Ann. Intern. Med. 92:351–356, March 1980.)

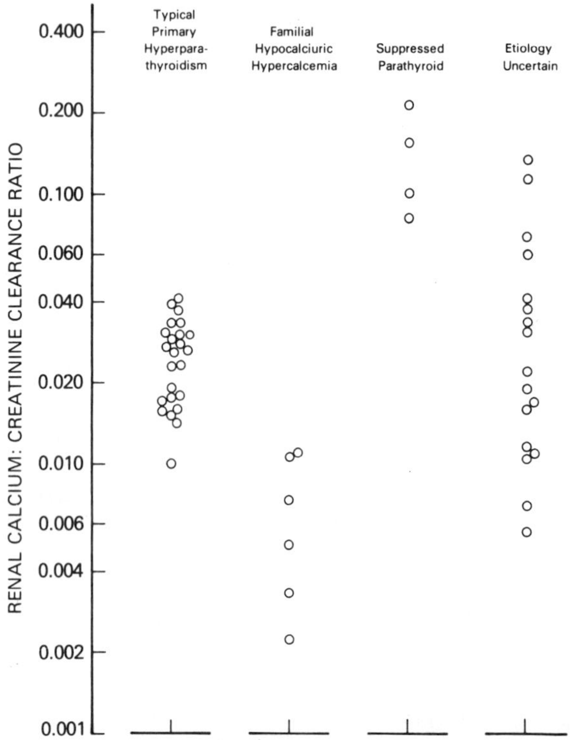

Six patients were index cases for kindreds with familial hypocalciuric hypercalcemia. Four patients had hypercalcemia with suppression of parathyroid hormone secretion. Thirty had typical primary hyperparathyroidism; only 1 with parathyroid carcinoma had recurrent hypercalcemia when last seen. Twenty patients could not be classified, and 7 were not hypercalcemic when evaluated. Eight of 24 patients with parathyroid hyperplasia had first-degree relatives with hypercalcemia, and 1 of these kindreds had familial multiple endocrine neoplasia type I. In the 6 kindreds with familial hypocalciuric hypercalcemia, asymptomatic hypercalcemia at all ages was a common feature. Only 1 proband had been aware of a hypercalcemic relative before family screening. No nephrolithiasis was encountered. Six hypercalcemic relatives have had 10 parathyroidectomies done elsewhere; 4 remain hypercalcemic, and 2 have developed chronic hypocalcemia. The biochemical findings are given in the table. The calcium-creatinine clearance ratio nearly completely separated the kindreds from cases of typical primary hyperparathyroidism and parathyroid suppression (Fig 27–4).

Optimal management of patients with familial hypocalciuric hypercalcemia remains unclear, but standard subtotal parathyroidectomy appears inadequate, since a small remnant of parathyroid tissue can sustain hypercalcemia. Relative hypocalciuria should suggest the possibility of familial hypocalciuric hypercalcemia, while relative hypercalciuria may increase the likelihood of appropriately suppressed parathyroids.

▶ [Familial hypocalciuric hypercalcemia is an important entity because, as these authors emphasize, patients with this condition constitute almost 10% of patients seen after unsuccessful previous parathyroidectomy. Fully one third of the patients referred to this group after unsuccessful parathyroid operations elsewhere either had hypercalcemia for which no cause could be established definitively or were, in fact, normocalcemic. These figures are eloquent testimony to the fact that all of us must sharpen our diagnostic acumen.

The diagnosis of primary hyperparathyroidism still remains the most important feature of the workup of these patients. Parathyroid operations must not be undertaken to establish a diagnosis. There is rarely any real hurry to operate on a hyperparathyroid patient unless the hypercalcemia is causing a hypercalcemic crisis, an unusual event. Therefore, everyone—including the surgeon—must take sufficient time to establish without doubt the presence or absence of primary hyperparathyroidism before operation is undertaken. There is nothing more depressing to internists, surgeons, and patients alike than repeated operations in the absence of true hyperparathyroidism. I would like to emphasize that elevation of the peripheral parathyroid hormone level is not the definitive test that many think it is. We have seen many patients who have primary hyperparathyroidism proved at operation who do not have such elevation. In addition, many patients who have normal levels, and who are therefore thought to have an inappropriately low parathyroid hormone level for the value of the elevated serum calcium concentration, do not have primary hyperparathyroidism, as emphasized in this study and in our own experience. Furthermore, it should be made very clear that selective catheterizations of the venous drainage of the parathyroids is by no means a definitive method of diagnosis of hyperparathyroidism, because if a catheter is placed sufficiently close to a normal parathyroid, elevations of parathyroid hormone level may be detected in the absence of hyperparathyroidism. We have had that experience on more than a few occasions. The diagnosis of primary hyperparathyroidism depends on persistent hypercalcemia, usually with high urinary cyclic adenosine monophosphate levels in the absence of other demonstrable causes of hypercalcemia. The latter must be sought vigorously and repeatedly before operation is undertaken. It is incumbent on the surgeon to insist that the diagnostic criteria are followed as rigidly as possible.—W.S.] ◀

27–5 **Localization of Parathyroid Tissue by Ultrasound Scanning Prior to Surgery in Patients With Hyperparathyroidism.** Preoperative localization of parathyroid glands is desirable, preferably by an easily performed, accurate, noninvasive method. Ultrasonography has been used to assess thyroid nodules, and reports have stated that parathyroids above a certain size can be identified echographically. Bruce H. Barraclough, Thomas S. Reeve, Peter J. Duffy, and Richard H. Picker (Sydney) performed ultrasonography preoperatively in 24 patients with biochemically proved hyperparathyroidism. Scans were made at 5-mm intervals in the transverse and longitudinal planes in the supine patient. The longus colli muscle was used as a landmark.

Parathyroid tissue was visualized ultrasonically before surgery in 18 of 24 patients. The glands ranged in size from 5 to 12 mm. There were 3 false positive and 6 false negative studies. The false positive results represented follicular adenomas protruding from the posterior surface of the thyroid in patients with multinodular goiter. One true negative result was obtained in a patient with a parathyroid adenoma in the mediastinum. One false negative finding was due to low level echoes from an adenoma merged with the esophagus. Two hyperplastic glands and 1 adenoma over 5 mm in diameter were not visualized in 2 patients with multinodular goiter.

Echography may shorten the operating time and reduce the extent of neck exploration in patients with hyperparathyroidism. However, echography may not demonstrate parathyroid gland enlargement after neck dissection or thyroidectomy because of distortion of normal landmarks. A negative preoperative study might be followed by selective arteriography and venous sampling or computed tomography scanning. Mediastinal glands were not visualized echographically because of the acoustically dense overlying bone. Echography is a rapid, noninvasive, inexpensive procedure.

▶ [There is no doubt that echography is quick, easy to perform, noninvasive, and inexpensive. For those reasons, it is certainly worthwhile to examine a patient with hyperparathyroidism by ultrasonography prior to operation. However, unless the record improves somewhat, the surgeon who operates on the patient during the first cervical exploration still bears the responsibility for looking on both sides of the neck. Of 24 patients examined by ultrasonographic scanning in this study, 3 had false positive and 6 had false negative results. The operative procedure might have been facilitated if the findings had been clear-cut, but in many instances this was not the case.

The most difficult patients of all are those who have had previous cervical explorations. An experienced parathyroid surgeon rarely fails to find the offending lesion during an initial cervical exploration. On the other hand, the authors point out that ultrasonography may be limited in detecting lesions in areas that were previously operated on and in the mediastinum because of overlying bone. Therefore, I think that other means of localizing parathyroid tissue will be required for difficult patients who have been given prior surgical treatment. There were no such patients in this series, as far as I can ascertain. In the mediastinum and perhaps even in the neck, computerized tomography appears to offer some very real advantages. We must await further studies on the efficacy of that technique, also.—W.S.] ◀

(27–5) World J. Surg. 5:91–95, January 1981.

27–6 **Parathyroid "Double Adenomas": Fact or Fiction?** The existence of "multiple adenomas" of the parathyroid glands has long been debated. Carlos A. Verdonk and Anthony J. Edis (Mayo Clinic and Found.) attempted to determine whether selective removal of the enlarged glands will be curative when 2 enlarged and hypercellular parathyroids are associated with 2 normal-sized glands at surgery for primary hyperparathyroidism. The 38 patients seen in 1959–1977 with possible double adenomas constituted 1.9% of all patients with surgically proved hyperparathyroidism who were operated on. Two enlarged, hypercellular glands, each weighing more than 70 mg, were removed in these cases, whereas 2 other normal-sized glands were preserved.

The patients in the study were not clinically distinct from those with the usual forms of parathyroid disease. Five had multiple endocrine neoplasia, but none had familial hyperparathyroidism. Additional thyroid surgery was done in only 1 patient with a medullary carcinoma. All patients but 1 were eucalcemic in the early postoperative period and at follow-up. The exceptional patient belonged to a kindred with multiple endocrine neoplasia type I. Two patients had symptomatic hypocalcemia for less than 6 weeks after operation. The mean follow-up was 4.6 years; half the patients were followed up for 3 years or more after operation.

More than 1 parathyroid adenoma occasionally may be found coexisting with normal parathyroids in patients with primary hyperparathyroidism. Even if double adenomas are simply a variant of hyperplasia, exploration of both sides of the neck is necessary. In the absence of evidence of multiple endocrine neoplasia or familial hyperparathyroidism, double adenomas should be managed by selective excision of the enlarged glands rather than subtotal parathyroidectomy to avoid an unnecessary risk of hypoparathyroidism.

▶ [Some authors have suggested that double adenomas of the parathyroid are so rare that one can confine the exploration to one side of the neck if one large parathyroid and one normal or small parathyroid are found on that one side. Such a contention is based on the premise that double adenomas of the parathyroid do not exist, or are so rare as to be of no consequence. Verdonk and Edis show that this is not the case. We, too, have had similar experiences. Whether or not one regards the double adenoma as a variant of hyperplasia does not matter. What matters is that if a large parathyroid is left behind in the neck on the contralateral side in such a patient with double adenoma of the parathyroid gland, persistent hypercalcemia will occur. The favorable outcome in the series by Verdonk and Edis and the experiences of Harness et al. (*Arch. Surg.* 114:468, 1979) strongly support the practice of *bilateral* cervical exploration in all patients with hyperparathyroidism.

Some surgeons, but more particularly our endocrinologic colleagues, seem to have the strange idea that confining the exploration to one side of the neck is a wonderful goal to be attained and that such a procedure is far less traumatic to the patient. I submit that it takes very little time to explore the contralateral side of the neck once a classic cervical incision has been made and that failure to do so results in more harm than good.—W.S.] ◀

27–7 **Transcervical Thymectomy and Thymus Remnants.** Thymectomy through the sternum carries some risks and inconvenience.

(27–6) Surgery 90:523–526, September 1981.
(27–7) Br. Med. J. 282:1583–1584, May 16, 1981.

Therefore, a simpler procedure, transcervical thymectomy, was proposed by Kirschner et al. in 1969. Moises Rosenberg and Aquiles J. Roncoroni (Buenos Aires) reviewed findings in 61 patients having this procedure to determine whether thymic remnants were present in those in whom myasthenia had progressed unfavorably. Lateral anterior mediastinal tomography, done after air injection, showed a typical thymic shadow in 14 of the 19 patients studied. Typically, a second operation, transsternal thymectomy, yielded thymic tissue.

These findings are not attributed to inadequate initial exploration or lack of surgical experience. Probably these patients have small pieces of thymic tissue not connected with the main body of the gland, which become hypertrophic following initial operation. Residual or recurrent thymoma causes myasthenia following removal of an asymptomatic tumor, and thymic remnants have been found at reexploration and autopsy. Patients undergoing transcervical thymectomy for thymic hyperplasia should be evaluated postoperatively for the presence of thymic tissue. If worsening disease is due to hypertrophy of thymic remnants, the transcervical approach might best be abandoned. It is possible, however, that no surgical approach can assure complete removal of all thymic tissue.

▶ [This is an interesting and provocative study. It suggests what many surgeons have suspected for a long time, namely, that total thymectomy via a transcervical approach is very difficult. Whether the presence of a remnant of thymus leads to a higher incidence of recurrent myasthenia gravis is really the most important issue at hand. The findings in this article suggest that this might be the case, although we are not provided with sufficient data to be certain of this. If further studies prove that we can expect a higher incidence of recurrence when thymectomy is done by the cervical route, then the technique should, of course, be abandoned for myasthenia gravis patients. It remains useful however, when done carefully for patients who may have a parathyroid adenoma. We need further studies on the long-term question of the results of transcervical thymectomy for myasthenia.—W.S.] ◀

27–8 **Factors Affecting Response to Thymectomy for Myasthenia Gravis.** Joseph W. Rubin, Robert G. Ellison, H. Victor Moore, and Ganesh P. Pai (Med. College of Georgia, Augusta) reviewed the findings in 97 patients with myasthenia gravis followed for up to 15 years, 22 of whom underwent thymectomy. All but one of these procedures were done by transsternal incision with removal of all the mediastinal thymus. Currently, radical exenteration of anterior mediastinal soft tissues is carried out. The pericardium is left intact, but all fatty tissue is removed with attached parietal pleura and thymus from the diaphragm to the pharyngeal origins. The 17 female and 5 male patients had a mean age of 24 years.

All but 1 of the 22 patients are alive; there were no operative deaths. No patient had thymectomy for nonprogressive ocular myasthenia gravis (class I disease). Five of 6 patients with generalized weakness (class II disease) had complete remission. Seven patients had acute fulminating myasthenia (class III disease), and 2 achieved complete remission, although 1 died of lupus erythematosus 2½ years after thymectomy. Only 3 of 8 patients with late severe disease (class IV) are presently in remission. One patient had muscular atrophy

---

(27–8) J. Thorac. Cardiovasc. Surg. 82:720–728, November 1981.

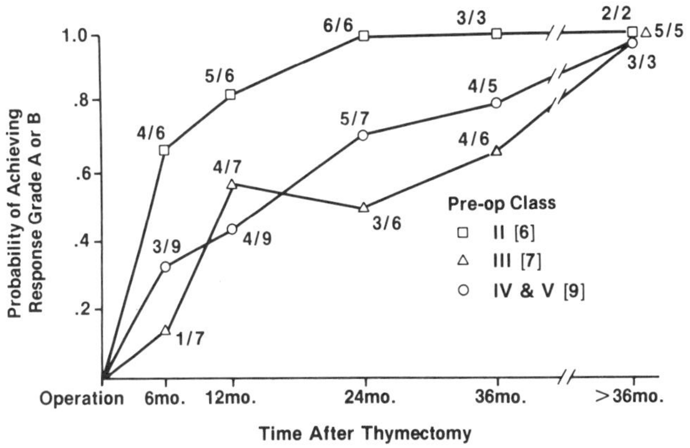

Fig 27–5.—Preoperative symptoms and response to thymectomy. (Courtesy of Rubin, J.W., et al.: J. Thorac. Cardiovasc. Surg. 82:720–728, November 1981.)

(class V disease). Ten patients in all are in complete remission without anticholinesterase medication, 10 are functioning normally with minimal symptoms on decreased doses of medication. Probability of recovery according to preoperative class is shown in Figure 27–5. Class II and III disease was associated with hyperplasia and abundant germinal centers. Four of the 22 patients had serious morbidity after operation. The class V patient was ventilator dependent for several months after operation.

More than 90% of patients in this series are in remission or only minimally symptomatic after thymectomy. Remission appears to depend more on the duration and progression of symptoms before thymectomy than on the pathologic changes in the thymus. Wide excision of anterior mediastinal soft tissues should be performed in order to achieve ideal results. Persistent minimal symptoms and a need for medication may be caused by residual or regenerated thymic tissue.

▶ [This is a very nice review of the surgical treatment of myasthenia gravis. The results are excellent. It appears that there is a swing away from transcervical thymectomy, and an analysis of the series of patients who underwent this operation suggests that the good results may be related to the fact that disease in these patients generally was very mild. The authors suggest that extensive anterior mediastinal dissection for removal of all possible traces of thymic tissue is more effective than a less radical procedure. This contention is not completely proved, but it would appear that the trend is moving away from the transcervical approach.—W.S.] ◀

Subject Index

A

B

D

E

F

G

M

Q

R

T